1998
YEAR BOOK OF
MEDICINE®

Statement of Purpose

The YEAR BOOK Service

The YEAR BOOK series was devised in 1901 by practicing health professionals who observed that the literature of medicine and related disciplines had become so voluminous that no one individual could read and place in perspective every potential advance in a major specialty. In the final decade of the 20th century, this recognition is more acutely true than it was in 1901.

More than merely a series of books, YEAR BOOK volumes are the tangible results of a unique service designed to accomplish the following:

- to *survey* a wide range of journals of proven value
- to *select* from those journals papers representing significant advances and statements of important clinical principles
- to provide *abstracts* of those articles that are readable, convenient summaries of their key points
- to provide *commentary* about those articles to place them in perspective

These publications grow out of a unique process that calls on the talents of outstanding authorities in clinical and fundamental disciplines, trained literature specialists, and professional writers, all supported by the resources of Mosby, the world's preeminent publisher for the health professions.

The Literature Base

Mosby and its Editors survey more than 1,000 journals published worldwide, covering the full range of the health professions. On an annual basis, the publisher examines usage patterns and polls its expert authorities to add new journals to the literature base and to delete journals that are no longer useful as potential YEAR BOOK sources.

The Literature Survey

The publisher's team of literature specialists, all of whom are trained and experienced health professionals, examines every original, peer-reviewed article in each journal issue. More than 250,000 articles per year are scanned systematically, including title, text, illustrations, tables, and references. Each scan is compared, article by article, to the search strategies that the publisher has developed in consultation with the 270 outside experts who form the pool of YEAR BOOK editors. A given article may be reviewed by any number of editors, from one to a dozen or more, regardless of the discipline for which the paper was originally published. In turn, each editor who receives the article reviews it to determine whether or not the article should be included in the YEAR BOOK. This decision is based on the article's inherent quality, its probable usefulness to readers of that YEAR BOOK, and the editor's goal to represent a balanced picture of a given field in each volume of the YEAR BOOK. In addition, the editor indicates when to include figures and tables from the article to help the YEAR BOOK reader better understand the information.

Of the quarter million articles scanned each year, only 5% are selected for detailed analysis within the YEAR BOOK series, thereby assuring readers of the high value of every selection.

The Abstract

The publisher's abstracting staff is headed by a seasoned medical professional and includes individuals with training in the life sciences, medicine, and other areas, plus extensive experience in writing for the health professions and related industries. Each selected article is assigned to a specific writer on this abstracting staff. The abstracter, guided in many cases by notations supplied by the expert editor, writes a structured, condensed summary designed so that the reader can rapidly acquire the essential information contained in the article.

The Commentary

The YEAR BOOK editorial boards, sometimes assisted by guest commentators, write comments that place each article in perspective for the reader. This provides the reader with the equivalent of a personal consultation with a leading international authority—an opportunity to better understand the value of the article and to benefit from the authority's thought processes in assessing the article.

Additional Editorial Features

The editorial boards of each YEAR BOOK organize the abstracts and comments to provide a logical and satisfying sequence of information. To enhance the organization, editors also provide introductions to sections or individual chapters, comments linking a number of abstracts, citations to additional literature, and other features.

The published YEAR BOOK contains enhanced bibliographic citations for each selected article, including extended listings of multiple authors and identification of author affiliations. Each YEAR BOOK contains a Table of Contents specific to that year's volume. From year to year, the Table of Contents for a given YEAR BOOK will vary depending on developments within the field.

Every YEAR BOOK contains a list of the journals from which papers have been selected. This list represents a subset of the more than 1,000 journals surveyed by the publisher and occasionally reflects a particularly pertinent article from a journal that is not surveyed on a routine basis.

Finally, each volume contains a comprehensive subject index and an index to authors of each selected paper.

The 1998 Year Book Series

Year Book of Allergy, Asthma, and Clinical Immunology: Drs. Rosenwasser, Borish, Boguniewicz, Nelson, Routes, and Spahn

Year Book of Anesthesiology and Pain Management®: Drs. Tinker, Abram, Chestnut, Roizen, Rothenberg, and Wood

Year Book of Cardiology®: Drs. Schlant, Collins, Gersh, Graham, Kaplan, and Waldo

Year Book of Chiropractic®: Dr. Lawrence

Year Book of Critical Care Medicine®: Drs. Parrillo, Balk, Calvin, Franklin, and Shapiro

Year Book of Dentistry®: Drs. Meskin, Berry, Jeffcoat, Leinfelder, Roser, Summitt, and Zakariasen

Year Book of Dermatologic Surgery®: Drs. Greenway, Barrett, Papadopoulos, and Whitaker

Year Book of Dermatology®: Dr. Thiers

Year Book of Diagnostic Radiology®: Drs. Osborn, Groskin, Dalinka, Maynard, Pentecost, Rebner, Ros, Smirniotopoulos, and Young

Year Book of Drug Therapy®: Drs. Lasagna and Weintraub

Year Book of Emergency Medicine®: Drs. Wagner, Dronen, Davidson, King, Niemann, and Roberts

Year Book of Endocrinology®: Drs. Bagdade, Braverman, Horton, Kannan, Landsberg, Molitch, Morley, Nathan, Odell, Poehlman, Rogol, and Ryan

Year Book of Family Practice®: Drs. Berg, Bowman, Davidson, Dexter, and Scherger

Year Book of Gastroenterology®: Drs. Aliperti and Fleshman

Year Book of Geriatrics and Gerontology®: Drs. Burton, Beck, Ostwald, Rabins, Reuben, Roth, Shapiro, and Whitehouse

Year Book of Hand Surgery®: Drs. Amadio and Hentz

Year Book of Hematology®: Drs. Spivak, Bell, Ness, Quesenberry, Wiernik, and Horowitz

Year Book of Infectious Diseases: Drs. Keusch, Barza, Bennish, Poutsiaka, Skolnik, and Snydman

Year Book of Medicine®: Drs. Cline, Frishman, Jett, Klahr, Malawista, Mandell, McCallum, and Utiger

Year Book of Neonatal and Perinatal Medicine®: Drs. Fanaroff, Maisels, and Stevenson

Year Book of Nephrology, Hypertension, and Mineral Metabolism: Drs. Schwab, Bennett, Emmett, Hostetter, Kumar, and Toto

Year Book of Neurology and Neurosurgery®: Drs. Bradley and Gibbs

Year Book of Nuclear Medicine®: Drs. Gottschalk, Blaufox, Neumann, Strauss, and Zubal

Year Book of Obstetrics, Gynecology, and Women's Health: Drs. Mishell, Herbst, and Kirschbaum

Year Book of Occupational and Environmental Medicine®: Drs. Emmett, Frank, Gochfeld, and Hessl

Year Book of Oncology®: Drs. Ozols, Eisenberg, Glatstein, Loehrer, and Tallman

Year Book of Ophthalmology®: Drs. Wilson, Augsburger, Cohen, Eagle, Grossman, Laibson, Maguire, Nelson, Penne, Rapuano, Sergott, Spaeth, Tipperman, Ms. Gosfield, and Ms. Salmon

Year Book of Orthopedics®: Drs. Morrey, Beauchamp, Currier, Tolo, Trigg, and Swiontkowski

Year Book of Otolaryngology–Head and Neck Surgery®: Drs. Paparella and Holt

Year Book of Pathology and Laboratory Medicine®: Drs. Raab, Cohen, Olson, Sirgi, and Stanley

Year Book of Pediatrics®: Dr. Stockman

Year Book of Plastic, Reconstructive, and Aesthetic Surgery®: Drs. Miller, Bartlett, Garner, McKinney, Ruberg, Salisbury, and Smith

Year Book of Psychiatry and Applied Mental Health®: Drs. Talbott, Ballenger, Frances, Lydiard, Meltzer, Schowalter, and Tasman

Year Book of Pulmonary Disease®: Drs. Jett, Maurer, Ryu, Strollo, and Wenzel

Year Book of Rheumatology®: Drs. Panush, Hadler, LeRoy, Liang, Reichlin, Simon, and Weinblatt

Year Book of Sports Medicine®: Drs. Shephard, Drinkwater, Eichner, Torg, Alexander, and Mr. George

Year Book of Surgery®: Drs. Copeland, Bland, Deitch, Eberlein, Howard, Luce, Seeger, Souba, and Sugarbaker

Year Book of Thoracic and Cardiovascular Surgery®: Drs. Ginsberg, Wechsler, and Williams

Year Book of Urology®: Drs. Andriole and Coplen

Year Book of Vascular Surgery®: Dr. Porter

1998

The Year Book of MEDICINE®

Editors

Martin J. Cline, M.D.
William H. Frishman, M.D.
James Jett, M.D.
Saulo Klahr, M.D.
Stephen E. Malawista, M.D.
Gerald L. Mandell, M.D.
Richard W. McCallum, M.D., F.A.C.P., F.A.C.G.
Robert D. Utiger, M.D.

Mosby

St. Louis Baltimore Boston Carlsbad Naples New York Philadelphia Portland London
Madrid Mexico City Singapore Sydney Tokyo Toronto Wiesbaden

Mosby

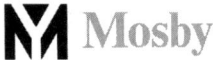

Dedicated to Publishing Excellence

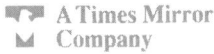

A Times Mirror
Company

Publisher: Gretchen Murphy
Developmental Editor: Marcy Reed
Manager, Periodical Editing: Kirk Swearingen
Production Editor: Amanda Maguire
Project Supervisor, Production: Joy Moore
Production Assistant: Karie House
Manager, Literature Services: Idelle L. Winer
Illustrations and Permissions Coordinator: Phyllis K. Thompson

1998 EDITION
Copyright © August, 1998 by Mosby, Inc.

Printed in the United States of America
Composition by Reed Technology and Information Services, Inc.
Printing/binding by Maple-Vail

Mosby, Inc.
11830 Westline Industrial Drive
St. Louis, MO 63146
Customer Service: customer.support@mosby.com
www.mosby.com/Mosby/CustomerSupport/index.html

International Standard Serial Number: 0084-3873
International Standard Book Number: 0-8151-3156-9

Editors

Martin J. Cline, M.D.
Bowyer Professor of Medical Oncology, Emeritus, Department of Medicine, University of California School of Medicine, Los Angeles, California

William H. Frishman, M.D.
Professor and Chairman, Department of Medicine, New York Medical College; Chief of Medicine, Westchester County Medical Center, Valhalla, New York

James Jett, M.D.
Professor of Medicine, Mayo Medical School, Consultant in Thoracic Diseases and Medical Oncology, Mayo Clinic, Rochester, Minnesota

Saulo Klahr, M.D.
Simon Professor of Medicine, Department of Internal Medicine, Washington University, Barnes-Jewish Hospital, St. Louis, Missouri

Stephen E. Malawista, M.D.
Professor of Medicine, Department of Internal Medicine, Yale University School of Medicine, New Haven, Connecticut

Gerald L. Mandell, M.D.
Professor of Medicine, Owen R. Cheatham Professor of the Sciences; Chief, Division of Infectious Diseases, University of Virginia Health Sciences Center, Charlottesville, Virginia

Richard W. McCallum, M.D., F.A.C.P., F.A.C.G.
Professor of Medicine, Chief of Gastroenterology and Hepatology, Director of Center for GI Motility Disorders, University of Kansas Medical Center, Kansas City, Kansas and Kansas City Veterans Administration Medical Center, Kansas City, Missouri

Robert D. Utiger, M.D.
Clinical Professor of Medicine, Harvard Medical School, Boston, Massachusetts; Deputy Editor, The New England Journal of Medicine

Contributors

Janet R. Maurer, M.D.
Head, Section of Lung Transplantation, Department of Pulmonary and Critical Care Medicine, Cleveland Clinic Foundation, Cleveland, Ohio

Jay H. Ryu, M.D.
Associate Professor of Medicine, Mayo Medical School, Consultant in Pulmonary and Critical Care Medicine, Mayo Clinic, Rochester, Minnesota

Patrick J. Strollo, Jr., M.D.
Associate Professor of Medicine, University of Pittsburgh; Director, Pulmonary Sleep Evaluation Laboratory, University of Pittsburgh Medical Center, Pittsburgh, Pennsylvania

Sally E. Wenzel, M.D.
Associate Professor of Medicine, National Jewish Medical and Research Center and The University of Colorado Health Sciences Center, Denver, Colorado

Table of Contents

JOURNALS REPRESENTED   xv

PUBLISHER'S PREFACE   xix

INFECTIOUS DISEASES   1
Gerald L. Mandell, M.D.

   INTRODUCTION   3

1. Mechanisms of Disease   5

   Introduction   5

2. Human Immunodeficiency Virus (HIV)   9

   Introduction   9

3. AIDS Opportunistic Infection   19

   Introduction   19

4. Viral Infections   29

   Introduction   29

5. Respiratory Infections   41

   Introduction   41

6. Bacterial and Fungal Infections   47

   Introduction   47

7. Gastrointestinal Infections   59

   Introduction   59

8. Chlamydia Pneumoniae and Cardiovascular Disease   67

   Introduction   67

9. Biologic Terrorism and Warfare   71

   Introduction   71

HEMATOLOGY AND ONCOLOGY   77
Martin J. Cline, M.D.

   INTRODUCTION   79

10. Red Cells, White Cells, and Hemostasis   81

11. Leukemia and Myeloproliferative Disorders   95

12. Lymphoproliferative Disorders and Multiple Myeloma   107

13. Bone Marrow Transplantation and Gene Therapy   123

14. Cancer 141

THE HEART AND CARDIOVASCULAR DISEASE 157
William H. Frishman, M.D.

INTRODUCTION 159

15. Risk Factors for Coronary Artery Disease 163

16. Acute Coronary Syndromes 173

17. Chronic Coronary Artery Disease 185

18. Coronary Interventional Procedures 199

19. Cardiomyopathy/Heart Failure 207

20. Valvular Heart Disease 221

21. Noninvasive Testing 227

22. Arrythmias 233

23. Other Topics 247

ENDOCRINOLOGY, DIABETES, AND METABOLISM...... 257
Robert D. Utiger, M.D.

INTRODUCTION 259

24. The Pituitary Gland 265

25. Adrenal Glands 275

26. The Thyroid Gland 293

27. The Parathyroid Glands and Bone 305

28. The Reproductive System 325

29. Carbohydrate Metabolism and Diabetes Mellitus 335

30. Obesity and Lipid Metabolism 351

KIDNEY, WATER, AND ELECTROLYTES 357
Saulo Klahr, M.D.

INTRODUCTION 359

31. Glomerular Disease 363

32. Other Diseases of the Kidney 381

33. Acute Renal Failure 399

34. Chronic Renal Failure 405

35. Hypertension 415

36. Transplantation 425

37. Dialysis 429

38. Water, Electrolytes, and Acid-Base 439

39. Calcium, Phosphorus, and Bone 443

RHEUMATOLOGY 449
   Stephen E. Malawista, M.D.

40. Rheumatoid Arthritis 451

   Introduction 451

41. Systemic Lupus Erythematosus 465

   Introduction 465

42. Spondyloarthropathy and Reactive Arthritis 477

   Introduction 477

43. Sclerosing Syndromes 483

   Introduction 483

44. Crystal-associated Arthritis 487

   Introduction 487

45. Vasculitis 491

   Introduction 491

46. Infectious Arthritis 499

   Introduction 499

47. Other Topics 509

   Introduction 509

THE CHEST 513
   James R. Jett, M.D.

INTRODUCTION 515

48. Nicotine 517

49. Lung Cancer 523

50. Malignant Effusion 529

51. Chronic Obstructive Pulmonary Disease 531

Cystic Fibrosis 536

52. Lung Volume Reduction Surgery 539

53. Asthma 543

54. Interstitial Lung Disease 555

55. Pleural Emboli/Pulmonary Hypertension 563

56. Tuberculosis 571

57. Tuberculosis and the Human Immunodeficiency Virus 575

58. Human Immunodeficiency Virus 577

59. Bacterial Infections 581

60. Intensive Care Medicine 585

61. Sleep 591

THE DIGESTIVE SYSTEM 595
Richard W. McCallum, M.D.

62. Diagnostic Testing 597

63. Inflammatory Bowel Disease 605

64. Hepatology—Hepatitis 611

65. Hepatology—General 617

66. Helicobacter Pylori 629

67. Gastrointestinal Motility 641

68. Gastroesophageal Reflux Disease 661

SUBJECT INDEX. 673

AUTHOR INDEX 721

Journals Represented

Mosby and its Editors survey more than 1,000 journals for its abstract and commentary publications. From these journals, the Editors select the articles to be abstracted. Journals represented in this YEAR BOOK are listed below.

American Journal of Cardiology
American Journal of Clinical Pathology
American Journal of Gastroenterology
American Journal of Kidney Diseases
American Journal of Medicine
American Journal of Pathology
American Journal of Physiology
American Journal of Respiratory and Critical Care Medicine
American Journal of Roentgenology
American Journal of Surgery
American Surgeon
Annals of Allergy, Asthma, & Immunology
Annals of Internal Medicine
Annals of Oncology
Annals of Surgery
Archives of Internal Medicine
Archives of Surgery
Arthritis and Rheumatism
Blood
Bone Marrow Transplantation
British Journal of Obstetrics and Gynaecology
British Journal of Surgery
British Medical Journal
Cancer
Chest
Circulation
Clinical Endocrinology (Oxford)
Clinical Infectious Diseases
Critical Care Medicine
Diabetes
Diabetes Care
Diabetologia
Digestive Diseases and Sciences
Diseases of the Colon and Rectum
European Heart Journal
European Journal of Cancer
European Journal of Haematology
European Journal of Nuclear Medicine
European Respiratory Journal
Fertility and Sterility
Gastroenterology
Gastrointestinal Endoscopy
Gut
Hepatology
Human Pathology
Infection Control and Hospital Epidemiology
International Journal of Epidemiology

International Journal of Radiation, Oncology, Biology, and Physics
Journal of Clinical Endocrinology and Metabolism
Journal of Clinical Epidemiology
Journal of Clinical Investigation
Journal of Clinical Microbiology
Journal of Clinical Oncology
Journal of Clinical Pathology
Journal of General Internal Medicine
Journal of Infectious Diseases
Journal of Internal Medicine
Journal of Rheumatology
Journal of Thoracic and Cardiovascular Surgery
Journal of Urology
Journal of Women's Health
Journal of the American Academy of Dermatology
Journal of the American College of Cardiology
Journal of the American Medical Association
Journal of the American Society of Nephrology
Journal of the National Cancer Institute
Kidney International
Lancet
Mayo Clinic Proceedings
Medicine
Medicine and Science in Sports and Exercise
Nature
Nephrology, Dialysis, Transplantation
Neurogastroenterology Motility
New England Journal of Medicine
Pediatric Infectious Disease Journal
Pediatric Pathology & Laboratory Medicine
Pediatric Research
Pediatrics
Proceedings of the National Academy of Sciences
Radiology
Science
Stroke
Surgery
Thorax
Transplantation
Urology
Western Journal of Medicine

STANDARD ABBREVIATIONS

The following terms are abbreviated in this edition: acquired immunodeficiency syndrome (AIDS), cardiopulmonary resuscitation (CPR), central nervous system (CNS), cerebrospinal fluid (CSF), computed tomography (CT), deoxyribonucleic acid (DNA), electrocardiography (ECG), health maintenance organization (HMO), human immunodeficiency virus (HIV), intensive care unit (ICU), intramuscular (IM), intravenous (IV), magnetic resonance (MR) imaging (MRI), and ribonucleic acid (RNA).

NOTE

The YEAR BOOK OF MEDICINE is a literature survey service providing abstracts of articles published in the professional literature. Every effort is made to assure the accuracy of the information presented in these pages. Neither the editors nor the publisher of the YEAR BOOK OF MEDICINE can be responsible for errors in the original materials. The editors' comments are their own opinions. Mention of specific products within this publication does not constitute endorsement.

To facilitate the use of the YEAR BOOK OF MEDICINE as a reference tool, all illustrations and tables included in this publication are now identified as they appear in the original article. This change is meant to help the reader recognize that any illustration or table appearing in the YEAR BOOK OF MEDICINE may be only one of many in the original article. For this reason, figure and table numbers will often appear to be out of sequence within the YEAR BOOK OF MEDICINE.

Publisher's Preface

With the publication of this year's volume of the YEAR BOOK OF MEDICINE, we bid farewell to editors Martin Cline, M.D., Richard McCallum, M.D., and Robert Utiger, M.D. Each spent many, many hours reviewing thousands of articles for possible inclusion in the YEAR BOOK. Then came the job of authoring editorial comments and compiling usable manuscripts. Their dedication cannot be overstated.

We are especially honored to have enjoyed so many years of valued expertise from Dr. Cline and Dr. Utiger. Their tremendous contributions to the YEAR BOOK will be greatly missed.

We extend our thanks to all of the editors for their insightful commentaries and editorial expertise, and we wish them well in the years ahead.

PART ONE

INFECTIOUS DISEASES
GERALD L. MANDELL, M.D.

Introduction

Progress in understanding and managing infectious diseases continues at an astounding pace. New information on the pathogenesis of various infections is largely due to advances in basic sciences. Of special note are the projects, often industry-based, focused on identification of the entire genome of pathogenic microbes. Elucidation of the genome indicates new targets for chemotherapy and vaccine development. It is clear that disease manifestations are produced by the interaction of the microbe with the host's immune system. Study of the disease process and the role of host immunity also suggests therapeutic roles for immunomodulators and inhibitors of immune activators.

International travel and the availability of foodstuffs in our supermarkets grown in faraway places adds new dimensions to the epidemiology of infectious diseases. It has been said that when we shop in a gleaming, clean supermarket we should approach the fresh fruit and vegetable area just as if we are partaking of these splendid foods in a developing country. The recent approval of irradiation of red meat to eliminate pathogens is a logical and timely response to the problem of microbial contamination of meat.

There are very few "new" pathogens but newly recognized and newly emerging pathogens continue to excite and frighten both the scientific community and the public at large.

HIV infection continues to infect and kill patients worldwide. Advances in our knowledge are spectacular but the big breakthrough is still elusive. Triple (and soon quadruple drug) therapy can be remarkably effective in selected patients. However, this therapy is expensive, difficult to tolerate and requires meticulous compliance. It is also clear that it is not a cure. Because we cannot eliminate the ravages of HIV on the immune system, much work is focused on preventing and treating opportunistic infections; some of these are covered in this section.

More mundane infections are still a major problem. Advances in diagnosis, prevention and therapy are of interest.

We must conclude on an ominous note. The threat of biologic terrorism and warfare is very real. In comparison to nuclear weapons, which require tremendously expensive and technologically advanced procedures to manufacture, biologic products can be produced simply and cheaply. Materials and equipment used for legitimate purposes can easily be subverted to produce these dangerous agents of disease.

Gerald L. Mandell, M.D.

3

1 Mechanisms of Disease

Introduction

Therapy of sepsis continues to be elusive and there is a long list of failed therapies. Although not clinically effective, the study of ibuprofen does shed some light on the physiology of the syndrome. When several people are exposed to a pathogen, why do some get ill and others not? Studies of the interferon gamma receptor gene are adding important new pieces of data to this puzzle. Fever continues to fascinate infectious diseases physicians, and the article by Alcami and Smith supplies an ingenious new wrinkle to the discussion.

Gerald L. Mandell, M.D.

The Effects of Ibuprofen on the Physiology and Survival of Patients With Sepsis
Bernard GR, for the Ibuprofen in Sepsis Study Group (Vanderbilt Univ, Nashville, Tenn; Univ of British Columbia, Vancouver, Canada; Univ of Miami, Fla; et al)
N Engl J Med 336:912–918, 97   1–1

Introduction.—Several previous studies involving small groups of patients with sepsis reported some benefits of ibuprofen, but it is uncertain whether this agent can reduce physiologic abnormalities and improve survival. The effects of ibuprofen in patients with the sepsis syndrome were determined in a randomized trial.

Methods.—The multicenter trial employed a double-blind, placebo-controlled design. Patients recruited from ICUs had a diagnosis of sepsis, defined as fever, tachycardia, tachypnea, and acute failure of at least 1 organ system. The 455 patients enrolled in the study were given intravenous ibuprofen in a dose of 10 mg/kg (maximum dose 800 mg) over a period of 30–60 minutes every 6 hours for 8 doses, or placebo, administered in the same volume and at the same times. Data on the patient's condition were obtained at study entry, every 4 hours for the first 44 hours, and then at 72, 96, and 120 hours. Ibuprofen and placebo groups were compared for rates of organ failure and 30-day mortality.

Results.—Ibuprofen and placebo groups were similar in mean age, gender distribution, and variables known to affect morbidity and mortality. The predominant site of infection was the lung. Although rates of organ dysfunction were similar at study entry in the 2 groups, renal dysfunction was significantly more common in the placebo group. Only the ibuprofen group showed significant declines in urinary levels of prostacyclin and thromboxane, both of which are elevated in sepsis syndrome. Temperature, heart rate, oxygen consumption, and lactic acidosis were also reduced with ibuprofen treatment, and patients in this group had no increased incidence of renal dysfunction, gastrointestinal bleeding, or other adverse events. The 2 groups did not differ, however, in the incidence or duration of shock or acute respiratory distress syndrome. Thirty-day mortality was 37% with ibuprofen and 40% with placebo, not a significant difference.

Conclusion.—Treatment with nonsteroidal anti-inflammatory drugs has improved survival and reduced physiologic abnormalities in animal models of sepsis. In this large series of patients, however, ibuprofen failed to prevent the development of shock or the acute respiratory distress syndrome or to improve 30-day survival, despite the drug's beneficial effects on certain clinical indicators.

▶ I am afraid this is another agent in a long line of those that have failed in clinical trials for sepsis. Ibuprofen is a potent anti-inflammatory agent by virtue of its significant inhibition of cyclooxygenase and thereby synthesis of prostaglandins and thromboxane. As would be expected, ibuprofen decreased temperature, heart rate, and minute ventilation as compared to placebo in septic patients. However, there was no change in the incidence or duration of shock, acute respiratory distress syndrome, or survival. Sepsis is so complicated, with so many interacting factors, that our attempts at therapy now appear to be overly simplistic.

G.L. Mandell, M.D.

A Mutation in the Interferon-γ-Receptor Gene and Susceptibility to Mycobacterial Infection

Newport MJ, Huxley CM, Huston S, et al (Imperial College, London; Erasmus Univ, Rotterdam, The Netherlands)
N Engl J Med 335:1941–1949, 1996   1–2

Objective.—Only a small percentage of those infected with *Mycobacterium tuberculosis* ever demonstrate clinically evident disease. Studies have shown that genetic factors play a role in susceptibility. Studies of 4 children from Malta with an autosomal recessive disorder predisposing them to infection with a range of mycobacteria identified the chromosomal location of a recessive gene responsible for the increased susceptibility.

Methods.—The 4 children demonstrated disseminated atypical mycobacterial infection in the absence of a known immunodeficiency. Three of the children are related, but the genetic link to the fourth has not been determined. Each child was infected with a different strain or species of mycobacterium. Deoxyribonucleic acid from peripheral blood lymphocytes of patients, unaffected family members, and controls was amplified using polymerase chain reaction. The ability of interferon-γ to upregulate the production of tumor necrosis factor-α (TNF-α) by monocytes was determined.

Results.—After typing of 360 microsatellite markers, a single 5-cm region was found on chromosome 6q in the 3 affected related children homozygous for the same alleles for 8 microsatellites. Parents and unaffected siblings were heterozygous. The gene for interferon-γ receptor 1 is found in this region, and expression of this receptor was defective in the children but not in a control or an unaffected parent. The cDNA-sequencing showed a substitution of A for C at position 395, which resulted in a stop codon in all affected children. These children were homozygous for the mutation. Production of TNF-α was dramatically decreased in the surviving affected child compared to the controls. His parents' response was intermediate.

Conclusion.—A mutation in the gene coding for interferon-γ receptor, that, in turn, is supposed to upregulate production of TNF-α, was found in 4 children with severe mycobacterial infections.

▶ The human genome and infectious agents have co-evolved. We are just learning to understand why, with equal exposure to pathogens, some patients become ill and others do not. The chemokine receptor data, with HIV infection, is a recent case in point. Individuals with certain abnormalities in the chemokine receptor appear to be completely or relatively resistant to infection with HIV, which uses the receptor to enter cells.

Instead of focusing on patients who did not get ill, these authors studied 4 related children who had severe disseminated atypical mycobacterial infection. They identified a mutation that inhibited the normal macrophage response to interferon-γ. The old name for interferon-γ was "macrophage activating factor," and if macrophages are not normally activated by this molecule, they have a decreased ability to kill intracellular pathogens. This seems to be mediated, at least in part, by TNF upregulation induced by the interferon-γ. Perhaps more subtle genetic changes will be identified in the near future that will explain the marked variations seen in susceptibility to mycobacterial and other infections.

G.L. Mandell, M.D.

TABLE 3.—Frequency and Duration of Signs and Symptoms Reported for 5% or More of 218 Patients at the Time of Acute HIV-1 Disease

Percentage of patients, sign or symptom	No. (%) of patients	Average duration in d (no. of patients)	Median duration in d (range)
>50%			
Fever (temperature of ≥38°C)	168 (77.1)	16.9 (162)	14.0 (3.0–184.0)
Lethargy	143 (65.6)	23.7 (139)	18.0 (1.0–184.0)
Cutaneous rash	123 (56.4)	15.0 (117)	11.0 (1.0–73.0)
Myalgia	119 (54.6)	17.7 (112)	11.0 (2.0–184.0)
Headache	111 (50.9)	25.8 (108)	13.0 (2.0–continuing*)
>25%–50%			
Pharyngitis or sore throat	96 (44.0)	12.2 (90)	8.0 (1.0–51.0)
Cervical adenopathy	85 (39.0)	15.1 (8)	12.0 (3.0–32.0)
Arthralgia	67 (30.7)	22.6 (64)	15.0 (3.0–184.0)
Oral ulcer	63 (28.9)	13.4 (63)	8.0 (1.0–85.0)
Odynophagia	61 (28.0)	16.3 (58)	14.0 (2.0–48.0)
5%–25%			
Axillary adenopathy	53 (24.3)	164.1 (6)	13.5 (1.0–continuing*)
Weight loss	52 (23.9)	29.0 (49)	19.0 (3.0–continuing*)
Nausea	52 (23.9)	17.8 (50)	14.0 (2.0–109.0)
Diarrhea	50 (22.9)	12.5 (47)	8.0 (1.0–39.0)
Night sweats	48 (22.0)	14.8 (45)	10.0 (3.0–57.0)
Cough	48 (22.0)	18.4 (48)	12.5 (2.0–184.0)
Anorexia	46 (21.1)	14.6 (44)	10.0 (2.0–68.0)
Inguinal adenopathy	44 (20.2)	8.5 (2)	8.5 (7.0–10.0)
Abdominal pain	42 (19.3)	15.1 (40)	12.0 (1.0–73.0)
Oral candidiasis	37 (17.0)	10.4 (34)	7.5 (1.0–34.0)
Vomiting	27 (12.4)	9.8 (27)	10.0 (1.0–31.0)
Photophobia	26 (11.9)	11.2 (25)	10.0 (2.0–39.0)
Sore eyes	25 (11.5)	13.2 (24)	11.5 (3.0–36.0)
Genital ulcer	15 (6.9)	13.5 (15)	12.0 (3.0–35.0)
Tonsillitis	15 (6.9)	13.3 (13)	10.0 (1.0–41.0)
Depression	14 (6.4)	22.8 (9)	7.0 (3.0–76.0)
Dizziness	12 (5.5)	10.7 (10)	9.5 (1.0–26.0)

*The treating physician considered that the sign or symptom became a chronic feature.
(Courtesy of Vanhems P, Allard R, Cooper DA, et al: Acute human immunodeficiency virus type 1 disease as a mononucleosis-like illness: Is the diagnosis too restrictive? *Clin Infect Dis* 24:965–970, 1997. Published by the University of Chicago.)

nucleosis-type illness. Nine percent had a meningitis-like syndrome (Table 3).

Conclusion.—Patients with acute HIV-1 have a broad array of symptoms and signs when first seeking medical care. Less than 20% have the classical features of a mononucleosis-type illness. The possibility of HIV-1 seroconversion should be considered in patients with a febrile syndrome, especially one associated with gastrointestinal or mucocutaneous features and risk factors for HIV infection.

▶ It is very important to identify the acute HIV infection syndrome, as intensive triple-drug treatment of these patients may result in an excellent response with an undetectable viral load; a seemingly normal immune system; and, perhaps, even a "cure." The authors emphasize that the syndrome does not have to include a mononucleosis-like illness. Only a minority of their patients had sore throat and cervical adenopathy. In my view, an unexplained febrile illness in an adult with HIV risk factors should prompt testing for HIV infection. The table shows that the findings seen in 50% or more of the patients are very nonspecific.

G.L. Mandell, M.D.

Reduction of Concentration of HIV-1 in Semen After Treatment of Urethritis: Implications for Prevention of Sexual Transmission of HIV-1
Cohen MS, and the AIDSCAP Malawi Research Group (Univ of North Carolina, Chapel Hill; Lilongwe Central Hosp, Malawi; John Snow Inc, Boston; et al)
Lancet 349:1868–1873, 1997   2–2

Introduction.—There is strong epidemiologic evidence that sexually transmitted diseases (STDs) significantly increase the risk of acquiring HIV-1, but the biological mechanism has yet to be determined. In a study conducted in Malawi, where transmission of HIV-1 is predominantly by heterosexual contact, the hypothesis that STDs increase concentration of the virus in semen, leading to increased infectiousness and a greater possibility of disease transmission, was investigated.

Methods.—The study was designed as a prospective, sequential comparison of 2 cohorts, both of which included men who were HIV-positive. Men in one cohort were seen at an STD clinic and had urethritis; those in the control cohort, selected from a dermatology clinic, did not have urethritis. The main hypothesis of the study was that antibiotic therapy for urethritis would decrease the concentration of HIV-1 in semen. Concentrations of HIV-1 RNA in cell-free seminal plasma were measured at study entry and after men with urethritis received antibiotic therapy.

Results.—The STD and control groups had similar proportions of men who were HIV-positive (55% and 48%, respectively). Baseline semen samples were provided by 86 HIV-1-seropositive men in the STD group and 49 seropositive controls; baseline blood samples were available for 69 and 35 men, respectively. The HIV-positive patients from STD and control groups were similar in age, CD4 counts, and blood-plasma viral burden. Median seminal plasma HIV-1 RNA concentrations were 8 times higher in the STD group than in the control group at baseline. The concentrations of viral RNA in semen were higher in men with gonorrhea than in those with nongonococcal urethritis (median 15.8 vs. 2.52 × 10⁴ copies/mL). Those with nongonococcal urethritis did not differ significantly from controls in baseline seminal HIV-1 RNA concentrations. Antimicrobial treatment of STDs led to a significant decrease in the concentration of HIV-1 RNA in semen, whereas blood plasma viral RNA concentrations remained unchanged. Seminal plasma HIV-1 RNA concentrations did not change significantly in the control group during the 2-week study period.

Conclusion.—The presence of urethritis, particularly gonococcal urethritis, increases the infectiousness of HIV-1-seropositive men. Identification and treatment of seropositive men with STDs may reduce the transmission rate of HIV-1 infection.

▶ Factors affecting efficiency of transmission of HIV-1 are being unraveled. It is well accepted that ulcerogenic genital diseases such as chancroid, herpes genitalis, and syphilis increase the likelihood of acquiring infection. This is probably because the virus has easier access to host cells. This study shows, in a convincing manner, that coexistent urethritis in men markedly increases HIV-1 RNA in semen, both in comparison to patients without urethritis and in comparison to the same patient after treatment. Although studies have not documented an effect on transmission, one would anticipate that treatment of coexistent urethritis would reduce the efficiency of transmission. This has important public health implications.

G.L. Mandell, M.D.

Differential Regulation of HIV-1 Fusion Cofactor Expression by CD28 Costimulation of CD4⁺ T Cells

Carroll RG, Riley JL, Levine BL, et al (Henry M. Jackson Found, Rockville, Md; Walter Reed Army Inst for Research, Rockville, Md; Naval Med Research Inst, Bethesda, Md; et al)
Science 276:273–276, 1997   2–3

Introduction.—Human immunodeficiency virus-type 1 (HIV-1) is influenced by the chemokine receptor family and by the host T-cell activation state. Commitment to T-cell activation needs T-cell receptor (CD3) engagement and a costimulatory signal; CD28 with its ligands CD80 or CD86 offer a needed costimulus to induce an immune response. Activation with immobilized antibodies to CD3 (anti-CD3) and CD28 (anti-CD28) causes a potent anti-HIV effect. The intrinsic CD3–CD28-specific antiviral effect was evaluated by comparing the HIV-1 infection process in cells stimulated with either immobilized anti-CD3 and anti-CD28 or with the mitogenic lectin, phytohemagglutinin (PHA), and interleukin-2 (IL-2).

Findings.—A virus-resistant state was caused by activation of CD4⁺ T lymphocytes from donors with HIV-1 and immobilized antibodies to CD3 and CD28. This effect was specific for macrophage-tropic HIV-1. Transcripts encoding CXCR-4–Fusin (the fusion cofactor used by T-cell linetropic isolates) were plentiful in CD3–CD28-stimulated cells. The transcripts encoding CCR5 (the fusion cofactor used by macrophage-tropic viruses) were not capable of being distinguished.

Conclusion.—The CD3–CD28 costimulation causes an HIV-1-resistant phenotype similar to that observed in some highly exposed individuals who are not infected with HIV.

Potent Inhibition of HIV-1 Infectivity in Macrophages and Lymphocytes by a Novel CCR5 Antagonist

Simmons G, Clapham PR, Picard L, et al (Inst of Cancer Research, London; Centre Médical Universitaire, Geneva; Geneva Biomedical Research Inst)

Science 276:276–279, 1997   2–4

Introduction.—It has recently been demonstrated that the chemokine receptors CXCR-4 and CCR5 act as coreceptors together with CD4 for HIV type 1 (HIV-1) infection. Regulated upon activation normal T-cell expressed and secreted (RANTES) and other chemokines that interact with CCR5 to prevent infection of peripheral blood mononuclear cell cultures also inhibit infection of primary macrophages but do so ineffectively. These chemokines could fail to influence HIV replication in nonlymphocyte compartments and promote unwanted side effects if used to treat patients infected with HIV-1. Reported are results of a RANTES receptor antagonist evaluated for its capability to inhibit HIV-1 infection of different cell types.

Findings.—A derivative of RANTES created by chemical modification of the amino terminus, aminooxypentane (AOP)-RANTES did not cause chemotaxis and was a subnanomolar antagonist of CCR5 function when exposed to monocytes. It potently inhibited infection of diverse cell types that included macrophages and lymphocytes by nonsyncytium-inducing, macrophage-tropic strains of HIV-1.

Conclusion.—Activation of cells by chemokines is not necessary for inhibition of viral uptake and replication. The use of chemokine receptor antagonists like AOP-RANTES that reach full receptor occupancy at nanomolar concentrations are likely candidates for the therapy of individuals infected with HIV-1.

▶ The interaction of chemokine receptors with HIV is important but complex. These 2 articles (Abstract 2–3 and Abstract 2–4) help to unravel the story and to further progress toward using these receptors for chemotherapy or chemoprophylaxis. Chemokines are cytokines (substances produced by cells that activate or influence other cells) and serve as attractants or activators for a variety of cells of the immune system. Chemokine receptors on the surface of lymphocytes are important for fusion of HIV-1 with the cells. The CD4 receptor on lymphocytes and macrophages also is responsible for the initial binding of the virus to the cell. Human immunodeficiency virus-1 has different phenotypes. These phenotypes preferentially infect either macrophages or T lymphocytes and use different chemokine receptors as cofactors for fusion. Carroll et al. showed that they could induce a virus-resistant state in lymphocytes by down-regulating a certain chemokine receptor (CCR5) that is used by macrophage-tropic viruses. This mechanism mimicked that seen in some patients who have mutations in CCR5 and who appeared to be resistant to HIV infection despite repeated exposure. Simmons et al. were able to inhibit infectivity by using a chemokine receptor antagonist that occupied the receptor and precluded HIV-1 from using this receptor for cell fusion.

Thus, both groups of investigators are targeting the important CCR5 molecule. The therapeutic potential is exciting.

G.L. Mandell, M.D.

Rational Interleukin 2 Therapy for HIV Positive Individuals: Daily Low Doses Enhance Immune Function Without Toxicity
Jacobson EL, Pilaro F, Smith KA (New York Hosp Cornell Med Ctr)
Proc Natl Acad Sci U S A 93:10405–10410, 1996   2–5

Background.—High doses of interleukin-2 (IL-2) cause extreme toxicity and markedly increased plasma HIV levels in HIV-positive persons. The nontoxic, effective dose levels of IL-2 and whether IL-2 could be given safely to asymptomatic, HIV-positive patients without promoting viral replication were investigated.

Methods and Findings.—Interleukin-2 doses of 62,500–250,000 IU/m²/ day were administered subcutaneously for 6 months to 16 HIV-positive patients with 200–500 CD4+ T cells/mm³. Before treatment, IL-2 was detectable in the plasma of most HIV-positive patients. In 10 patients receiving the maximum nontoxic dose, ranging from 187,500 to 250,000 IU/m²/day, peak plasma IL-1 levels were near saturating for high-affinity IL-2 receptors. The plasma levels of proinflammatory cytokines remained undetectable during 6 months of treatment in this dose range. Plasma HIV RNA levels did not significantly change. However, delayed type hypersensitivity responses to common recall antigens were augmented markedly. Furthermore, IL-2 dose-dependent increases in circulating natural killer cells, eosinophils, monocytes, and CD4+ T cells were observed.

Conclusions.—Asymptomatic HIV-positive persons can self-administer very low doses of IL-2 safely, with no evident toxicity, for 6 months. Such doses effectively stimulate immune reactivity. Thus IL-2 immunotherapy may now be considered an adjuvant to antiviral chemotherapy in this patient population.

Controlled Trial of Interleukin-2 Infusions in Patients Infected With the Human Immunodeficiency Virus
Kovacs JA, Vogel S, Albert JM, et al (Natl Inst of Allergy and Infectious Diseases, Bethesda, Md; Science Applications Internatl Corp, Frederick, Md; Chiron Corp, Emeryville, Calif)
N Engl J Med 335:1350–1356, 1996   2–6

Background.—In patients with HIV infection, the number or percentage of CD4 cells provides the best single indicator of the immune system's ability to prevent the development of opportunistic infections. An uncontrolled pilot study of patients infected with HIV found that intermittent interleukin-2 therapy led to sustained increases in the number of CD4 cells.

The long-term effects of intermittent interleukin-2 therapy on the HIV load were examined in a randomized controlled study.

Methods.—Study participants were 60 HIV-infected patients with baseline CD4 counts above 200 cells per cubic millimeter. In the pilot study, patients with CD4 counts of this level were most likely to respond to interleukin-2. Thirty-one patients were randomly assigned to interleukin-2 plus antiretroviral therapy and 29 to antiretroviral therapy alone. Interleukin-2, started at a dosage of 18 million IU/day, was administered every 2 months for 6 cycles of 5 days each. Evaluations were conducted monthly for 14 months after randomization. In addition to CD4 counts, patients were assessed for changes in plasma HIV load, level of p24 antigenemia, and percentage of CD4 cells.

Results.—The 2 groups were similar in age and weight, HIV-risk group, and laboratory findings at baseline. Antiviral regimens at enrollment and during the study were also comparable for interleukin-2 and placebo groups. Patients in the interleukin-2 group increased their mean CD4 count from 428 cells per cubic millimeter at entry to 916 at 12 months. The placebo group, in contrast, showed a decrease in CD4 counts from a mean of 406 cells per cubic millimeter at baseline to 349. Serial measurements of the plasma HIV RNA or p24 antigen concentration did not differ between groups during the 12-month treatment period. In an extended phase of the study, with all patients eligible to receive interleukin-2, the mean CD4 count increase was sustained in the patients randomly allocated to interleukin-2. Administration of interleukin-2 was associated with moderate and severe clinical side effects (commonly fever, malaise, and fatigue) and laboratory abnormalities (most frequently asymptomatic hyperbilirubinemia). Toxic effects decreased as the dosage was reduced in later cycles.

Summary.—Intermittent infusions of interleukin-2 produced substantial and sustained increases in CD4 counts in patients with HIV infection and baseline counts greater than 200 cells per cubic millimeter. The treatment did not lead to long-term increases in the plasma viral load, and toxicity was substantially lower than in previous reports.

▶ Interleukin-2 (IL-2) is a cytokine made by T cells, which promotes the growth and differentiation of lymphocytes including CD cells. It was originally known as T-cell growth factor and was important in the studies by Gallo et al.[1] in their first isolation of HIV. Lymphocytes would not support the growth of HIV unless they were stimulated with T-cell growth factor now known as IL-2. Kovacs et al. (Abstract 2–6) report that IL-2 caused sustained and significant increases in CD4 counts with no associated increase in plasma HIV-RNA levels and thus they felt that this was a promising therapy. Patients did, however, have significant constitutional symptoms. Note that the doses used in the Kovacs study were 18 million IU/day. Jacobson (Abstract 2–5) used much lower doses (62,500 to 250,000 IU/day) and found decreased toxicity but enhancement of immune status. This was defined by increases in natural killer cells, CD4 cells, and delayed type hypersensitivity responses. Both groups suggest further studies, especially coupled with potent antiviral therapy. We anxiously await the results of such studies.

G.L. Mandell, M.D.

Reference

1. Gallo RC, Salahuddin SZ, Popovic M et al: Human T-lymphotropic retrovirus. HTLV-III, isolated from AIDS patients and donors at risk for AIDS. *Science* 224:500–503, 1984.

Decay Characteristics of HIV-1–infected Compartments During Combination Therapy

Perelson AS, Essunger P, Cao Y, et al (Los Alamos Natl Lab, New Mexico; Rockefeller Univ, New York; Univ of Tampere, Finland)
Nature 387:188–191, 1997   2–7

Background.—When HIV-infected patients are treated with antiretroviral agents, plasma levels of HIV drop rapidly. The authors show that, with combination chemotherapy, this initial decrease is followed by a slower second-phase decay of plasma viremia.

Study Design.—Eight HIV-infected patients, with no prior antiretroviral treatment and CD4 lymphocyte counts from 26 to 505/µL, were treated with a triple-therapy regimen consisting of nelfinavir, zidovudine, and lamivudine. Plasma HIV RNA concentration was assessed weekly for the first month of treatment and then every other week using the branched DNA assay.

Results.—Each patient responded to therapy with a similar pattern of decrease in viral load: an initial rapid exponential decline of about 2-logs (first phase), followed by a slower exponential decline (second phase), suggesting the existence of only 1 major secondary virion source. Plasma virus levels fell below the standard detection threshold of 500 copies/mL by the eighth week of therapy and below 25 copies/mL by week 20. No infectious virus could be detected in 10^7 peripheral blood mononuclear cells (PBMC) from any patient after 8 weeks of therapy. The second phase was probably the result of infected tissue macrophages or dendritic cells, activation of latently infected lymphocytes, or the release of trapped virus particles. These secondary sources of virus were incorporated into a mathematical model of the decline of viral load and used to analyze data from these 8 patients. Additional viral load data were obtained from measuring the infectivity titer of latent HIV in PBMC by limiting dilution at each time point. These data were also incorporated into the model. The rate of proviral decay was significantly slower than plasma virus or PBMC infectivity decay, suggesting that long-lived infected cells are the major reservoir for virus in the second phase of plasma viremia decay. The principle contributor to this second phase has a half life of 5.8 to 24.8 days and may consist of infected tissue macrophages or virus trapped on follicular dendritic cells in lymphoid tissue.

Conclusion.—This model suggests that if antiretroviral therapy completely inhibits new infection, HIV virus could be completely eliminated from all known compartments after 2.3 to 3.1 years of therapy. However, other sources of virus may be present for life, such as minor reservoirs of virus or sanctuary sites that are not penetrated by antiretroviral drugs or viral DNA within mononuclear cells that could become activated to produce infectious virus. Despite these caveats, recent advances in both treatment and understanding of HIV infection suggest that the possibility of eliminating HIV from an infected person should be seriously considered.

▶ Perelson and colleagues continue to dazzle us with kinetic models described by complex differential equations. Despite the difficulty in interpreting the mathematics, the conclusions are profound and sobering. They postulate a long-lived infected cell compartment that will require completely successful therapy for at least 2–3 years for eradication. However, they also emphasize the fact that there may be longer-lived sanctuary sites that can never be eradicated, and, thus, treatment of HIV infection may have to be for life. We know, from reports of sad clinical experience, that stopping therapy in patients with an undetectable viral load after about a year of therapy has resulted in rapid rebound of the virus.

G.L. Mandell, M.D.

Antiretroviral Therapy for HIV Infection in 1997: Updated Recommendations of the International AIDS Society–USA Panel
Carpenter CCJ, Fischl MA, Hammer SM, et al (Brown Univ, Providence, RI; Univ of Miami, Fla; Harvard Med School, Boston; et al)
JAMA 277:1962–1969, 1997   2–8

Introduction.—In mid-1996, the International AIDS Society–USA published its recommendations for antiretroviral therapy in patients with HIV infection. Since then, developments in several areas have necessitated updating of the recommendations, with a focus on incorporating increased understanding of the pathogenesis of HIV disease into treatment approaches. New recommendations for antiretroviral therapy for HIV were reported.
Methods.—An expert panel considered various sources of data in making their updated recommendations. These included new study results, including phase-3 controlled trials; data on clinical, virologic, and immunologic end points; interim analysis of ongoing studies; studies of HIV pathophysiology; and expert opinions. The panel met on a quarterly basis to discuss new data and how this information altered the recommendations. All recommendations were reached by consensus.
Recommendations.—The available data support the use of earlier and more aggressive antiretroviral therapy for HIV disease than previously recommended. Treatment is now recommended for all patients with HIV RNA levels greater than 5,000–10,000 copies/mL of plasma. The data also

underscore the importance of choosing the initial drug regimen—it should be individualized to the patient for the purposes of maximizing clinical benefit and adherence. Specific combinations are proposed for use in certain groups of patients. Preferably, the initial regimen should be the one most likely to reduce and maintain plasma HIV RNA levels below the current level of detection using the most sensitive available assays.

The patient must be willing to commit to a complex, expensive, and potentially toxic triple-drug regimen. It is essential to perform proper plasma viral load testing, because this information is essential for establishing prognosis and monitoring the effectiveness of therapy. When the plasma HIV RNA level is increasing, it is a sign of treatment failure. Such a rise should be documented before the treatment regimen is changed. Other indications for changing therapy include unacceptable toxicity, drug intolerance, nonadherence, or current use of a suboptimal treatment regimen. Alternative combinations are proposed for patients in whom different initial regimens have failed; when a regimen has failed, the new regimen should include at least 2 or preferably 3 new drugs. The new recommendations also include updated recommendations for treatment of acute HIV infection, postexposure prophylaxis, and perinatal transmission. In the case of primary infection, aggressive treatment should be given as soon as possible in an attempt to eradicate the virus from the host.

Summary.—The latest recommendations for antiretroviral drug therapy for HIV infection are based on data suggesting that HIV replication should be suppressed to the greatest extent possible throughout the course of infection. Further updates to the recommendations are expected as new data become available.

▶ An expert panel came up with very sensible recommendations for antiretroviral therapy. I am especially pleased to see that thinking about HIV therapy has moved to be in line with other infectious diseases, i.e., early treatment is better than late treatment and optimal therapy is better than suboptimal therapy. It took us a while to get to that point and depended on the development of potent drugs where the efficacy clearly exceeds the toxicity. There are still many questions related to therapy. I feel that every infected patient should be offered optimal therapy with the hope that prolonged suppression has the potential for cure. As the experts point out, these recommendations are subject to change as new data accrue.

G.L. Mandell, M.D.

3 AIDS Opportunistic Infection

Introduction

Prophylaxis clearly is important. In addition to effective antiretroviral therapy it is the most important thing that we can do to keep our patients well for as long as possible. Development of resistance can be a problem and the physician has to weigh the risks of promoting resistance against the advantage of decreasing the numbers of infections.

Gerald L. Mandell, M.D.

Low-dose Fluconazole as Primary Prophylaxis for Cryptococcal Infection in AIDS Patients With CD4 Counts of ≤100/mm³: Demonstration of Efficacy in a Prospective, Multicenter Trial
Singh N, Barnish MJ, Berman S, et al (Univ of Pittsburgh, PA; Kennedy Mem Hosp, Stratford, NJ; Veterans Affairs Med Ctr, Long Beach, CA; et al)
Clin Infect Dis 23:1282–1286, 1996   3–1

Background.—Five to ten percent of patients with HIV infection have disseminated cryptococcal infections. Such infections are associated with a 10% to 20% mortality rate, despite treatment. The efficacy of low-dose fluconazole as primary prophylaxis for cryptococcal infection was assessed prospectively.

Methods.—Two hundred eighteen patients were enrolled at 4 centers between April 1993 and September 1995. All had HIV infection and CD4 cell counts of 100/mm³ or less. At baseline, median CD4 cell count was 29/mm³. Fifty-eight percent of the patients had an AIDS-defining illness or infection before enrollment. Fluconazole, 200 mg, was taken orally 3 times a week.

Findings.—The incidence of cryptococcal meningitis was 0.4% (developing in 1 patient). The breakthrough isolate was susceptible to fluconazole. Kinetic study showed adequate drug absorption and serum fluconazole levels. Noncompliance was a possibility in this patient. Eighteen percent of the patients had mucocutaneous and/or esophageal candidiasis. The only factor independently associated with breakthrough candidiasis was noncompliance with fluconazole treatment.

Conclusions.—This dosage of fluconazole was an effective primary prophylaxis against cryptococcosis in these HIV-infected patients with CD4 cell counts of 100/mm³ or less. The cost of this treatment was notably lower than that of daily drug administration, and patient convenience was increased.

Detection and Significance of Fluconazole Resistance in Oropharyngeal Candidiasis in Human Immunodeficiency Virus–infected Patients
Revankar SG, Kirkpatrick WR, McAtee RK, et al (Univ of Texas, San Antonio)
J Infect Dis 174:821–827, 1996   3–2

Background.—Oropharyngeal candidiasis (OPC), the most common fungal infection in patients with HIV, can result in significant morbidity. Fluconazole has been widely used to treat acute episodes of OPC and for prophylaxis. However, yeast species that are not very susceptible to fluconazole are being increasingly isolated from patients with OPC. The epidemiology and clinical significance of fluconazole-resistant yeasts in OPC were studied.

Methods.—Fifty patients with recurrent OPC were included in the prospective study. A novel technique for detecting fluconazole resistance with chromogenic media containing fluconazole was used. Findings were confirmed by macrobroth assessment. Resistant yeasts were defined as MICs of 8μg/ml or greater.

Findings.—Thirty-two percent of the patients were found to have resistant yeasts. The yeast isolated was resistant *Candida albicans* in 14%, resistant non-*C. albicans* in 14%, and mixed resistant yeasts in 4%. In 11 of 16 isolates, MICs were 32 or greater. Risk factors associated with resistance included previous fluconazole use and severe immunosuppression. Despite this high prevalence of resistance, 48 patients responded clinically to fluconazole therapy.

Conclusions.—Fluconazole-resistant *C. albicans* and non-*C. albicans* yeast infections occur commonly in severely immunosuppressed patients. However, fluconazole is still very effective clinically.

▶ These two articles (Abstracts 3–1 and 3–2) present a good-news, bad-news pair concerning fluconazole prophylaxis in patients with AIDS. The article by Singh et al. has no control group. Previous studies have shown that 200 mg of fluconazole per day reduced the incidence of cryptococcal infection from 7.1% to .9% in HIV-infected patients with CD4 counts of less than 200. Revankar et al. used 200 mg of fluconazole thrice weekly and treated patients with CD4 counts of less than 100 and found an infection rate of only 0.4%. Nearly all cases of cryptococcal meningitis occur in patients with less than 100 CD4 cells. Most of those occur in patients with CD4s of less than 50 per cubic millimeter. The bad news is related to *Candida albicans* resistance. The data are somewhat confusing because clinical resistance appears to be different from laboratory-defined resistance. One has to question the meanings of the in vitro assay. My fungal-expert colleagues are now working on in vitro assays that will allow laboratories to report data that are meaningful in the clinical context.

G.L. Mandell, M.D.

Weekly Fluconazole for the Prevention of Mucosal Candidiasis in Women With HIV Infection
Schuman P, for the Terry Beirn Community Programs for Clinical Research on AIDS (Wayne State Univ, Detroit)
Ann Intern Med 126:689–696, 97   3–3

Background.—Candidiasis is a common complication of HIV infection. As the immune system becomes more suppressed, the risk of developing oropharyngeal and esophageal candidiasis rises. Vaginal candidiasis is also common in women with HIV infection. There is little information on the natural history, treatment, and prevention of mucosal candidiasis in women. Fluconazole is effective in treating candidiasis in patients with HIV infection or AIDS, and may also prevent mucosal candidiasis in women with HIV infection.

Methods.—Fluconazole, 200 mg/wk, or placebo was administered to 323 female patients with HIV infection and CD4+ cell counts of 300 cells/mm^3 or less. Median treatment periods were 17 months for fluconazole and 10 months for placebo.

Results.—After a median of 29 months, at least 1 episode of candidiasis occurred in 72 of 162 patients given fluconazole and 93 of 161 patients given placebo. Fluconazole prevented oropharyngeal candidiasis and vaginal candidiasis, but not esophageal candidiasis. The relative risks did not differ among women with a history of mucosal candidiasis and women who did not have that history. For patients with a history of infection, the absolute risk reduction was 25.6 per 100 person-years; this was more than twice the reduction in patients with no history of infection and reflects the higher risk of patients with previous infection. Under clinical and in vitro conditions, *Candida albicans* was resistant to fluconazole in vaginal specimens in less than 5% of patients.

Discussion.—Weekly fluconazole (200 mg) was safe and effective in the female patients with HIV infection in preventing oropharyngeal and vaginal candidiasis. Prophylaxis with fluconazole should be considered only for individuals with a high risk of recurrence and should not be used routinely in all patients.

Infection Due to Fluconazole-resistant *Candida* in Patients With AIDS: Prevalence and Microbiology

Maenza JR, Merz WG, Romagnoli MJ, et al (Johns Hopkins Univ, Baltimore, Md)

Clin Infect Dis 24:28–34, 1997   3–4

Background.—Up to 90% of patients with AIDS have mucosal candidiasis. Infection rates from azole-resistant *Candida* are on the rise because the use of oral azoles for preventing and treating mucosal candidiasis and invasive fungal infections is becoming more common. Fluconazole resistance is associated with advanced immunosuppression and extended exposure to azoles, but fluconazole can lower the rate of cryptococcosis, esophageal candidiasis, and superficial fungal infections. The benefits of antifungal prophylaxis and the risks of drug resistance must be evaluated against rates of fluconazole resistance in *Candida* isolates from patients with AIDS.

Methods.—Oral specimens were obtained from 100 consecutive patients with AIDS and CD4 cell counts of less than 200/mm³. The following information was collected for all patients: presence or absence of pseudomembranous thrush, symptoms of oral or esophageal candidiasis, history of infections, and dosage of previous and current antifungal therapy.

Results.—From 26 of 64 patients with positive cultures, at least 1 fungal organism with in vitro fluconazole resistance was isolated. In vitro resistance correlated with clinical thrush when fluconazole-resistant *C. albicans* was isolated. Ten patients had only non-*albicans* species of *Candida*, and none of these patients had active thrush. Patients with fluconazole-resistant *C. albicans* had lower CD4 cell counts, more treated episodes of thrush, and longer previous treatment with fluconazole than patients with fluconazole-susceptible *C. albicans*. Multivariate analysis showed that the number of episodes and length of previous treatment with fluconazole were independent predictors of fluconazole-resistance.

Discussion.—A high rate of fluconazole-resistant candidiasis was seen in these patients with HIV infection. The relative importance of various risk factors for infection from azole-resistant *Candida* is unknown. The role of non-*albicans* species of *Candida* in oral candidiasis is also unknown. Treatment of oral thrush with topical agents may prevent or delay the development of resistance.

▶ Ann Landers says "use it *or* lose it." Infectious diseases physicians say "use it *and* lose it" when it comes to antimicrobials. Maenza et al. (Abstract 3–4) showed that fluconazole-resistant strains of *Candida albicans* were surprisingly common in patients with AIDS treated with the agent. On the other hand, Shuman et al. (Abstract 3–3) showed that HIV-infected women appeared to benefit from 200 mg of fluconazole per week. They had approximately 50% fewer episodes of both oropharyngeal candidiasis and vaginal candidiasis. Present recommendations for patients with AIDS should take into account the potential for development of pathogenic resistant strains of

Candida albicans. Thus, most superficial mucosal disease should be treated topically, e.g., clotrimazole troches for pharyngitis and topical agents for vaginitis. Oral therapy with fluconazole should be reserved for topical treatment failures and patients with more invasive disease. Prophylactic use of fluconazole should be limited to those patients who have had recurrent mucosal candidiasis and who are at high risk for recurrence (i.e., CD4 counts below 50). Unfortunately those patients at greatest risk for recurrence are also at greatest risk for harboring resistant organisms.

G.L. Mandell, M.D.

Intravenous Cidofovir for Peripheral Cytomegalovirus Retinitis in Patients With AIDS
Lalezari JP, Stagg RJ, Kuppermann BD, et al (Quest Clinical Research, San Francisco; Gilead Sciences, Inc, Foster City, Calif; Univ of California, Irvine, Calif; et al)
Ann Intern Med 126:257–263, 1997   3–5

Background.—The most common intraocular infection associated with AIDS is cytomegalovirus (CMV) retinitis. Left untreated, CMV retinitis may progress to retinal tissue destruction and blindness. The efficacy of IV cidofovir in delaying the progress of previously untreated CMV retinitis was investigated.

Methods.—Forty-eight patients with AIDS and previously untreated peripheral CMV retinitis were randomly assigned to immediate or deferred treatment. Cidofovir was given intravenously in a dosage of 5 mg/kg body weight once a week for 2 weeks and then once every other week. Each infusion was given with oral probenecid and IV hydration with normal saline solution to minimize nephrotoxicity.

Findings.—Median times to CMV retinitis progression in the immediate- and deferred-treatment groups were 120 days and 22 days, respectively. The most serious adverse events possibly associated with cidofovir were neutropenia, occurring in 15%; and proteinuria, occurring in 12%. Both conditions were asymptomatic. However, cidofovir had to be discontinued in 24% of patients because of nephrotoxicity. Fifty-six percent of the patients had transient reactions to probenecid, including mild to moderate constitutional symptoms or nausea. These reactions were dose limiting in 7% (Fig 1).

Conclusions.—Cidofovir effectively delays progression of previously untreated CMV retinitis. Drug-related nephrotoxicity may be minimized by strict adherence to kidney function monitoring before cidofovir administration and by concomitant treatment with probenecid and saline-solution hydration.

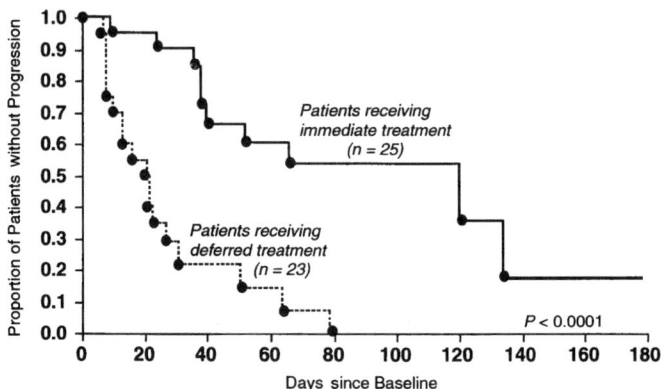

FIGURE 1.—Kaplan-Meier plot of time to progression of cytomegalovirus (*CMV*) retinitis in the immediate- and deferred-cidofovir treatment groups. The estimated median time to progression of CMV retinitis was 22 days (95% confidence interval [*CI*], 10 to 27 days) in the deferred-treatment group and 120 days (CI, 40 to 134 days) in the immediate-treatment group (*p* < 0.001, log-rank test). (Courtesy of Lalezari JP, Stagg RJ, Kuppermann BD, et al: Intravenous cidofovir for peripheral cytomegalovirus retinitis in patients with AIDS. *Ann Intern Med* 126:257–263, 1997.)

Parenteral Cidofovir for Cytomegalovirus Retinitis in Patients With AIDS: The HPMPC Peripheral Cytomegalovirus Retinitis Trial—A Randomized, Controlled Trial

Lewis RA, and the Studies of Ocular Complications of AIDS Research Group in Collaboration With the AIDS Clinical Trials Group (Baylor College of Medicine, Houston)

Ann Intern Med 126:264–274, 1997   3–6

Background.—Cytomegalovirus (CMV) retinitis, common in patients with AIDS, is a major cause of visual loss. The efficacy of IV cidofovir was evaluated in a multicenter, phase II/III, randomized, controlled clinical trial.

Methods.—Sixty-four patients with AIDS and previously untreated small peripheral CMV retinitis lesions (at low risk for loss of visual acuity) were assigned to 1 of 3 groups. In the deferral group, treatment was deferred until retinitis progressed. In the low-dose cidofovir group, 5 mg/kg/body weight cidofovir was given once a week for 2 weeks, followed by maintenance therapy with 3 mg/kg once every 2 weeks. In the high-dose group, 5 mg/kg cidofovir was given once a week for 2 weeks, followed by maintenance therapy with cidofovir, 5 mg/kg once every 2 weeks. Hydration and probenecid were administered along with cidofovir to minimize nephrotoxicity.

Results.—In the low-dose group, median time to progression was 64 days. Patients deferred from low-dose treatment had progression at a median 21 days. Median time to progression was not reached in the high-dose group by the end of the study. In those for whom high-dose treatment was deferred, median time to progression was 20 days. The rates of visual loss were comparable among the groups. Proteinuria of 2+ or more occurred at rates of 2.6, 2.8, and 6.8 per person-year in the deferral, low-dose, and high-dose groups, respectively. None of the patients had proteinuria of 4+. However, persistent increases of serum creatinine levels exceeding 177 μmol/L developed in 2 patients receiving cidofovir. The rate of probenecid reactions was 0.70 person-year.

Conclusions.—Low- and high-dose IV cidofovir effectively slows the progression of CMV retinitis. The risk of nephrotoxicity may be minimized (but not eliminated) by the administration of probenecid and hydration, intermittent dosing, and monitoring for proteinuria.

▶ Infectious-diseases physicians were used to quantitating "cures." In HIV-infected patients it is often difficult to achieve a cure. Lifetime therapy is the rule for certain infections. These two reports Abstracts 3–4 and 3–5 demonstrate marked prolongation in the time to progression in patients treated with cidofovir, a new cytosine nucleotide analogue (Figure 1, Lalezari et al). The drug is given intravenously, and maintainance can be achieved with intravenous doses once every 2 weeks. Kidney function must be monitored, and hydration and probenecid are effective in reducing nephrotoxicity. It is difficult to compare the efficacy of cidofovir with that of daily IV ganciclovir or daily intravenous foscarnet but the clear advantage of cidofovir therapy is that indwelling catheters are not necessary because a dose every 2 weeks is effective in delaying progression of CMV retinitis.

G.L. Mandell, M.D.

Coccidioidomycosis in Patients Infected With Human Immunodeficiency Virus: Review of 91 Cases at a Single Institution
Singh VR, Smith DK, Lawerence J, et al (Maricopa Med Ctr, Phoenix, Ariz)
Clin Infect Dis 23:563–568, 1996   3–7

Introduction.—Although coccidioidomycosis is usually subacute and self-limited in otherwise healthy individuals, this fungal disease often involves extrapulmonary dissemination in patients with poor T cell-mediated immunity. Extrathoracic coccidioidomycosis has been considered an AIDS-defining illness since 1987. The clinical manifestations, diagnosis, treatment, and outcome of the fungal illness were examined in a retrospective study of 91 patients with HIV infection and coccidioidomycosis.

Methods.—The 91 patients had been treated at a single institution, a county hospital in Phoenix, Arizona. Hospital charts and other records were reviewed for clinical information and dates of death. The diagnosis of coccidioidomycosis was based on culture of *Coccidioides immitis* from respiratory secretions or other biological materials, recognition of the organism in histopathologic or Papanicolaou-stained cytologic specimens, or positivity of coccidioidal serologic tests in the setting of a compatible clinical illness.

Results.—In 37 of 91 HIV-infected patients with coccidioidomycosis, this fungal infection was the AIDS-defining illness. The patient group was 93% male; 51% were white, 46% were homosexual, and 24% were IV drug users. Common signs and symptoms of the illness were fever and chills (68%), cough (64%), weight loss (50%), night sweats (36%), and enlarged lymph nodes (24%). Chest radiographs revealed diffuse reticulonodular infiltrates in 65% and focal abnormalities in 14%. Pulmonary involvement was present in 80% of patients and the meninges were involved in 14%.

The radiographic finding of diffuse reticulonodular infiltrates, a common presentation of coccidioidomycosis in patients with AIDS, was associated with a lower mean CD4 lymphocyte count. Eight of 14 patients with coccidioidal meningitis had diffuse pulmonary involvement. Results of serologic tests for antibodies to *C. immitis* were negative for 21 patients, including 17 with diffuse pulmonary disease. Overall mortality was 60%, but patients with diffuse pulmonary disease had the highest mortality (68%) and lowest median duration of survival (54 days).

Conclusion.—Coccidioidomycosis is an important opportunistic infection in patients with HIV who live in an area where the fungus is endemic. Mortality is increased when diffuse pulmonary disease is present and/or CD4 lymphocyte count is less than 50/μL.

▶ Unfortunately, HIV-infected patients may serve as human canaries, signifying infections prevalent in their home community. There are areas in Texas where the most common AIDS-defining illness is histoplasmosis. Likewise, where tuberculosis is prevalent, that becomes a common infection in AIDS patients. The present report from Phoenix, Arizona, indicates that coccidioidomycosis is commonly seen in their patients. The infection has a high mortality and diffuse pulmonary infiltrates are an especially ominous finding. Those of us who don't live and practice in the Southwest should be aware that travel through this part of the country can put patients at risk, and this is especially important to remember in HIV-infected patients.

G.L. Mandell, M.D.

Thalidomide for the Treatment of Oral Aphthous Ulcers in Patients With Human Immunodeficiency Virus Infection
Jacobson JM, Greenspan JS, Spritzler J, et al (Bronx Veterans Affairs Med Ctr, NY; Univ of California at San Francisco; Harvard School of Public Health, Boston; et al)
N Engl J Med 336:1487–1493, 1997   3–8

Background.—Aphthous ulceration in the mouth and oropharynx can be extensive and debilitating in patients with advanced HIV infection. Preliminary studies suggest that thalidomide may facilitate oral aphthous ulcer healing.

Methods.—Fifty-seven patients completed a double-blind, randomized, placebo-controlled study of thalidomide treatment for oral aphthous ulcers. Thalidomide, 200 mg, or placebo was taken orally for 4 weeks.

Findings.—Fifty-five percent of the patients in the thalidomide group and only 7% in the placebo group showed complete healing of ulcers after 4 weeks. Active treatment decreased pain and improved ability to eat. Adverse effects included somnolence and the presence of a rash, in 7 patients each. Six of the 29 thalidomide recipients quit treatment because of toxicity. Levels of HIV RNA were increased in the active treatment group, and there were unexpected increases in the plasma levels of tumor necrosis factor α (TNF-α) and soluble TNF-α receptors.

Conclusions.—Although severe aphthous ulcers are not common in individuals infected with HIV, they can be devastating when they do occur. Thalidomide is an effective treatment for this condition.

▶ Aphthous ulcers are seen in immunocompetent individuals but can be a severe problem in patients with HIV infection. The cause of the ulcers is unknown. Thalidomide is a sedative that causes severe teratogenic effects on the fetus. Recent data have suggested that thalidomide is a potent inhibitor of the production of TNF, and anecdotes have suggested that it would be effective for aphthous ulcers in patients with AIDS. Thalidomide was effective for the treatment of the aphthous ulcers, but there were 2 markedly unexpected results: (1) treated patients had elevated levels of TNF instead of the expected decreased levels and (2) treated patients had increased levels of HIV in the blood instead of decreased levels as expected. The side effects were significant, and about 20% of the patients had to discontinue treatment. Nonetheless, this is something to consider in patients with debilitating aphthous ulcers.

G.L. Mandell, M.D.

4 Viral Infections

Introduction

It is nice to have a new pathogen that does not seem to cause much disease; this appears to be the case with hepatitis G virus. We continue to learn more about hepatitis B. Dengue is an increasing problem and perhaps will become a greater danger to the United States as global warming proceeds. The link between bovine spongioform encephalopathy and disease in humans is now very firm.

Gerald L. Mandell, M.D.

Influence of Hepatitis G Virus Infection on the Severity of Liver Disease and Response to Interferon-α in Patients With Chronic Hepatitis C
Martinot M, Marcellin P, Boyer N, et al (Hôpital Beaujon, Clichy, France; Chiron Corp, Emeryville, Calif)
Ann Intern Med 126:874–881, 1997   4–1

Background.—Infections with hepatitis G virus (HGV) and hepatitis C virus (HCV) commonly occur together. However, the effect of HGV infection on chronic hepatitis C infection has not been thoroughly studied.
Methods.—Two hundred twenty-eight patients with chronic hepatitis C infection were studied retrospectively. All had been treated with interferon-α. Before treatment was begun, serum HGV RNA and serum HCV RNA were assessed with branched-DNA assays. A line probe assay was used to determine HCV genotype. Polymerase chain reaction at the end of treatment and 6 months later determined levels of serum HGV RNA and serum HCV RNA.
Findings.—Twenty-one percent of the patients had HGV infection, including 32% of IV drug users. The median serum HGV RNA concentration was 33×10^6 genome equivalents/mL. Hepatitis G virus infection was more common among men with a history of IV drug use and was associated with HCV genotype 3a, independent of the infection source. Patients with and without HGV infection did not differ in serum HCV RNA levels, liver histologic findings, or response to interferon-α treatment. Loss of serum HGV RNA was unassociated with the biochemical response, in contrast to loss of serum HCV RNA.

Conclusion.—Hepatitis G virus was common in these patients with chronic hepatitis C, especially those with HCV genotype 3a infection. Compared with the level of HCV viremia, the level of HGV viremia was high. Liver disease severity and response to interferon-α therapy were not influenced by HGV infection.

▶ We don't really know very much about HGV infection, except that it is caused by an RNA virus that can be transmitted parenterally. Hepatitis G virus does not seem to be very pathogenic, and this article documents the fact that, even in conjunction with HCV, there does not seem to be a contribution to liver damage by HGV.

G.L. Mandell, M.D.

Transmission of Hepatitis B to Patients From Four Infected Surgeons Without Hepatitis B e Antigen
Heptonstall J (Public Health Lab Service Communicable Disease Surveillance Centre, London)
N Engl J Med 336:178–184, 1997   4–2

Introduction.—The transmission of hepatitis B virus (HBV) to patients from surgeons who carry hepatitis B e antigen (HBeAg) has been documented in numerous reports. Four unconnected instances of transmission of HBV to patients by 4 infected surgeons whose serum did not show HBeAg were identified.

> *Case Reports.*—All 4 patients were female and were seen for acute onset of jaundice. None of them received blood transfusions. Each patient had surgery within the past 6 months. An investigation was begun and members of each surgical team were tested for HBV carrier status. Three surgeons were positive for HBsAg and negative for anti-HBc IgM. One surgeon was known to be an HBeAg-negative carrier of HBV and continued to operate within existing guidelines. All other members of the 4 surgical teams were immune to HBV or uninfected. All patients recovered completely and no patients experienced fulminant hepatitis.

Methods.—Serum HBV DNA was amplified by a nested polymerase chain reaction from serum of the 4 infected surgeons and infected patients. Direct sequencing of the 2 regions of the HBV genome was executed. Patients who underwent surgeries by the infected surgeons were offered testing.
Results.—All 4 surgeons were carriers of HBV and none of them had detectable levels of HBeAg. It was not possible to distinguish the nucleotide sequences of HBV DNA from the surgeons and their corresponding infected patients. At least 2 other exposed patients who were offered screening probably acquired hepatitis B from their respective infected

surgeons. All surgeons made career changes that did not put patients at risk of exposure to the virus.

Conclusion.—Surgeons who are carriers of HBV with no detectable serum HBeAg can transmit the hepatitis B virus to their patients. Surgeons in the United Kingdom are presently allowed to perform procedures within guidelines if their serum contains HBsAg, but not HBeAg.

▶ Hepatitis B is one of our most transmissable blood infections. In addition to hepatitis B surface antigen, it appears that HBeAg is closely associated with transmissability. Prior data strongly suggest that the presence of HBeAg correlates with higher levels of viremia and a greater risk for transmission. The present article provides proof that infection from surgeon to patient can occur in the absence of HBeAg.

G.L. Mandell, M.D.

Dengue Fever in US Military Personnel in Haiti
Trofa AF, DeFraites RF, Smoak BL, et al (Walter Reed Army Inst of Research, Washington, DC; US Army Med Research Inst of Infectious Diseases, Fort Detrick, Frederick, Md)
JAMA 277:1546–1548, 1997   4–3

Objective.—Dengue fever (DF) is a tropical disease caused by a flavivirus and spread by mosquitoes. It causes a fever, a headache, myalgia, and malaise, sometimes with a rash, and ranges in severity from a mild febrile illness to severe complications such as hemorrhaging and shock. Outbreaks commonly occur in Caribbean countries and can occur among Americans traveling in that region. An outbreak of DF among U.S. military personnel stationed in Haiti is reported.

Methods.—Medical surveillance personnel were sent to Haiti in 1994, in support of more than 20,000 troops stationed there to restore the democratically elected government. Routine medical surveillance was performed in 22 military clinics across Haiti. All patients with a temperature higher than 38.1°C, especially those without focal clinical findings, were referred to the combat support hospital. There the patients were assessed according to standard clinical and laboratory protocols, and daily follow-up was conducted by the surveillance team. Testing included arbovirus isolation and specific antibody determination.

Results.—During the first 6 weeks in Haiti, there were 406 admissions to the combat support hospital. Twenty-five percent of these were for febrile illness; all 103 patients admitted with fevers recovered. There were 30 cases of DF, but there were no apparent cases of malaria. Twenty-two patients had dengue virus serotypes 1, 2, and 4, whereas the other 8 had IgM antibodies to dengue virus. The clinical signs alone were insufficient to differentiate between patients with DF and other febrile illnesses. Dengue virus was the only arbovirus identified.

Conclusions.—An outbreak of DF among U.S. troops stationed in Haiti was identified by active surveillance under the direction of an epidemiologic team. The diagnosis of DF must be confirmed by viral isolation and serologic studies. People traveling to Haiti and other tropical countries are at significant risk for DF, which they could then carry back to the United States. Most cases of DF will resolve without serious complications. Signs of impending dengue hemorrhagic fever or dengue shock syndrome include thrombocytopenia and associated petechiae, hemoconcentration, or hemorrhaging.

▶ Dengue fever has been reported in many tropical countries, including those in the Caribbean. Tourists are at risk, and the best prevention is avoidance of mosquito bites. This report indicates that severe "breakbone" fever is unusual, and that a fever, a conjunctival infection, and a rash (nonpetechial) are the most common signs. Although hemorrhagic fever has been described in tourists, it is usually seen in patients who sustain repeated infections with different serotypes.

G.L. Mandell, M.D.

Frequent Genital Herpes Simplex Virus 2 Shedding in Immunocompetent Women
Wald A, Corey L, Cone R, et al (Univ of Washington, Seattle; Glaxo Wellcome Company, Durham, NC)
J Clin Invest 99:1092–1097, 1997   4–4

Introduction.—Herpes simplex virus (HSV) type 2 (HSV-2) is the leading cause of genital ulcer disease and an independent risk factor for acquisition of HIV infection in industrialized countries. In the United States, the prevalence of HSV-2 increased 32% between 1978 and 1990. Because reactivation of HSV-2 occurs intermittently, management emphasizes episodic therapy of symptomatic reactivation. The frequency and pattern of HSV-2 reactivation were evaluated using both viral isolation and HSV polymerase chain reaction (PCR) assay.

Methods.—Study participants were in good health and not receiving immunosuppressive medication. Daily samples of genital secretions were obtained from women who were HSV-2 seropositive and from a subset receiving oral acyclovir (400 mg twice a day). Because the in vivo inhibition of PCR positivity by acyclovir would indicate the presence of replicating and potentially infectious virus on mucosal surfaces, detection rates of HSV DNA were compared when patients were receiving the antiviral therapy and when no therapy was given.

Results.—Herpes simplex virus DNA was detected in genital secretions in 19 of 20 women during 42–85 consecutive sampling days; HSV was isolated by culture in 15 women. Overall, HSV DNA was detected on 28% of days sampled, compared to 8.1% of days on which HSV was isolated by culture from the same specimens (Fig 1). None of the women shed on

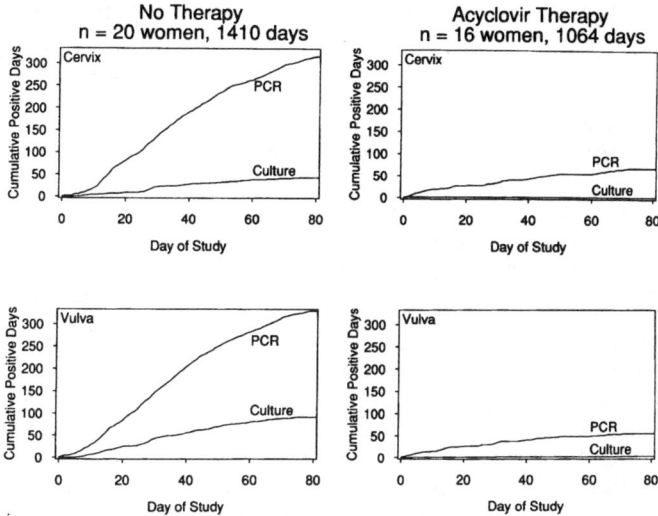

FIGURE 1.—The cumulative culture and polymerase chain reaction-positive days from samples of genital secretions from women receiving placebo or acyclovir therapy. The cumulative number of days is illustrated both for the cervix and the vulva. *Abbreviation:* PCR, polymerase chain reaction. (Reproduced from Wald A, Corey L, Cone R, et al: Frequent genital herpes simplex virus 2 shedding in immunocompetent women. *J Clin Invest* 99:1092–1097, 1997 by copyright permission of the Rockefeller University Press.)

more than 21% of days by viral isolation, whereas 11 of 20 women had HSV DNA detected on more than 20% of days, 4 of 20 on more than 50%, and 2 of 20 on 75% of days. Oral acyclovir treatment promptly reduced the frequency of HSV DNA detection by a median of 80%. Within 3–4 days of discontinuing oral acyclovir, however, HSV DNA reappeared in the genital area. Lesions consistent with herpes were observed on 40% of days on which HSV DNA was detected. The geometric mean HSV copy number was significantly higher in samples obtained on days with lesions.

Discussion.—Genital HSV-2 reactivation occurs much more frequently than previously realized. The sensitive PCR assay found HSV-2 shedding on an average of 28% of days sampled among healthy immunocompetent women who were HSV-2 seropositive. Reactivation was more frequent in women with recent acquisition of genital herpes, occurred in clusters of days or episodes, was associated with higher copy numbers and longer duration of shedding when genital lesions were present or viral cultures were positive, and was reduced with antiviral therapy.

▶ A study of Figure 1 will illustrate important points of this report. Polymerase chain reaction is much more sensitive than culture in detecting genital HSV-2. The virus could be detected in genital swab specimens in 28% of the days and in only 40% of those days were lesions seen. Oral acyclovir treatment markedly reduced the frequency of HSV DNA detection. The presence of virus is necessary but not sufficient to predict transmission.

Other factors such as viral titer, immunity of the contact, and type of sexual activity must also be important.

G.L. Mandell, M.D.

Acyclovir With and Without Prednisone for the Treatment of Herpes Zoster
Whitley RJ, and the National Institute of Allergy and Infectious Diseases Collaborative Antiviral Study Group (Univ of Alabama, Birmingham)
Ann Intern Med 125:376–383, 1996   4–5

Purpose.—Herpes zoster is a common problem in elderly and immuno-compromised patients. Antiviral treatment can promote healing of the cutaneous lesions and relief of pain. Despite the lack of adequate scientific data, prednisone has come into widespread use in the treatment of herpes zoster, in the hope of preventing persistent or chronic pain. The effects of acyclovir and prednisone on chronic pain and quality of life for patients with herpes zoster were assessed in a randomized, double-blind trial.

Methods.—The study included 208 immunocompetent patients older than 50 years. All had localized herpes zoster developing within 72 hours before study enrollment. They were randomly assigned in a 2 × 2 factorial design to receive both active treatments, acyclovir plus prednisone pla-cebo, prednisone plus acyclovir placebo, or both placebos. Acyclovir dos-age was 800 mg orally 5 times a day for 21 days. Prednisone treatment started at 60 mg/day for the first 7 days, then 30 mg/day for days 8–14 and 15 mg/day for days 15–21. Every day for 4 weeks, the patients were monitored for healing of cutaneous lesions, pain resolution, return to normal activity, and return to normal sleep. Monthly monitoring contin-ued for 6 months thereafter. Other outcomes measured were analgesic use, adverse events, and laboratory studies. The results were analyzed by intention to treat.

Results.—The 4 groups were similar demographically. Patients receiving both active treatments had a shorter time to total crusting and healing than patients receiving both placebos—risk ratios (RRs) were 2.27 for total crusting and 2.07 for healing (Table 2). Patients in the acyclovir plus placebo group also had a faster cessation of acute neuritis, RR 3.02; return to uninterrupted sleep, RR 2.21; return to normal activity, RR 3.22; and need for analgesic medications, RR 3.15. Healing was faster with acyclovir plus prednisone than with prednisone plus acyclovir placebo; for patients receiving prednisone plus acyclovir placebo, healing was no faster than in the double-placebo group. Resolution of pain in the 6 months after disease onset was similar for all 4 groups. There were no serious adverse clinical events or laboratory abnormalities.

Conclusions.—The combination of prednisone and acyclovir is better than either drug alone for the treatment of herpes zoster in immunocom-petent older adults. Benefits are seen in terms of pain, time to healing, and

TABLE 2.—Disease Resolution According to Cox Regression Model*

	Risk Ratio (95% CI)				
	Acyclovir plus Prednisone Compared with Placebo	Acyclovir plus Prednisone Placebo Compared with Placebo	Prednisone plus Acyclovir Placebo Compared with Placebo	Main Effect of Acyclovir; Acyclovir Compared with No Acyclovir	Main Effect of Virus: Prednisone Compared with No Prednisone
One-month evaluation of cutaneous healing					
Time to total crusting	2.27 (1.46 to 3.55)†	1.51 (0.98 to 2.33)	1.04 (0.67 to 1.63)	1.81 (1.32 to 2.48)†	1.25 (0.90 to 1.74)
Time to total healing	2.07 (1.26 to 3.38)†	1.57 (0.97 to 2.53)	0.90 (0.53 to 1.52)	1.88 (1.32 to 2.67)†	1.11 (0.78 to 1.59)
One-month evaluation of quality of life					
Time to cessation of acute neuritis	3.02 (1.42 to 6.41)†	1.47 (0.67 to 3.21)	2.54 (1.22 to 5.31)†	1.29 (0.79 to 2.10)	2.28 (1.35 to 3.86)†
Time to uninterrupted sleep	2.12 (1.25 to 3.58)†	1.18 (0.68 to 2.05)	1.52 (0.90 to 2.58)	1.29 (0.88 to 1.89)	1.65 (1.14 to 2.41)†
Time to return to 100% usual activity	3.22 (1.92 to 5.40)†	1.63 (0.96 to 2.76)	1.50 (0.89 to 2.53)	1.90 (1.33 to 2.71)†	1.74 (1.21 to 2.51)†
Time to no use of analgesic agents	3.15 (1.69 to 5.89)†	1.27 (0.66 to 2.49)	2.02 (1.06 to 3.85)†	1.44 (0.95 to 2.15)	2.25 (1.42 to 3.54)†
Six-month evaluation of pain					
Time to cessation of zoster-associated pain	1.56 (0.92 to 2.66)	1.39 (0.84 to 2.32)	1.26 (0.72 to 2.21)	1.29 (0.94 to 1.77)	1.26 (0.91 to 1.75)

*Prognostic variables included in the model were sex, race, age, number and duration of lesions before enrollment, surface area of lesions, and severity of pain at baseline.
†P < 0.05.
(Courtesy of Whitley AJ, and the National Institute of Allergy and Infectious Diseases Collaborative Antiviral Study Group: Acyclovir with and without prednisone for the treatment of herpes zoster. *Ann Intern Med* 125:376–383, 1996.)

quality of life. The authors emphasize that not all patients can take high-dose prednisone.

▶ The results were clear-cut. Acyclovir plus prednisone is better than acyclovir alone for the therapy of herpes zoster. Table 2 shows the odds ratio for a good outcome markedly in favor of acyclovir plus prednisone. The authors speculate that therapy with famciclovir and valaciclovir probably would also benefit by the addition of adjunctive corticosteroid therapy.

G.L. Mandell, M.D.

Diagnosis of Viral Infections of the Central Nervous System: Clinical Interpretation of PCR Results
Jeffery KJM, Read SJ, Peto TEA, et al (John Radcliffe Hosp, Oxford, England; Oxfordshire Health Authority, England; Imperial College, London)
Lancet 349:313–317, 1997   4–6

Objective.—Diagnosis of viral infections of the CNS is complicated by the lack of satisfactory viral culture and serologic methods for culturing organisms from CSF. Polymerase chain reaction (PCR) would be clinically useful for such diagnoses if a gold standard existed. A protocol for PCR amplification of CSF for viruses associated with CNS disease was developed.

Methods.—All CSF samples received at the diagnostic virology laboratory of John Radcliffe Hospital, Oxford, England, between May 1994 and May 1996 were prospectively examined by nested PCR for viral CNS infections. The data obtained were used to classify CSF from 410 patients examined between May 1994 and May 1995 into 4 groups: definite, probable, possible, and no viral CNS infection. The probable group was subdivided into group A (meningitis), group B (encephalitis), group C (acute ascending polyneuropathy or myelopathy consistent with Guillain-Barré syndrome, Miller Fisher syndrome, or transverse myelopathy), and group D (space-occupying lesions in immunocompromised patients). Clinical factors independently associated with a positive PCR result were identified using logistic regression analysis.

Results.—There were 143 positive PCR results in 2,233 consecutive samples from 2,162 patients. Enteroviruses, herpes simplex virus, varicella zoster virus, and Epstein-Barr virus were the most common viruses detected. Independent predictors of a positive PCR test result included fever, virus-specific rash, and a CSF white cell count of 5/μL or more. Patients with a positive PCR test result were 88.2 times more likely than patients with a negative PCR test result to have a viral infection. There was only a 10% chance that patients with a negative PCR test result would have a viral infection.

Conclusion.—Patients with a positive PCR test result were 88.2 times more likely to have a viral infection than patients with a negative PCR test result. Patients with a negative PCR test result have only a 10% chance of having a viral infection.

▶ It appears that PCR is the best technique for identifying viruses in the central nervous system. One of the strengths of this report is the observation that PCR was nearly always negative in patients with a low clinical probability of a viral central nervous system infection. Note that 96% of all the positive PCRs were either enteroviruses, herpes simplex virus, varicella zoster virus, or Epstein-Barr virus.

G.L. Mandell, M.D.

Health Effects of Human T-Lymphotropic Virus Type I (HTLV-I) in a Jamaican Cohort
Murphy EL, Wilks R, Morgan OSC, et al (Univ of California, San Francisco)
Int J Epidemiol 25:1090–1097, 1996   4–7

Background.—The health effects of human T-lymphotrophic virus type 1 (HTLV-1) infection, unlike those of adult T-cell leukemia (ATL) and HTLV-1–associated myelopathy (HAM), have not been clearly defined. The health effects of this infection were investigated in a Jamaican cohort.

Methods.—A cohort of 201 Jamaican food service workers with confirmed HTLV-1 seropositivity and 225 seronegative control subjects of comparable age and sex from the same population were included. At study enrollment in 1987 and 1988, the subjects completed a health questionnaire and underwent a physical examination and laboratory testing.

Findings.—The prevalence of HAM was 0.5% among the seropositive patients and 0 in the control subjects. None of the subjects had ATL. Though current symptoms did not differ between groups, the seropositive subjects were more likely to have a medical history of hepatitis or jaundice, malaria, and dengue fever. However, these differences were only borderline significant. Body weight and body mass index were lower in low-income seropositive women than in their seronegative counterparts. Similar differences were noted in the smaller groups of men. There was a trend toward greater prevalence of severe anemia and a significantly lower prevalence of eosinophilia in HTLV-1–seropositive subjects compared with control subjects.

Conclusions.—Though most HTLV-1–seropositive individuals are free of symptoms, about 0.5% of these carriers may have HAM. Chronic HTLV-1 infection may have subtle effects on body mass and hematologic variables.

▶ In this country HTLV-1 questions usually relate to patients who are found to be serologically positive during routine blood donor evaluation. Information about prognosis is hard to come by, so this study from Jamaica is useful. The comparison of HTLV-1–seropositive adults with matched seronegative control subjects showed very few differences. There was one case of

HTLV-1–associated myelopathy in the positive group and no cases in the negative group, and no patients had adult T-cell leukemia-lymphoma. There were some unexplained differences in weight and body mass index and anemia but the relationship with HTLV-1 is unclear. Other reports confirm that HTLV-1–associated myelopathy is uncommon, even in patients with long-term infections (probably well under 1%). It has been reported that the lifetime risk of developing T-cell leukemia-lymphoma is 4% to 5%.

G.L. Mandell, M.D.

Severe Cytomegalovirus Infection in Immunocompetent Patients
Eddleston M, Peacock S, Juniper M, et al (Univ of Oxford, England)
Clin Infect Dis 24:52–56, 1997   4–8

Background.—Severe cytomegalovirus (CMV) infection occurs rarely in previously healthy immunocompetent persons. The literature on severe CMV disease in such patients was reviewed to determine the natural history of the disorder and its response to specific antiviral therapy.

Methods and Findings.—In a search of the worldwide literature from 1966 to 1995, 34 patients were identified. Fifteen patients died. Multiorgan involvement was associated with a high mortality rate. Clinical involvement of the liver or lungs only was potentially fatal. None of the patients with isolated CNS infection died. Few patients received specific antiviral treatment. Five of 6 patients with severe infection recovered after treatment with ganciclovir or foscarnet. The poor prognosis in the absence of specific antiviral treatment suggests that prompt diagnosis and early initiation of such treatment may be important in patients with CMV disease.

Conclusions.—Cytomegalovirus can cause severe, multiorgan infection in immunocompetent individuals. Early diagnosis is essential. Clinicians encountering such cases should report them to provide more information on which to base treatment guidelines.

▶ Most adults show evidence of having been infected with cytomegalovirus. This infection is usually not apparent, but a mononucleosis-like illness has been described (usually without pharyngitis). The authors have put together an excellent review of 34 cases of severe infections in apparently immunocompetent adults. The patients could be divided into two general groups: those with encephalitis who did relatively well and those with disseminated disease, especially involving the liver, who had a relatively high mortality rate. The authors conclude that specific therapy with ganciclovir or foscarnet appeared to be beneficial.

G.L. Mandell, M.D.

Transmissions to Mice Indicate That 'New Variant' CJD Is Caused by the BSE Agent

Bruce ME, Will RG, Ironside JW, et al (Inst for Animal Health, Edinburgh, Scotland; Western Gen Hosp, Edinburgh, Scotland; Inst for Animal Health, Compton, Newbury, UK; et al)

Nature 389:498–501, 1997   4–9

Introduction.—Transmissible spongiform encephalopathies, or "prion," diseases are caused by many strains, which are distinguishable by their disease characteristics in experimentally infected animals. There have been cases of a clinically and pathologically atypical form of Creutzfeldt-Jakob disease, known as new variant Creutzfeldt-Jakob disease that has been recognized in very young people in the United Kingdom with 1 case reported in France. The interim results of transmission of sporadic Creutzfeldt-Jacob disease and new variant Creutzfeldt-Jacob disease are reported.

Methods.—Six typical sporadic cases of Creutzfeldt-Jacob disease and 3 cases of new variant Creutzfeldt-Jacob disease were used to set up transmissions to mice. Two dairy farmers who had bovine spongiform encephalopathy in their herds, 2 controls with no known occupational exposure to bovine spongiform encephalopathy and 2 historical patients who had died before the onset of bovine spongiform encephalopathy had Creutzfeldt-Jacob disease. Patients with the new variant disease also were included. Isolates from these brains were transmitted to the mice.

Results.—A characteristic pattern of disease in mice that is retained after experimental passage through a variety of intermediate species is produced by a strain of agent from cattle affected by bovine spongiform encephalopathy. The first direct evidence for the accidental spread of transmissible spongiform encephalopathies has been shown with the bovine spongiform encephalopathy signature being identified in transmissions to mice of transmissible spongiform encephalopathies of domestic cats and 2 exotic species of ruminant.

Conclusion.—There is strong evidence that the same agent strain involved in bovine spongiform encephalopathy also is involved in the new variant Cruetzfeldt-Jakob disease. Variant Cruetzfeldt-Jacob disease appears to be a new condition that is appearing almost exclusively in the United Kingdom. There are serious concerns that bovine spongiform encephalopathy has spread to humans through dietary exposure.

▶ Prions are not viruses but this important article is included in the viral infections section. This study appears to have firmly established the relationship between bovine spongiform encephalopathy (BSE) seen in cattle and the new variant of Creutzfeldt–Jakob disease (CJD). The outbreak of BSE in cattle, which appears to be related to the inclusion of animal parts in cattle feed was followed by a new variant of CJD in which the patients were younger and had a distinct CNS pathology. Investigators found that disease induced in mice by injection of brain homogenates from patients with the new variant CJD appeared to be identical to disease induced by brain homogenates from cattle dying of BSE. This was distinct from disease induced by brain tissue from patients dying of sporadic CJD. These results strongly indicate the identity of the BSE agent and the new variant CJD agent.

G.L. Mandell, M.D.

5 Respiratory Infections

Introduction

There are many areas in medicine that are common but puzzling. In this section we have addressed the problem of sinusitis and the sputum gram stain in pneumonia. It is interesting that pneumonia caused by *Chlamydia pneumoniae* can be indistinguishable from that caused by the pneumococcus. Other reports have shown that respiratory syncytial virus can look very much like influenza virus in nursing home patients.

Gerald L. Mandell, M.D.

Effect of a Rhinovirus-caused Upper Respiratory Illness on Pulmonary Function Test and Exercise Responses

Weidner TG, Anderson BN, Kaminsky LA, et al (Ball State Univ, Muncie, Ind)
Med Sci Sports Exerc 29:604–609, 1997   5–1

Background.—It has been suggested that viral upper respiratory infections (URIs) are the most frequent cause of acute disability among athletes. The risk of rhinovirus infections may be increased by heavy exercise. There are few data on the physiologic consequences during exercise in athletes with a rhinovirus-caused URI. The effects of rhinovirus-caused URIs on the submaximal exercise response, maximal exercise functional capacity, and resting pulmonary function were studied in active volunteers.

Methods.—The study included 45 young men and women. Although fitness levels varied, all research subjects exercised at least 3 times a week. The 35 research subjects assigned to the experimental group were all free of antibody to human rhinovirus 16 on serologic screening. After baseline pulmonary function testing and a graded exercise test, the experimental research subjects were inoculated with human rhinovirus 16 on 2 consecutive days. On the third day, the infected research subjects repeated the pulmonary function and graded exercise tests. The 10 control patients performed the same tests on 2 occasions 1 week apart. The data were analyzed to see how the rhinovirus illness affected the research subjects' exercise performance and pulmonary function.

Results.—In both groups, no significant differences in physiologic responses between the pre-exercise and postexercise tests were noted on analysis of variance. Neither were there any significant differences between maximal exercise performance between trials. The pulmonary function test results showed no significant interactions between treatment and group assignment.

Conclusions.—Surprisingly, rhinovirus-caused URIs do not seem to have any effect on resting pulmonary function or acute submaximal and maximal exercise capacity. However, this is the first study of the effects of URIs of known cause on the physiologic response to exercise. An effect might be seen during longer bouts of submaximal exercise or in a different age group.

▶ This study detected no impairment in exercise capacity by a rhinovirus cold. Influenza, which affects the lower airways, does cause impairment in pulmonary function.

G.L. Mandell, M.D.

The Ten-day Mark as a Practical Diagnostic Approach for Acute Paranasal Sinusitis in Children
Ueda D, Yoto Y (Sapporo Higashi Tokushukai Hosp, Japan)
Pediatr Infect Dis J 15:576–579, 1996   5–2

Introduction.—Acute sinusitis may complicate up to 10% of upper respiratory infections in children and is often overlooked by the primary care physician. A group of pediatric outpatients with upper respiratory infections was evaluated to determine the usefulness of the 10-day mark in diagnosing acute sinusitis.

Methods.—The study group included 2,013 children with respiratory complaints. Those whose symptoms persisted for more than 10 days without signs of improvement were suspected of having sinusitis and underwent a radiographic projection of maxillary sinuses (Water's view). Sinusitis was diagnosed if radiography revealed diffuse opacification, mucosal thickening of at least 4 mm, or air-fluid level. All patients were treated with cefaclor (40 mg/kg/24 hr, divided into 3 doses) for 2 weeks. Adjunctive treatment included decongestants and anti-inflammatory agents. Patients were examined again at 2 weeks and had repeat radiographic imaging.

Results.—Use of the 10-day mark identified 146 children with a possible diagnosis of sinusitis. The radiographic examination yielded abnormal findings of maxillary sinuses in 135 (92.5%) children, 88 boys and 47 girls who ranged in age from 2 to 15 years. Thirty-five of these children had allergic respiratory diseases. Sinusitis was classified according to duration of symptoms: acute, less than 3 weeks (124 cases); subacute, 3 weeks to 3 months (9 cases); and chronic, more than 3 months (2 cases). The overall incidence of maxillary sinusitis in the group of children with respiratory symptoms was 6.7%. Most children with sinusitis were between the ages of 3 and 6 years. The most common radiographic findings were mucosal thickening and bilateral opacified sinus; no films showed an air-fluid level.

Two-week antimicrobial treatment brought about complete improvement in 61% of nonallergic patients, but in only 11% of those with allergy.

Discussion.—Inadequate treatment of sinusitis in children can result in the development of chronic sinusitis, and intracranial complications can be life-threatening. The 10-day mark was confirmed to be a simple and practical method for identifying sinusitis in children with respiratory symptoms. Water's view radiographs can then confirm the diagnosis.

Primary-care-based Randomised Placebo-controlled Trial of Antibiotic Treatment in Acute Maxillary Sinusitis
van Buchem FL, Knottnerus JA, Schrijnemaekers VJJ, et al (St Elisabeth Hosp, Tilburg, The Netherlands; Univ of Limburg, Maastricht, The Netherlands)
Lancet 349:683–687, 1997   5–3

Introduction.—The presence of acute maxillary sinusitis in patients seeking treatment for symptoms of the common cold is thought to indicate a need for antibiotics. Although antibiotic therapy appears to be effective in those referred to ear, nose, and throat (ENT) clinics after the discovery of empyema, its usefulness in primary-care patients is uncertain. This question was examined in a double-blind, randomized, placebo-controlled trial of adult patients with suspected acute maxillary sinusitis.

Methods.—The patients were referred by general practitioners for radiographs of the maxillary sinus. Acute maxillary sinusitis was suspected on the basis of case history and physical examination. Radiographs with Caldwell and Waters' projections were assessed by 1 radiologist and classified as: (1) normal, (2) mucosal swelling of 5 mm or less, (3) mucosal swelling greater than 5 mm, (4) complete shadowing, or (5) fluid level. Patients with findings 1 and 2 were treated by their general practitioner as normal; the remaining patients were referred to an ENT specialist. Of 488 patients referred for radiography, 272 had abnormal findings and 214 were randomly assigned to amoxycillin or placebo. Clinical course was assessed after 1 and 2 weeks, and patients were studied for 1 year for relapses and complications.

Results.—After 2 weeks, symptoms had greatly decreased or disappeared in 83% of patients in the amoxycillin group vs. 77% of those in the placebo group. Both the clinical picture after 1 and 2 weeks and the mean differences between baseline and follow-up symptoms scores were essentially similar in the 2 groups. The antibiotics and placebo groups were also similar in mean radiographic improvement at 2 weeks. During the follow-up year, relapses occurred in 17% of patients treated with placebo and in 21% of those treated with antibiotics; no complications were reported in either group.

Discussion.—Patients with acute maxillary sinusitis have a good prognosis whether or not antibiotic therapy is prescribed. Because antibiotic treatment does not improve their clinical course, these patients do not require an initial radiographic examination. Whether antibiotics should be given when symptoms persist beyond 2–3 weeks remains to be determined.

▶ Sinusitis continues to puzzle me. Everybody with a cold has a runny nose. This discharge frequently turns purulent and may be associated with "sinus symptoms." Gwaltney et al.[1] showed that the majority of patients with colds have abnormalities in their CT scans that are indicative of sinusitis. The article by Ueda et al. (Abstract 5–2) attempts to support 10 days of symptoms as a cutoff for the diagnosis of sinusitis in children. They show that most of the children who had symptoms longer than 10 days have abnormal radiographic findings (which might be expected from the Gwaltney study). After antibiotic treatment, most patients improved.

The Buchem study (Abstract 5–3) challenges the effect of antibiotics. Adult patients with maxillary sinusitis diagnosed by symptoms and radiography were divided into 2 groups: placebo and amoxicillin treatment. There was no effect of treatment.

I remain confused and I am not sure when antibiotics are indicated in patients with sinus symptoms. The old rules suggested sinus tenderness, fever, and air-fluid levels on radiographs as definitive indicators for those who need treatment. Recently, experts have been adding chronicity to the equation, that is, patients who have sinus symptoms for more than a given period, somewhere between 10 days and 2 weeks, as in the Ueda study, should be treated. I'm not convinced. This is an evolving field and an important one.

G.L. Mandell, M.D.

Reference

1. Gwaltney JM, Phillips CD, Miller RD, et al: Computed tomographic study of the common cold. *N Engl J Med* 330:25–30, 1994.

Sputum Gram's Stain in Community-acquired Pneumococcal Pneumonia
Reed WW, Byrd GS, Gates RH Jr, et al (Fitzsimons Army Med Ctr, Aurora, Colo; Walter Reed Army Med Ctr, Washington, DC)
West J Med 165:197–204, 1996   5–4

Objective.—Although the sputum Gram's stain has been widely used to identify etiologic agents in community-acquired pneumococcal pneumonia, its usefulness has been questioned. A meta-analysis was conducted to evaluate the sensitivity and specificity of Gram's stain and the effect of stain interpreter, definition of positive Gram's stain, or control for antibiotic on the results.

Methods.—A summary receiver-operator characteristic (ROC) curve was generated from data obtained from a MEDLINE search that yielded 12 articles which were included in the analysis. Articles were graded for quality by 3 blinded reviewers.

Results.—Almost one third of patients were unable to produce sufficient sputum, but only 4 studies noted this. The definition of positive Gram's stain was clear in only 6 studies. Reference standards used varied from study to study, and blood cultures were not evaluated in 11 studies because of poor sensitivity. Sensitivities and specificities ranged from 15% to 100% and 11% to 100%, respectively.

Conclusion.—Because of the lack of a consistent standard of reference, widely varying sensitivities and specificities, unclear definitions, and inconsistent test characteristics, results of the sputum Gram's stain may be misleading.

▶ Older physicians, and especially infectious diseases specialists, prided themselves on the information that could be obtained by simple examination of a Gram stain of the sputum. This meta-analysis casts doubt on the usefulness of the procedure. This is somewhat of a moot issue because my understanding is that the Clinical Laboratory Improvement Act prohibits individual physicians from examining and interpreting Gram stain results. Despite this, I have a strong bias that a Gram stain of the sputum that shows many neutrophils and a predominant flora of gram-positive lancet-shaped diplococci is a strong indicator for pneumococcal infection and allows one to design treatment accordingly. In addition, the rarer pneumonias, such as staphylococcal pneumonia, may be first identified on a Gram stain of the sputum.

G.L. Mandell, M.D.

***Chlamydia Pneumoniae* as a New Source of Infectious Outbreaks in Nursing Homes**
Troy CJ, Peeling RW, Ellis AG, et al (Ontario Ministry of Health, Toronto; Health Canada, Ottawa, Ont; Windsor Regional Public Health Laboratory Ont, Canada)
JAMA 277:1214–1218, 1997   5–5

Introduction.—The highest incidence of *Chlamydia pneumoniae* occurs in the elderly. Outbreaks of acute respiratory illness were reported among residents of 3 nursing homes in Ontario from September to November 1994. The extent and severity of illness and the mode of transmission of *C. pneumoniae* within these 3 facilities are reported.

Methods.—The 3 homes were owned and operated by the same private companies and shared many of the same volunteers who were involved in organized social events. Disease surveillance forms, patient medical charts, and a self-administered questionnaire for staff members were reviewed to determine the morbidity and mortality of residents in the 3 nursing homes. Single and paired serum samples underwent *C. pneumoniae* serologic testing, nasopharyngeal swabs were cultured for *C. pneumoniae*, and direct fluorescent antibody assays were done to confirm *C. pneumoniae* infection.

Results.—The attack rates for confirmed and suspected incidences of infection were 68% in nursing home A, 46% in nursing home B, and 44% in nursing home C and 34% among staff members of nursing home C. In nursing home C, the incidence of new coughs was 100%, the incidence of fevers was 64%, the incidence of sore throats was 24%, and the incidence of hoarseness in patients was 14%. Staff members in nursing home C were significantly more likely to report hoarseness and sore throats. Residents who smoked were significantly more likely to have earlier onsets of illness than nonsmokers. This may be related to airborne transmission in a designated smoking room.

Conclusion.—Findings indicate that *C. pneumoniae* was a source of infection in 3 nursing home outbreaks. The optimal treatment and prevention of future outbreaks requires further investigation.

▶ *C. pneumoniae* has recently made headlines because of its association with coronary artery disease. This report emphasizes the organism's role in causing respiratory infections in nursing home residents. Coughs, fevers, sore throats, and hoarseness were the most common clinical manifestations, and a number of patients had pneumonia, which resulted in some fatalities. Points to be emphasized are the very high attack rates, about 50%, and the potential serious nature of the infection. Because the organism is susceptible to tetracyclines and macrolides, treatment with these agents is recommended.

G.L. Mandell, M.D.

6 Bacterial and Fungal Infections

Introduction

The management of many of these infections is becoming more, rather than less, problematic. This is partly due to increasing resistance to antimicrobial agents. Fortunately, new antibiotics are being developed which have potential to be useful for some of these infections.

Gerald L. Mandell, M.D.

The Clinical Significance of Positive Blood Cultures in the 1990s: Comprehensive Evaluation of the Microbiology, Epidemiology, and Outcome of Bacteremia and Fungemia in Adults
Weinstein MP, Towns ML, Quartey SM, et al (Univ of Medicine and Dentistry of New Jersey, New Brunswick; Duke Univ, Durham, NC; Univ of Utah, Salt Lake City)
Clin Infect Dis 24:584–602, 1997   6–1

Introduction.—Articles published in 1983 and authored by 2 of the investigators of this study considered the clinical significance of positive blood cultures by analyzing 500 episodes of bacteremia and fungemia in adults. Two decades later, there have been many advances in medical practice, and new infections have appeared. To assess changes since the mid-1970s, investigators reviewed 833 episodes of positive blood cultures in 707 patients with septicemia.

Methods.—During a 12-month period (February 1992 through January 1993), all inpatients at 3 centers who were 18 years or older and had culture-positive blood were evaluated. All positive cultures were assessed critically, and isolates were categorized as true positives, contaminants, or of unknown clinical significance. Each episode of bacteremia, fungemia, or mycobacteremia was classified as either community- or hospital-acquired septicemia. Data were obtained on antimicrobial therapy and on patient outcome, and treatment was judged for adequacy.

Results.—During the study period, 1,585 blood culture-positive episodes occurred in 1,267 patients; there were 843 episodes of true bacter-

TABLE 1.—Microorganisms Isolated From Blood of Patients at Duke University Medical Center, Robert Wood Johnson University Hospital, and the Salt Lake City VA Medical Center, February 1992 Through January 1993

Microorganism (no. of isolates)	No. (%) of isolates per indicated category		
	True pathogen	Contaminant	Unknown
Aerobic and facultative bacteria			
Gram-positive			
Staphylococcus aureus (204)	178 (87.2)	13 (6.4)	13 (6.4)
Coagulase-negative staphylococci (703)	87 (12.4)	575 (81.9)	41 (5.8)
Enterococcus species (93)	65 (69.9)	15 (16.1)	13 (14.0)
Viridans streptococci (71)	27 (38.0)	35 (49.3)	9 (12.7)
Streptococcus pneumoniae (34)	34 (100)	0	0
Group A streptococci (3)	3 (100)	0	0
Group B streptococci (15)	10 (66.7)	3 (20.0)	2 (13.3)
Other streptococci (13)	8 (61.5)	3 (23.1)	2 (15.4)
Bacillus species (12)	1 (8.3)	11 (91.7)	0
Corynebacterium species (53)	1 (1.9)	51 (96.2)	1 (1.9)
Listeria monocytogenes (2)	1 (50.0)	0	1 (50.0)
Lactobacillus species (15)	6 (54.5)	2 (18.2)	3 (27.3)
Other gram-positive bacteria (15)	2 (13.3)	12 (80)	1 (6.7)
Gram-negative			
Escherichia coli (143)	142 (99.3)	0	1 (0.7)
Klebsiella pneumoniae (65)	65 (100)	0	0
Enterobacter cloacae (25)	25 (100)	0	0
Serratia marcescens (22)	22 (100)	0	0
Proteus mirabilis (16)	16 (100)	0	0
Other Enterobacteriaceae (45)	41 (91)	1 (2.2)	3 (6.7)
Pseudomonas aeruginosa (55)	53 (96.4)	1 (1.8)	1 (1.8)
Pseudomonas species (8)	6 (75)	0	2 (25)
Stenotrophomonas maltophilia (7)	5 (71.4)	0	2 (28.6)
Acinetobacter baumanii (16)	13 (81.2)	1 (6.2)	2 (12.5)
Haemophilus influenzae (3)	3 (100)	0	0
Other gram-negative bacteria (16)	10 (62.5)	3 (18.8)	3 (18.8)
Anaerobic bacteria			
Clostridium perfringens (13)	3 (23.1)	10 (76.9)	0
Clostridium species (15)	12 (80)	3 (20)	0
Propionibacterium species (48)	0	48 (100)	0
Other gram-positive anaerobic bacteria (7)	4 (57.1)	2 (28.6)	1 (14.3)
Bacteroides fragilis group (18)	16 (88.9)	0	2 (11.1)
Other gram-negative anaerobic bacteria (5)	2 (40)	2 (40)	1 (20)
Yeasts and fungi			
Candida albicans (30)	27 (90)	0	3 (10)
Other *Candida* species (15)	15 (100)	0	0
Cryptococcus neoformans (8)	8 (100)	0	0
Torulopsis glabrata (15)	14 (93.3)	0	1 (6.7)
Other yeasts and fungi (4)	2 (50)	1 (25)	1 (25)
Mycobacteria			
Mycobacterium avium complex (16)	16 (100)	0	0
M. tuberculosis (1)	1 (100)	0	0
All microorganisms (1,844)	944 (51.2)	791 (42.9)	109 (5.9)

(Courtesy of Weinstein MP, Towns ML, Quartey SM, et al: The clinical significance of positive blood cultures in the 1990s: Comprehensive evaluation of the microbiology, epidemiology, and outcome of bacteremia and fungemia in adults. *Clin Infect Dis* 24:584–602, 1997. University of Chicago, publisher.)

TABLE 5.—Sources and Confirmatory Evidence for Episodes of Unimicrobial Bacteremia and Fungemia, According to Microorganism

Microorganism(s) (no. of episodes)	No. of sources confirmed by Culture	No. of sources confirmed by Clinical evidence	Common source(s) (no. of episodes)
Staphylococcus aureus (159)	56	74	IV (56), skin (19), respiratory (18), bone/joint (10)
Coagulase-negative staphylococci (73)	16	45	IV (59), skin (5)
Streptococcus pneumoniae (34)	5	22	Respiratory (26)
Group B streptococci (8)	4	3	Skin (3), GU (3)
Viridans group streptococci (24)	3	10	Respiratory (3), skin (2)
Enterococcus species (38)	13	9	GU (15), IV (3)
Escherichia coli (116)	70	30	GU (67), biliary (11), peritoneal (10)
Klebsiella pneumonia (48)	15	15	Biliary (10), GU (8), peritoneal (5)
Enterobacter cloacae (12)	3	2	Biliary (2), respiratory (2)
Serratia marcescens (20)	11	6	GU (4), respiratory (4), IV (3)
Proteus mirabilis (13)	10	2	GU (9)
Pseudomonas aeruginosa (48)	25	12	Respiratory (19), GU (9)
Acinetobacter baumanii (12)	4	0	Respiratory (3)
Bacteroides fragilis group (9)	3	4	Abscess (6)
Candida albicans (21)	7	2	IV (5), peritoneal (2)
Candida tropicalis (7)	1	4	IV (1), GU (1), peritoneal (1)
Torulopsis glabrata (12)	1	4	GU (4)
Mycobacterium avium (15)	0	0	No sources identified

Note: The list of microorganisms includes all those isolated 5 times or more as causes of unimicrobial bacteremia or fungemia.

Abbreviations: abscess, intraabdominal abscess; GU, genitourinary tract; IV, intravascular device; respiratory, respiratory tract.

(Courtesy of Weinstein MP, Towns ML, Quartey SM, et al: The clinical significance of positive blood cultures in the 1990s: Comprehensive evaluation of the microbiology, epidemiology, and outcome of bacteremia and fungemia in adults. *Clin Infect Dis* 24:584–602, 1997. University of Chicago, publisher.)

emia or fungemia, 658 contaminant episodes, and 84 episodes of unknown clinical significance. The microorganism most frequently causing true bacteremia was *Staphylococcus aureus* (Table 1). Other common pathogens were *Escherichia coli,* coagulase-negative staphylococci (CNS), *Klebsiella pneumoniae,* and *Enterococcus* species. Overall, 52.1% of all episodes were nosocomial, and 73.5% occurred in patients hospitalized on the medical services of the hospitals. Leading identifiable sources of septicemia included IV catheters, the respiratory and genitourinary tracts, and intra-abdominal foci. Most *S. aureus* and CNS bacteremias were associated with intravascular devices (Table 5). Deaths attributed directly or indirectly to an episode of septicemia numbered 148 (17.5%). Mortality was lowest (13.3%) among patients who received appropriate antimicrobial therapy throughout the course of infection. Factors independently influencing outcome in multivariate analysis were age, microorganism, source of infection, predisposing factors, blood pressure, body temperature, and therapy.

Discussion.—Findings suggest that contaminants in blood cultures are more common in the 1990s than they were in the 1970s, and IV catheters have increased in importance as a source of infection. Isolation of CNS is more frequent, and there has been a proportionate increase in fungemia and a decrease in anaerobic bacteremia. In both periods, *S. aureus* and *E. coli* were the most frequent etiologic agents. Mortality appears to have been reduced.

▶ There is a wealth of data in this article. For example, Table 5 associates blood culture isolates with their source. There are some interesting associations. For example, the most common source for *Pseudomonas* bacteremia was the respiratory tract. The most lethal type of positive blood cultures were yeast and fungi, and they yielded a relative risk of death of 6.54 compared with 1.0 for CNS. This is probably not because of the virulence of the organisms but because the host must be significantly impaired before these organisms invade the bloodstream.

Table 1 is useful because it can help determine the likelihood of a given isolate being a true pathogen or a contaminant. For example, in a patient with *Pseudomonas aeruginosa* bacteremia, it is highly likely (96.4%) to be a true pathogen. In contrast, CNS appear to be true pathogens in only 12.4% of instances.

G.L. Mandell, M.D.

Diagnosis of Triple-lumen Catheter Infection: Comparison of Roll Plate, Sonication, and Flushing Methodologies

Sherertz RJ, Heard SO, Raad II (Bowman Gray School of Medicine, Winston Salem, NC; Univ of Massachusetts, Worcester; MD Anderson Cancer Ctr, Houston)
J Clin Microbiol 35:641–646, 1997   6–2

Objective.—Quantitative catheter culture techniques include the roll plate method, flushing with broth, centrifugation, swabbing and then vortexing the swab, vortexing, and sonication. This study compares the diagnostic capabilities of the sonication, roll plate, and flushing methods for culturing triple-lumen central catheters.

Methods.—The tips and subcutaneous segments of 254 triple-lumen catheters were cultured by the 3 methods. Catheter colonization and catheter-related bacteremia were determined and compared statistically among the 3 methods.

Results.—Of the 29 catheter segments positive by the roll plate method, only 18 (62.1%) were positive by the sonication method. Of the 57 catheters whose segments were positive by the sonication method, 46 (80.7%) consecutive catheter segments were also positive. Therefore, culture by sonication after culture by roll plate will underestimate the incidence of colonization. Sonication was significantly more sensitive in detecting colonization in the tip (53%) and subcutaneous segment (57%) than the roll plate method (Table 1). Catheters with culture-positive lumens were significantly more likely to have a positive culture after sonication (82%) than after the roll plate method (57%). When colonized catheters from patients with bacteremia were compared with colonized

TABLE 1.—Sensitivities of 7 Different Catheter Culture Methods With
89 Catheters

Catheter segment and culture method	No. (%) positive
Subcutaneous segment	
Roll plate	17 (37.8)*
Sonication	26 (57.8)*
Tip segment	
Roll plate	15 (33.3)†
Sonication	24 (53.3)†
Proximal lumen	17 (37.8)
Middle lumen	21 (46.7)
Distal lumen	12 (26.7)
Composite index‡	45 (100)

*Differences are statistically significant for the pair ($P < 0.05$).
†Differences are statistically significant for the pair ($P < 0.05$).
‡At least 1 of the 7 catheter cultures met the quantitative definitions described in the text for 45 of 89 catheter cultures.
(Courtesy of Sherertz RJ, Heard SO, Raad II: Diagnosis of triple-lumen catheter infection: Comparison of roll plate, sonication, and flushing methodologies. *J Clin Microbiol* 35:641–646, 1997.)

catheters from patients without bacteremia, 57.1% vs. 36.7% were positive. For catheters with only 1 of 3 sites showing a positive culture, 36.7% involved a subcutaneous segment, 26.7% involved the tip, and 36.7% involved the lumen. The duration of catheterization of these sites was 5.1, 8.6, and 13.1 days, respectively. Subcutaneous segments became contaminated significantly more quickly than either the tip or lumen. Failure to aspirate blood for culture indicated the presence of a lumen thrombosis. Culture-positive lumens (100 or more colony-forming units) had a 91% incidence of failed blood aspiration.

Conclusion.—Culturing 1 segment of a vascular catheter may be inadequate to determine catheter infection. Infection rates of catheter lumen and tip suggest that hematogenous colonization may be a more important source of infection than previously thought.

▶ Twenty years ago Maki et al.[1] described an innovative method for culturing IV catheters. Before Dr. Maki's studies, it was common practice to cut the tip off of a catheter and put it in a broth. There were many false positive results, probably related to skin contamination. His roll method was semiquantitative and involved rolling the catheter over the surface of an agar plate and counting colonies. He found a good correlation with a count of greater than 15 colony-forming units and true infection.

Triple-lumen catheters are now frequently used and it is time to reexamine the issue. It is important to emphasize that the current study uses catheter colonization as the end point; however, some patients with colonized catheters are not ill and do not have bacteremia. Table 1 indicates the different sensitivities of the methods and shows that no single method picks up more than half of colonized catheters. When the subset of patients with positive blood cultures was considered, the positivity rate went up, but roll plates, even at 2 sites, still missed 30% of the positive cultures. The useful points for the clinician are that catheter colonization is relatively common (about half of all catheters are colonized) and that a negative roll culture does not rule out the catheter as the source of the infection. As an aside, the authors postulate that because of the location of colonization it appears that catheters may frequently be infected secondarily from bacteremia originating at another site.

G.L. Mandell, M.D.

Reference

1. Maki DG, Weise CE, Sarafin HW: A semiquantitative culture method for identifying intravenous catheter-related infections. *N Engl J Med* 296:1305–1309, 1977.

Nasal and Cutaneous Carriage of *Staphylococcus aureus* in Hemodialysis Patients: The Effect of Nasal Mupirocin
Boelaert JR, Van Landuyt HW, Gordts BZ, et al (Brugge, Belgium)
Infect Control Hosp Epidemiol 17:809–811, 1996   6–3

Background.—Bacteremia is a major cause of morbidity and mortality in patients receiving hemodialysis, and *Staphylococcus aureus* is one of the most important infectious organisms. The risk of infection may be elevated for patients who are nasal carriers of *S. aureus*. Intranasal muciprocin can reduce the incidence of *S. aureus* infection among these patients. The link between *S. aureus* carriage in the nares and on the hands of patients receiving hemodialysis was investigated, including the effects of nasal muciprocin on carriage rates.

Methods.—Cultures were obtained from the nares and hands of patients starting hemodialysis. The study included 20 patients who did and 20 who did not carry *S. aureus* in their nares. All patients with nasal carriage received nasal calcium muciprocin. Isolates of *S. aureus* were compared by pulsed-field gel electrophoresis. Seventeen patients in each group were followed up for 17 months.

Results.—Seventy-five percent of patients who carried *S. aureus* in their nares also carried it on their hands, compared to 10% of patients who were not nasal carriers. Of patients who carried *S. aureus* in their nares and on their hands, 87% had the same strain at both sites. Treatment with intranasal muciprocin eliminated *S. aureus* at both sites.

Conclusions.—Patients receiving hemodialysis who carry *S. aureus* in their nares are likely to carry the same organism on their hands. Vascular access site infection may occur from either of these sites. Intranasal muciprocin treatment can eliminate *S. aureus* from both sites.

Emergence of High-level Mupirocin Resistance in Methicillin-resistant *Staphylococcus aureus* Isolated From Brazilian University Hospitals
dos Santos KRN, de Souza Fonseca L, Filho PPG (Instituo de Microbiologia, Rio de Janeiro, Brasil)
Infect Control Hosp Epidemiol 17:813–816, 1996   6–4

Background.—In Brazil, nosocomial infections caused by bacteria resistant to antibiotics are widespread. By 1986, more than half the *Staphylococcus aureus* isolates in Sao Paulo hospitals were resistant to methicillin. Mupirocin is a novel topical antibiotic with excellent activity against staphylococci. Mupirocin resistance in strains of methicillin-resistant *S. aureus* (MRSA) isolated from patients in 2 hospitals with different mupirocin policies was investigated.

Methods and Findings.—One hundred fourteen multiresistant MRSA strains were isolated from a total of 62 patients at a hospital in Rio de Janeiro and a hospital in Uberlandia. Forty-four isolates were resistant to mupirocin. Sixty-three percent of the strains in the Rio de Janeiro hospital were resistant to mupirocin, compared to only 6.1% in the Uberlandia hospital. At the former hospital, topical mupirocin was used extensively, whereas its use was rare in the latter.

Conclusions.—The development of mupirocin resistance is associated with its prior use, especially in patients in whom mupirocin treatment had been administered for several months. The judicious use of this antibiotic is important if it is to be used in the treatment and prevention of serious infections with MRSA.

▶ Mupirocin is a small molecule with a fatty acid side chain derived from products of *Pseudomonas* species. It is topically bactericidal for *Staphylococcus aureus*. The article by Boelaert (Abstract 6–3) reinforces some of our concepts of carriage of the organism. *Staphylococcus aureus* finds a reservoir in the nares and the other parts of the body are sporadically positive, but if the nasal sanctuary is eliminated, the organism is often completely eradicated. The authors find that intranasal mupirocin eliminated the staphylococci from the nares and the hands of most patients. This is important because it is a way of reducing staphylococcal infections in susceptible patients such as presurgical patients, and, in this case, patients undergoing hemodialysis. As one might expect, heavy use of mupirocin results in resistance to the agent. dos Santos et al. (Abstract 6–4) observed that resistance was very frequent at a hospital that used a lot of mupirocin. Mupirocin is especially useful in those instances where staphylococcal infection has been shown to originate from carriers of the organism. It should not be used in a routine fashion and it should not be used merely to convert positive cultures to negative cultures.

G.L. Mandell, M.D.

Staphylococcus aureus Prosthetic Joint Infection Treated With Debridement and Prosthesis Retention

Brandt CM, Sistrunk WW, Duffy MC, et al (Mayo Clinic/Mayo Found, Rochester, Minn)
Clin Infect Dis 24:914–919, 1997   6–5

Background.—Although not frequent, prosthetic joint infection (PJI) after total joint arthroplasty is a serious complication. Eradicating such infection without permanently removing the prosthesis is difficult. The micro-organism–specific probability of treatment failure for patients with *Staphylococcus aureus* PJI treated by debridement and prosthesis retention was determined.

Methods.—Thirty patients with 33 *S. aureus* PJIs were initially treated by debridement and prosthesis retention at the Mayo Clinic between 1980 and 1991. Treatment failure was strictly defined as a relapse of *S. aureus* PJI or occurrence of culture-negative PJI during continuous antistaphylococcal therapy.

Findings.—Treatment failure occurred in 21 of the infected prostheses. The cumulative probabilities of treatment failure at 1 and 2 years were 54% and 69%, respectively. The joints in which treatment failed required a median of 4 additional operations to control the infection. Prostheses debrided more than 2 days after symptom onset had a greater probability of treatment failure than prostheses debrided within 2 days of symptom onset (Fig 1).

Conclusion.—Debridement and prosthesis retention as the initial treatment for *S. aureus* PJI has a high cumulative probability of failure. The probability of treatment failure may be associated with the duration of symptoms.

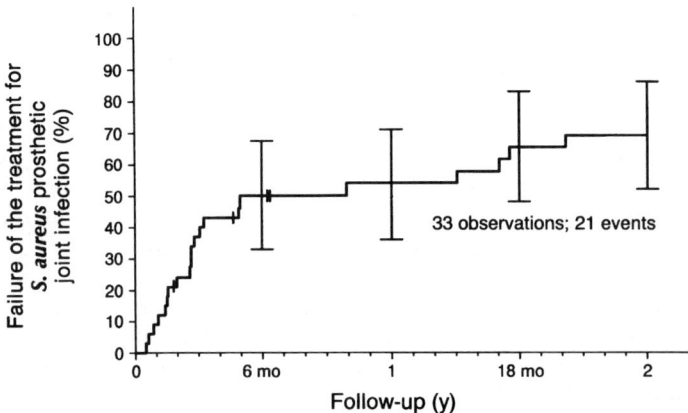

FIGURE 1.—Overall cumulative probability (and 95% confidence intervals) of failure of treatment of *Staphylococcus aureus* prosthetic joint infection within the first 2 years after debridement and prosthesis retention. *Short vertical marks* represent censored events. (Courtesy of Brandt CM, Sistrunk WW, Duffy MC, et al: *Staphylococcus aureus* prosthetic joint infection treated with debridement and prosthesis retention. *Clin Infect Dis* 24:914–919, 1997. Published by the University of Chicago.)

▶ A prosthetic joint infected with *S. aureus* has a poor prognosis. Figure 1 shows that at the end of 2 years, 69% of joints treated with debridement and antibiotics needed to be removed. The treatment of choice for infected prostheses remains a 2-stage revision arthroplasty in which the prosthesis is removed. The patient is treated intensively, usually for a period of 6–8 weeks, and if no sign of infection is evident, a new prosthesis is implanted. However, selected patients may respond favorably to debridement with retention of the prosthesis, and these seem to be those patients whose infected prosthesis can be debrided within 2 days of onset of symptoms.

G.L. Mandell, M.D.

Efficacy of Cefepime in the Treatment of Infections Due to Multiply Resistant *Enterobacter* Species
Sanders WE Jr, Tenney JH, Kessler RE (Creighton Univ, Omaha, Neb; Bristol Myers Squibb Pharmaceutical Research Inst, Wallingford, Conn)
Clin Infect Dis 23:454–461, 1996   6–6

Objective.—The new cephalosporin drug cefepime has a broader spectrum of antimicrobial activity and greater potency than other cephalosporins. Its unique characteristics include rapid penetration into many gram-negative bacilli, targeting of multiple penicillin-binding proteins, and resistance to inactivation by many β-lactamases. For these reasons, it is active against organisms that are resistant to other drugs, such as ceftazidime, cefotaxime, and ceftriaxone. Cefepime was assessed for use in treating *Enterobacter* infections with resistance to ceftazidime.

Patients.—The retrospective study included 16 patients with 17 infections caused by *Enterobacter* strains with reduced susceptibility or resistance to ceftazidime. Most of the organisms isolated were also resistant to other β-lactam drugs, though all were susceptible to cefepime. The infections included pneumonia, urinary tract infection, intra-abdominal infection, and bacteremia.

Outcomes.—All infections responded clinically to IV cefepime. The infecting organism was thought to have been eradicated in 88% of the sites. Cefepime was effective even in chronic infections that had failed to respond to previous treatment with imipenem, aminoglycosides, or ciprofloxacin. There were no cases of cefepime resistance.

Discussion.—Cefepime appears to be effective in the treatment of infections caused by *Enterobacter* strains with multiple β-lactam resistance. Cefepime treatment can succeed in chronic infections in which all previous treatments have failed. Although more research is needed, cefepime may also be useful in the treatment of patients infected with multiply resistant strains of other genera with group 1 β-lactamases.

▶ Cefepime has been called a fourth generation cephalosporin. It can be thought of simply as having the in vitro activity of cefotaxime or ceftriaxone plus ceftazidime. In addition, the agent resists inactivation by β-lactamases that may be active against the third generation cephalosporins. This is important because certain *Enterobacter* and *Citrobacter* species are resistant to third generation cephalosporins as a result of β-lactamase production. This paper reports 16 patients with organisms that were relatively resistant to ceftazidime who responded to cefepime therapy. Of course some of these patients may have responded to long-term therapy with the other agents, but the good results suggest that cefepime will be a useful therapeutic agent.

G.L. Mandell, M.D.

Evaluation of a Novel Endoluminal Brush Method for In Situ Diagnosis of Catheter Related Sepsis

Kite P, Dobbins BM, Wilcox MH, et al (Univ of Leeds, England)
J Clin Pathol 50:278–282, 1997   6–7

Purpose.—Catheter-related sepsis (CRS) is an important problem that can be difficult to diagnose. When a central venous catheter is removed because of suspected infection, a subsequent line tip culture is negative 75% to 85% of the time. A new endoluminal brush technique could permit in situ diagnosis of CRS without the need for removal of the central venous line. The endoluminal brush method for diagnosis of catheter-related infection is studied prospectively.

Methods.—The study included 230 central venous catheters removed from 216 patients. One hundred twenty-eight catheters were removed because of suspected CRS or colonization. No line-associated infection was suspected in the remaining 102 catheters. Ninety percent of the catheters had been used for total parenteral nutrition. Before removal, each catheter was studied by in situ endoluminal brush sampling, in which a nylon brush was passed all the way to the distal end of the line and then withdrawn for processing. The catheter was then removed and studied by the Maki roll technique of extraluminal sampling and a modified Cleri flush technique of endoluminal sampling. The findings of the 3 techniques were compared.

TABLE 4.—Relation Between Significant Extraluminal or Endoluminal Growth of Microorganisms and the Diagnosis of Catheter-related Sepsis (CRS) and Catheter Colonization

Site(s) of significant bacterial growth	% of catheters associated with	
	CRS	Colonization
Extraluminal only	5	41
Extra- and endoluminal	77	53
Endoluminal only	18	7

(Courtesy of Kite P, Dobbins BM, Wilcox MH, et al: Evaluation of a novel endoluminal brush method for in situ diagnosis of catheter-related sepsis. *J Clin Pathol* 50:278–282, 1997 by permission of the BMJ Publishing Group.)

Results.—The presence of CRS was confirmed in 16% of catheters in which it was clinically suspected, as well as in 2% of catheters in which infection was not suspected. The frequency of line colonization was 92% with the Maki roll technique vs. 43% with both the Cleri flush and endoluminal brush techniques. On culture of colonized catheters, mixed growth was twice as likely to be seen with the Maki roll technique than with the 2 endoluminal techniques. Patients with CRS rarely had either endoluminal or extraluminal organisms, whereas 59% of catheters classified as being colonized showed only significant extraluminal growth. Relying on endoluminal brush sampling alone, just 1 case of CRS would have been missed. In contrast, relying on extraluminal sampling alone, 4 cases of CRS would have been missed. The sensitivity was 95% with the endoluminal brush method vs. 82% with the Maki roll technique; the specificity was 82% with the brush method and 66% with the Maki roll technique.

Conclusions.—The new endoluminal brush technique is a sensitive and specific test for CRS. It can recognize the presence of sepsis without the need for line removal. The technique is simple and appears to be safe and cost-effective. Most patients with CRS have both extraluminal and endoluminal organisms (Table 4).

▶ Intravascular CRS is a common problem. When patients have positive blood cultures and an obviously infected line, we make the diagnosis of CRS and remove the line. When patients have positive blood cultures and are febrile but the line looks good, the course of action is not so clear. These investigators brushed the inside of the catheter and used their results to determine whether the catheter was infected; this can be done leaving the catheter in place. They reported no problems with dislodged organisms entering the bloodstream; however, that has to remain a concern. They conclude that infected catheters are infected on both the endoluminal surface and the extraluminal surface simultaneously in most patients; therefore, they concluded that their endoluminal sampling was accurate (Table 4). I await more data.

G.L. Mandell, M.D.

7 Gastrointestinal Infections

Introduction

Raspberries; hamburgers; ice cream; all are related to severe gastrointestinal infection. In addition, our kids and grandkids have been forbidden to play with those cute little reptile pets which seem so innocuous. It is amazing how hard it is to eradicate microbes and that is why terminal sterilization via radiation is attractive (but not for turtles and iguanas).

Gerald L. Mandell, M.D.

An Outbreak in 1996 of Cyclosporiasis Associated With Imported Raspberries
Herwaldt BL, and the Cyclospora Working Group (Natl Ctr for Infectious Diseases, Atlanta, Ga)
N Engl J Med 336:1548–1556, 1997   7–1

Background.—*Cyclospora cayetanensis*, recently established as a coccidian parasite, causes gastroenteritis. Before 1996, cyclosporiasis in North America occurred primarily in overseas travelers. However, a large outbreak was reported at that time.

Methods and Findings.—In 1996, 1,465 cases of cyclosporiasis were reported by 20 states, the District of Columbia, and 2 Canadian provinces. Sixty-seven percent were confirmed by laboratory findings. Nearly half the cases were associated with 55 social events held between May 3 and June 14. At 50 of these events, raspberries were known to have been served, and at another 4, raspberries may have been served. Adequate data were available for 41 events. At 27 of these, the associations between berry consumption and cyclosporiasis were significant. The raspberries were known to come from Guatemala for 21 of the 29 events for which good data existed and may have come from Guatemala for another 8 events. Five Guatemalan farms may have been the source of the raspberries for 25 events. The mode of the raspberry contamination was not clear.

Conclusion.—The large 1996 outbreak of cyclosporiasis in North America was found to be associated with the consumption of Guatemalan raspberries. These findings show that a local cluster of food-borne illness may be part of a widespread outbreak. In such an outbreak, the source of the implicated vehicle needs to be pursued.

▶ *Cyclospora* was first recognized as a cause of diarrheal illness in Nepal. Cases in the United States were very uncommon. This outbreak from Guatamalan-grown raspberries highlights the fact that when we go to the supermarket, we must recognize the risks of imported fruits and vegetables. Some have argued that the only safe fresh fruit and vegetable supply is that which is irradiated at some point in the distribution chain. However, this raises a whole new set of problems related to the safe and secure transport, utilization, and disposal of radioactive materials.

G.L. Mandell, M.D.

Escherichia coli O157:H7 Diarrhea in the United States: Clinical and Epidemiologic Features
Slutsker L, for the *Escherichia coli* O157:H7 Study Group (Natl Ctr for Infectious Diseases, Atlanta, Ga)
Ann Intern Med 126:505–513, 1997   7–2

Background.—*Escherichia coli* O157:H7 is increasingly recognized as an important cause of bloody diarrhea, and infection with the pathogen is a major cause of postdiarrheal hemolytic syndrome in children in the United States and Canada. The frequency of isolation of *E. coli* O157:H7 was determined, and the clinical and epidemiologic features of infection were identified in a population prevalence study in 10 U.S. hospitals.

Methods.—The 10 hospitals selected represented all 4 census divisions in the United States. Nine served general patient populations, and 1 was a pediatric center. Each institution screened a median of 1,300 stool specimens annually. A clinical data form was completed for all patients from whom *Campylobacter, Salmonella* or *Shigella* species or *E. coli* O157:H7 were isolated and from every 25th patient from whom no pathogen was isolated.

Results.—Overall, 1,708 specimens (5.6%) examined during the study period (October 1990–October 1992) yielded at least 1 of the 4 major bacterial enteric pathogens. Dual infections were present in 11 patients. *E. coli* O157:H7 was isolated from 0.39% of 30,463 tested fecal specimens, found most frequently during the summer months, and exhibited the highest isolation proportions in hospitals in Maine and Wisconsin. In addition, *E. coli* was more likely to be isolated from visibly bloody stool specimens than from specimens without visible blood and was the pathogen isolated from 39% of visibly bloody stool specimens that yielded a bacterial enteric pathogen. The largest number of *E. coli* O157:H7 isolates was obtained from children aged 1–4 years (18 specimens) and adults aged 60–69 years (17 specimens). All 118 *E. coli* O157:H7 isolates produced at least 1 Shiga toxin, and 10 (8.5%) were resistant to at least 1 antimicrobial

TABLE 2.—History and Physical and Laboratory Findings in Patients From Whom *Escherichia coli* O157:H7, *Campylobacter* Species, *Salmonella* Species, or *Shigella* Species Were Isolated at 10 Hospitals in the United States, 1990 to 1992

Characteristic*	Patients with *Escherichia coli* O157:H7 (n = 104)	Patients with *Campylobacter* Species (n = 568)	Patients with *Salmonella* Species (n = 389)	Patients with *Shigella* Species (n = 232)	Patients with Any of the Four Pathogens
			%		
History					
Diarrhea	98.0	96.9	95.2	96.4	96.3
Bloody diarrhea	91.3	37.0	33.8	54.3	44.1
Abdominal cramps	90.5	79.5	69.7†	77.9	77.7
Reported fever	35.0	58.7	72.0	78.6	64.2
≥7 bowel movements per day†	65.5	61.1	54.8	53.6	58.3
Vomiting	35.6	34.4	41.0	49.0	39.0
Hospitalization	47.1	20.7	38.2	20.6	28.1
Physical and laboratory findings					
Objective fever	41.4	50.9	69.4	69.4	56.6
Abdominal tenderness	72.0	45.4	28.8	33.5	40.8
Visible blood in stool specimen	63.0	7.8	4.8	14.7†	11.8
Stool specimen positive for occult blood†	82.8	52.0	43.4	59.1	53.5
Any fecal leukocytes in stool specimens	70.5	42.9	29.4	37.8	39.5
≥10 fecal leukocytes per high-power field in stool specimen	23.9	16.0	10.2	11.1	13.9
Peripheral leukocyte count > 10 × 10^9/L	70.9	42.0	45.3†	58.0†	49.0

*Denominator for each characteristic includes only patients for whom information was available.
†This information was available for less than 65% of patients.
(Courtesy of Slutsker L, for the *Escherichia coli* O157:H7 Study Group: *Escherichia coli* O157:H7 diarrhea in the United States: Clinical and epidemiologic features. *Ann Intern Med* 126:505–513, 1997.)

agent. Diarrhea was an almost universal finding with each pathogen (Table 2), but bloody diarrhea was significantly more common among those with *E. coli* O157:H7 infections. Other clinical signs or symptoms independently associated with *E. coli* compared with the remaining 3 pathogens were visibly bloody stool specimens, no reported fever, a peripheral leukocyte count greater than $10 \times 10^9/L$, and abdominal tenderness.

Conclusion.—Isolation proportions from fecal specimens for *E. coli* O157:H7 surpassed those of other common enteric pathogens in certain geographic areas and age groups. Patients with a history of acute bloody diarrhea should have their fecal specimens cultured for *E. coli* O157:H7 because infection with this organism may result in serious disease.

▶ This pathogen has emerged as a major cause of bacterial diarrhea, but physicians should be especially concerned about the association of infection with *E. coli* O157:H7 and the hemolytic uremic syndrome. It is informative to note the low positive rate of stool cultures in patients with acute diarrhea. Of about 30,000 stool specimens, only 5.6% yielded a pathogen. As can be seen in Table 2, *Campylobacter, Salmonella, Shigella* and *E. coli* O157:H7 were isolated in that order.

The data support the concept that all bloody stool specimens should be cultured because 20% of those yielded a pathogen. *E. coli* O157:H7 was by far the most common isolate in visibly bloody stools. Of those cultures of bloody stools that did grow a pathogen, 39% grew *E. coli* O157:H7.

This article does not address the current debate concerning the treatment of acute diarrhea caused by *E. coli* O157:H7. Early data suggested that patients who received trimethoprim-sulfamethoxazole had a higher incidence of hemolytic uremic syndrome, but this association has been questioned because those patients were initially sicker. In adults it seems reasonable to offer treatment with a quinolone for the syndrome that involves acute fever and bloody diarrhea. Therapeutic choices in children are more difficult, and some would choose not to offer treatment.

G.L. Mandell, M.D.

Iguanas and *Salmonella* Marina Infection in Children: A Reflection of the Increasing Incidence of Reptile-associated Salmonellosis in the United States

Mermin J, Hoar B, Angulo FJ (Ctrs for Disease Control and Prevention, Atlanta, Ga)
Pediatrics 99:399–402, 1997   7–3

Introduction.—The incidence of *Salmonella* infections caused by exposure to reptiles is increasing in the United States, especially among infants. This increase reflects the growing popularity of reptiles, particularly iguanas, as pets. The demographic and risk factors associated with a single *Salmonella* serotype—*Salmonella* Marina, which was first isolated in 1964 from a marine iguana—were explored.

TABLE.—Recommendations for Preventing Transmission of *Salmonella* From Reptiles to Humans

Reptile owners should always wash their hands after handling reptiles and reptile cages

Persons at increased risk for infection or serious complications of salmonellosis, eg, children <5 years of age and immunocompromised persons, should avoid contact with reptiles

Reptiles should be kept out of households in which children <1 year of age and persons with weak immune systems live. Families expecting a new child should give away their pet reptiles before the infant arrives

Reptiles should not be kept in child-care centers

Reptiles should not be allowed to roam freely throughout the house

Reptiles should be kept out of kitchens and other food-preparation areas to prevent contamination. Kitchen sinks should not be used to bathe reptiles or to wash their dishes, cages, or aquariums. If bathtubs are used for these purposes, they should be thoroughly cleaned afterwards.

(Reproduced by permission of Pediatrics, from Mermin J, Hoar B, Angulo FJ: Iguanas and *Salmonella*. Marina infection in children: A reflection of the increasing incidence of reptile-associated salmonellosis in the United States. *Pediatrics* 99:399–402, copyright 1997.)

Methods.—All isolates of *S.* Marina reported in 1994 to the National *Salmonella* Surveillance System as of February 1995 were identified. Attempts were made to contact all patients by telephone and to have these patients or an adult member of the household complete a questionnaire. Items included in the survey were demographic data, clinical course, diet, travel history, and contact with reptiles during the week before illness onset.

Results.—The number of reported isolates of *S.* Marina rose from 1 in 1989 to 67 in 1995, an increase that paralleled changes in iguana importation. Interviews were completed with 32 patients infected with *S.* Marina. Twenty-six of 32 isolates were from infants younger than 1 year; ages of the remaining 6 patients were 13 months, 14 months, and 9, 12, 15, and 91 years. Twenty-four patients (75%) were male. Diarrhea was present in 97% and bloody diarrhea in 59%. Eleven patients were hospitalized for a median of 3.5 days. One patient, a 91-year-old woman, died of a myocardial infarction that occurred at the same time as the infection. No patient had traveled away from home in the 7 days before onset of illness. In 28 cases (88%), exposure to an iguana had occurred during the week before the illness; only 4 of these patients, however, reported touching the iguana. More than half of the respondents did not recognize the iguana as the source of infection and approximately one third of the families continued to keep the animal as a pet. Bacteremia occurred in 4 cases and was associated with antibiotic use during the 30 days before *S.* Marina infection.

Conclusion.—Many parents are unaware of the risk of reptile-associated salmonellosis. Because *S.* Marina infection is a potentially serious illness, pediatricians, veterinarians, and pet store owners should advise patients and customers of the risk and of preventive measures (Table).

▶ The banning of baby pet turtles in the 1970s was remarkably effective in reducing the number of cases of salmonellosis in children. The new association is with another reptile, iguanas. The train of infection appears to be clear. *Salmonella* can be normal flora in reptiles and handling by young children results in the organisms being transmitted. See the table for recommendations for preventing transmission of *Salmonella* from reptiles to humans.

G.L. Mandell, M.D.

An Outbreak of Gastroenteritis and Fever Due to *Listeria Monocytogenes* in Milk
Dalton CB, Austin CC, Sobel J, et al (Ctrs for Disease Control and Prevention, Atlanta, GA; Illinois Dept of Public Health, Springfield; Bureau of Public Health, Wisconsin, Madison)
N Engl J Med 336:100–105, 1997   7–4

Background.—In 1994, an outbreak of gastroenteritis and fever occurred among attendees of a picnic in Illinois. Complaints about the taste of commercial pasteurized milk served at the picnic prompted investigations that resulted in the culture of *Listeria monocytogenes* in milk samples.

Methods.—Picnic attendees were interviewed, and surveillance for invasive listeriosis was implemented in the states receiving milk from the dairy implicated. Stool, milk, and serum samples were analyzed.

Findings.—The symptoms of 45 individuals met the case definition for illness from *L. monocytogenes*. Stool cultures from 11 individuals were found to contain the organism. Illness occurring in the week after the picnic was associated with chocolate milk intake. Diarrhea and fever were the most common symptoms. Four patients were admitted to the hospital. The median infection incubation period was 20 hours. Levels of antibody to listeriolysin O were increased in individuals who became ill. Isolates from stool specimens from patients who became ill after the picnic, from sterile sites in another 3 patients found by surveillance, from the milk samples, and from a tank drain at the dairy were all serotype 1/2b. These isolates were indistinguishable on multilocus enzyme electrophoresis, ribotyping, and DNA macrorestriction analysis.

Conclusions.—*L. monocytogenes* can cause gastroenteritis with fever. Sporadic cases of invasive listeriosis may be related to unrecognized outbreaks caused by contaminated food.

▶ We take the food chain for granted until we are faced with an outbreak such as that described here. Consider the logistics in collecting milk and transporting it, and it is not surprising that every once in a while things break down. *Listeria monocytogenes* waits for that opportunity, and a number of outbreaks have been associated with milk, ice cream, and other dairy products. In addition to the gastroenteritis described here, *Listeria* species may cause bacteremia, meningitis, and a characteristic rhombencephalitis. Pregnant women in the third trimester and neonates are especially susceptible to infection with *Listeria* species.

G.L. Mandell, M.D.

8 Chlamydia Pneumoniae and Cardiovascular Disease

Introduction

We must watch this development with some skepticism but also with excitement. The atherosclerosis scientific community is convinced that atherosclerosis is, at least in part, an inflammatory disease. It is my working hypothesis that several microbes, *Chlamydia pneumonia,* cytomegalovirus or herpes simplex virus for example, may initiate or aggravate the inflammation which results in disease in susceptible hosts.

Gerald L. Mandell, M.D.

Specificity of Detection of *Chlamydia Pneumoniae* in Cardiovascular Atheroma: Evaluation of the Innocent Bystander Hypothesis
Jackson LA, Campbell LA, Schmidt RA, et al (Univ of Washington, Seattle)
Am J Pathol 150:1785–1790, 1997   8–1

Background.—*Chlamydia pneumonia* in atherosclerotic plaque has been reported, suggesting that detection of this organism is specific to atheromatous tissue. This possibility was further investigated.

Methods.—Cardiovascular and noncardiovascular tissue samples obtained from 38 persons at autopsy were examined by polymerase chain reaction and immunocytochemistry. Thirty-three granuloma biopsy specimens were also tested.

Findings.—*Chlamydia pneumoniae* was detected in 34% of coronary artery tissue samples, in 13% from lung, in 10% from liver, and in 5% from spleen. Twenty-one cases had at least 1 positive tissue sample. Of these, 11 had only a positive cardiovascular tissue, 7 had both cardiovas-

TABLE 1.—Detection of *Chlamydia pneumoniae* by Polymerase Chain Reaction and Immunocytochemistry in Tissues Obtained From 38 Autopsy Cases

Tissue	Number of cases with tissue available for testing	Number (%) positive by PCR	Number (%) positive by ICC	Number (%) positive by ICC and/or PCR
Cardiovascular				
Coronary artery	38	6 (16)	8 (21)	13* (34)
Venous bypass graft	2	0	1 (50)	1 (50)
Myocardium	17	3 (18)	2 (12)	5 (29)
Lung	38	3 (8)	2 (5)	5 (13)
Liver	38	0	4 (10)	4 (10)
Spleen	38	0	2 (5)	2 (5)
Bone marrow	20	2 (10)	0	2 (10)
Lymph node	12	0	1 (8)	1 (8)

*One sample positive by both polymerase chain reaction (PCR) and immunocytochemistry (ICC).
(Courtesy of Jackson LA, Campbell LA, Schmidt RA, et al: Specificity of detection of *chlamydia pneumoniae* in cardiovascular atheroma: Evaluation of the innocent bystander hypothesis. *Am J Pathol* 150:1785–1790, copyright 1997 by the American Society for Investigative Pathology.)

cular- and noncardiovascular-positive tissues, and 3 had only a noncardiovascular positive tissue (Table 1).

Conclusion.—*Chlamydia pneumoniae* was detected relatively infrequently in noncardiovascular tissues. Its detection in such tissues was usually associated with its detection in cardiovascular tissue from the same patient. *Chlamydia pneumoniae* was also found infrequently in granulomatous tissue. The data, thus, support the hypothesis that *C. pneumoniae* plays a role in the pathogenesis of atherosclerosis.

▶ Evidence mounts solidifying the association of infection with *C. pneumoniae* and atherosclerotic cardiovascular disease. The association is strong but causality is still conjectural. The table shows that when infection is identified, it is most commonly a cardiovascular infection. Note that 34% of the 38 coronary artery tissue specimens tested positive for the organism in this Seattle study.

G.L. Mandell, M.D.

Chlamydia Pneumoniae **Antibodies and Serum Lipids in Finnish Men: Cross Sectional Study**
Laurila A, Bloigu A, Näyhä S, et al (Natl Public Health Inst, Oulu, Finland; Regional Inst of Occupational Health, Oulu, Finland)
BMJ 314:1456–1457, 1997   8–2

Background.—*Chlamydia pneumoniae* infection has been associated with atherosclerosis and has recently been found in atherosclerotic lesions. Acute infections are known to interfere with lipid metabolism. The effect of *C. pneumoniae* infection on serum lipid concentrations was investigated.

Methods and Findings.—A total of 1,053 men, aged 20 to 87 years, participating in a Finnish reindeer herders' health survey between 1986 and 1989 were studied. Thirty-two percent were current smokers. Smokers had significantly greater antibody prevalence and age-adjusted geometric mean antibody titers compared with nonsmokers. Eighty-three percent of smokers and 77% of nonsmokers had IgG antibodies. In nonsmokers, triglyceride levels increased and high-density lipoprotein cholesterol–to–total cholesterol ratios declined significantly according to IgG antibody titers. These values were comparable in the smokers. Men who were positive for IgG had significantly greater triglyceride concentrations and lower high-density lipoprotein cholesterol–to–total cholesterol ratios. The association between IgA antibodies and lipid concentrations was minor.

Conclusion.—The specific IgG antibodies noted in this study suggest that these men had been infected by *C. pneumoniae* or had a persistent *C. pneumoniae* infection. Thus, the changes in serum lipid values may reflect disturbances in liquid metabolism caused by infection.

▶ Here is a different and confusing slant on the *C. pneumoniae*–coronary artery disease story. Smokers have a "worse" lipid profile as compared with nonsmokers. Among the nonsmokers, those infected with *C. pneumoniae* have a lipid profile that resembles that of smokers; i.e., it presumably puts the patients at higher risk for cardiovascular disease. It is logical to assume that infection of cells in atherosclerotic lesions leads to local inflammatory changes resulting in deposition of cholesterol. It is harder to imagine, as the authors postulate, that this very localized infection leads to production of systemic cytokines that alter the lipid profile.

G.L. Mandell, M.D.

9 Biologic Terrorism and Warfare

Introduction

In addition to utilizing this information in instances of known terrorist activities physicians should remember that unusual clusters of disease may have been induced with evil intent.

Gerald L. Mandell, M.D.

Clinical Recognition and Management of Patients Exposed to Biological Warfare Agents
Franz DR, Jahrling PE, Friedlander AM, et al (US Army Med Research Inst of Infectious Disease, Fort Detrick, Md; Walter Reed Army Inst of Research, Washington, DC)
JAMA 278:399–411, 1997   9–1

Purpose.—This article reviews and summarizes information on 10 important biological warfare (BW) agents (Table 1) to increase the ability of physicians to recognize these agents and consider them during differential diagnosis.

Anthrax.—Aerosol delivery of anthrax spores as BW agents would result in inhalational anthrax, which leads to necrotizing hemorrhagic mediastinitis. The prodrome features fever, malaise, and fatigue. There may be a brief symptomatic improvement, or the disease may progress directly to an abrupt onset of severe respiratory distress with dyspnea, stridor, diaphoresis, and cyanosis. Bacteremia, septic shock, metastatic infection, and death follow within 36 hours. Once the symptoms appear, treatment is usually ineffective. Physical findings are usually nonspecific, but an immunoassay to detect the toxin is available. Treatment should be initiated with IV ciprofloxacin as soon as possible. A licensed vaccine is available for prophylaxis.

Brucellosis.—Brucellosis usually manifests itself with fever, chills, and malaise. Respiratory symptoms are common. Endocarditis and CNS infections are rare but account for most of the fatalities. Symptoms can last for months, and relapses are common. Symptoms and signs are nonspecific. A serum tube agglutination test is the standard method for diagnosis. Patients should be treated with antibiotic combinations. There is no approved human vaccine.

Plague.—Pneumonic plague would be the most likely BW presentation. Patients would develop pneumonia plus malaise, fever, chills, headache, myalgia, cough with a bloody sputum, and sepsis. Pneumonic plague progresses rapidly, with dyspnea, stridor, and cyanosis. Respiratory failure, shock, and ecchymoses may precede death. A presumptive diagnosis can be based on safety-pin bipolar staining and the identification of a gram-negative coccobacillus. Immunofluorescent staining for the capsule is diagnostic. The F1 capsule also can be detected by immunoassay. A four-fold rise in antibody titer is also diagnostic. Streptomycin sulfate, tetracycline, chloramphenicol, and gentamicin sulfate are effective therapies, but only if treatment is initiated within 24 hours of symptom onset. A licensed vaccine is available.

Q Fever.—The onset of Q fever may be abrupt or insidious, with fever, chills, and headache. Diaphoresis, malaise, fatigue, anorexia, and myalgia are also common symptoms. Temperature tends to fluctuate. Neurologic symptoms are not uncommon. Liver function tests may be abnormal. Case fatality is low, but malaise may persist for months. Serologic testing is necessary for diagnosis. Tetracyclines are standard therapy, and macrolide antibiotics also are effective.

Tularemia.—Typhoidal tularemia manifests with fever, prostration, and weight loss. Untreated disease has a 35% fatality rate. The signs and symptoms of this disease are nonspecific, and it is difficult to culture. Serologic testing can be used to establish a retrospective diagnosis. Streptomycin is the preferred treatment, but gentamicin also is effective. Laboratory-related infections are common. A vaccine is available as an Investigational New Drug (IND).

Smallpox.—Variola infection leads to viremia and a rash, with malaise, fever, rigors, vomiting, headache, and backache. Delirium is not uncommon. The rash spreads with the most abundant lesions on the extremities and face. Lesions are generally synchronous. The pustules form scabs that leave depressed, depigmented scars. Patients should be considered infec-

---

*Information on diagnostics, medical management, and vaccines is available by contacting Commander, USAMRIID, at 301-619-2833 (phone) or 301-619-4625 (fax). Readers are advised to consult product literature before administering drugs or vaccines.

BSL, biosafety level; *Rx*, chemotherapy; *Px*, chemoprophylaxis; *Ag*, antigen; *ELISA*, enzyme-linked immunosorbent assay; *IV*, intravenously; *q*, every; *IM*, intramuscular; *qd*, each day; *bid*, twice a day; *PO*, by mouth; *IFA*, immunofluorescent assay; *IND*, investigational new drug; *SC*, subcutaneous; *EM*, electron microscopy; *PCR*, polymerase chain reaction; *VIG*, vaccinia immune globin; *DOD*, Department of Defense; *VEE*, Venezuelan equine encephalitis; *EEE*, eastern equine encephalitis; *WEE*, western equine encephalitis; *NA*, not available; *RVF*, Rift Valley Fever; *KHF*, Korean hemorrhagic fever; *YF*, yellow fever; *RT-PCR*, reverse transcriptase polymerase chain reaction; *Ab*, antibody; *CCHF*, Congo-Crimean hemorrhagic fever; *AHF*, Argentine hemorrhagic fever; *BHF*, Bolivian hemorrhagic fever; *CDC*, Centers for Disease Control and Prevention.

(Courtesy of Franz DR, Jahrling PE, Friedlander AM, et al: Clinical Recognition and Management of Patients Exposed to Biological Warfare Agents *JAMA* 278:399–411, copyright 1997, American Medical Association.)

(Continued)

TABLE 1.—Summary of Biological Warfare Agents*

Agent	Infective Dose (Aerosol)	Incubation Period	Diagnostic Samples (BSL)*	Diagnostic Assay
Anthrax	8000 to 50 000 spores	1–5 d	Blood (BSL-2)	Gram stain Ag-ELISA, Serology: ELISA
Brucellosis	10–100 organisms	5–60 d (occasionally months)	Blood, bone marrow, acute and convalescent sera (BSL-3)	Serology: agglutination Culture
Plague	100–500 organisms	2–3 d	Blood, sputum, lymph node aspirate (BSL-2/3)	Gram or Wright-Giemsa Stain Ag-ELISA, Culture, Serology: ELISA, IFA
Q fever	1–10 organisms	10–40 d	Serum (BSL-2/3)	Serology: ELISA, IFA
Tularemia	10–50 organisms	2–10 d	Blood, sputum, serum EM of tissue (BSL-2/3)	Culture Serology: agglutination
Smallpox	Assumed low (10–100 organisms)	7–17 d	Pharyngeal swab, scab material (BSL-4)	ELISA, PCR, virus isolation
Viral encephalitides	10–100 organisms	VEE, 2–6 d EEE/WEE, 7–14 d	Serum VEE (BSL-3) EEE (BSL-2) WEE (BSL-2)	Viral isolation Serology: ELISA or hemogglutination inhibition
Viral hemorrhagic fevers	1–10 organisms	4–21 d	Serum, blood Most viral hemorrhagic fevers (BSL-4) RVF, KHF, and YF (BSL-3)	Viral isolation Ag-ELISA RT-PCR Serology: Ab-ELISA
Botullnum	0.001 µg/kg (type A)	1–5 d	Nasal swab (possibly) (BSL-2)	Ag-ELISA, Mouse neutral
Staphylococcal enterotoxin B	30 ng/person (incapacitating); 1.7 µg/person (lethal)	1–6 h	Nasal swab, serum, urine (BSL-2)	Ag-ELISA Serology: Ab-ELISA

(Continued)

TABLE 1.—Summary of Biological Warfare Agents*

Agent	Patient Isolation Precautions	Chemotherapy (Rx)
Anthrax	Standard precautions	Ciprofloxacin 400 mg IV q 8–12 h Doxycycline 200 mg IV, then 100 mg IV q 8–12 h Penicillin 2 million units IV q 2 h plus streptomycin 30 mg/kg IM qd (or gentamicin)
Brucellosis	Standard precautions Contact isolation if draining lesions present	Doxycycline 200 mg/d PO plus rifampin 600–900 mg/d PO×6 wk
Plague	Pneumonic: droplet precautions until patient treated for 3 d	Streptomycin 30 mg/kg IM qd in 2 divided doses ×10 d (or gentamicin) Doxycycline 200 mg IV then 100 mg IV q 12 h×10–14 d Chloramphenicol 1 g IV q 6 h×10–14 d
Q fever	Standard precautions	Tetraacycline 500 mg PO q 6 h×5–7 d Doxycycline 100 mg PO q 12 h×5–7 d
Tularemia	Standard precautions	Streptomycin 30 mg/kg IM qd ×10–14 d Gentamicin 3–5 mg/kg/d ×10–14 d
Smallpox	Airborne precautions	Cidofovir (effective in vitro)
Viral encephalitides	Standard precautions (mosquito control)	Supportive therapy analgesics anticonvulsants as needed
Viral hemorrhagic fevers	Contact precautions Consider additional precautions if massive hemorrhage	Supportive therapy Ribavirin (CCHF/arenaviruses) 30 mg/kg IV initial dose 15 mg/kg IV q 6 h×4 d 7.5 mg/kg IV q 8 h×6 d Antibody passive for AHF, BHF, Lassa fever, and CCHF
Botullnum	Standard precautions	DOD heptavalent antitoxin for (Serotypes A-G) (IND): equine despeciated 1 vial (10 mL) IV CDC Trivalent equine antitoxin for Serotypes A, B, E (licensed)
Staphylococcal enterotoxin B	Standard precautions	Ventilatory support and supportive care

(Continued)

TABLE 1.—Summary of Biological Warfare Agents*

Chemoprophylaxis (Px)	Vaccine Availability	Comments
Ciprofloxacin 500 mg PO bid×4 wk if unvaccinated, begin initial doses of vaccine Doxycycline 100 mg PO bid×4 wk plus vaccination	Michigan Biological Products Institute vaccine (licensed): 0.5 mL SC at 0, 2, 4 wk and 6, 12, 18 mo, then annual boosters	Vaccine: boost at-risk annually Alternates for Rx: gentamicin, erythromycin, and chloramphenicol
Doxycycline and rifampin for 3 wk in inadvertently inoculated persons	No vaccine available for human use	Trimethoprim-sulfamethoxazole may be substituted for rifampin; however, relapse rate with this drug may be up to 30%
Tetracycline 500 mg PO qid×7 d Doxycycline 100 mg PO q 12 h×7 d	Greer inactivated vaccine (licensed): 1.0 mL, then 0.2 mL boost at 1–3 and 3–6 mo	Boost at-risk 12, 18 mo & yearly. Plague vaccine not protective against aerosol in animal studies Alternate Rx: chloramphenicol or trimethoprim-sulfamethoxazole Rx: chloramphenicol for plague meningitis
Tetracycline start 8–12 d postexposure ×5 d Doxycycline start 8–12 d postexposure ×5 d	IND 610-inactivated whole cell vaccine given as single 0.5 mL SC	Recommend skin test before vaccination
Doxycycline 100 mg PO q 12 h×14 d Tetracycline 2 g/d PO×14 d	Live attenuated vaccine (IND): scarification	Culture difficult and potentially dangerous
Vaccinia immune globulin 0.6 mL/kg IM (within 3 d of exposure); best within 24 h	Wyeth calf lymph vaccinia vaccine (licensed) DOD cell-culture derived vaccinia vaccine (IND): scarification	Preexposure and postexposure vaccination recommended if >3 y since last vaccination
NA	VEE DOD TC-83 live attenuated vaccine (IND): 0.5 mL SC×1 dose VEE DOD C-84 (formalin inactivated TC-83)(IND): 0.5 mL SC for up to 3 doses EEE inactivated (IND): 0.5 mL SC at 0 & 28 d WEE inactivated (IND): 0.5 mL SC at 0, 7, and 28 d	TC-83 reactogenic in 20% No seroconversion in 20% Only effective against subtypes 1A, 1B, and 1C Vaccine used for nonresponders to TC-83 EEE and WEE inactivated vaccines are poorly immunogenic, and multiple immunizations are required
NA	AHF Candid #1 vaccine (x-protection for BHF)(IND) RVF inactivated vaccine (IND)	Aggressive management of secondary infections and hypotension is important
NA	DOD pentavalent Toxoid for serotypes A–E (IND): SC at 0, 2, & 12 wk, then yearly boosters	Skin testing for hypersensitivity before equine antitoxin administration Ventilatory assistance
NA	No vaccine available	Vomiting and diarrhea may occur if toxin is swallowed

tious until all scabs separate. As smallpox has been eradicated, heightened awareness will be necessary for diagnosis. Any confirmed case of smallpox should be considered an international emergency. Strict quarantine for 17 days should be imposed on all contacts. Vaccine is available and may even be protective after exposure.

Viral Encephalitides.—The majority of these infections manifest with fever, headache and myalgia and can include confusion, obtundation, dysphasia, seizure, paresis, ataxia, myoclonus or palsy. Diagnosis is through virus isolation or serologic testing. There is no specific therapy. Vaccines are available but are reactogenic.

Viral Hemorrhagic Fevers.—VHF usually presents with fever, myalgia, and prostration, which can evolve to shock and mucous membrane hemorrhage. Diagnosis requires identification of the virus. Ribavirin and antibody therapy are useful for the treatment of VHF.

Botulinum Toxins.—These are the most toxic compounds that have been identified. Early symptoms include palsies and paralysis. Progression to respiratory failure, the usual cause of death, can occur within 24 hours. Diagnosis would depend on the occurrence of an epidemic of cases of paralysis in afebrile patients. Laboratory tests are of limited value. An antitoxin is available from the CDC.

Staphylococcal Enterotoxin B.—Inhaled SEB can induce septic shock. Use of SEB in BW would present as an epidemic of respiratory illness over a short period. Laboratory tests are of limited value. Serologic testing may be useful in retrospective diagnosis. Therapy is limited to supportive care.

Conclusions.—Health care professionals need to be aware of the threat of biological warfare and have an an understanding of the types of agents that can be used as weapons. Through heightened awareness, a BW agent can be identified early, and action can be taken to save lives.

▶ Biological warfare and terrorism have been called "the poor man's nuclear weapon." Some of these biological agents have been used as weapons in the past, and some will certainly be used in the future. It is distressingly easy for terrorists to produce and distribute these agents, and therefore physicians must be aware of the possibility that a cluster of illness is related to evil deeds. Accordingly, I have asked the publisher to reprint Table 1 which lists the 10 microbes or toxins likely to be deployed against civilian populations in its entirety. Innovative and potentially effective detection and defense strategies are being formulated for the future. For now, we must depend on classic strategies of epidemiology, diagnosis, treatment, and prevention.

G.L. Mandell, M.D.

HEMATOLOGY AND ONCOLOGY

MARTIN J. CLINE, M.D.

Introduction

This year marks both the 20th anniversary of my association with the YEAR BOOK OF MEDICINE and my farewell to this venerable publication. "Tho' age cannot wither," etc., my joints tell me it is time to take down my shingle and turn from diseases of man to those of the rose garden. My consolations are two: First, I no longer have to witness the struggles to survive of an academic institution in today's medical market place, and second, the treatment of powdery mildew is considerably easier than the administration of MACOP-B chemotherapy.

As I leave, I cannot resist the temptation to review the changes in my field of medicine over two decades and to contrast the contents of the 1978 YEAR BOOK with those of the 1998 edition.

Twenty years ago, the literature provided our first insights that idiopathic aplastic anemia might be mediated by immunological mechanisms, and I reviewed an article on recovery of hematologic function after treatment with chemotherapy. I sagely observed that "all the facts are not in (about pathogenesis)". Although some of the facts are still outside and wandering about, today we think that many cases respond to anti-lymphocyte or anti-thymocyte globulin or to the immunosuppressive effects of bone marrow transplantation because immunological mechanisms are critical in marrow suppression. Parenthetically, in 1978 I also reviewed two of the early articles on allogeneic bone marrow transplantation in aplastic anemia; one from Seattle and one from UCLA. This, of course, is now the standard therapy for cases of aplastic anemia under the age of 50 years and with a matched donor. I also included the first large series of patients (one hundred cases) with acute leukemia treated by bone marrow transplantation. Now, of course, tens of thousands of patients have been so treated.

Twenty years ago I also spent a great deal of time on the management of polycythemia vera and various disorders of iron metabolism. These days the management of these disorders is so well defined that they rarely merit comment in the YBOM. On the other hand, in 1978 I talked about splenectomy in chronic lymphocytic leukemia, endomyocardiopathy in eosinophilia and the best therapy for aggressive lymphoma, and in 1998 I am still talking about these topics. Some things never change—or, at least, they change very slowly.

The intriguing thing to me is that in 1978 we could not have conceived of discussing (as we do in 1998) the molecular basis of paroxysmal nocturnal hemoglobinuria, the gene defect in familial colon cancer and the potential treatment of hemophilia by gene therapy. Some things do change—and change very rapidly.

I am certain that you will enjoy Neal Young, M.D., the new editor of the hematology/oncology Section of the YEAR BOOK OF MEDICINE. He is imaginative, articulate, and well informed. Good luck to all of you.

Martin J. Cline, M.D.

10 Red Cells, White Cells, and Hemostasis

Primary Treatment of Acquired Aplastic Anemia: Outcomes With Bone Marrow Transplantation and Immunosuppressive Therapy
Doney K, Leisenring W, Storb R, et al, for the Seattle Bone Marrow Transplant Team (Univ of Washington, Seattle; Seattle VA Med Ctr)
Ann Intern Med 126:107–115, 1997   10–1

Background.—In the last 25 years, bone marrow transplantation has become established as treatment for aplastic anemia. Bone marrow transplantation is the preferred treatment for individuals with severe aplasia and genotypically or phenotypically HLA-identical, related donors. Bone marrow transplantation is not always an option for patients older than 50 years because of the morbidity and mortality associated with older age. For these patients, immunosuppressive therapy is often the recommended treatment.

Methods.—The medical records of 395 patients with aplastic anemia treated with bone marrow transplantation from an HLA-identical related donor or immunosuppressive therapy were reviewed. Survival rates, complications, and predictive factors of survival were analyzed.

Results.—Of 168 patients who underwent bone marrow transplantation, sustained engraftment was seen in 89%. Grade II to IV acute graft-versus-host disease developed in 46 patients. Of 227 patients given immunosuppressive therapy, a complete, partial, or minimal response was seen in 44%; 54% had no response or died. At 15 years, survival was 69% in patients who underwent bone marrow transplantation and 38% in patients given immunosuppressive therapy. Factors associated with improved survival were bone marrow transplantation as primary therapy, younger age, no transfusion before transplantation, and a higher absolute neutrophil count. Survival was not significantly affected by length of disease, year of treatment, sex of patient, lack of response to platelet transfusions, or previous treatment with androgens or corticosteroids.

Conclusions.—Bone marrow transplantation is associated with significantly improved survival in patients with severe aplastic anemia aged 40 years or younger and who have an HLA-identical, related donor compared with survival after immunosuppressive therapy. Survival rates are similar after these treatments in patients older than 40 years.

▶ The alternative therapies for aplastic anemia are allogeneic bone marrow transplantation and immunosuppressive treatment. Several factors influence the choice of therapy: the age of the patient, the history of transfusions up to the time of treatment, and the availability of an HLA-matched bone marrow donor. The authors of this study compared the results of the two modalities of therapy in a population of nearly 400 patients with aplastic anemia. There were few surprises, but the results are worth noting. Actuarial survival at 15 years was 69% for bone marrow transplantation and 38% for patients given immunosuppressive treatment. Note, however, that there may have been a bias in the selection of patients for immunosuppressive treatment in that such patients may be older, may have a history of more transfusions, or may be in physical shape too poor to permit transplant. In the bone marrow transplantation group, 89% had sustained engraftment, but a substantial number—nearly 40%—had chronic graft-vs-host disease. In contrast, only 44% of patients with immunosuppressive treatment had a complete, partial, or minimal response.

It was believed that allogeneic bone marrow transplantation, when feasible and available, was best therapy for aplastic anemia. Apparently it is.

M.J. Cline, M.D.

Resistance to Apoptosis Caused by *PIG-A* gene Mutations in Paroxysmal Nocturnal Hemoglobinuria
Brodsky RA, Vala MS, Barber JP, et al (Johns Hopkins Med Institutions, Baltimore, Md; Case Western Reserve Univ, Cleveland, Ohio)
Proc Natl Acad Sci U S A 94:8756–8760, 1997   10–2

Background.—Paroxysmal nocturnal hemoglobinuria (PNH) is a clonal hematopoietic stem cell disorder that results from mutations in an X-linked gene, *PIG-A*. This gene encodes for an enzyme needed for the first step in the biosynthesis of glycosylphosphatidylinositol (GPI) anchors. Mutations in *PIG-A* result in absent or reduced cell surface expression of all GPI-anchored proteins. Although many of the clinical manifestations of PNH can be explained by a deficiency of GPI-anchored complement regulatory proteins, such as CD59 or CD55, it is not clear why the PNH clone dominates hematopoiesis and why it tends to evolve into acute leukemia.

Methods and Findings.—The possibility that *PIG-A* mutations contribute to clonal expansion by inducing cellular resistance to apoptosis was studied. *PIG-A* mutations were found to confer a survival advantage by making cells relatively resistant to apoptotic death. Granulocytes and affected CD34+ (CD59⁻) cells from PNH patients were placed in serum-free medium and were found to survive longer than their normal counterparts. In addition, PNH cells were relatively resistant to apoptosis induced by ionizing irradiation. Replacing the normal *PIG-A* gene in PNH cell lines reversed cellular resistance to apoptosis.

Conclusion.—The main mechanism by which PNH cells maintain a growth advantage over normal progenitors appears to be inhibited apoptosis resulting from *PIG-A* mutations. This may play a role in the propensity of PNH to transform into more aggressive hematologic disorders. Also, GPI anchors seem important in regulating apoptosis.

▶ Paroxysmal nocturnal hemoglobinuria is a disorder with an acquired defect in the red cell membrane that increases the sensitivity of the cell to complement-mediated lysis. The clinical consequence is a hemolytic anemia of an intermittent or "paroxysmal" nature. Dark urine, as a consequence of nocturnal hemolysis, is sometimes seen. This phenomenon, which gives its name to the disorder, is thought to be the result of a slight nocturnal fall in blood pH with secondary complement activation.

The anemia is usually intermittent in nature but may be continuous. It may be complicated by the development of iron deficiency, as iron is lost in the urine as hemosiderin. Thrombosis is a major complication of PNH. Venous thrombi may occur anywhere in the body, and bowel infarction or occlusion of hepatic veins may be fatal. The mechanism of the thrombotic tendency is not known but is probably linked to the abnormal platelet surface.

The basic defect in PNH arises in a multipotent stem cell, as abnormalities are seen in leukocytes and platelets as well as red cells. The cause was identified in 1994 as an abnormality of the so-called PIG-A gene. The defect results in incomplete synthesis of GPI which serves as an "anchor" that attaches certain proteins to the red cell membrane. Associated with this is deficient anchoring of a protein called decay-accelerating factor (DAF). Decay-accelerating factor functions to accelerate the inactivation of C3b, a key intermediate in the complement activation cascade. A deficiency of DAF results in the accumulation of C3b on the surface of the PNH red cell. This leads to further activation of the cascade and accumulation of the "membrane attack complex" of C5b,6,7,8, and 9. When sufficient attack complex is accumulated, it bores holes in the cell membrane and the cell lyses.

The defective stem cell that gives rise to the complement-sensitive red cells is monoclonal. It may exist side by side with normal erythropoietic stem cells so that the red cells in the peripheral blood consist of a mixed population of normal and abnormal. There may even be several monoclonal populations differing in complement sensitivity and derived from different abnormal stem cells. It has never been understood as to why the abnormal PNH cells should have a growth advantage over normal hematopoietic cells and become the dominant population in the marrow. This study suggests that the mechanism is based on the fact that the mutation interferes with programmed cell death (apoptosis), so that the PNH population continues to expand.

M.J. Cline, M.D.

High-dose Intravenous Immune Globulin and the Response to Splenectomy in Patients With Idiopathic Thrombocytopenic Purpura

Law C, Marcaccio M, Tam P, et al (McMaster Univ, Hamilton, Ont, Canada)
N Engl J Med 336:1494–1498, 1997   10–3

Objective.—For patients with idiopathic thrombocytopenic purpura, treatment with high-dose IV immune globulin causes a temporary increase in platelet count, perhaps through blockade of macrophage Fc receptors in the spleen and elsewhere. Splenectomy is sometimes effective as well, though it has not been possible to predict which patients will respond to splenectomy. Response to IV immune globulin therapy was assessed as an indicator of response to splenectomy in patients with idiopathic thrombocytopenic purpura.

Methods.—The retrospective study included 30 patients with idiopathic thrombocytopenia who had undergone first treatment with IV immune globulin and then splenectomy. The patients' responses to the 2 treatments were compared. Responses were assessed in terms of platelet count: less than 50,000/mm^3, poor response; 50,000 to 150,000 mm^3, good response; and greater than 150,000/mm^3, excellent response.

Results.—Nine patients had a poor response to IV immune globulin. One year postoperatively, these patients all had a poor response to splenectomy as well. The remaining 21 patients all had a good or excellent response to IV immune globulin. All but 2 of this group also had a good or excellent response to splenectomy. As a predictor of response to splenectomy, response to IV immune globulin had a sensitivity of 100%, specificity of 82%, and positive and negative predictive value of 91% and 100%, respectively.

Conclusions.—In patients with idiopathic thrombocytopenic purpura, the response to IV immune globulin is a sensitive and specific predictor of response to splenectomy. For patients with a good or excellent response to IV immune globulin, early splenectomy may be considered as an alternative to prolonged steroid therapy. This prognostic indicator may also be helpful in groups in whom splenectomy is frequently deferred, such as young and elderly patients.

▶ Idiopathic thrombocytopenic purpura [ITP] is a disorder in which antibody binding to platelets results in shortening of their survival in the blood, with consequent thrombocytopenia and bleeding. In small children, ITP is usually acute and self-limited and often results from antibody to a viral antigen which reacts with the platelet. In adults, ITP is more often chronic and the origin of the antiplatelet antibody is unknown.

Clinically, the disease may be seen as a petechial rash, easy bruising or bleeding without other systemic symptoms. In some cases, bleeding is severe and intracranial hemorrhage is feared. There is no palpable splenomegaly or lymphadenopathy and no history of administration of a drug associated with thrombocytopenia. The blood smear is normal, except for the lack of platelets and the bone marrow contains abundant megakaryocytes, many of them young. The diagnosis of ITP is based on the typical clinical and hematologic picture and the exclusion of other known causes of thrombocytopenia.

Platelet transfusions are generally ineffective in ITP because of their short half-life in the circulation. The available treatments include corticosteroids, splenectomy, IV IgG preparation, immunosuppressives, vincristine and danazole. Corticosteroids decrease binding of antibody and interfere with phagocytosis of platelets by mononuclear phagocytes. They are effective in about one half of cases.

When corticosteroids fail or when the platelet count falls as they are being tapered, splenectomy is often considered. Splenectomy removes the principal organ in which antibody-coated platelets are trapped. It works in about one half of cases, although about three quarters of cases have a good initial response.

Intravenous gamma globulin in large doses (400–500 mg/kg daily) often elevates the platelet count in ITP by blocking platelet ingestion by mononuclear phagocytes. Although it is frequently effective, the benefits are transient. Intravenous gamma globulin is particularly useful when rescuing a patient from a deteriorating situation or in preparing for a surgical procedure such as splenectomy. This article provides evidence that the response to IV gamma globulin is a good prognostic guide to the likelihood of response to splenectomy.

M.J. Cline, M.D.

Administration of Pegylated Recombinant Human Megakaryocyte Growth and Development Factor to Humans Stimulates the Production of Functional Platelets That Show no Evidence of In Vivo Activation
O'Malley CJ, Rasko JEJ, Basser RL, et al (Centre for Developmental Cancer Therapeutics, Melbourne, Victoria, Australia; Austin Repatriation Med Centre; Ludwig Inst for Cancer Research, Australia; et al)
Blood 88:3288–3298, 1996   10–4

Background.—The hematopoietic growth factor *mpl*-ligand, also known as megakaryocyte growth and development factor (MGDF), stimulates the production of Meg-CFC, increases the ploidy of human megakaryocytes, and generates functional platelets in vitro. The inverse correlation between endogenous thrombopoietin levels and the platelet mass found in several models of thrombocytopenia is further evidence of the importance of *mpl*-ligand in regulating platelets. The effect of pegylated recombinant human MGDF (PEG-rHuMGDF) on platelet production and platelet function in humans was investigated.

Methods and Findings.—Patients with advanced-stage solid tumors were given PEG-rHuMGDF daily for up to 10 days. Circulating platelet counts did not increase at doses of 0.03 or 0.1 µg/kg/day by day 12 of the study. However, doses of 0.3 and 1 µg/kg/day were associated with a three-fold median increase in platelet count by day 16. In in vitro assays, aggregation and adenosine triphosphate (ATP)-release responses were unchanged in the platelets produced in vivo in response to PEG-rHuMGDF. Aspirin given to a patient with a platelet count of $1,771 \times 10^9/L$ resulted in the typical aspirin-induced ablation of the normal aggregation and ATP-release response to stimulation with arachidonic acid, collagen, and adenosine diphosphate. The expression of the platelet-surface activation marker CD62P and induction of the fibrinogen-binding site on glycoprotein IIb/IIIa were unchanged. Increased reticulated platelets were noted after 3 days of treatment with PEG-rHuMGDF, preceding the increase in circulating platelet count by 5–8 days. This reflected the production of new platelets in response to PEG-rHuMGDF. Mean platelet volume subsequently declined in a manner inversely proportional to the platelet count. Plasma glycocalicin levels increased 3 days after the initial increase in the peripheral platelet count. Plasma glycocalicin levels were proportional to the total platelet mass, which suggests that platelets generated in response to PEG-rHuMGDF were not destroyed more actively (Fig 1).

Conclusions.—Administration of PEG-rHuMGDF to humans appears to increase the circulating platelet count, resulting in fully functional platelets. The platelets showed no detectable increase in reactivity or changes in activation status.

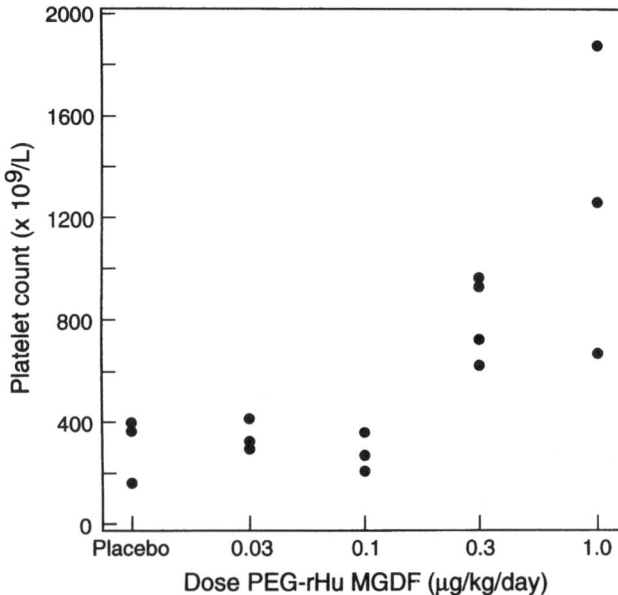

FIGURE 1.—Individuals were randomized to receive placebo or pegylated recombinant human megakaryocyte growth and development factor (PEG-rHuMGDF) (0.03, 0.1, 0.3, and 1.0 µg/kg/day) at a ratio of 1:3. The maximum platelet count ($\times 10^9/L$) for individual patients is shown for each patient cohort. (Courtesy of O'Malley CJ, Rasko JEJ, Basser RL, et al: Administration of pegylated recombinant human megakaryocyte growth and development factor to humans stimulates the production of functional platelets that show no evidence of in vivo activation. *Blood* 88:3288–3298, 1996.)

▶ We are beginning to see the first reports of clinical trials in man of thrombopoietin (also known as megakaryocyte growth factor). As this article demonstrates, cloned thrombopoietin works. It increases the platelet count and the platelets are fully functional. Not surprising, but very exciting. We shall soon see thrombopoietin in routine use.

M.J. Cline, M.D.

Stimulation of Megakaryocyte and Platelet Production by a Single Dose of Recombinant Human Thrombopoietin in Patients With Cancer
Vadhan-Raj S, Murray LJ, Bueso-Ramos C, et al (Univ of Texas, Houston; SyStemix Inc, San Francisco; Genentech Inc, South San Francisco; et al)
Ann Intern Med 126:673–681, 1997   10–5

Introduction.—Thrombocytopenia often develops in patients with cancer. This carries a risk of bleeding, which may lead to the need for platelet transfusion. There is a need for treatments to increase platelet production or to prevent or reduce the problem of thrombocytopenia. Recombinant human thrombopoietin, a recently cloned cytokine, was tested for use in the prevention and treatment of thrombocytopenia.

Methods.—The phase I and II clinical trial included 12 patients with sarcoma at high risk of severe chemotherapy-induced thrombocytopenia. Three weeks before starting chemotherapy, each patient received a single IV dose of thrombopoietin, 0.3 to 2.4 µg/kg. The hematopoietic response was assessed by study of peripheral blood and bone marrow samples taken before and after treatment. Clinical tolerance was evaluated as well.

Results.—Thrombopoietin treatment produced a dose-related increase in platelet count (from a mean of 61% to 213%). The rise in platelet count was apparent by day 4 and peaked at a median of day 12. Occurring along with the rise in platelet count was a prolongation of serum thrombopoietin half-life, from 20 to 30 hours. On evaluation, the platelets looked morphologically normal and had normal aggregation responses to agonists. Bone marrow megakaryocytes also increased by up to fourfold in dose-related fashion. The response was also marked by expansion of bone marrow progenitors of the myeloid, erythroid, multipotential, and megakaryocytic lineages, and by a sixfold to tenfold increase in mobilization of multiple cell lineage progenitors in the peripheral blood. There were no serious adverse events.

Conclusion.—A single IV dose of recombinant human thrombopoietin stimulates platelet production in humans. The response is sustained and is dose dependent. In addition to its lineage-dominant effect on peripheral blood counts, thrombopoietin has a multilineage effect on bone marrow progenitor cells and mobilizes progenitor cells of multiple lineages into the peripheral blood. This agent must be further studied for use in the prevention and treatment of thrombocytopenia.

▶ The authors note that the use of platelet transfusions doubled in the decade from 1982 to 1992, reflecting an increase in use for cardiac surgery, aggressive chemotherapy, and organ transplantation. Platelets are produced by fragmentation of the cytoplasm of mature megakaryocytes in the bone marrow. This process appears to be primarily under the control of the hormone thrombopoietin. Under certain conditions, the body can increase platelet production threefold to fivefold above normal.

It was anticipated that the cloning of thrombopoietin would lead to a clinically useful agent for the stimulation of platelet production in conditions of thrombocytopenia. Previous studies have shown that the platelets produced under stimulation of thrombopoietin are functionally intact. This study shows (remarkably) that a single IV dose of thrombopoietin is sufficient to increase megakaryocyte counts in the bone marrow by as much as fourfold and to augment platelet counts by 60% to 200% percent. The effect is enhanced by the long half-life of thrombopoietin. Clearly, we have an important new therapeutic agent.

M.J. Cline, M.D.

Activated Protein C Resistance Caused by Factor V Gene Mutation: Common Coagulation Defect in Chronic Venous Leg Ulcers?
Peus D, Heit JA, Pittelkow MR (Mayo Clinic, Rochester, Minn)
J Am Acad Dermatol 36:616–620, 1997   10–6

Introduction.—As many as one fourth of the patients with venous leg ulcers may have activated protein C resistance (APCR), which is most often caused by a point mutation of the factor V gene. Activated protein C resistance is now thought to be the major cause of venous thrombosis because it commonly occurs before deep venous insufficiency. Deep venous thrombosis is a major pathogenetic factor in venous leg ulcers. Evidence for APCR as a genetic risk factor for venous leg ulcers is reviewed.

APCR and Venous Leg Ulcers.—When the balance of procoagulant and anticoagulant mechanisms is disturbed, the result is either bleeding or thromboembolic disorders. The most common mutation causing APCR is a single nucleotide change of guanine to adenine at position 1691 of the factor V gene. This mutation is frequent among patients with venous leg ulcers. Given that APCR carries a 10-fold increase in risk of venous thrombosis, the mutation probably plays an important role in the development of leg ulcers. A clot-based test can be used to diagnose APCR, and a polymerase chain reaction assay is available to identify mutation of the factor V gene. These tests may be considered for patients with a history of venous thrombosis in the absence of malignancy, those with a family history of thrombosis, and those with chronic venous leg ulcers.

Testing and Management of APCR.—Knowing that APCR is present, the physician may choose to administer anticoagulant therapy to prevent additional thrombosis and disease progression. The benefits of anticoagulation depends on the degree of certainty that the venous ulcer was caused by venous thrombosis. Prophylactic anticoagulation is indicated for patients who are heterozygous for the fV R506Q allele when they are placed at increased risk of thrombosis, such as during surgery. Also, patients who are heterozygous with active thrombosis should receive heparin followed by oral anticoagulation therapy. Long-term anticoagulant therapy may be considered for those with recurrent thrombosis. Patients who are homozygous for the mutation or heterozygous for fV R506Q but who have another coagulation defect are at high risk of recurrent thrombosis and therefore should receive long-term oral anticoagulation therapy. Information on hereditary risk factors for thrombophilia will be useful in determining the need for anticoagulant therapy. Patients with the fV R506Q mutation will remain at elevated risk of thrombosis throughout their lives, especially if additional coagulation defects or other risk factors are present.

Discussion.—Activated protein C resistance is an important genetic risk factor for venous leg ulcers. Large, long-term clinical studies are needed to identify the best approach for the prevention of venous thrombosis in subjects with APCR. If thrombosis can be prevented, the result may be a marked reduction in the occurrence of chronic venous ulcers and other consequences of venous insufficiency.

▶ Before Factor V Leiden was discovered it was unusual to be able to identify an inherited abnormality of the coagulation system in patients with venous thromboembolic disease. Factor V Leiden is known to confer resistance to activated protein C. Protein C destroys activated factors V and VIII and thus acts as a negative regulator of blood clotting.

Since the discovery of Factor V Leiden, the percentage of identifiable defects in patients with venous thromboembolic disease has increased dramatically. The incidence of Factor V Leiden is about 5% in populations of European origin, but is rare in Black Africans or non-Western Asian or Japanese populations. Diagnosis of the defect has been made easier by the development of a simple screening test.[1]

This article provides us with lots of statistics and the insight that resistance to activated protein C is not infrequently the cause of chronic venous leg ulcers.

Statistics of note in this article: (1) 1% of the population is affected by chronic venous leg ulcers. (2) Abnormalities of protein C, protein S, antithrombin III and fibrinogen account for approximately 10% of venous thromboses. (3) Abnormality of Factor V with resistance to activated protein C is 10 times more common than any other genetic coagulation defect. (4) Abnormality of Factor V with resistance to activated protein C accounts for 12–21% of venous thromboses in unselected patients.

M.J. Cline, M.D.

Reference

1. Blasczyk R, Ritte M, Thiede C, et al: Simple and rapid detection of Factor V Leiden by allele-specific PCR amplification. *Thromb & Haemostasis* 75:757–759, 1996.

Mortality and Causes of Death in Families With the Factor V Leiden Mutation (Resistance to Activated Protein C)
Hille ETM, Westendorp RGJ, Vandenbroucke JP, et al (Univ Hosp Leiden, The Netherlands)
Blood 89:1963–1967, 1997   10–7

Objective.—Activated protein C (APC) resistance is a common autosomal hereditary abnormality and is associated with a mutation at the APC cleavage site in the factor V gene (factor V Leiden). Activated protein C resistance is also associated with a risk of venous thrombosis, which is 8 times higher in unselected carriers of the mutation. There is concern that this condition may shorten life expectancy. Mortality from all causes was examined in 171 parents whose children carried the mutation for APC resistance.

Results.—After adjustment for age, sex, and calendar period, no excessive mortality in the parents was found compared to the general population. There was no difference in the cause-specific standardized mortality ratio for malignant neoplasms, diseases of the circulatory system, or cerebrovascular disease. There was a small increase in standardized mortality ratios for diseases of the respiratory system and ischemic heart diseases. Individuals younger than 45 years were 9 times more likely to die of ischemic heart disease. Thromboembolic complications were listed once on death certificates as a primary cause of death and 3 times as a secondary cause of death.

Conclusions.—Activated protein C resistance does not appear to shorten life expectancy. These findings suggest that, on the basis of carrier state alone, long-term anticoagulation in individuals who are carriers of factor V Leiden is not indicated.

▶ Under normal conditions, APC destroys activated factors V and VIII and thus acts as a negative regulator that restrains the blood clotting process. Factor V Leiden is a mutated form of factor V, which occurs in some families and which is resistant to APC. Because this mutated form of factor V is not destroyed by protein C, the clotting process is not regulated normally in individuals with the mutation, and they are at increased risk of thromboembolic events.

Factor V Leiden is an extremely common genetic abnormality and several studies have found an incidence of factor V Leiden of about 5% in Western populations. All individuals with the mutation do not suffer from repeated or unusual thromboembolism so that a decision about prophylactic anticoagulation is not always obvious. This study found a ninefold increased risk of dying of ischemic heart disease in affected individuals younger than 45 years; however, in a large number of affected individuals there was no major effect of the mutation on life-expectancy. The authors conclude that anticoagulation on the basis of carrier state alone is not warranted.

The diagnosis of factor V Leiden has been made easier by the development of a simple screening test.[1]

M.J. Cline, M.D.

Reference

1. Blasczyk R, Ritte M, Thiede C, et al: Simple and rapid detection of Factor V Leiden by allele-specific PCR amplification. *Thromb & Haemost* 75:757–759, 1996.

Hypereosinophilic Syndrome and Myocardial Infarction in a 15-Year-Old
Rauch AE, Amyot KM, Dunn HG, et al (Albany Med College, NY; Bellvue Hosp, Niskayana, NY)
Pediatr Pathol Lab Med 17:469–486, 1997   10–8

Introduction.—Hypereosinophilic syndrome (HES) is a rare disorder in adults that is even more rare in children. The leading cause of death for both adults and children with HES is cardiac dysfunction. Described was an adolescent with HES who died of myocardial infarction.

Case Report.—Girl, 15 years, was referred because of a white blood cell (WBC) count of 138,000/mm³ with a differential of 90% eosinophils and mild anemia. Her platelet count was 240,000/mm³. Results of a complete blood count taken 6 months earlier during a routine physical examination were normal. On admission, acneiform lesions were detected on the patient's face and she had several darkly pigmented, vertical nonblanching streaks in her nails. She complained of left-side weakness on hospital day 3 that could not be consistently reproduced. Her WBC count increased to 153,000/mm³ (133,110/mm³, absolute eosinophils). Numerous bilateral cortical and subcortical infarcts were observed on MRI. Administration of hydroxyurea had a marginal effect on the WBC count. On hospital day 15, the patient required intubation for shortness of breath and findings consistent with adult respiratory distress syndrome. Granulocyte apheresis was performed, but her condition continued to deteriorate. She had a cardiac arrest and was successfully resuscitated but had terminal arrest after several hours.

A limited postmortem examination revealed a massive subendocardial infarct over the left ventricle and septum. Light microscopy of the left ventricular myocardium showed evidence of acute necrosis with coagulative necrosis, edema, and an inflammatory infiltrate consisting primarily of eosinophils and neutrophils. Char-

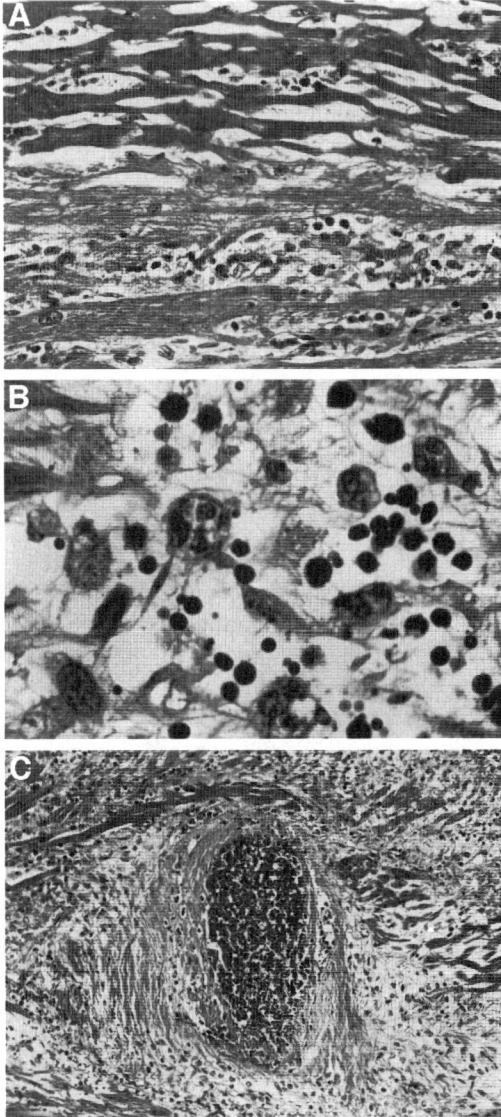

FIGURE 3.—**A**, sections through the left ventricular septum showing recent myocardial infarct. Junction area between necrotic and viable myocardium is shown. Hematoxylin-eosin; original magnificates, ×200. **B**, detail of eosinophilic myocardial infiltrate with associated Charcot-Leyden crystals; hematoxylin-eosin; original magnification, ×400. **C**, example of a thrombosed small vessel within ventricular septum; hematoxylin-eosin; original magnification, ×100. All reproduced at 50%. (From Rauch AE, Amyot KM, Dunn HG, et al: Hypereosinophilic syndrome and myocardial infarction in a 15-year-old. *Pediatr Pathol Lab Med* 17:469–486, 1997. Reproduced with permission. All rights reserved.)

cot-Leyden crystals were abundant in the necrotic areas. These findings were consistent with injury occurring within a matter of days. Thrombosis of small vessels was detected, indicating microvascular occlusion as a possible cause of myocardial necrosis (Fig 3). Selective extracellular major basic protein deposition was observed in the adrenal cortex and the glomerular mesangium of the kidneys.

Conclusion.—This patient with HES and a rapid downward course died with heart failure secondary to a subendocardical myocardial infarction. The glomerular and adrenal gland lesions have not been previously reported.

▶ Eosinophils develop in the bone marrow and are normally released into the blood as mature bi-lobed cells. They circulate for only a few hours before entering the tissues. The exact life span of the eosinophil is unknown, but it is probably considerably longer than the few days that the neutrophil lives. It is estimated that only about 1% of the body's eosinophil population is in the blood at any given time; the rest is in the bone marrow and tissues.

Eosinophils degranulate with a variety of inflammatory stimuli. The products released by degranulation may injure normal tissues as well as parasites. Tissue injury and fibrosis are frequently seen in disorders in which very high levels of eosinophils persist for prolonged periods.

The HESs may be defined as disorders in which the concentration of blood eosinophils is greater that 1500 per μL for more than 6 months without evidence of parasitism or allergy. In most cases, the cause is unknown. In a few cases, the eosinophilia is associated with lymphoma, clonal expansion of helper T cells, eosinophilic leukemia or other myeloproliferative disorders.

The table below lists the organs involved in the HESs. Involvement of the heart or lungs is most ominous. Glucocorticoid or myelosuppressive drugs are often used, but treatment is generally not very satisfactory. At least 1 case has been treated by bone marrow transplantation.

HYPEREOSINOPHILIC SYNDROMES

	ORGAN INVOLVED	*% OF CASES*
•	BLOOD	100
•	HEART	50–70
•	SKIN	50–70
•	NERVOUS SYSTEM	35–70
•	LUNGS	40–60
•	SPLEEN	30–60

M.J. Cline, M.D.

11 Leukemia and Myeloproliferative Disorders

Molecular Remission in PML/RARα-Positive Acute Promyelocytic Leukemia by Combined All-*trans* Retinoic Acid and Idarubicin (AIDA) Therapy
Mandelli F, for the Gruppo Italiano Malattie Ematologiche Maligne dell' Adulto and Associazione Italiana di Ematologia ed Oncologia Pediatrica Cooperative Groups (Univ "La Sapienza," Rome; Univ of Milano-Monza, Italy; Ospedali Riuniti de Bergamo, Italy; et al)
Blood 90:1014–1021, 1997   11–1

Background.—Acute promyelocytic leukemia (APL), a type of acute myeloid leukemia, is characterized by a specific t(15;17) chromosome translocation in the leukemic blasts, the frequent association at diagnosis of a severe hemorrhagic diathesis, and in vitro and in vivo sensitivity to the differentiating agent all-*trans* retinoic acid (ATRA). The mainstay of APL treatment is anthracycline-based chemotherapy (CHT) and ATRA. The response to a new protocol combining ATRA and idarubicin (AIDA protocol) was investigated.

Methods.—Two hundred fifty-three patients with newly diagnosed APL were enrolled in the AIDA trial between July 1993 and February 1996. All patients had genetic evidence of the specific t(15;17) lesion in their leukemic cells. Induction treatment consisted of oral ATRA, 45 mg/m²/day until complete remission, given with IV idarubicin, 12 mg/m²/day on days 2, 4, 6, and 8. Consolidation treatment consisted of 3 polychemotherapy cycles. Hematologic and molecular response was assessed by reverse transcription–polymerase chain reaction (RT-PCR) after induction and after consolidation.

Findings.—Of 240 patients evaluable for induction, 5% died of early complications. The remainder achieved hematologic remission. There were no cases of resistant leukemia. Of 139 patients assessed by RT-PCR after induction, 60.5% were PCR negative, and 39.5% were PCR positive. At the end of consolidation, 162 patients were evaluable by RT-PCR.

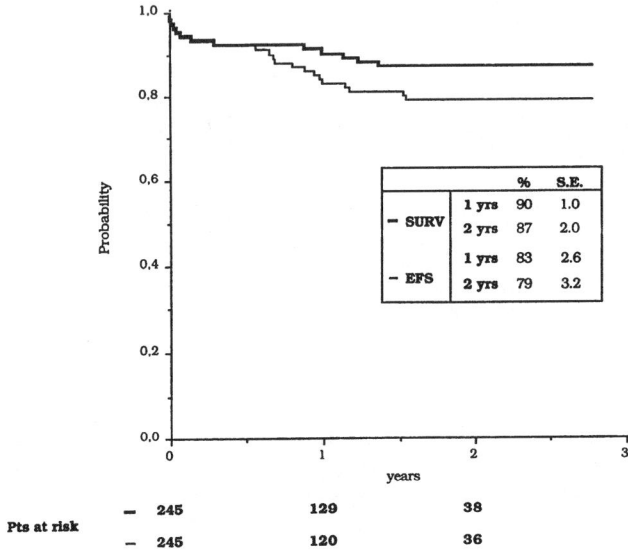

FIGURE 1.—Kaplan-Meier estimates of overall survival and event-free survival (*EFS*). (Courtesy of Mandelli F, for the Gruppo Italiano Malattie Ematologiche dell' Adulto and Associazione Italiana di Ematologia ed Oncologia Pediatrica Cooperative Groups: Molecular remission in PML/RARα-positive acute promyelocytic leukemia by combined all-*trans* retinoic acid and idarubicin (AIDA) therapy. *Blood* 90:1014–1021, 1997.)

Ninety-eight percent were PCR negative, and 2%, PCR positive. After a median 12 months of follow-up, overall estimated actuarial event-free survival was 83% at 1 year and 79% at 2 years (Fig 1).

Conclusions.—The AIDA protocol is well tolerated and induces molecular remission in nearly all patients with PML/RARα-positive APL. These preliminary survival data suggest a remarkable cure rate with this treatment.

▶ Acute promyelocytic leukemia (also known as AProL or M3 acute myeloid leukemia) is a form of acute myeloid leukemia in which the predominant cell type is the promyelocyte. In nearly 100% of cases a characteristic translocation of chromosomes 15 and 17 (t[15:17]) is found. This translocation involves a gene known as PML and the gene for the α-retinoic acid receptor.

Bleeding is often a striking feature of acute promyelocytic leukemia because the blast cells contain procoagulant material which, when released into the circulation, can trigger disseminated intravascular coagulation. In treating acute promyelocytic leukemia, attention is paid to the prevention of this complication.

The other notable feature of acute promyelocytic leukemia is that it is very often responsive to a form of retinoic acid known as ATRA. This drug induces maturation of the immature leukemic cells.

All-*trans* retinoic acid and an anthracycline drug such as daunorubicin or idarubicin have been the mainstays of treatment of acute promyelocytic leukemia; however, they have some problems. Although ATRA induces remissions in more than 90% of patients, disease ultimately relapses in all unless chemotherapy is added. Chemotherapy alone induces remissions in 70% to 80% of patients, but there is often a high mortality rate in the early phases of treatment—up to 20%.

This study examined the combination of ATRA and idarubicin as initial induction therapy followed by 3 cycles of multidrug consolidation therapy. More than 95% of 253 patients achieved hematologic remission of leukemia with a 5% early mortality rate. After consolidation therapy, 98% of patients were negative for leukemic cells by a specific PCR reaction. The initial data suggest that a large percentage of these patients may be cured of their disease—a remarkable achievement.

M.J. Cline, M.D.

Randomized Comparison of DAT Versus ADE as Induction Chemotherapy in Children and Younger Adults With Acute Myeloid Leukemia: Results of the Medical Research Council's 10th AML Trial (MRC AML10)
Hann IM, Stevens RF, Goldstone AH, et al (Med Research Council, London)
Blood 89:2311–2318, 1997   11–2

Background.—In United Kingdom Medical Research Council (MRC) trials, standard therapy for acute myeloid leukemia (AML) has been DAT (daunorubicin, cytarabine, and thioguanine). Etoposide has been claimed to be more effective in the treatment of monocytic and myelomonocytic types of AML. The MRC AML10 study compared the relative efficacy and toxicity of thioguanine with those of etoposide for induction chemotherapy in patients with AML who were younger than 56 years of age.

Study Design.—Between May 1988 and April 1995, 1,966 patients from 163 centers in 3 countries entered the MRC AML 10 trial. Of those 1,966 patients, 1,857 were assessable. Patients were randomized: 929 to DAT and 928 to ADE (daunorubicin, cytarabine, and etoposide). There were no significant differences in presentation features between these 2 groups.

Results.—The complete remission rate was 81% with DAT and 83% with ADE. Among those who achieved remission, the percentage who achieved remission after 1 course of DAT was 70%, after 2 courses was 22%, and after more than 2 was 8%. The percentage who achieved remission after 1 course of ADE was 74%, after 2 was 21%, and after more than 2 was 5%. The percentage failing to achieve complete remission was 11% with DAT and 9% with ADE. The death rate during consolidation chemotherapy was 9% with ADE and 6% with DAT. The median hospital stay was the same for both groups. Patients receiving ADE had slightly more severe nonhematologic toxicity. There were no significant differences between these 2 treatment groups in disease-free survival, relapse rate, and survival at 6 years. No benefit of etoposide could be demonstrated for patients with monocytic or myelomonocytic disease.

Conclusions.—In this large clinical trial of chemotherapy for AML, the etoposide-containing regimen (ADE) was equivalent to the standard thioguanine-containing regimen (DAT) in both toxicity and efficacy, with high remission rates and good long-term survival rates. Whether the addition of either etoposide or thioguanine to daunorubicin-cytarabine induction therapy is beneficial should be addressed in future randomized clinical trials.

▶ A combination of daunorubicin, cytarabine, and 6-thioguanine (DAT or 'TAD' as it was first called) in one schedule or another has been standard induction therapy for AML for nearly 2 decades. Various alternatives have been examined but none has consistently proved superior.

This study compares DAT with a combination in which etoposide is substituted for 6-thioguanine. This substitution is logical because when used, as single agents, etoposide is more effective than 6-thioguanine. Surprisingly, however, the 2 treatment programs were similar or identical in every parameter that one can think of measuring—remission induction, number of courses of therapy necessary to achieve remission, therapy-related deaths, duration of stay in hospital, and so forth.

One should note that although treatment has not changed, the results of treatment *have* improved over the decades—largely as a result of better supportive facilities with improved antibiotics, the availability of hematopoietic growth factors and perhaps also with experience. Thus, in this series more than 80% of patients achieved a remission and more than 40% of those who achieved remission were alive and free of disease at 6 years, i.e., presumably cured of their AML. This is a remarkable achievement.

M.J. Cline, M.D.

Treatment of Refractory Chronic Lymphocytic Leukemia With Fludarabine Phosphate via the Group C Protocol Mechanism of tht National Cancer Institute: Five-Year Follow-up Report
Sorensen JM, Vena DA, Fallavollita A, et al (NIH, Bethesda, Md; EMMES Corp, Potomac, Md)
J Clin Oncol 15:458–465, 1997   11–3

Background.—Fludarabine phosphate is a nucleoside analog with antitumor activity against hematologic malignancies. The Cancer Therapy Evaluation Program organized a group C treatment protocol in 1989 to allow patients with refractory chronic lymphocytic leukemia (CLL) to be treated with fludarabine in a clinical practice setting. This report describes the results of this trial after 5 years of follow-up.

Methods.—Adult patients with a diagnosis of intermediate- or high-risk Rai stage CLL and active disease were eligible to participate in this trial. They were registered by their physicians, who then received the study protocol. Treatment involved administration of 25 mg/m² daily of fludarabine by infusion for 5 days, repeated every 28 days for 6 cycles. Complete responders received 2 more cycles, and partial responders received 6 more cycles. Of the 724 patients who received fludarabine from 634 physicians in 14 countries, 703 were evaluated for this study.

Results.—Of the 703 patients assessed for this study, 32% responded. Of these responders, 3% had a complete response (CR), and 205 had a partial response (PR). The median response duration was 13.1 months, and the median survival time from registration was 12.6 months. Age, performance status, and Rai stage were all prognostic factors for survival. Grade 4 hematologic toxicity was reported in 43% of these patients and was associated with infection in 22%. Neurotoxicity was reported in 14% and was associated with age.

Conclusions.—A group C protocol was initiated to examine the long-term efficacy of fludarabine in the treatment of CLL in clinical practice. Fludarabine had acceptable toxicity, but there was a low response rate in patients with advanced disease.

▶ Fludarabine was first evaluated in clinical trials in 1983. Since then, it has been used in thousands of patients, primarily those with indolent lymphocytic malignancies. Last year we reviewed a French study,[1] which compared fludarabine with a standard treatment protocol in CLL. The study directly compared fludarabine with the CAP regimen, consisting of cyclophosphamide, doxorubicin, and prednisone in the treatment of patients with advanced-stage CLL. The patients were about equally divided between those who had received prior treatment and those who were untreated.

In that study, fludarabine was somewhat superior to CAP in overall response rate but was statistically better only in those patients who had received prior treatment. The important point for me was that in previously untreated patients who did get a remission with fludarabine, the remissions were of significantly longer duration than they were with CAP. The median duration of remission with fludarabine was more than 208 days. This achievement appeared to be at no greater cost in toxicity.

The present U.S. study is a five-year follow-up of fludarabine treatment of patients with advanced refractory CLL. The results of fludarabine treatment are not as impressive as they were in the earlier French study. Only 32% of patients responded to the drug, and the median survival from registration in the study protocol was only 12 months. Complete remission was obtained in only 3% of cases.

These results should be compared with another French study,[2] which examined the use of fludarabine as initial therapy for low grade follicular lymphomas. In a group of 54 patients with untreated low-grade follicular lymphomas, fludarabine induced complete remission of disease in 37% of cases, and 65% of patients had a useful response to the drug. These results were achieved at moderate cost in toxicity. Treatment was stopped in 9 of the 54 patients because of drug toxicity.

It would seem that fludarabine is most effective when used early in disease process.

M.J. Cline, M.D.

References

1. The French Cooperative Group on Chronic Lymphocytic Leukemia: Multicentre prospective randomized trial of fludarabine. *Lancet* 347:1432, 1996.
2. Solal-Celigny P, Brice P, Brousse N, et al: Phase II trial of fludarabine monophosphate as first-line treatment in patients with advanced follicular lymphoma: a multicenter study by the Groupe d'Etude des Lymphomes de l'Adulte. *J Clin Oncol* 14:514–519, 1996.

Case/Control Study of the Role of Splenectomy in Chronic Lymphocytic Leukemia

Seymour JF, Cusack JD, Lerner SA, et al (Royal Melbourne Hosp, Australia; Univ of Texas, Houston)

J Clin Oncol 15:52–60, 1997
11–4

Background.—Many reports have suggested that surgical removal of the enlarged spleen can be beneficial for patients with chronic lymphocytic leukemia. However, the chances of clinically significant hematologic improvement after splenectomy remain unknown. The morbidity, mortality, and chances of hematologic response in patients with chronic lymphocytic leukemia undergoing splenectomy were studied. The potential survival benefit was evaluated as well.

Methods.—The retrospective study included 55 patients with chronic lymphocytic leukemia who underwent splenectomy over a 22-year period. The morbidity and mortality of splenectomy were evaluated, along with the probability of hematologic response. In addition, a case-control study was performed to assess the effects of splenectomy on survival. The patients were matched to 55 fludarabine-treated controls for age, serum albumin level, sex, hemoglobin level, Rai stage, number of previous treatments, and time since diagnosis.

Results.—The patients undergoing splenectomy had only modest bloodproduct requirements in the postoperative period. Eighteen percent of patients had minor infections, and 25% had pneumonia/atelectasis. There were 3 cases of septicemia and 2 of intestinal perforation. Perioperative mortality was 9%. All deaths were related to septic complications and occurred in patients with a performance status of 2 or greater and treatment-refractory Rai stage III or IV disease. Splenic weight was the only factor significantly predicting increases in hemoglobin and neutrophil count. No factor was associated with increased platelet count.

Thirty-day mortality and overall mortality were similar for the splenectomy patients and the fludarabine-treated controls. Survival tended to be better for patients with Rai stage IV disease who underwent splenectomy. For patients with stage IV disease, 2-year actuarial survival was 51% with splenectomy versus 28% with fludarabine.

Conclusions.—In patients with advanced chronic lymphocytic leukemia, splenectomy is associated with modest morbidity, mortality, and resource use. Most patients demonstrate major hematologic improvement after surgery, with hemoglobin and neutrophil count increasing in relation to splenic weight. Overall survival is similar to that in nonsplenectomized controls. Hematologic benefit and, possibly, improved survival are most likely for patients with thrombocytopenia. The authors propose a randomized trial of splenectomy for thrombocytopenic patients with chronic lymphocytic leukemia.

▶ Chronic lymphocytic leukemia (CLL) is by far the most common of the chronic lymphoid leukemias. It is almost always a malignancy of B cells. CLL is usually a disease of older people, and cases in patients younger than 40 years are rare. The onset is often insidious, with a gradually increasing blood lymphocytosis followed after months or years by increasing generalized lymphadenopathy and splenomegaly. At presentation, many patients are asymptomatic, and the diagnosis is often made at the time of a routine blood count, which reveals lymphocytosis. If the disease is left untreated, the WBC count may eventually exceed 500,000 cells/mL, and the lymph nodes and spleen may be massively enlarged. With time, manifestations of immunodeficiency and autoimmune phenomena often develop. This study was undertaken to evaluate the morbidity and mortality and the possible therapeutic benefits of splenectomy in CLL. An analysis of the influence of splenectomy on survival was undertaken. The patients all had advanced disease. Perioperative mortality was 9%; in all cases death was the result of sepsis. Patients with severe thrombocytopenia were most likely to benefit from splenectomy, but improvement in hemoglobin levels and granulocyte counts were also noted.

Clearly splenectomy is a reasonable approach in selected patients with CLL and cytopenias; however, because of the relatively high mortality associated with the procedure, it should be reserved for patients unresponsive to other measures.

M.J. Cline, M.D.

Interferon Alfa-2b Combined With Cytarabine Versus Interferon Alone in Chronic Myelogenous Leukemia

Guilhot F, for the French Chronic Myeloid Leukemia Study Group (Hôpital Jean Bernard, Poitiers, France; Hôpital Saint-Louis, Paris; Hôpital Edouard Herriot, Lyons, France; et al)
N Engl J Med 337:223–229, 1997   11–5

Background.—Chronic myelogenous leukemia (CML) has a poor response to hydroxyurea or busulfan therapy. Treatment with interferon prolongs survival. Cytarabine has been shown to have antileukemic activity. A multicenter, sequential, randomized trial was initiated to compare interferon alone with interferon plus cytarabine in the treatment of patients with CML.

Methods.—Patients with CML who were younger than 70 years old were eligible for inclusion if they had been diagnosed within 6 months,

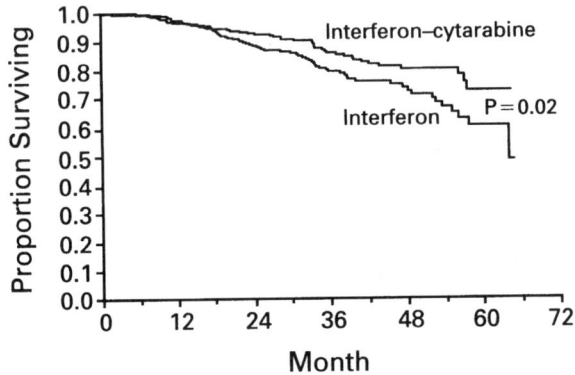

FIGURE 1.—Kaplan–Meier estimates of overall survival among the patients with chronic myelogenous leukemia, according to treatment group. $P = 0.02$ for the comparison of the groups by the log-rank test. Data are based on an intention-to-treat analysis. (Courtesy of Guilhot F, for the French Chronic Myeloid Leukemia Study Group: Interferon Alfa-2b Combined With Cytarabine Versus Interferon Alone in Chronic Myelogenous Leukemia. *N Engl J Med* 337:223–229, 1997. Reprinted by permission of *The New England Journal of Medicine.* Copyright 1997, Massachusetts Medical Society.)

were in the chronic phase, and had been treated only with hydroxyurea. From January 1991 to May 1996, 745 patients without bone marrow donors were randomized to receive hydroxyurea and interferon α-2b, with or without monthly courses of cytarabine. The study end points were overall survival, hematologic response at 6 months and cytologic response at 12 months.

Results.—Sequential analysis revealed significant improvement in survival in the interferon–cytarabine group, compared with the interferon group (Fig 1). After 3 years, the survival rate was 85.7% in the interferon–cytarabine group and 79.1% in the interferon group. The rate of hematologic response at 6 months was significantly higher in the interferon–cytarabine group. Cytogenetic responses were detected at 12 months in 41% of the interferon–cytarabine group and in 24% of the interferon group.

Conclusions.—This multicenter, sequential, randomized trial demonstrated that interferon in combination with cytarabine increased the rate of cytogenetic response and increased survival in patients in the chronic phase of CML.

▶ The initial studies of interferon were carried out in the early 1980s at the MD Anderson Hospital. At the time interferon was hailed as a potentially curative agent—a breakthrough in the treatment of CML. Now, some 15 years later, we are still waiting for the cures, and it is not absolutely certain that it is much superior to chemotherapeutic drug treatment.

Reports from both sides of the Atlantic Ocean have been published in the past 10 years both confirming and denying the superiority of interferon. An overview of 7 randomized trials suggests that interferon is probably better than chemotherapy—57% versus 42% survival at 5 years—but it is rarely curative.

α-Interferon generally has been reported to produce remissions in about 70% of patients with CML—about the same rate or a little less than that achieved with hydroxyurea. It also has been reported that those patients who achieve cytogenetic responses (disappearance of the Philadelphia chromosome) with α-interferon treatment survive longer than those who do not achieve such a remission—not surprising. However, with intensive interferon therapy, only 10% to 20% of patients have such a cytogenetic response, and they often still have the molecular abnormality of the disease in their blood, as determined by the polymerase chain reaction (PCR), and are therefore likely to have residual disease, which will ultimately relapse.

This study compares interferon alone with interferon plus cytarabine. The authors conclude that the combination of drugs was superior in patient survival at 3 years and in the induction of both hematologic and cytogenetic responses. However, before you start treating your patients with interferon, remember 4 things: (1) Interferon therapy is a lot harder on the patient than hydroxyurea; (2) interferon rarely cures disease; (3) interferon therapy may adversely affect the outcome of subsequent bone marrow transplantation; (4) allogeneic bone marrow transplantation is the only known cure for CML.

M.J. Cline, M.D.

Outcome of Allogeneic Bone Marrow Transplantation With Lymphocyte-depleted Marrow Grafts in Adult Patients With Myelodysplastic Syndromes
Mattijssen V, Schattenberg A, Schaap N, et al (Univ Hosp Nijmegen, The Netherlands)
Bone Marrow Transplant 19:791–794, 1997   11–6

Background.—Myelodysplastic syndromes (MDSs) are a group of clonal hematopoietic disorders characterized by refractory cytopenia and dysplastic changes in blood and bone marrow. These syndromes show a tendency to progress to AML. The clinical course of MDS ranges from indolent to rapidly fatal disease, with patients dying from infection or bleeding, transfusion complications, or acute leukemia. Although conventional treatment does not provide a cure, allogeneic bone marrow transplantation (BMT) may be curative in younger patients with MDS. The outcomes of this treatment with lymphocyte-depleted marrow grafts in adults with MDS were reported.

Methods.—Thirty-five patients, aged 23 to 60 years, with MDS underwent BMT between 1986 and 1994. Thirteen patients had transfusion-dependent refractory anemia, and 22 had a more advanced stage of MDS (15 of whom were in complete remission after chemotherapy). In 31 patients, pretransplant conditioning consisted of cyclophosphamide and total body irradiation with or without the addition of idarubicin. Four patients were conditioned with other schedules. The donors for 32 patients were genotypically HLA-identical and MLC-negative siblings. All patients were given a graft depleted of 98% of T lymphocytes by counterflow centrifugation.

Findings.—At a median follow-up of 20 months, 14 patients are alive and in continuous remission. Seven patients experienced relapses between 3 and 18 months after BMT and subsequently died. In addition, there were 14 transplantation-related deaths. Patients younger and older than 40 years had comparable outcomes. The probability of disease-free survival (DFS) 2 years after BMT was 39%. The probabilities of DFS were 73% in patients with HLA-identical and MLC-negative sibling donors transplanted for refractory anemia and 42% for those with more advanced stages of MDS in complete remission.

Conclusion.—Bone marrow transplantation with lymphocyte-depleted grafts can cure a substantial number of older patients with MDS, especially when grafts from HLA-identical and MLC-negative siblings are used. Patients with RA, especially, had a good probability of DFS.

▶ Myelodysplasia or myelodysplastic syndromes is the name given to a group of disorders characterized by morphologically abnormal and often ineffective hematopoiesis. Myelodysplastic syndrome usually occurs in older individuals and is characterized by anemia refractory to therapy and a variable decrease in other cell types.

Most patients with MDS have anemia which is usually associated with some other evidence of marrow failure. In all types of MDS, abnormal red cell morphology is common. Giant platelets and abnormal monocytes and granulocytes are also frequent. The bone marrow is typically hypercellular, with grossly abnormal erythropoiesis. In most cases, the molecular defect causing the abnormal hematopoiesis has not been identified, although chromosomal abnormalities are common.

Five groups of MDS cases are recognized in the FAB classification as follows:

1. Refractory anemia
2. Refractory anemia with ring sideroblasts (greater than 15%),
3. Refractory anemia with excess blasts (5% to 20%) (RAEB),
4. Chronic myelomonocytic leukemia, and
5. RAEB in transformation (20% to 30% blasts).

Although this classification, which combines malignant and nonmalignant diseases, is not very logical, it is today's standard. The disorders have diverse clinical manifestations and are probably of diverse etiologies. Some cases of MDS progress to acute myeloid leukemia and some are frankly leukemic at the outset. These are usually poorly responsive to chemotherapy, hence this study on allogeneic BMT in 35 patients with MDS.

In some ways, this is a strange study in that 13 of the patients had refractory anemia, which rarely progresses to leukemia and which can usually be managed by transfusions for many years. If we look only at those patients with more advanced stages of MDS, according to the authors, their chance of DFS after allogeneic BMT from an HLA-matched sibling is 42%. This is not bad, considering the seriousness of these disorders.

M.J. Cline, M.D.

12 Lymphoproliferative Disorders and Multiple Myeloma

Comparison in Low–Tumor-Burden Follicular Lymphomas Between an Initial No-Treatment Policy, Prednimustine, or Interferon Alfa: A Randomized Study From the Groupe D'Etude des Lymphoms Folliculaires
Brice P, for the Groupe d'Etude des Lymphoms de l'Adulte (Hôpital Saint-Louis, Paris)
J Clin Oncol 15:1110–1117, 1997   12–1

Background.—Follicular lymphoma is one of the most common subgroups of non-Hodgkin's lymphoma, accounting for 25% to 40% of non-Hodgkin's lymphomas. At diagnosis, most patients with follicular lymphoma have widespread disease, mainly involving the lymph nodes. However, some patients are found to have a low tumor burden at diagnosis. Therapeutic options for such patients have not been established. The effects of 3 options for patients with low–tumor-burden follicular lymphoma were determined: treatment delayed until clinically meaningful progression, immediate treatment with an oral alkylating agent, or treatment with the biological response modifier, interferon α-2b.

Methods.—One hundred ninety-three patients with newly diagnosed low–tumor-burden follicular lymphoma were assigned randomly to no initial treatment (arm 1); prednimustine, 200 mg/m^2/day, for 5 days a month for 18 months (arm 2); or interferon α-2b, 5 MU/day for 3 months, followed by 5 MU 3 times a week for 15 months (arm 3).

Findings.—The overall response rate was 78% in arm 2 and 70% in arm 3. Deferred therapy yielded a similar response rate—70%. At a median follow-up of 45 months after randomization, the median freedom-from-treatment interval was 24 months in arm 1. The intervals of freedom from treatment failure in arms 2 and 3 were 40 months and 35 months, respectively. Median overall survival time was not reached. The overall survival rates at 5 years were 78%, 70%, and 84% in arms 1, 2, and 3, respectively. Patients with disease progression within 1 year of enrollment had a significantly shorter survival duration.

Conclusion.—For patients with low–tumor-burden follicular lymphoma, delaying treatment is a feasible policy that does not adversely affect 5-year survival. More intensive treatment should be considered for patients with early disease progression.

▶ Follicular lymphomas are considered to be low grade malignancies of B cells. In this disease the pattern of the lymph nodes is primarily follicular, suggesting a germinal center origin. The predominant cell population is a mixture of small lymphocytes with cleaved nuclei and large blastlike cells. The normal cellular counterpart is thought to be germinal center cells. In most of these lymphomas the unique feature is a chromosomal translocation, t(14;18), involving the *bcl*-2 gene.

Follicular center cell lymphomas constitute between 25% and 40% of lymphomas in the United States. Generally, they affect adults. The disease tends to be indolent and localized mainly to lymph nodes and spleen, but transformation to a more aggressive histology is frequent sometime in the course of the disease. Generally these lymphomas are not cured by therapy.

This study examined 3 options for initial treatment of follicular lymphoma patients with a low tumor burden defined as small nodes in fewer than 3 sites and the absence of splenomegaly or systemic symptoms. The options were (1) no therapy, (2) an oral alkylating agent, or (3) interferon α. The most noteworthy observation of the study was that overall survival at 5 years was more-or-less the same in all groups: between 70% and 84%. Consequently, delaying treatment did not adversely affect outcome and it reduced the long-term toxicity of alkylating agents. It is recommended, however, that treatment be initiated as soon as there is evidence of disease progression.

M.J. Cline, M.D.

2-Chlorodeoxyadenosine (2-CDA) Therapy in Previously Untreated Patients With Follicular Stage III-IV Non-Hodgkin's Lymphoma
Betticher DC, Zucca E, von Rohr A, et al (Inst of Med Oncology, Inselspital, Berne, Switzerland; Ospedale San Giovanni, Bellinzona, Switzerland; Christie Hosp, Manchester, England; et al)
Ann Oncol 7:793–799, 1996   12–2

Introduction.—Follicular lymphoma is a common subtype of malignant lymphoma and is associated with a median survival range of 5 to 10 years. With advanced disease, current treatment options are not effective in providing a prolonged relapse-free survival period. In recent years, new drugs such as purine analogs have shown promise in the treatment of low-grade lymphomas. A study was done to evaluate the effectiveness of 2-chlorodeoxyadenosine (2-CDA) in the treatment of advanced follicular non-Hodgkin's lymphoma (NHL) in non-pretreated patients. In addition, bone marrow and peripheral blood were examined by polymerase chain reaction (PCR) to assess the prognostic value of residual disease.

Methods.—Patients with recently diagnosed stage III-IV follicular NHL were treated with 2-CDA, 0.1 mg/kg daily, for 7 days, given as a continuous intravenous or subcutaneous infusion. Response to therapy was assessed after 3 and 5 treatment cycles. Response was categorized as a complete remission (complete absence of disease), partial remission (reduction in disease by 50%), no change in disease, or progressive disease (25% or greater increase in measurable disease). Whole blood and bone marrow samples were obtained before, during, and after treatment; and PCR analyses were performed for assessment of bcl-2/JH rearrangement.

Results.—Thirty-seven patients received a total of 167 cycles of 2-CDA, with a median of 5 cycles. Therapy was stopped early in 11 patients because of death, metabolic disorder, progressive disease, toxicity, or patient choice. Complete remission was achieved in 14% of patients and partial remission in 70%, for an overall response rate of 84%. After 5 cycles of 2-CDA, the median time to relapse was 15.7 months. The overall survival rate was 89%; 27 patients (73%) remained event-free for 1 year. At study entry, 10 of 25 patients were found to have bcl-2JH rearrangement in bone marrow or peripheral blood. After 2-CDA therapy, 5 of these patients had negative results and have shown no progression of disease. Of 3 patients who remained positive, 1 had relapse of disease 8 months after treatment. Eight of 37 patients experienced grade 3 or 4 neutropenia, and 4 experienced grade 3 or 4 thrombocytopenia. Delayed, persistent thrombocytopenia occurred in 6 patients.

Conclusion.—2-Chlorodeoxyadenosine was found to be effective in the treatment of previously untreated follicular lymphoma. However, there appeared to be no gain in response rates or remission duration as compared with standard treatments.

▶ Follicular lymphomas are the most common type of malignant lymphoma. They are of B-cell origin. The B-cell lymphomas fall into the seven main categories, of which approximately 40% are follicular and another 40% are diffuse. A follicular pattern means that there is some preservation of nodal architecture, whereas a diffuse pattern means that the architecture is destroyed.

The great majority of follicular lymphomas have a characteristic chromosomal translocation and an abnormality of the bcl-2 gene. This gene is involved in apoptosis (i.e., controlled cell death) of lymphoid cells.

Follicular lymphomas tend to be indolent and localized mainly to lymph nodes and spleen. Occasionally extranodal sites are involved, and transformation to more aggressive disease is frequent late in the disease. These lymphomas generally have a more favorable natural history then the more aggressive diffuse lymphomas; however, in contrast to diffuse lymphomas, the follicular lymphomas rarely enter complete remission with chemotherapy. Consequently, most patients with follicular lymphomas are treated in a manner aimed at reducing the mass of malignant tumor and improving their quality of life rather than achieving a complete remission (i.e., readication of all clinically detectable tumor).

Cyclophosphamide, vincristine, and prednisone (CVP) is probably the most commonly used drug combination in follicular lymphomas. This study examined the efficacy of 2-CDA as possible first-line therapy for advanced follicular lymphomas. This relatively new drug proved no better than conventional therapy but did produce a surprisingly high rate of complete remissions of disease (14%). This is noteworthy and suggests that 2-CDA should be examined in combination with other drugs.

M.J. Cline, M.D.

CHOP vs. ProMACE-CytaBOM in the Treatment of Aggressive Non-Hodgkin's Lymphomas: Long-term Results of a Multicenter Randomized Trial
Montserrat E, García-Conde J, Viñolas N, et al (Univ of Barcelona)
Eur J Haematol 57:377–383, 1996   12–3

Background.—In 1985, the PETHEMA Group initiated a randomized, multicenter study to determine whether a regimen of alternating courses of prednisone, cyclophosphamide, doxorubicin, and etoposide (ProMACE) and cytarabine, bleomycin, vincristine, and methotrexate (CytaBOM) was more effective than cyclophosphamide, doxorubicin, vincristine, and prednisone (CHOP) in aggressive non-Hodgkin's lymphomas. The final, long-term results of that study were reported.

Methods.—One hundred seventy-five patients with previously untreated aggressive non-Hodgkin's lymphoma were assigned randomly to CHOP or ProMACE-CytaBOM treatment. All had follicular large-cell, diffuse small cleaved-cell, diffuse mixed, diffuse large-cell, or immunoblastic lymphoma with an Ann Arbor stage of II, III, or IV. The final analysis included 148 assessable patients.

Findings.—Response rates were 83.5% in the CHOP group and 88% in the ProMACE-CytaBOM group, a nonsignificant difference. The 2 groups were also comparable in treatment failures (29% and 31%, respectively, at 5 years) and overall survival (42% in both groups at 5 years). The 2 regimens were also comparable when response rates and outcomes were analyzed in different prognostic subgroups. Significant differences also did not occur in toxicity, though only 1 patient died of CHOP-related toxicity, whereas 6 died of ProMACE-CytaBOM-related toxicity.

Conclusions.—These data indicate that proMACE-CytaBOM is not superior to CHOP therapy in patients with aggressive lymphomas. Thus CHOP continues to be the standard chemotherapy in such patients. New treatment approaches for these lymphomas should be compared with CHOP.

▶ As noted in previous YEAR BOOKS OF MEDICINE, the CHOP regimen (cyclophosphamide, doxorubucin, vincristine, and prednisone) has been the standard multi-agent chemotherapy regimen for aggressive non-Hodgkin's lymphoma. It is certainly the best known and is probably the most effective of the so-called first generation chemotherapy regimens. Studies over nearly 2 decades found that CHOP produced approximately 50% complete remissions in patients with high-grade non-Hodgkin's lymphomas, and that approximately 25% to 30% of patients were cured of their disease.

More intensive regimens of combination chemotherapy are a favorite theme of investigation in high-grade non-Hodgkin's lymphoma, with the expectation or hope that they would cure a greater proportion of patients. In general, the initially reported results of these intensive regimens have been excellent, with claimed cure rates of up to 55% or 65%. However these intensive programs were more difficult to use, and were more toxic than the original CHOP program. Moreover, subsequent data failed to demonstrate that they were convincingly more effective than CHOP.

This study examined CHOP vs. a complex and aggressive multi-agent chemotherapy program in 175 patients studied for 7–11 years. The conclusion: CHOP is still the standard chemotherapy program. But do look at Abstract No. 12–11 for a different approach.

M.J. Cline, M.D.

Benefit of Autologous Bone Marrow Transplantation Over Sequential Chemotherapy in Poor-risk Aggressive Non-Hodgkin's Lymphoma: Updated Results of the Prospective Study LNH87-2
Haioun C, for the Groupe d'Etude des Lymphomes de l'Adulte (Hôpital Henri Mondor, Créteil, France; Hôpital Saint Louis, Paris; Hôpital Laënnec, Paris; et al)
J Clin Oncol 15:1131–1137, 1997   12–4

Background.—The superiority of high-dose chemotherapy and autologous bone marrow transplantation over standard salvage therapy for patients with aggressive non-Hodgkin's lymphoma that remains sensitive to chemotherapy has recently been reported. Early analysis of 464 patients with lymphoma and unfavorable characteristics who responded to induction treatment showed no advantage to consolidative high-dose chemotherapy and autologous bone marrow transplantation over sequential chemotherapy.

Methods.—There were 916 patients given induction treatment with the LNH84 protocol who were randomly assigned to treatment with anthracycline. In further randomization, 541 patients in complete remission received consolidation therapy by sequential chemotherapy or autotransplantation. Of higher risk patients, 236 patients in complete remission were evaluated for the consolidation phase; 111 of these received sequential chemotherapy and 125 received autotransplantation.

Results.—In the 541 patients who were randomly allocated, disease-free survival and survival were similar in the 2 consolidative treatment groups. In the higher risk group, the 5-year disease-free survival was 59% in patients treated with cyclophosphamide, carmustine, and etoposide and 39% in patients treated with sequential chemotherapy. The 5-year survival was 65% in patients treated with cyclophosphamide, carmustine, and etoposide and 52% in patients treated with sequential chemotherapy.

Discussion.—In patients with aggressive non-Hodgkin's lymphoma in complete first remission, sequential chemotherapy was superior to transplantation. Dose-intensive consolidation therapy may be a good alternative for higher risk patients in complete remission after induction treatment.

▶ Over the past 7 years, I have reviewed for the YEAR BOOK OF MEDICINE a number of studies that examine high-dose chemotherapy combined with either autologous bone marrow transplantation or peripheral stem cell transplantation in patients with non-Hodgkin's lymphoma of high or intermediate histologic grade. In most studies, transplantation was compared with conventional chemotherapy and, in most studies, survival without relapse was approximately 50% in both treatment groups. My conclusion was that autologous bone marrow transplantation or stem cell transplantation is a valid treatment option but is probably not superior to conventional chemotherapy. Last year, I reviewed a large study that also examined the extensive literature on autologous bone marrow transplantation in refractory non-Hodgkin's lymphoma.[1] The conclusion was much the same, i.e., that autologous bone marrow transplantation is probably not superior to conventional chemotherapy.

This study comes to a different conclusion—that autologous bone marrow transplantation *is* superior to chemotherapy in high-risk aggressive non-Hodgkin's lymphoma when the transplant is performed in the first complete remission of disease. In this study nearly 60% of more than 900 patients achieved a remission. Of these, over 200 patients with aggressive disease were assigned to either sequential chemotherapy or bone marrow transplantation. Both groups did surprisingly well, but 5-year disease-free survival was considerably better in the autologous bone marrow transplantation group (59%) than in the chemotherapy group (39%). It looks like we shall have to change our views of the utility of autologous bone marrow transplantation in non-Hodgkin's lymphoma, at least for those cases in the worst prognostic category.

M.J. Cline, M.D.

Reference

1. Meehan KR, Pritchard RS, Leichter JW, et al: Autologous bone marrow transplantation versus chemotherapy in relapsed/refractory non-Hodgkin's lymphoma. (1997 YEAR BOOK OF MEDICINE, p. 209–210.)

Late Relapse in Patients With Diffuse Large-Cell Lymphoma Treated With MACOP-B

Lee AYY, Connors JM, Klimo P, et al (Britich Columbia Cancer Agency, Vancouver, Canada; Univ of British Columbia, Vancouver, Canada)

J Clin Oncol 15:1745–1753, 1997   12–5

Background.—Patients considered cured of aggressive lymphoma may experience relapses with diffuse or follicular lymphoma for up to 26 years after treatment. Few data on the clinical course and treatment outcomes of these late-relapse patients have been published.

Methods.—One hundred twenty-seven patients with de novo advanced-stage diffuse large-cell lymphoma treated by 12 weeks of chemotherapy between 1981 and 1986 were studied. The 10-year overall survival rate was 52%. Of the 106 patients (83%) entering complete remission, 43 relapsed. The median follow-up was 146 months. Twenty-six patients had early relapses, and 17 had relapses after a continuous complete remission of more than 24 months. All of the latter patients had B-cell lymphoma.

Outcomes.—The mean rate of late relapse (at 24 months or more after diagnosis) was 2.2% per year, reaching a projected 22% actuarial risk of late relapse after 10 years. Late relapses occurred at 38 to 141 months; the median was 69 months. Ten patients had relapses of aggressive histologic subtypes. These patients were treated with curative intent by anthracycline-based chemotherapy. Four are currently in second complete remission, 1 is alive with disease, and 5 died from disease or while receiving treatment. These 10 patients had an overall survival rate of 42% 6 years from the time of relapse. Another 6 patients had relapses with low-grade follicular lymphoma and received various treatments intended to control (but not necessarily cure) disease. One of these patients is in second complete remission, and 1 is alive with disease. The remaining 4 have died from disease or while receiving treatment. This patient group had a 6-year overall survival-from-relapse rate of 40%. The type of late relapse could not be predicted by *bcl*-2 translocation or Bcl-2 protein expression at diagnosis. One patient, who did not have a repeat biopsy at relapse, died 9 months later despite aggressive treatment.

Conclusion.—Patients who relapse late with aggressive-histology lymphoma should be treated with curative intent. Palliative treatment may benefit patients who relapse with follicular histology. Late-relapse lymphoma behaves similarly to de novo lymphoma, with outcome depending on histologic subtype at relapse.

▶ In an article on lymphomas and autologous bone marrow transplantation reviewed earlier this year,[1] the authors made the point that patients with high-grade disease who are in remission at 2 years are apt to be cured of their disease, whereas those with intermediate and low-grade non-Hodgkin's lymphoma are still at risk of relapse after 2 years in remission. This article presents data contrary to that view.

Lee et al, treated 127 patients with diffuse large cell lymphoma with methotrexate, doxorubicin, cyclophosphamide, vincristine, prednisone, and bleomycin (MACOP-B), a standard aggressive multiagent regimen, between 1981 and 1986. They observed a complete remission rate of 83% and an overall survival rate at 10 years of 52%—results that are really quite good. They observed that 17 patients with B-cell lymphomas had late relapses which occurred between 3½ and approximately 12 years after initial therapy remission.

Interestingly, 2 types of relapse were observed. Patients relapsed either with lymphomas of "aggressive" histology or with lymphomas of "benign" follicular histology. The former often responded to aggressive treatment, and the latter responded to palliative treatment as if they were de novo lymphomas. The results of this study are consistent with those of other reports which have documented that patients considered cured of aggressive lymphomas can relapse with diffuse or follicular lymphomas up to 26 years later.[2]

M.J. Cline, M.D.

References

1. Bowell B, et al: Durability of remission after autologous bone marrow transplantation for non-Hodgkin's lymphoma. *Bone Marrow Transplant* 19:443, 1997.
2. Marazuela M, Yerba M, Giron JA, et al: Late relapse with nodular lymphoma after treatment for diffuse non-Hodgkin's lymphoma. *Cancer* 67: 1950–1953, 1991.

Elderly Patients With Aggressive Non-Hodgkin's Lymphoma: Disease Presentation, Response to Treatment, and Survival—A Groupe d'Etude des Lymphones de l'Adulte Study on 453 Patients Older Than 69 Years
Bastion Y, Blay J-Y, Divine M, et al (Centre Hospitalier Lyon-Sud, Pierre-Bénite, Centre Léon-Bérard, France; Hôpital Edouard-Herriot, Lyon, France; et al)
J Clin Oncol 15:2945–2953, 1997   12–6

Background.—The incidence of non-Hodgkin's lymphoma (NHL) has been increasing by 8% to 10% annually, with more than half of new cases occurring in elderly patients. It is not known whether the characteristics and outcomes of NHL in older patients differ from those in younger patients. Disease characteristics and optimal therapy for elderly patients with NHL were investigated in the current randomized study.

Methods.—A total of 453 patients with NHL who were older than 69 years and had aggressive lymphoma were enrolled in the trial. Median age was 75 years. A total of 220 were given cyclophosphamide, 750 mg/m^2; teniposide (VM 26), 75 mg/m^2; and prednisone, 40 mg/m^2/d for 5 days (CVP). The remaining 233 patients were given CVP plus pirarubicin (THP-doxorubicin), 50 mg/m^2 (CTVP), each for 6 courses every 3 weeks.

Findings.—The 2 treatment groups were similar, except that more patients on the CTVP arm had an increased lactic dehydrogenase (LDH) level. Treatment with CTVP was more often associated with leukopenia, thrombocytopenia, and infectious complications. Of the patients on the CVP arm, 16%, and 21% on the CTVP arm died during chemotherapy (a nonsignificant difference). A complete response (CR) was achieved in 40% of the patients overall, including 47% on CTVP and 32% on CVP. Median time to treatment failure was 7 and 5 months in the CTVP and CVP groups, respectively. Both groups had a median survival time of 13 months. However, the 5-year survival was 26% in the CTVP group, compared with 19% in the CVP group. The main cause of death was lymphoma progression.

Conclusions.—Aggressive lymphoma in elderly patients is associated with adverse prognostic parameters at the time of diagnosis. Patients treated with an anthracycline-containing regimen appear to have a slightly longer survival.

▶ This study examined the results of 2 moderately intense treatment programs for aggressive non-Hodgkin's lymphoma in 400 patients over the age of 69 years, which is, I suppose, a fair definition of elderly.

Complete remission was achieved in 40% of patients, but it was at a high cost. About 20% of patients died during the chemotherapy. Furthermore, the remissions were brief—between 5 and 7 months in duration.

One must tread cautiously in recommending aggressive treatment for elderly patients with non-Hodgkin's lymphoma considering that median survival was only 13 months from the time of initiating treatment, and that for at least half of that time the patients were ill from the chemotherapy as well as from disease. However, the therapeutic options are limited. Without treatment more than 90% of patients will be dead within a year. With aggressive treatment about 1 patient in 5 will be alive at 5 years.

M.J. Cline, M.D.

Durability of Remission After ABMT for NHL: The Importance of the 2-Year Evaluation Point
Bolwell B, Goormastic M, Andresen S (Cleveland Clinic Found, Ohio)
Bone Marrow Transplant 19:443–448, 1997   12–7

Background.—Few reports of autologous bone marrow transplantation (ABMT) for the treatment of non-Hodgkin's lymphoma include mature follow-up. One large series of patients undergoing autologous bone marrow/peripheral progenitor cell transplantation for non-Hodgkin's lymphoma between 1988 and 1993 was reviewed.

Patients and Findings.—One hundred ten adults were included in the series. Overall survival was 50%, and relapse-free survival, 35%, with an estimated median relapse-free survival of 16 months. Neither relapse-free nor overall survival differed significantly according to low-, intermediate-, or high-grade histologic type. Increased lactic dehydrogenase at the time of transplant was the strongest negative prognostic variable. Two years after transplantation, 47 patients were in complete remission. Extended follow-up showed that all patients with high-grade histologic subtypes remained in complete remission, whereas patients with intermediate- and low-grade histologic subtypes continued to be at risk for relapse over time. All 8 patients with immunoblastic histologic findings remain in remission, whereas 4 of 14 with diffuse large cell lymphoma had relapses 24–48 months after ABMT.

Conclusions.—Patients with high-grade histologic subtypes of non-Hodgkin's lymphoma in complete remission 2 years after ABMT are probably cured. However, those with intermediate- and low-grade histologic subtypes continue to be at risk for relapse and need appropriate clinical surveillance for at least 48 months after ABMT.

▶ This abstract continues the theme of ABMT in cases of non-Hodgkin's lymphoma. It makes the point that patients with high-grade disease who are in remission at 2 years are apt to be cured of their disease, whereas those with intermediate- and low-grade non-Hodgkin's lymphoma are still at risk of relapse after two years in remission. This finding is consistent with the slower pace of disease and the refractoriness to complete ablation of tumor in low- and intermediate-grade of non-Hodgkin's lymphoma.

M.J. Cline, M.D.

Posttransplant T-Cell Lymphoproliferative Disorders—An Aggressive, Late Complication of Solid-Organ Transplantation
Hanson MN, Morrison VA, Peterson BA, et al (Univ of Minnesota, Minneapolis; Veteran's Affairs Med Ctr, Minneapolis; Hennepin County Med Ctr, Minneapolis; et al)
Blood 88:3626–3633, 1996 12–8

Background.—T-cell non-Hodgkin's lymphomas sometimes develop in solid-organ transplant recipients. The occurrence of a morphologically and immunophenotypically distinct group of T-cell lymphoproliferative disorders late in the course of 6 such patients was described.

Methods and Findings.—The 6 patients were 3 women and 3 men, aged 31 to 56 years. All had undergone splenectomy. Lymphoma was diagnosed 4 to 26 years after transplantation. Initial symptoms were associated with sites of involvement. Five patients had pulmonary involvement; 4, marrow; and 1, CNS. None of the patients had lymphadenopathy. In 5 patients, lactate dehydrogenase levels were increased. Five had a leukoerythroblastic reaction. Histologic assessment indicated large-cell type in all patients. Cytoplasmic granules were often observed. In the patients tested, CD2, CD3, and CD8 were expressed; and B-cell antigens were negative. T-cell receptor β- and τ-chain genes were rearranged clonally in 3 of 3 cases and in 1 of 3 cases, respectively. The findings of all T-cell posttransplant lymphoproliferative disorders (T-PTLDs) determined to be negative for Epstein-Barr virus (EBV), human T-cell leukemia/lymphoma virus

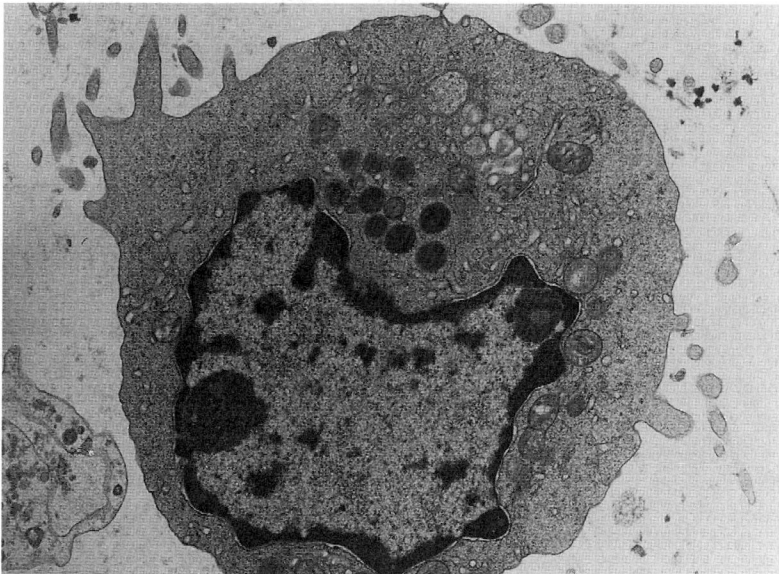

FIGURE 4.—Electron micrograph of a granulated lymphoma cell from patient 3. Note the electron-dense granules. Parallel tubular arrays noted in the cells of typical large granular lymphocytosis of the T-cell type were not noted in these cells. (Uranyl acetate and lead citrate, original magnification × 10,000.) (Courtesy of Hanson MN, Morrison VA, Peterson BA, et al: Posttransplant T-cell lymphoproliferative disorders—an aggressive, late complication of solid-organ transplantation. *Blood* 88:3626–3633, 1996.)

types 1 and 2 (HTLV-1 and 2), and human herpes virus 8 (HHV-8) genomes. Two of six patients treated with acyclovir or chemotherapy responded. Overall median survival was 5 weeks (Fig 4).

Conclusions.—Clinically aggressive T-PTLD may be a late complication of solid-organ transplantation. This disorder does not appear to be associated with EBV, HTLV-1 or 2, or HHV-8 infection.

▶ The development of lymphomas is a well recognized, albeit relatively infrequent, complication of transplantation of "solid" organs such as kidney and heart. These lymphomas, which presumably arise at least in part as a consequence of immunosuppression related to the transplant procedure, are almost always B-cell lymphomas. Now these authors have identified a unique subset of post transplantation lymphomas, which are of T-cell origin and which appear to be unusually agressive. Chemotherapy was generally ineffective, and most patients died within a few weeks. Another unusual feature of these tumors is their late development after organ transplantation—a median of 15 years after transplantation with a range of 4 to 26 years. The pathogenetic mechanism underlying T-cell lymphoma development is not known.

M.J. Cline, M.D.

Outcome of Patients With Hodgkin's Disease Failing After Primary MOPP-ABVD

Bonfante V, Santoro A, Viviani S, et al (Istituto Nazionale Tumori, Milano, Italy)
J Clin Oncol 15:528–534, 1997   12–9

Introduction.—The impact of conventional salvage therapy is dismal in patients with Hodgkin's disease who fail to achieve a complete response or are in relapse after a short-term complete remission. The long-term results, response to salvage treatments, and prognostic factors were analyzed in 115 patients with Hodgkin's disease who were resistant to or relapsed after first-line treatment with mechlorethamine, vincristine, procarbazine, and prednisone-adriamycin, bleomycin, vinblastine, and dacarbazine (MOPP-ABVD).

Methods.—Of 415 patients with Hodgkin's disease who underwent first-line treatment of MOPP-ABVD and radiotherapy, 115 were assessable for the impact of second-line treatments. Median patient follow-up was 91 months. Thirty-nine of 115 patients (34%) had disease progression during primary treatment, 48 relapsed after complete remission up to 12 months, and 28 relapsed after complete remission more than 12 months after all treatments.

Results.—The 8-year rate of freedom from second progression was 44% for patients with initial complete remission longer than 12 months and 22% for patients with complete remission shorter than 12 months. The overall 8-year total survival rate was 27%. No patients with initial induction failure were free of disease beyond 3 years. The median duration of freedom from second progression was 13 months. Median survival duration was 38 months. Freedom from second progression was significantly influenced by response to first-line chemotherapy and disease extent at progression. Degree of nodal involvement was of borderline significance. Overall survival was significantly influenced by response to first-line chemotherapy, extent of lymphoma at progression, and age at lymphoma progression. Twelve patients experienced second malignancies.

Conclusion.—Retreatment with initial chemotherapy seems to be the treatment of choice for patients with Hodgkin's disease who relapse after initial complete remission that lasts longer than 12 months. Treatment strategies have to be balanced against the risk of causing second malignancies and severe late sequelae.

▶ In this study, 115 patients "failing" combination chemotherapy with alternating MOPP-ABVD were evaluated. Of this group, 34% were "induction failures" and the rest had disease relapse after entering a remission. The latter group were further divided into those with relapse within 12 months of completing therapy and those with relapse after 12 months of completing therapy.

The results are rather disappointing. At 8 years, the survival was only 8% in those classified as "induction failures" and only 28% in those whose disease recurred within 12 months of achieving remission. The outcome in the latter group is similar to that of patients whose disease relapses after a single 4-drug combination [MOPP OR ABVD alone]. Clearly, we need better therapy for resistant Hodgkin's disease. Unfortunately, autologous bone marrow transplantation with intensive therapy does not seem to work in this situation.

M.J. Cline, M.D.

A Trial of Three Regimens for Primary Amyloidosis: Colchicine alone, Melphalan and Prednisone, and Melphalan, Prednisone, and Colchicine
Kyle RA, Gertz MA, Greipp PR, et al (Mayo Clinic and Mayo Found, Rochester, Minn)
N Engl J Med 336:1202–1207, 1997   12–10

Introduction.—Primary systemic amyloidosis is a rare disease characterized by accumulation in vital organs of a fibrillar protein consisting of monoclonal light chains. Patients with primary systemic amyloidosis were stratified according to their dominant clinical manifestation, then randomly assigned to receive either colchicine; melphalan and prednisone; or a combination of the 3 drugs.

Methods.—Two-hundred twenty patients were stratified according to their chief clinical manifestations of disease: 105, renal disease; 46, cardiac involvement; 19, peripheral neuropathy; and 50, other. They were randomly assigned to receive either: colchicine (72), melphalan and prednisone (77), or melphalan, prednisone, and colchicine (71). Outcome was determined by duration of survival, improvement in renal or liver function, and disappearance or decrease of more than 50% of urinary monoclonal protein.

Results.—Median duration of patient survival was 8.5 months in the colchicine group, 18 months in the melphalan and prednisone group, and 17 months in the melphalan, prednisone, and colchicine group. Patients with reduced serum or urine monoclonal protein at 12 months had an overall length of survival of 50 months, compared to 36 months in patients without a reduction at 12 months. Thirty-four patients (15%) were alive at 5-year follow-up.

Conclusion.—Patients who received melphalan and prednisone had objective responses and prolonged survival, compared to patients who received colchicine. Despite these findings, treatment for primary systemic amyloidosis remains inadequate.

▶ Primary amyloidosis is an uncommon paraprotein disorder in which aggregates of monoclonal immunoglobulin light chain are deposited in various organs including the heart, kidneys, and peripheral nerves.

Among the paraprotein disorders, primary amyloidosis has been the least well defined with respect to therapy, and it is often frustrating to manage patients with organ involvement. Colchicine has been used in this disease because of its benefit in patients with Mediterranean fever and secondary amyloidosis. Anecdotal cases have been reported of response to cytotoxic immunosuppressive agents, but response to therapy has been difficult to assess because of the indolent nature of the disease process and its reversal with treatment. In an earlier study by this group from the Mayo Clinic, the combination of melphalan (a cytotoxic drug) and prednisone was superior to colchicine.

This study reviews a randomized treatment program involving 220 patients with primary amyloidosis—an extraordinarily large number for this uncommon disorder. The findings appear to be clear-cut: in primary amyloidosis, the combination of melphalan and prednisone is superior to colchicine in objective responses and duration of survival.

M.J. Cline, M.D.

Fas Gene Mutations in the Canale-Smith Syndrome, an Inherited Lymphoproliferative Disorder Associated With Autoimmunity
Drappa J, Vaishnaw AK, Sullivan KE, et al (Cornell Univ, New York; Univ of Pennsylvania, Philadelphia)
N Engl J Med 335:1643–1649, 1996   12–11

Background.—The Canale-Smith syndrome, a childhood disorder characterized by lymphadenopathy and autoimmunity, is similar to lymphoproliferation (*lpr*) phenotype or the generalized-lymphoproliferative-disease (*gld*) phenotype in mice. Whether Canale-Smith syndrome is also caused by mutations of the *Fas* gene (as in *lpr* mice) or the Fas ligand (as in *gld* mice) was investigated.

Methods and Findings.—Four affected patients and their families were studied. The patients had increased numbers of circulating double-negative T cells and profoundly impaired apoptosis of activated T cells incubated with an anti-Fas antibody. Three novel *Fas* mutations were identified. All were heterozygous and predicted to impair signal transduction by Fas. Autoimmune manifestations of the Canale-Smith syndrome, including hemolytic anemia and thrombocytopenia, persisted into adolescence. Intermittent lymphadenopathy was noted in 2 patients studied into adulthood, though this declined with time. Both of these patients subsequently had neoplasms. One died of hepatocellular carcinoma at the age of 43 years.

Conclusions.—In this study, mutations in the *Fas* gene were documented in patients with the Canale-Smith syndrome. This implicates the *Fas* gene in the accumulation of lymphocytes and the autoimmunity characteristic of the syndrome.

▶ The Canale-Smith syndrome, first described in 1967, is a rare familial disorder characterized by lymphadenopathy, hepatosplenomegaly, thrombocytopenia, and hemolytic anemia. The lymph nodes are hyperplastic but do not contain malignant cells.

On the basis of the observation that abnormalities of the *Fas* gene may be associated with a lymphoproliferative disorder and autoimmunity in mice, Drappa and his colleagues investigated 4 patients with the Canale-Smith syndrome and their families and found mutations in the *Fas* gene.

The *Fas* gene codes for a membrane receptor. Part of that receptor known (dramatically) as the death domain transduces signals for programmed cell death (apoptosis) in activated lymphocytes and macrophages. All 4 patients had mutations in the region of the gene that codes for this domain. The presumption is that the defect leads to accumulation of a subpopulation of lymphocytes that would otherwise have died. These lymphocytes may have autoreactive characteristics that result in the autoimmune hemolysis and thrombocytopenia.

I am truly amazed by the rapid accumulation in recent years of knowledge about the molecular mechanisms of familial immunodeficiency and lympho-proliferative disorders.

M.J. Cline, M.D.

13 Bone Marrow Transplantation and Gene Therapy

Treatment-related Mortality in 1000 Consecutive Patients Receiving High-Dose Chemotherapy and Peripheral Blood Progenitor Cell Transplantation in Community Cancer Centers
Weaver CH, Schwartzberg LS, Hainsworth J, et al (Response Oncology Inc, Memphis, Tenn; Sarah Cannon Cancer Ctr, Nashville, Tenn)
Bone Marrow Transplant 19:671–678, 1997   13–1

Background.—High-dose chemotherapy (HDC) with peripheral blood progenitor cell (PBPC) support is being used increasingly to treat chemotherapy-sensitive diseases. This report describes the 100-day treatment-related mortality (TRM) of 1,000 consecutive patients receiving 1 of 5 regimens of HDC with PBPC support in a multicenter, community-based clinical trial.

Study Design.—A retrospective analysis was conducted of the first 1,000 consecutive adult patients with leukemia, non-Hodgkin's lymphoma, Hodgkin's disease, multiple myeloma, sarcoma, ovarian cancer, or breast cancer, who were treated between February 1989 and September 1994 with one of 5 published HDC regimens, followed by PBPC support in 28 community medical centers under the care of 159 oncologists. Of these 1,000 patients, 707 were treated with cyclophosphamide, thiopeta, and carboplatin (CTCb); 173 were treated with carmustine, etoposide, cytarabine, and cyclophosphamide (BEAC); 56 were treated with busulfan, melphalan, and thiopeta (BuMelT); 35 were treated with ifosfamide, carboplatin, and etoposide (ICE); and 29 were treated with busulfan and cyclophosphamide (BuCy). Treatment-related mortality was analyzed in this group of patients.

Findings.—Of the 1,000 patients treated with HDC with PBPC support in community medical centers, 5.9% died within 100 days of PBPC infusion. Of these 59 patients, 25 died predominantly of disease progression, whereas 34 died of TRM. Of the 34 TRM deaths, 15 were from infection and 19 were from regimen-related toxicities (RRT). Logistic regression demonstrated that increasing age and lower number of CD34[+] cells/kg were significantly associated with an increased risk of TRM within 100 days. The high-dose CTCb regimen was associated with a lower mortality risk than the other 4 high-dose regimens used in this study.

Conclusions.—This study examined the treatment-related mortality of 1,000 adult patients treated in community health centers with high-dose chemotherapy and peripheral blood progenitor cell support. This type of therapy was administered successfully from community-based health programs, with no apparent increase in treatment-related mortality. Patient age, the type of high-dose chemotherapeutic regimen used, and the number of CD34[+] infused were significant prognostic factors.

▶ Over the past several years, we have reviewed the results of peripheral blood stem cell transplantation in a variety of diseases - acute and chronic leukemias, aggressive and indolent lymphomas, multiple myeloma and a variety of solid tumors. In some of these disorders, particularly selected aggressive lymphomas, high-dose chemotherapy combined with peripheral blood stem cell transplantation appears to convey some benefit. In other disorders, for example advanced Hodgkin's disease and advanced breast cancer, the procedure seems to be of little value. In many instances, and in both responsive and unresponsive diseases, the procedure has been widely applied in many different medical settings—in part because it is technically rather simple, and in part because it (unlike allogeneic bone marrow transplantation) has a low associated mortality. This article examines the mortality rate in a large group of patients treated at community cancer centers. Mortality was about 3.5% and was influenced by the age of the patient, the drug program, and the number of stem cells collected and infused.

My guess is that it will take thousands more patients and another 10 years before we have clearly defined those situations in which high-dose therapy combined with peripheral blood stem cell transplantation has real usefulness.

M.J. Cline, M.D.

Results of Allogeneic Bone Marrow Transplants For Leukemia Using Donors Other Than HLA-Identical Siblings

Szydlo R, Goldman JM, Klein JP, et al (Hammersmith Hosp, London; Med College of Wisconsin, Milwaukee; Salick Health Care Inc, Los Angeles; et al)
J Clin Oncol 15:1767–1777, 1997   13–2

Background.—Because most patients with leukemia who may benefit from a bone marrow transplant have no HLA-identical sibling, the outcomes of transplants from alternative donors need to be investigated. There have been no large studies comparing HLA-mismatched–related with unrelated donor transplants.

Methods.—The study included 2,055 recipients of allogeneic bone marrow transplants for chronic myelogenous leukemia, acute myelogenous leukemia, and acute lymphoblastic leukemia. Donors were 1,224 HLA-identical siblings; 238 haploidentical relatives mismatched for 1 HLA-A, HLA-B, or HLA-DR antigen; 102 haploidentical relatives mismatched for 2 HLA-A, HLA-B, or HLA-DR antigen; 383 unrelated persons HLA-matched, and 108 unrelated persons mismatched for 1 HLA-A, HLA-B, or HLA-DR antigen.

Findings.—Recipients of alternative donor transplant tissue had significantly greater transplant-related mortality than recipients of HLA-identical sibling tissue. Transplant-related mortality at 3 years in patients with early leukemia was 21% after HLA-identical sibling transplants and more than 50% after all types of alternative donor transplants. In patients with early leukemia, the relative risks of treatment failure, using HLA-identical sibling transplants as the reference, were 2.43 after 1-HLA-antigen–mismatched related donors, 3.79 after 2-HLA-antigen–mismatched related donors, 2.11 after HLA-matched unrelated donors, and 3.33 after 1-HLA-antigen–mismatched unrelated donors. Differences in treatment failure were less marked among patients with more advanced leukemia. The corresponding relative risks of such failure were 1.22, 1.81, 1.39, and 1.63, respectively.

Conclusion.—Although alternative donor transplants are effective in some patients, treatment failure is higher after such transplantation than after HLA-identical sibling transplants. Outcomes depend on how advanced the leukemia is, the relationship between the donor and the recipient, and the degree of HLA matching. Patients with early leukemia have a more than twofold greater risk of treatment failure after alternative donor transplantation than patients receiving HLA-identical sibling tissue.

▶ The objective of this study was to compare the results of allogeneic bone marrow transplantation in leukemia using various categories of donors—HLA-identical siblings, HLA-mismatched relatives, and unrelated donors. The results are not surprising, but they are instructive and provide data on which to base decisions when one is contemplating allogeneic bone marrow transplantation with a donor who is less than ideal, i.e., a donor who is not an HLA-identical sibling.

As anticipated, allogeneic bone marrow transplantation from an HLA-identical sibling had the best results and was used as the standard of comparison for transplants from other types of donors. For patients treated for "early" leukemia, transplant-related mortality was over twice as high when donors other than HLA-identical siblings were used, and treatment failure was 2 to 4 times higher. For patients with more advanced leukemia, the differences between "perfect" and "imperfect" donors were less striking, but this was largely the result of the fact that these patients do poorly under all conditions, even when an HLA-identical sibling is used as the donor.

M.J. Cline, M.D.

Influence of Age on the Outcome of 500 Autologous Bone Marrow Transplant Procedures for Hematologic Malignancies

Kusnierz-Glaz CR, Schlegel PG, Wong RM, et al (Stanford Univ, Calif)
J Clin Oncol 15:18–25, 1997   13–3

Background.—Although age has a major role in the outcome of alloge-neic bone marrow transplantation, the effect of age on the outcome of high-dose therapy and autologous bone marrow transplantation is unclear. Results of autologous bone marrow transplantation in individuals older than 50 years are important because diseases such as acute myelogenous leukemia, non-Hodgkin's lymphoma, and multiple myeloma are more common in older individuals.

Methods.—A retrospective analysis was conducted of 500 consecutive patients who had autologous bone marrow transplantation for Hodgkin's disease, non-Hodgkin's lymphoma, multiple myeloma, or acute myeloge-nous leukemia. Patients were categorized into minimal or advanced disease groups. Patients were between 1 year and 65 years old.

Results.—At 5 years, the event-free survival rate was 44%, the relapse rate was 47%, and regimen-related mortality was 8.6%. The strongest predictor of event-free survival and relapse was disease status at the time of transplantation. In patients with minimal disease, the event-free survival rate was 48% and the relapse rate was 43%. In patients with advanced disease, the event-free survival rate was 30% and the relapse rate was 72%. The rate of event-free survival was 46% in patients younger than 50 years and 34% in patients 50 years or older (Fig 2). Age was predictive of

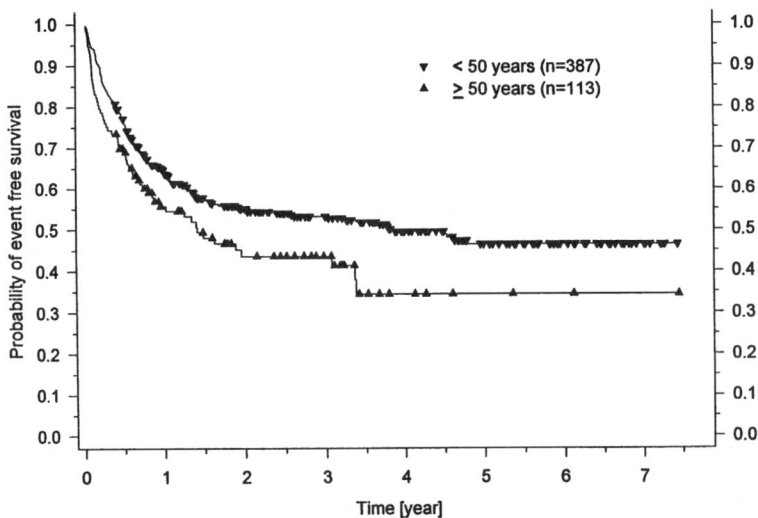

FIGURE 2.—Probability of event-free survival after autologous transplantation in 500 patients youn-ger than 50 years and 50 years or older (P < 0.03). (Courtesy of Kusnierz-Glaz CR, Schlegel PG, Wong RM, et al: Influence of age on the outcome of 500 autologous bone marrow transplant procedures for hematologic malignancies. *J Clin Oncol* 15:18–25, 1997.)

event-free survival. The regimen-related mortality rate was 7.4% in patients younger than 50 years and 12.7% in patients 50 years or older. The factors most predictive of regimen-related mortality were age and period of transplantation.

Discussion.—Although older patients have a lower long-term event-free survival rate after autologous bone marrow transplantation, a high percentage of patients have a disease-free outcome. This treatment should not be limited based only on the age of the patient. The upper age limit for autologous bone marrow transplantation remains to be determined.

▶ Autologous bone marrow transplantation is being used increasingly in hematologic malignancies such as high-grade lymphoma, multiple myeloma, and acute leukemia. Autologous bone marrow transplantation or its allied procedure, peripheral blood stem cell transplantation, is widely used in medical centers throughout the world. It is popular, in part, because most patients with hematologic malignancies survive the procedure of *autologous* bone marrow transplantation, whereas at least 20% of patients undergoing *allogeneic* bone marrow transplantation die of transplant-related complications.

This study examines the effect of age of the patient on the outcome of autologous bone marrow transplantation. A large number of cases from a single medical center were examined. Not surprisingly, patients younger than 50 years did better than those older than 50 years; however, many patients up to age 65 years did well. It appears, therefore, that we should not exclude patients between ages 50 and 65 years. Interestingly, the actuarial 5-year disease-free survival in the group as a whole was a remarkable 44%. The strongest predictor of outcome was disease status (minimal vs. advanced) at the time of autologous bone marrow transplantation.

M.J. Cline, M.D.

Donor Leukocyte Infusions in 140 Patients With Relapsed Malignancy After Allogeneic Bone Marrow Transplantation
Collins RH Jr, Shpilberg O, Drobyski WR, et al (Texas Oncology, Dallas; Baylor Univ, Dallas; Chaim Sheba Med Ctr, Tel-Hashomer, Israel; et al)
J Clin Oncol 15:433–444, 1997   13–4

Background.—Allogeneic bone marrow transplantation (BMT) has antileukemic, or graft-versus-leukemia (GVL), activity. In an effort to enhance this activity, leukocytes from the original donor have been reinfused into relapsed recipients. To understand the benefits and toxicities associated with this donor leukocyte infusion (DLI), data from 140 patients from 25 North American BMT centers were analyzed retrospectively.

Study Design.—Of the 100 North American BMT centers contacted, 50 had performed the DLI procedures, and 25 of these returned a complete questionnaire evaluating the following: patient demographics, diagnosis, BMT procedure, post-BMT relapse, DLI, response to DLI, post-DLI com-

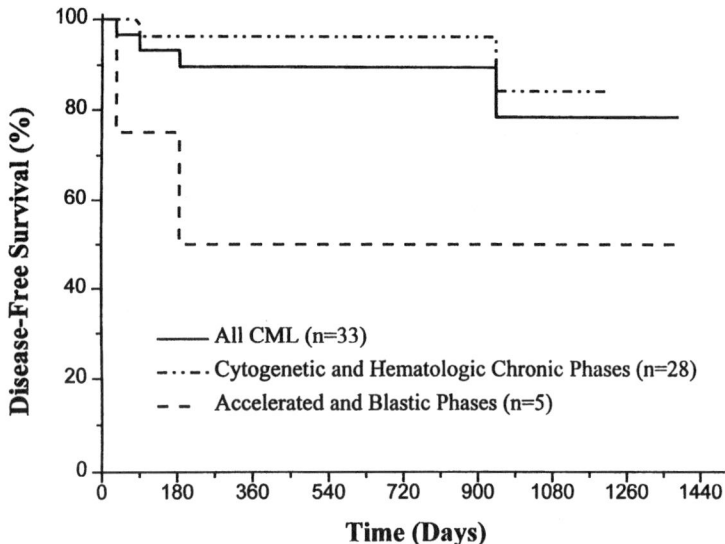

FIGURE 2.—DFS in CML patients who achieved CR after DLI. (Courtesy of Collins RH Jr, Shpilberg O, Drobyski WR, et al: Donor leukocyte infusions in 140 patients with relapsed malignancy after allogeneic bone marrow transplantation. *J Clin Oncol* 15:433–444, 1997.)

plications, and follow-up. The study group consisted of 140 patients who had received DLI. Patients were categorized as follows: 56 chronic myelogenous leukemia (CML) 46 with acute myelogenous leukemia (AML), 15 with acute lymphoblastic (ALL), 6 with myelodysplastic syndrome (MDS), 6 with non-Hodgkin's lymphoma (NHL), 5 with myeloma, 2 with Hodgkin's disease, 2 with juvenile CML, 1 with chronic lymphocytic leukemia (CLL), and 1 with Fanconi's anemia and myelodysplasia.

Findings.—A complete response (CR) was achieved by 60% of the CML patients who received DLI without chemotherapy. The response rate was higher in patients with cytogenetic or chronic-phase relapse, than in patients with accelerated-phase or blastic-phase relapse. The actuarial probability of remaining in CR at 2 years for these CML patients was over 89% (Fig 2). The complete remission rate for AML was 15.4%, and for ALL it was 18.2%. Complete response also was achieved by 2 of 4 assessable myeloma patients and 2 of 5 assessable myelodysplasia patients. The complications of DLI included both acute and chronic graft-versus-host (GVH) disease and pancytopenia. Prognostic factors included post-BMT chronic GVH disease, chronic phase disease status, and less than 2 years between BMT and DLI. After DLI, both acute and chronic GVH disease were significantly associated with disease response.

Conclusions.—A retrospective study was performed of 140 patients who underwent donor leukocyte infusion after relapse following allogeneic BMT. This study confirmed a high rate of complete, durable remission in patients with relapsed cytogenetic or chronic-phase CML. Complete remission did not occur with as high a frequency in patients with other hematologic malignancies in this study group. Side effects of DLI included pancytopenia and GVH disease. The occurrence of GVH disease following DLI was strongly associated with disease response.

▶ The graft-versus-leukemia effect of allogeneic bone marrow transplantation has been documented by a large number of observations of various types. The presumed mechanism is an attack on leukemic cells by immunologically competent cells in the donor bone marrow.

A few years ago this concept was used in designing a program in which donor leukocytes were infused into patients whose chronic leukemia had relapsed after an allogeneic bone marrow transplant. It was recognized that GVH disease (i.e., an immune attack on other tissues of the marrow recipient) would be an undesirable side effect of such therapy.

This article summarizes the recent experience with donor leukocyte infusion in transplant patients with relapsed leukemia. The results are surprisingly good in chronic myelocytic leukemia and not so good in other types of leukemia.

Donor leukocyte infusion in transplant patients with relapsed chronic myelocytic leukemia was associated with an overall complete response rate of 60% and an actuarial 2-year survival rate of nearly 90% in responders. In acute myelocytic leukemia and acute lymphocytic leukemia, the response rate was only 15%.

Antileukemic response to donor leukocyte infusion was highly correlated with GVH disease, and so many of the patients were quite sick, and some may well die, as a result of the treatment itself. Nevertheless, donor leukocyte infusion may be a valid option when everything else looks bleak after bone marrow transplantation for leukemia.

M.J. Cline, M.D.

Allogeneic Peripheral Blood Stem Cell Transplantation in Patients With Advanced Hematologic Malignancies: A Retrospective Comparison With Marrow Transplantation
Bensinger WI, Clift R, Martin P, et al (Univ of Washingotn, Seattle)
Blood 88:2794–2800, 1996   13–5

Background.—Preliminary studies indicate that HLA-identical allogeneic peripheral blood stem cells (PBSCs) produce prompt, complete hematopoietic engraftment without increasing the incidence or severity of acute graft-versus-host disease (GVHD). However, there have been no formal comparisons of HLA-identical allogeneic PBSC transplants and bone marrow (BM) transplants. A formal, retrospective case-control design was used to compare outcomes in one group receiving HLA-identical allogeneic PBSC transplants and another group previously transplanted with BM.

Methods.—Thirty-seven patients with advanced hematologic malignancies undergoing allogeneic PBSC transplants from HLA-identical siblings were included. The historical control group consisted of 37 similar patients with advanced hematologic malignancies undergoing BM transplants from HLA-identical donors. The patients undergoing BM transplants were treated between 1989 and 1994.

Findings.—Engraftment, determined by time to a peripheral neutrophil count exceeding 500/L and a platelet count of more than 20,000/μL without transfusions, occurred on days 14 and 11, respectively, in the patients transplanted with PBSC. In the patients receiving BM, engraftment occurred on days 16 and 15, respectively. The median red blood cell and platelet requirements were 8 and 24 U, respectively, in the PBSC group compared with 17 and 118 U in the BM transplant group. The estimated risks of developing grades 2 to 4 acute GVHD in the PBSC and BM groups were 37% and 56%, respectively. The estimated risks of grades 3 to 4 acute GVHD were 14% and 33% for the PBSC and BM groups, respectively. Chronic GVHD developed in 7 of the 18 patients receiving PBSC and in 6 of the 23 patients undergoing BM transplantation who could be evaluated. The estimated risks of transplant-related death at 200 days were 27% in the PBSC group and 45% in the BM group. Estimated risks of relapse were 70% and 53%, respectively, in the PBSC and BM groups. Overall survival rates were 50% and 41%, respectively.

Conclusions.—Allogeneic PBSC transplantation from HLA-identical donors appears to be associated with faster engraftment and fewer transfusions than BM transplantation from HLA-identical donors. The incidence of acute or chronic GVHD is no greater with allogeneic PBSC transplantation from HLA-identical donors.

▶ This study compares peripheral blood with bone marrow as a source of hematopoietic stem cells in allogeneic transplantation of patients with hematologic malignancy. The bottom line is that peripheral blood stem cells are no worse and are probably better than bone marrow as a resource for hematopoietic reconstitution after intensive therapy.

From the donor's perspective it is a tossup whether donating blood cells is superior to donating bone marrow. Most prefer the white cell collection technique, but some prefer the marrow donation (despite the anesthesia) to sometimes multiple sessions on a white cell separator.

M.J. Cline, M.D.

Outcome of Cord-Blood Transplantation From Related and Unrelated Donors
Gluckman E, for the Eurocord Transplant Group and the European Blood and Marrow Transplantation Group (Hôpital Saint-Louis, Paris; et al)
N Engl J Med 337:373–381, 1997   13–6

Background.—Cord blood banks have been developed worldwide so that cord blood can be used as a source of hematopoietic stem cells. This report describes an analysis of 143 cord blood transplantations performed between October 1988 and December 1996 at 45 European centers.

Study Design.—Questionnaires concerning disease, outcome, cord blood origin, number of cells collected and infused, HLA typing and hematologic reconstitution were sent to 45 transplantation centers. The study group consisted of 78 patients who received cord blood from a related donor and 65 patients who received cord blood from an unrelated donor. These 2 groups were analyzed separately.

Findings.—Among the patients who received cord blood from related donors, the Kaplan-Meier estimate of survival at 1 year was 63%. Favorable prognostic factors in the recipient included younger age, lower weight, transplants from HLA-identical donors and cytomegalovirus-negative serologic test results. Graft-versus-host disease of grade II or higher occurred in only 9% of the 60 recipients of HLA-matched, but in 50% of the 18 recipients of HLA-mismatched cord blood. Neutrophil engraftment occurred in 85% of patients receiving at least 37 million nucleated cells per kg, and was associated with younger age and lower weight. Among the 65 recipients who received cord blood from unrelated donors, the 1-year Kaplan-Meier survival estimate was 29%. The most important predictor of graft-versus-host disease in this subset of patients was cytomegalovirus serologic status.

Conclusions.—Cord blood can be a useful alternative source of hematopoietic stem cells for children and some adults with hematologic diseases, especially if the donor and recipient are related.

▶ Cord blood transplantation is a relatively new approach to the treatment of those diseases that may be benefited by the infusion of allogeneic stem cells. Such cells are usually obtained from the bone marrow or by leukopheresis of peripheral blood of a suitable donor. They are then used either in bone marrow transplantation or in peripheral blood stem cell infusion. Several centers have set up "banks" of frozen stored cord-blood cells for use in patients with aplastic anemia, leukemia, and other congenital or malignant diseases.

This report examines the results of 143 transplants with cord blood cells. When the cord blood came from *related* donors, the 1-year survival was 63%. When the cord blood came from *unrelated* donors, the 1-year survival was only 29%.

When the cord blood cells were from HLA-matched related donors, significant graft-versus-host disease occurred in only 9% of recipients—a small percentage.

These figures must be considered as crude because patients with a large variety of different diseases were being transplanted. Nevertheless, they do show that cord blood transplantation is feasible in some patients, especially those in the pediatric age range where the requirement for the number of stem cells is not as high as it is in adult patients.

M.J. Cline, M.D.

Extensive Amplification and Self-Renewal of Human Primitive Hematopoietic Stem Cells From Cord Blood

Piacibello W, Sanavio F, Garetto L, et al (Univ of Torino, Italy; Ospedale Mauriziano, Torino, Italy; Inst for Cancer Research and Treatment, Candiolo, Italy)
Blood 89:2644–2653, 1997   13–7

Introduction.—Cord blood is a possible alternative to bone marrow or growth factor mobilized peripheral blood cells as a source of transplantable hematopoietic tissue. The limited amount of hematopoietic stem cells may be adequate to reconstitute children but not adults. Ex vivo manipulations may be needed to engraft an adult. Described is an in vivo system in which the growth of cord blood CD34+ cells is sustained and greatly expanded for more than 6 months by a combination of 2 hematopoietic growth factors.

Methods.—Progenitors and cells belonging to all hematopoietic lineages were continuously and increasingly produced using extensive amplification and self-renewal.

Results.—At the end of 6 months of culture, the number of colony-forming unit–granulocyte-macrophage [CFU-GM] were well over 2,000,000-fold the CFU-GM present when the culture was created (Fig 2). After 20 weeks of liquid culture, even the very primitive hematopoietic progenitors—including the long-term culture-initiating cells (LTC-ICs) and blast cell colony-forming units—were greatly expanded to over 200,000 the original number.

Conclusion.—The remarkable prolonged maintenance and the massive expansion of these progenitors—which share many qualities of murine long-term repopulating cells—suggest that extensive renewal and little differentiation occur. This system may be of use in diverse clinical settings that involve treatment of grown-up children and adults with transplantation of normal genetically manipulated hematopoietic stem cells.

▶ Cord blood has been considered as a source of hematopoietic stem cells. It has many obvious advantages over the more common sources—bone marrow and peripheral blood. Some blood banks are stockpiling cord blood

FIGURE 2.—Different stages of hematopoiesis in stroma-free LTC of cord blood (CB) CD34+ cells. (A), expansion of hematopoietic cells in stroma-free cultures stimulated by thrombopoietin (TPO) (10 U/mL) alone (*solid circles*), by FLT3 (FL) (50 ng/mL) alone (*open circles*), and by the combination of TPO (10 U/mL) plus FL (50 ng/mL) (*solid squares*). The starting population was represented by 2×10^3 CD34+ CB cells in 1 mL in 24–well plates. Fresh growth factors were added twice a week. Cells were counted weekly from quadruplicate wells and the fold increase was obtained by dividing the number of cells of each well counted each week by the number of the starting population. Represented here is the mean ± SEM of 4 different experiments (each performed in quadruplicate). (B), expansion of the CD34+ (*solid squares*) and the CD34+ CD38− (*solid circle*) cell populations during LTC with FL plus TPO. Cord blood CD34+ cells were grown for 25 weeks. Every 2 to 3 weeks the cells harvested were stained with fluorescein isothiocyanate and phycoerythrin-conjugated anti-CD34 and anti-CD38 monoclonal antibody. The total number of each subpopulation was obtained by multiplying the percentage of each subset by the number of cells contained in each well. Results are expressed as the fold increase (compared with the starting subpopulation) and represent the mean ± SEM of analyses performed on quadruplicate wells in 4 separate experiments. (*open squares*) CD34+ cells in LTC grown in the presence of FL alone. (*open circles*)
(*Continued*)

FIGURE 2 (cont.)

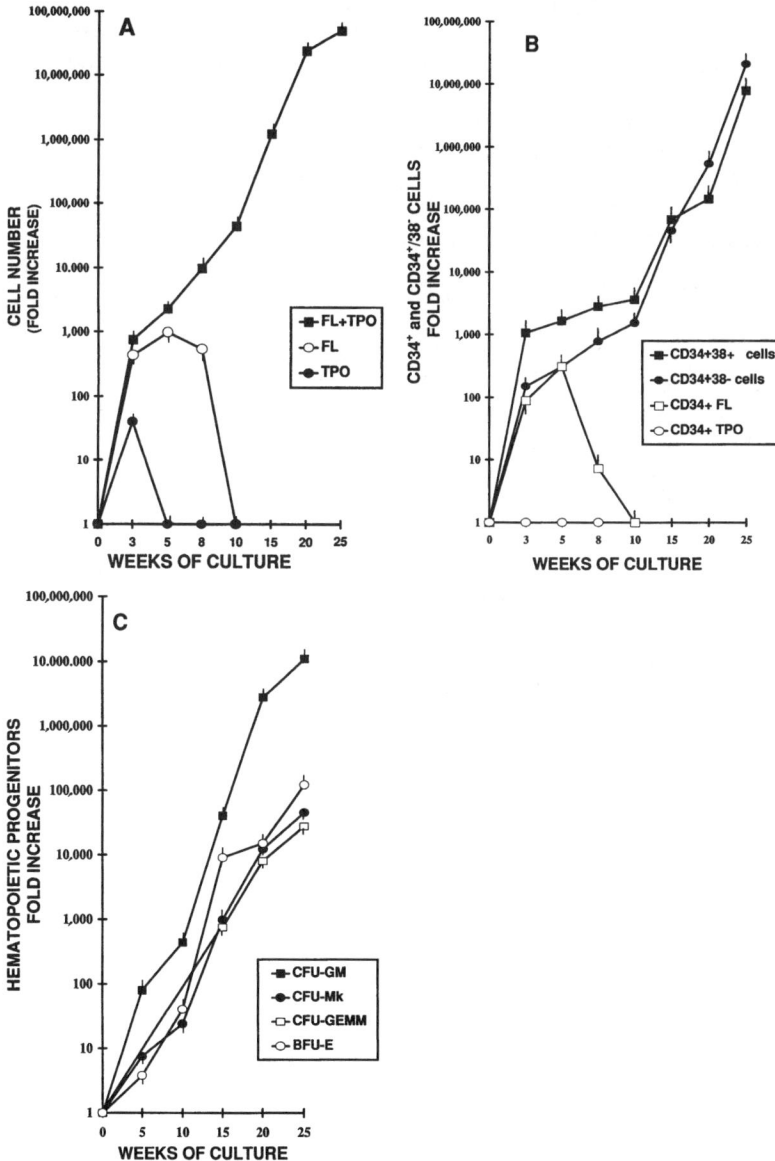

CD34+ cells in LTC grown in the presence of TPO alone. (C), production of hematopoietic progenitors in LTC in the presence of FL plus TPO. CD34+ CB cells were grown for 25 weeks. *Abbreviations*: CFU-GM, colony forming units–granulocyte-macrophage; *CFU-MK*, colony-forming units–megakaryocyte; *BFU-E*, burst-forming units–erythroid; *CFU-GEMM*, colony-forming units–granulocyte, erythroid, monocyte, megakaryocyte. Results represent the fold increase of each class of progenitors present in each well in determined periods of LTC, compared with the number of progenitors of the beginning of the cultures. Mean ± SEM of 4 wells per point in 4 separate experiments. (Courtesy of Piacibello W, Sanavio F, Garetto L, et al: Extensive amplification and self-renewal of human primitive hematopoietic stem cells from cord blood. *Blood* 89:2644–2653, 1997.)

for use in allogeneic bone marrow transplantation. One of the main limitations on the use of cord blood is the limited volume and relatively limited number of stem cells available from any 1 pregnancy. Investigators have considered that these numbers may be adequate for pediatric bone marrow transplantation but inadequate for the procedure in adults.

This article describes a remarkable expansion of hematopoietic stem cells from cord blood by cultivation in vitro with growth factors. Primitive stem cells increased by 200,000-fold over the course of several months. A technological advance such as this may open the way for widespread use of hematopoietic stem cells in cancer treatment and gene therapy.

M.J. Cline, M.D.

Solid Cancers After Bone Marrow Transplantation
Curtis RE, Rowlings PA, Deeg HJ, et al (Natl Cancer Inst, Bethesda, Md; Med College of Wisconsin, Milwaukee; Fred Hutchinson Cancer Research Ctr, Seattle; et al)
N Engl J Med 336:897–904, 1997   13–8

Background.—Bone marrow transplantation (BMT) is an effective treatment for leukemia and other disorders, but may be associated with late effects, such as new cancers, potentiated by compromised immune system function and the severe conditioning regimens used for transplantation. The risk of new solid cancers after BMT was investigated using a multi-institution data base.

Methods.—Data were derived from the International Bone Marrow Transplantation Registry (IBMTR) which includes the record of 234 transplantation centers from 1964 to 1990 and the Fred Hutchinson Cancer Research Center records from 1969 to 1992, for a total of 19,229 BMT recipients in the study population. The median age of participants at the time of transplant was 25.5 years.

Results.—Among the 19,229 transplant recipients in this series, there were 80 cases of new solid cancers. This was significantly higher than the rate expected for the general population. The cumulative incidence rate was 2.2% at 10 years and 6.7% at 15 years. The risk of malignant melanoma and cancer of the buccal cavity, liver, central nervous system, thyroid, bone and connective tissue was elevated for the study group. The cancer risk was significantly higher for patients who were younger at the time of transplantation. Multivariate analysis indicated that higher doses of total-body irradiation were associated with increased risk of solid cancer. Chronic graft-vs.-host disease and male sex were associated with squamous-cell cancers of the buccal cavity and skin.

Conclusions.—Bone marrow transplanation prolongs survival in many patients with life-threatening conditions, but is also associated with a significantly increased risk of new solid cancers later in life. This risk is higher for those who receive transplants at a younger age and increases over time. These results indicate that transplant recipients should be followed continually to detect precursor or early cancerous lesions and should be counseled to avoid exposure to carcinogens which may increase their risk of developing solid cancers.

▶ The risk of solid tumors in those surviving 10 or more years after bone marrow transplantation is over eightfold above that in the general population, and the risk continues to increase at 15 years. As the authors point out, the increasing risk with increasing time and the greater risk among young patients signals the need for lifelong surveillance for solid tumors. As I look back to the early days of bone marrow transplantation—which, for me, began in the late 1960s—I find it startling to consider that a retrospective survey of the years 1964 to 1992 encompasses over 19,000 transplanted patients.

M.J. Cline, M.D

Posttransplantation Lymphoproliferative Disorders in Bone Marrow Transplant Recipients Are Aggressive Diseases With a High Incidence of Adverse Histologic and Immunobiologic Features
Orazi A, Hromas RA, Neiman RS, et al (Indiana Univ, Indianapolis; Univ of Nebraska, Omaha)
Am J Clin Pathol 107:419–429, 1997   13–9

Introduction.—In organ transplant recipients receiving immunosuppressive therapies, posttransplantation lymphoproliferative disorders (PT-LPDs) are a well-documented complication. Reports focusing on the characteristics of these disorders following allogeneic bone marrow transplantation are few. The overall incidence of PT-LPDs varies from 0.6% to 7.4%, with a higher incidence (16% to 20%) in transplants from unrelated or mismatched donors. Bone marrow transplant recipients have a high incidence of extensive dissemination of this disorder at presentation, an aggressive course, and a high fatality rate when compared to recipients of solid organs. A group of patients receiving bone marrow transplants were examined for the clinical characteristics, the histologic and immunohistologic features, the proliferative fraction, and the genotypic status of their PT-LPDs.

Methods.—Ten patients with PT-LPDs were studied after T-cell–depleted allogeneic bone marrow transplantation. The morphological characteristics of the lesions and their clonality based on immunoglobulin heavy-chain gene rearrangement by polymerase chain reaction analysis and immunohistochemistry were studied. The proliferative activity of the lesions was measured by immunoperoxidase staining for the proliferating cell nuclear antigen (PCNA) and p53 gene product overexpression was studied. Epstein-Barr virus (EBV) was evaluated by anti-EBV latent membrane protein and by polymerase chain reaction analysis for the EBV genome (Fig 1).

Results.—Seven patients had polymorphic B-cell lymphoma and 3 had malignant immunoblastic lymphoma. Four of the patients with polymor-

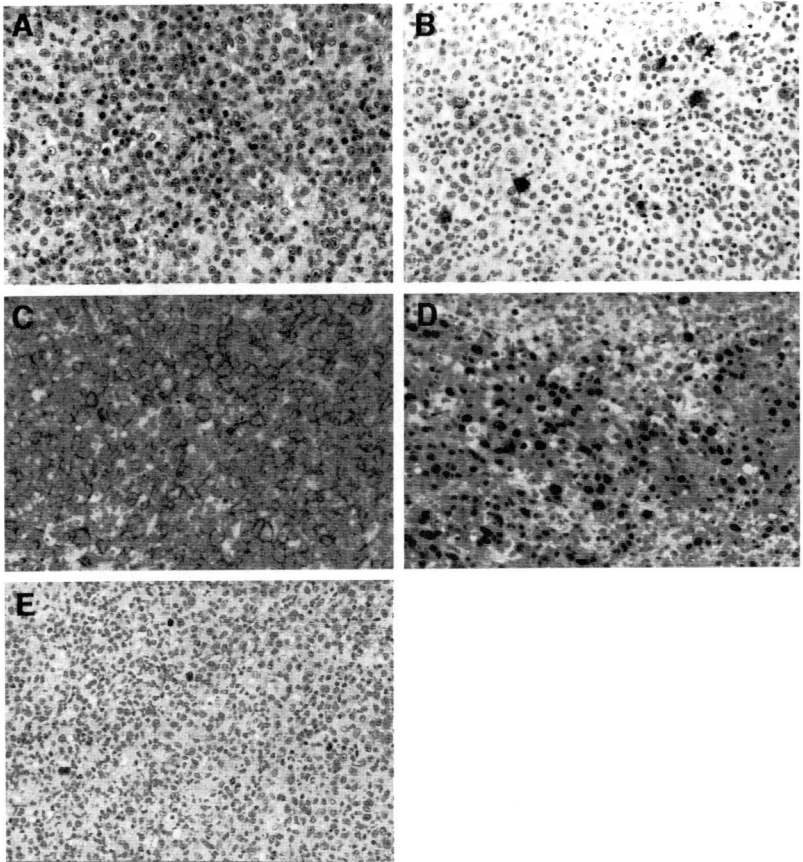

FIGURE 1.—Histopathology and immunohistochemical staining of the posttransplantation lympho-proliferative disorders in bone marrow transplant recipients. **A,** polymorphic B-cell lymphoma is characterized by a polymorphic cell infiltrate lacking prominent plasmacytic differentiation and large cells showing cytologic atypia; hematoxylin-eosin; original magnification, ×480. **B,** Epstein-Barr virus latent membrane protein positive expression in a proportion of the cells, mostly large cells. **C,** CD20 strongly expressed in numerous cells. **D,** proliferating cell nuclear antigen nuclear positivity in approximately 60% of the lymphoid cells. **E,** p53 expression in a small proportion of the nuclei (**B–E,** immunoperoxidase, diluted hematoxylin counterstain, original magnification, ×480). (Reprinted with permission, from Orazi A, Hromas RA, Neiman RS, et al: Posttransplantation lymphoproliferative disorders in bone marrow transplant recipients are aggressive diseases with a high incidence of adverse histologic and immunobiologic features. *Am J Clin Pathol* 107:419–429, 1997. Copyright © 1997 by the American Society of Clinical Pathologists. Reprinted with permission.)

phic B-cell lymphoma had B-cell monoclonality by immunologic or genotypic criteria or both. All 3 of the patients with malignant immunoblastic lymphoma had B-cell clonality by genotypic analysis, but 2 were polyclonal by immunologic analysis. All 10 patients had the EBV genome, the expression of EBV-LMP, or both. The patients with polymorphic B-cell lymphoma averaged PCNA expression of 58%, and the patients with malignant immunoblastic lymphoma averaged PCNA expression of 84%. Five patients tested positive for p53. With the administration of donor leukocytes, 2 of 4 cases of polymorphic B-cell lymphoma resolved; the rest of the patients died of PT-LPD within a short time of diagnosis.

Conclusion.—A high frequency of high-grade histologic subtypes, high proliferative activity, frequent monoclonality, frequent overexpression of p53 gene product, and poor prognosis are the characteristics of PT-LPDs after T-cell–depleted bone marrow transplantation.

▶ Lymphoproliferative disorders occur as a complication of both solid organ transplantation and bone marrow transplantation. They are frequent after transplantation of the heart or heart and lungs. After allogeneic bone marrow transplantation, lymphoproliferative syndromes are most frequent when the donor marrow is not a perfect match with the recipient and is depleted of T cells in an effort to prevent graft-vs.-host disease.

Lymphoproliferative syndromes that follow allogeneic bone marrow transplantation tend to be aggressive, multi-focal at their outset and have a high mortality rate. Most commonly the onset is between 2 and 6 months posttransplantation. Fever, rash, and lymphadenopathy are frequent, with variable involvement of other organ systems.

The histologic patterns of these lymphoproliferative syndromes are those of lymphomas with either (1) loss of nodal architecture with a mixture of B lymphocytes at various stages of differentiation (polymorphic B cell lymphoma) or (2) loss of nodal architecture with a uniform population of primitive lymphoid cells (immunoblastic lymphoma). In this study, only 3 of 7 cases of polymorphic B cell lymphoma arose from a single abnormal cell, i.e., were monoclonal, whereas all 3 cases of immunoblastic lymphoma were monoclonal. This observation suggests that in the polymorphic B cell syndrome there is a general stimulation of proliferation of many B cell clones. The fact that 2 of 4 cases resolved with administration of donor leukocytes further suggests that the source of the lymphocyte proliferation is the host, i.e., the patient recipient.

M.J. Cline, M.D.

HSV-TK Gene Transfer Into Donor Lymphocytes for Control of Allogeneic Graft-Versus-Leukemia
Bonini C, Ferrari G, Verzeletti S, et al (Istituto Scientifico HS Raffaele, Milan, Italy)
Science 276:1719–1724, 1997   13–10

Background.—Allogeneic bone marrow transplantation (allo-BMT) is the treatment of choice for many hematologic malignancies but is limited by the occurrence of the potentially life-threatening complication of graft-versus-host (GVH) disease. There is no specific treatment for GVH disease. The genetic manipulation of donor lymphocytes was attempted to incorporate a "suicide gene" that could be activated in the event of GVH disease, to make allo-BMT safer and more effective for a wider range of patients.

Methods.—Donor lymphocytes were transduced with a viral vector carrying a selectable marker and the herpes simplex virus thymidine kinase (HSV-TK) "suicide gene," which confers sensitivity to ganciclovir. After transduction, the cells were subjected to 1 round of selection to ensure that virtually 100% were carrying the "suicide gene." Twelve patients participated in this study, and this report describes follow-up on 8 of them.

Results.—The transduced cells survived for at least 12 months and could be detected in the patients' circulation, marrow aspirates, and tissue biopsies. In 5 of the 8 patients, graft-versus-leukemia (GVL) activity could be detected, with 3 patients having complete responses. Three patients developed GVH disease and were treated with ganciclovir. Treatment with ganciclovir resulted in elimination of all symptoms and signs of GVH disease, without any toxicity. Two of these patients who had achieved complete remission before the development of GVH disease remained in complete remission after ganciclovir treatment. No toxicity was observed that was related to the gene transfer procedure or to ganciclovir treatment.

Conclusions.—This study demonstrates that the transfer of "suicide genes" to donor lymphocytes before allo-BMT provides a new therapeutic tool which combines the benefits of allo-BMT with the possibility of eliminating GVH disease without toxicity. Genetic manipulation of donor lymphocytes has the potential to increase the number of patients who can benefit from allo-BMT, as well as to increase its safety and efficacy.

▶ The lymphocytes in donor bone marrow used in allogeneic bone marrow transplantation are potentially 2-edged swords. On the one hand, they are necessary to reconstitute the immune system of the recipient of the transplant and to attack residual leukemic cells. On the other hand, they may induce GVH disease in the recipient, which can vary in severity from mild to lethal.

This article describes an ingenious use of gene therapy in preserving the positive attributes of donor lymphocytes, while controlling their potential to mediate severe GVH disease. The trick was to introduce a "suicide" gene into the donor lymphocytes that made them uniquely sensitive to a drug (ganciclovir) that has no effect on other cells of the recipient. With this "suicide" gene on board, the lymphocytes could be infused for their anti-tumor effect. Once they got too pesky and started attacking the host they could simply be eliminated by administering ganciclovir. Wonderful!

M.J. Cline, M.D.

Complete Short-Term Correction of Canine Hemophilia A by In Vivo Gene Therapy
Connelly S, Mount J, Mauser A, et al (Genetic Therapy Inc, Gaithersburg, Md; Auburn Univ, Al)
Blood 88:3846–3853, 1996   13–11

Background.—Canine hemophilia A is a well-documented model of hemophilia A in human beings. The bleeding disorder in factor VIII

(FVIII)–deficient dogs has been shown to be corrected by plasma-derived and recombinant human FVIII protein. Also, FVIII inhibitors frequently develop in treated dogs. The utility of an adenoviral vector expressing a human FVIII complementary DNA in correcting the hemophilia A phenotype was determined in the canine model.

Methods and Findings.—Mixed-breed dogs were given adenoviral vector through the peripheral vein. Within 48 hours, the hemophilic phenotype was corrected, as demonstrated by activated clotting time, activated partial thromboplastin time, and cuticle bleeding time. Direct measures of human FVIII in the plasma demonstrated FVIII expression in amounts that far exceeded human therapeutic levels. The expression of FVIII in treated dogs lasted only 1 to 2 weeks because of the development of a human FVIII-specific inhibitor antibody response.

Conclusions.—Canine hemophilia A was corrected effectively with noninvasive, peripheral vein administration of a human FVIII adenoviral vector. Further advances in vector design are needed to enable sustained expression.

▶ This study is an illustration of the real progress being made, at least in the laboratory, in the field of gene therapy. The investigators address hemophilia A, an important human disease for which there is a valid animal model.

Instead of the more widely used retroviral gene vector, they used a modified adenovirus as the vector to introduce a human factor VIII gene into factor VIII–deficient dogs. Within the remarkably brief time of 48 hours, therapeutic levels of human factor VIII were present in the blood of the dogs.

One measure of progress in the field is that this study, which would have been considered remarkable only a few years ago, was published in a specialty journal of limited readership rather than in a premier scientific journal, such as *Science* or *Nature*.

M.J. Cline, M.D.

High Prevalence of Hepatitis G Virus in Bone Marrow Transplant Recipients and Patients Treated For Acute Leukemia
Skidmore SJ, Collingham KE, Harrison P, et al (Birmingham Public Health Lab, England)
Blood 89:3853–3856, 1997   13–12

Background.—A new hepatitis virus has recently been identified, hepatitis G virus (HGV). This virus is associated with both acute and chronic hepatitis and can be transmitted by transfusion. The prevalence of HGV was examined in a group of multitransfused patients with hematologic malignancy.

Methods.—The study was performed at a single adult bone marrow transplant center. All 60 patients who had been treated for acute leukemia or who had undergone a bone marrow transplant before September 1991 were included in the study group. Transfusion histories and serum aspartate aminotransferase (AST) levels were reviewed. A reverse transcription polymerase chain reaction technique was used to identify the virus in a patient's serum samples.

Results.—The HGV virus was detected in 48% of the 60 patients. There was no difference in viral detection rates based on AST levels. Although all the patients had similar transfusion histories, 61% of those who received bone marrow transplantation were HGV-positive compared to 33% of those treated with combination chemotherapy. There was no significant difference in infection rate before or after the introduction of blood donor screening for hepatitis C virus antibodies.

Conclusions.—Hepatitis G virus infection was extremely common in a group of multitransfused patients. The clinical significance of HGV infection was not clear from this study. The possibility that HGV infection is associated with chronic liver disease is a cause for concern. Further studies are required to understand the natural history of this newly identified virus.

▶ Hepatitis G virus (HGV) is a newly described virus that has been implicated in transfusion-associated hepatitis. It can cause both acute and chronic hepatitis.

Hepatitis G virus is rather similar to hepatitis C virus, which is responsible for more than 90% of cases of non-A, non-B transfusion-associated hepatitis. Interestingly, HGV was first detected in the serum of a surgeon who infected a number of his patients.

That HGV can cause hepatitis in bone marrow transplantation recipients is news to me.

M.J. Cline, M.D.

14 Cancer

The Detection of Micrometastases in the Peripheral Blood and Bone Marrow of Patients with Breast Cancer Using Immunohistochemistry and Reverse Transcriptase Polymerase Chain Reaction for Keratin 19
Schoenfeld A, Kruger KH, Gomm J, et al (Charing Cross and Westminster Med School, London; Charing Cross Hosp, London; St Georges Hosp, London, et al)
Eur J Cancer 33:854–861, 1997   14–1

Introduction.—Immunohistochemistry reveals micrometastases in the blood marrow of 20% to 30% of patients with operable breast cancer. Measurement of a tissue-specific gene transcript after polymerase chain reaction (PCR) amplification is far more sensitive than immunohistochemical methods, with no loss of specificity. A reverse transcriptase polymerase chain reaction (RT-PCR) for keratin 19 (K19) was studied for use in detecting micrometastases in the peripheral blood and bone marrow of patients with breast cancer.

Methods.—The study included 78 patients with breast cancer with no signs of distant metastases. After separation of the mononuclear fraction from blood and bone marrow samples, RT-PCR and immunohistochemistry for K19 were performed. The RT-PCR was performed in 2 40-cycle rounds using nested primers. Its ability to provide information in addition to that provided by immunohistochemistry was analyzed.

Results.—Initial experiments showed that the RT-PCR for K19 was at least 10 times more sensitive than immunohistochemistry, capable of detecting 1 tumor cell in 1 million normal bone marrow cells. On immunohistochemistry, K19-positive cells were found in 5% of peripheral blood specimens and 22% of bone marrow specimens. On RT-PCR, the rate of K19 positivity jumped to 25% in blood and 35% in bone marrow. The increase in detection frequency was significant. Detection of K19 by either method was unrelated to primary tumor size, presence of vascular invasion, lymph node involvement, or steroid receptor content.

Conclusions.—Reverse transcriptase-PCR using K19 primers is a sensitive and specific means of detecting micrometastases in the peripheral blood and bone marrow of patients with breast cancer. The prognostic significance of the results will require further follow-up. Technical improvements to quantify the RT-PCR assay should simplify the processing of large numbers of cases.

▶ Methods to detect microscopic metastases in breast cancer and many other malignancies have increased enormously in sensitivity in the past decade. First, we had simple microscopic observation of tissue sections stained with conventional histologic reagents. Then we had immunohistochemistry utilizing labeled antibodies directed against a specific tumor product. Now we have the PCR utilizing the messenger RNA of a specific tumor product. This last reaction has been used to detect tumor proteins in acute and chronic leukemias, lymphomas and some solid tumors. Its sensitivity, when pushed to the limit, is generally 1 malignant cell among 100,000–1,000,000 normal cells in bone marrow, lymph nodes, or blood.

This technology allows us to identify those patients in whom a relatively few malignant cells have escaped the primary tumor. The unanswered question is whether or not we should base therapy on the finding of a few metastatic cells. Are such cells always stem cells destined to proliferate at distant sites and create secondary tumors, or are they mostly "end" cells that will undergo apoptosis and die? Can such micrometastases be handled by the body's normal defense systems or do they inevitably mean that cancer has spread and will grow in new loci?

Clearly, in the future, new clinical trials will examine the prognostic significance of finding a few cellular escapees.

M.J. Cline, M.D.

National Treatment Trends for Ductal Carcinoma In Situ of the Breast
Winchester DJ, Menck HR, Winchester DP (Evanston Hosp, Ill; Northwestern Univ; American College of Surgeons, Chicago)
Arch Surg 132:660–665, 1997   14–2

Purpose.—The trend in management of ductal carcinoma in situ (DCIS) has been toward less radical surgery. There have been few randomized trials, however, leading to confusion over the management of an increasingly frequent type of cancer. Data from a large national cancer data base were reviewed to evaluate trends in the treatment of ductal carcinoma in situ, as they relate to demographics, individual patient characteristics, and time.

Methods.—The analysis included National Cancer Data Base data on 39,010 patients diagnosed as having DCIS between 1985 and 1993. The treatments provided were identified, including breast-preserving surgery, axillary lymph node dissection, and radiotherapy. Treatment delivered was analyzed for relationships to such variables as: patient age, income, and ethnicity; tumor size, grade, and site; year of diagnosis; treatment location; and hospital type and caseload.

Results.—From 1985 to 1993, the percentage of patients receiving breast-preserving therapy rose from 31% to 54%. All of the variables studied had some effect on treatment choice. Patients in the Northeast were most likely to receive breast-preserving therapy, while those in the south were least likely. Breast-preserving surgery was more likely and axillary lymph node dissection and radiotherapy less likely for patients with tumors of smaller size and lower grade. Adjuvant radiotherapy was given in only 45% of patients undergoing breast-preserving surgery, though the use of radiotherapy increased from 38% to 54% during the 8-year study period. The rate of axillary lymph node dissection decreased from 52% to 40% during the same time.

Conclusions.—The use of breast-preserving therapy for DCIS is rising. However, these data show a persistently high rate of axillary lymph node dissection and a persistently low rate of radiotherapy for patients with this form of breast cancer. Measures to optimize the management of DCIS in the United States should include dissemination of clinical trial results and professional education interventions.

▶ About 20% of breast cancers are very early cancers; i.e., carcinoma in situ. There are two types: One type is ductal carcinoma in situ = intraductal carcinoma. The other type is lobular carcinoma in situ which is not true cancer, but for the purpose of classification is called breast cancer in situ or stage 0 breast cancer.

For ductal carcinoma in situ, treatment may be one of the following: (1) Surgery to remove only the cancer (lumpectomy). (2) Surgery to remove only the cancer (lumpectomy) followed by radiation therapy. (3) Lumpectomy plus removal of the axillary lymph nodes. (4) Surgery to remove the whole breast (total mastectomy). (5) An experimental trial in which lumpectomy and radiation therapy is followed by hormone therapy.

There are few randomized trials comparing lumpectomy alone with lumpectomy plus radiation, hence best management is still controversial.

This study examines national trends for treating ductal carcinoma in situ and encompasses over 39,000 patients treated between 1985 and 1993. It notes that breast-conserving surgery accounted for more that 50% of cases during this period. By 1993, 12% of cases had total mastectomy and another 29% had modified radical mastectomy. The most frequently used procedure was partial mastectomy performed in 44% of patients. There is a trend for less lymph node dissection and increasing use of radiation therapy in the management of ductal carcinoma in situ.

M.J. Cline, M.D.

Five Versus More Than Five Years of Tamoxifen Therapy for Breast Cancer Patients With Negative Lymph Nodes and Estrogen Receptor-Positive Tumors
Fisher B, Dignam J, Bryant J, et al (Univ of Pittsburgh, PA)
J Natl Cancer Inst 88:1529–1542, 1996   14–3

Introduction.—Women with advanced breast cancer and those with primary operable breast cancer and positive axillary lymph nodes have been known to receive benefit from tamoxifen therapy. To assess the effectiveness of adjuvant tamoxifen therapy in women with histologically negative lymph nodes and estrogen receptor–positive tumors, the National Surgical Adjuvant Breast and Bowel Project began a randomized clinical trail (B-14) in 1982 with 2,800 women. Questions persisted on how long the benefits would be expected to last, the duration of tamoxifen administration necessary, and the adverse effects from prolonged therapy with tamoxifen. Findings are described after 10 years of follow-up of this study.

Methods.—In the original trial women received either tamoxifen at 20 mg/day or placebo. Those women who were treated with tamoxifen who remained free of disease after 5 years received either another 5 years of therapy or 5 years of placebo. The study evaluated the data to compare 5 years of therapy with more than 5 years of tamoxifen therapy.

Results.—A significant advantage was seen in women who received tamoxifen for the first 5 years. Their disease-free survival (69% vs. 58%), distant disease-free survival (76% vs. 67%), and relative risk and survival (80% vs. 76%) were significantly better than those of women who did not initially receive tamoxifen therapy. In the incidence of contralateral breast cancer, tamoxifen therapy was associated with a 37% reduction. For those who then discontinued tamoxifen therapy after the initial 5 years of therapy, there was more of an advantage in disease-free survival (92% vs. 86%) and distant disease-free survival (96% vs. 90%). For those who stopped using tamoxifen, survival was 96% compared with 94% for those who continued treatment. In the tamoxifen-treated women after 5 years, there was a higher incidence of thromboembolic events. The incidence of second cancers was not increased with tamoxifen therapy, except for endometrial cancer.

Conclusion.—After 10 years of follow-up, it was seen that the benefit from 5 years of tamoxifen therapy persisted. However, there was no additional benefit obtained from continuing therapy with tamoxifen for more than 5 years.

▶ This is an important study in breast cancer, which builds on earlier studies and previous knowledge. The salient points are these: (1) tamoxifen is superior to placebo in both young and old patients with estrogen-positive, node-negative breast cancer with respect to disease-free survival, (2) the beneficial effect of tamoxifen therapy is observed at both 5 and 10 years of follow-up, and (3) there is no advantage to administering tamoxifen for more than 5 years after the initial treatment of the breast cancer.

The disadvantages of using tamoxifen are a somewhat increased risk of thromboembolic events and of endometrial cancer in the receipients.

M.J. Cline, M.D.

Double Dose-Intensive Chemotherapy With Autologous Stem-Cell Support for Metastatic Breast Cancer: No Improvement in Progression-Free Survival by the Sequence of High-Dose Melphalan Followed by Cyclophosphamide, Thiotepa, and Carboplatin
Ayash LJ, Elias A, Schwartz G, et al (Dana Farber Cancer Inst, Boston; Harvard Med School, Boston)
J Clin Oncol 14:2984–2992, 1996   14–4

Background.—Previous research has shown that one fifth of patients with metastatic breast cancer responding to treatment remain free of progression a median of 50 months after 1 intensification cycle of cyclophosphamide, thiotepa, and carboplatin (CTCb) with autologous bone marrow transplantation (ABMT). Whether a sequence of high-dose melphalan followed by CTCb resulted in improved disease response and duration was investigated.

Methods.—Women with partial or better responses to induction therapy were given melphalan, 140 or 180 mg/m^2, with peripheral blood progenitor cell (PBPC) and granulocyte colony-stimulating factor (G-CSF) support. Women were monitored as outpatients, then received CTCb with marrow, PBPC, and G-CSF support in the hospital.

Findings.—Data on 67 women, a median of 25 months after CTCb treatment, were available for analysis. After administration of melphalan, 73% of the patients needed to be hospitalized for treatment of fever, mucositis, or infection. For the initial 33 patients receiving CTCb, the median interval between the start of melphalan treatment and CTCb treatment was 24 days. Liver toxicity developed in 11 patients during CTCb treatment, prompting an increase to a median of 35 days. Thereafter, no liver toxicity occurred. Thirty-four percent of the patients were free of progression at a median of 16 months after CTCb treatment. Overall, median progression-free survival (PFS) and survival times were 11 and 20 months, respectively.

Conclusions.—Compared with single-intensification CTCb, high-dose melphalan, followed by CTCb, did not yield superior PFS. Further research is needed.

▶ During the past few years, there has been a fad for the use of intensive chemotherapy followed by hematopoietic rescue with either autologous bone marrow or autologous peripheral blood stem cells. Convincing evidence that the procedure does much good has, however, been lacking.

In 1992 these investigators reported on a study begun in 1988 in which 62 women with advanced breast cancer received intensive therapy, followed by autologous hematopoietic rescue. Of those patients who responded to the treatment, 1 in 5 remained free of progressive disease for several years—a result that was not discouraging but could not be shouted from the roof tops. Undeterred, they have now tried doubling the intensity of the treatment with, unfortunately, no better results.

My conclusion is that intensive chemotherapy followed by hematopoietic rescue is a valid area for controlled clinical experimentation in breast cancer but that it has yet to be proved sufficiently effective to command entrance into the standard therapeutic armamentarium.

M.J. Cline, M.D.

High-dose Chemotherapy With Hematopoietic Rescue in Patients With Stage III to IV Ovarian Cancer: Long-term Results
Legros M, Dauplat J, Fleury J, et al (Centre Jean Perrin, Clermont-Ferrand, France; Maternité-Hôtel-Dieu, Clermont-Ferrand, France)
J Clin Oncol 15:1302–1308, 1997   14–5

Background.—Despite aggressive surgical and chemotherapeutic treatment, long-term survival of patients with stage III and IV epithelial ovarian carcinoma remains poor, even though this tumor is usually sensitive to chemotherapeutic agents. It is possible that this poor response is attributable to the resistance of some cells to conventional chemotherapeutic dosages. A pilot study was performed of high-dose chemotherapy (HDC) followed by hematopoietic rescue in 53 patients with poor-prognosis epithelial ovarian cancer.

Methods.—Between July 1984 and February 1995, 56 courses of HDC followed by hematopoietic rescue were performed in 53 patients with poor-prognosis epithelial ovarian cancer. Treatment consisted of surgery followed by high-dose melphalan in 23 patients and a combination of high-dose carboplatin plus cyclophosphamide in 30 patients. After HDC administration, autologous bone marrow transplantation or peripheral blood stem cell hematopoietic rescue was performed. Thirty-one of these patients were in complete remission and HDC was performed as consolidation therapy to prevent progression.

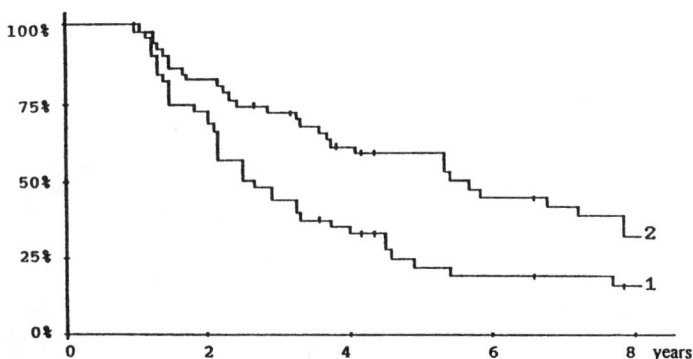

FIGURE 1.—Disease-free survival (*1*) and overall survival (*2*) from diagnosis for the entire patient cohort (N = 53) (Kaplan-Meier method). (Courtesy of Legros M, Dauplat J, Fleury J, et al: High-dose chemotherapy with hematopoietic rescue in patients with stage III to IV ovarian cancer: Long-term results. *J Clin Oncol* 15:1302–1308, 1997.)

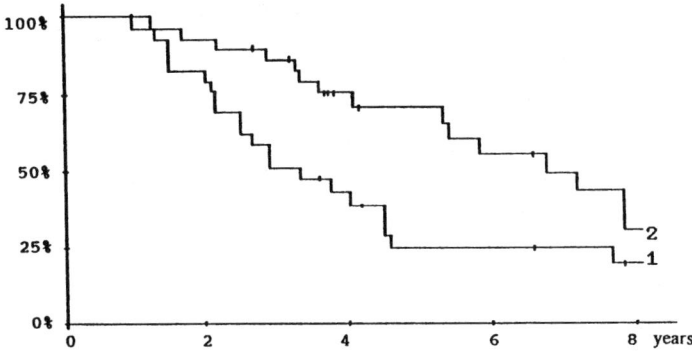

FIGURE 2.—Disease-free survival (*1*) and overall survival (*2*) from diagnosis for the consolidation group (group A, n = 31) (Kaplan-Meier method). (Courtesy of Legros M, Dauplat J, Fleury J, et al: High-dose chemotherapy with hematopoietic rescue in patients with stage III to IV ovarian cancer: Long-term results. *J Clin Oncol* 15:1302–1308, 1997.)

Results.—All patients in this study had severe bone marrow aplasia and neutropenic fevers that were treated with broad-spectrum antibiotics. The median time to recovery of a neutrophil count greater than $0.5 \times 10^9/L$ was 12 days. The median time to recovery of a platelet count greater than $50 \times 10^9/L$ was 22 days. One patient died of cardiac failure, but acute toxicity was acceptable for the remaining patients. These patients were observed for a median of 81.5 months, with a 5-year overall survival rate of 59.9% and a 5-year disease-free survival rate of 23.6% (Fig 1). At the end of the follow-up period in October 1995, 24 of the 53 patients were alive, and 12 had no evidence of disease. The best results occurred in 19 patients with pathologic complete response at second-look operation (consolidation group) (Fig 2). There was no difference in survival between patients treated with the 2 chemotherapeutic and hematopoietic rescue regimens.

Conclusions.—In this group of 53 patients with poor-prognosis advanced ovarian cancer, HDC followed by hematopoietic rescue was well tolerated. The 5-year 59.9% survival rate of this study compares favorably with the 20% to 30% survival rate for conventional therapy reported in the literature. The results of ongoing prospective randomized clinical trials will be useful in the evaluation of this treatment regimen.

▶ About three quarters of cases of ovarian carcinoma are disseminated at the time of diagnosis. The usual treatment for such tumors is a "debulking" surgical procedure followed by chemotherapy, usually with a combination of an alkylating agent such as cyclophosphamide and a platin compound such as cisplatin or carboplatin. The results of this therapy have been disappointing and most patients are dead of their disease within 2 years. More aggressive treatments and novel treatments, such as intraperitoneal infusion of anticancer drugs, have not provided much benefit, and we seem to be stuck at an impasse in the treatment of ovarian cancer. That is why this preliminary report seems so exciting.

The authors treated 53 patients with advanced ovarian cancer with high-dose chemotherapy supported by autologous stem cell rescue. A remarkable 60% of patients who underwent this treatment are alive at 5 years and a remarkable 24% of patients are said to be free of disease at 5 years. Almost unbelievable. As the authors say, "These results should be confirmed by an ongoing prospective randomized trial." I look forward to it. Maybe this is a breakthrough.

M.J. Cline, M.D.

Dose-Intense Therapy With Etoposide, Ifosfamide, Cisplatin, and Epirubicin (VIP-E) in 100 Consecutive Patients With Limited- and Extensive-Disease Small-Cell Lung Cancer

Fetscher S, Brugger W, Engelhardt R, et al (Univ of Freiburg, Germany; Univ of Tübingen, Germany)
Ann Oncol 8:49–56, 1997   14–6

Background.—The role of high-dose chemotherapy with peripheral stem cell transplantation (PBSCT) in patients with small-cell lung cancer (SCLC) has not yet been established. A phase I/II trial determined the feasibility and activity of the combination of ifosfamide, etoposide, cisplatin/carboplatin, and epirubicin (VIP-E/VIC-E) in patients with SCLC.

Methods.—One hundred consecutive patients with SCLC were given 2 cycles of combination chemotherapy followed by granulocyte colony-stimulating factor. They received etoposide, 500 mg/m²; ifosfamide, 4,000 mg/m²; cisplatin, 50 mg/m²; and epirubicin, 50 mg/m² (VIP-E). Thirty patients then proceeded to VIC-E high-dose chemotherapy with autologous PBSCT at a cumulative dose of etoposide, 1,500 mg/m², ifosfamide, 12,000 mg/m², carboplatin, 750 mg/m², and epirubicin, 150 mg/m². Surgical resection of the primary tumor was attempted as early as possible. After chemotherapy was completed, thoracic irradiation was given.

Outcomes.—Ninety-seven patients were evauable for response to conventional-dose VIP-E. Patients with limited disease had an objective response rate of 81%, and those with extensive disease, 77%. The treatment-related mortality rate was 2%. The median survivals for patients with limited and extensive disease were 19 months and 6 months, respectively. Two-year survivals were 36% and 0, respectively. All 30 patients receiving high-dose VIC-E had improved or maintained responses. Thirteen percent died of complications related to treatment. The median survivals in patients with limited and extensive disease were 26 months and 8 months, respectively, with 2-year survivals of 53% and 9%, respectively.

Conclusion.—Chemotherapy with VIP-E is an effective induction treatment for patients with SCLC. Among patients with limited disease, high-dose chemotherapy improved response rates and survival, especially for patients in surgical complete remission before high-dose treatment. However, in patients with estensive disease, higher response rates did not result in better survival. Selected patients with limited SCLC and good partial or complete remissions after previous treatment may benefit from high-dose chemotherapy and PBSCT.

▶ I decided to use this article as a point of departure for reviewing the status of therapy of SCLC. As the authors note, despite the development of many different and aggressive multiagent chemotherapy programs, the prognosis for SCLC has not changed much in the past 25 years. Patients with limited SCLC have a median survival of 12 to 16 months, and those with extensive disease have a median survival of only 6 to 11 months. Response to treatment rarely lasts more than 6 to 12 months.

Hematopoietic growth factor support has permitted the use of ever more intensive chemotherapy programs in recent years, but these have not been associated with improvements in survival. Similarly, extremely intensive therapy combined with autologous bone marrow or stem cell transplantation has not led to a cure of this disease.

A whole bagful of individual drugs can temporarily shrink this tumor. The authors of this article picked 4 of the most potent and combined them in an "alphabet soup" multiagent program. They found that 1 in 3 patients with limited SCLC and 1 in 5 with extensive SCLC had complete remissions in response to drug therapy. The median survivals were, respectively, 19 and 6 months—not much improvement over older programs. We still have a long way to go with this particular cancer. Fortunately, its incidence appears to be decreasing, at least in the Western world.

M.J. Cline, M.D.

The DCC Protein and Prognosis in Colorectal Cancer
Shibata D, Reale MA, Lavin P, et al (Harvard Med School, Boston; Yale Univ, New Haven, Conn; Boston Biostatistics Research Found, Farmingham, Mass; et al)
N Engl J Med 335:1727–1732, 1996   14–7

Objective.—Allelic loss of chromosome 18q is linked to a poor outcome in individuals with stage II of Dukes' stage B2 colorectal cancer. The DCC (deleted in colorectal cancer) gene is suspected of being the gene inactivated by this loss. The expression of the DCC protein in stage II and III colorectal cancers was studied histochemically to determine its importance as a prognostic marker of colon cancer.

Methods.—Antibody studies were performed on 132 formalin-fixed, paraffin-embedded samples from patients (66 female) with stage II or III colorectal cancers. Status of DCC was determined by immunohistochemical analysis. The Cox proportional-hazards model was used to determine the contributions of age, sex, tumor site, degree of differentiation of the tumor, presence of radiation or chemotherapy, TNM stage, and DCC status.

Results.—Positivity of DCC was found in 59% of sections from females and 41% from males. Tumors were well or moderately well differentiated in 86% of patients. The TNM stage and the DCC status were not related. Patients were studied for an average of 95.7 months for DCC-positive tumors and 85.1 months for DCC-negative tumors. Overall survival depended on disease stage and DCC-positivity or DCC-negativity. Tumor stage and DCC status were independent predictors of death.

Conclusion.—In patients with colorectal cancer, the absence of DCC is a marker for poor outcome. Patients with stage II colorectal cancer and no DCC expression have tumors that behave like stage III cancers. Determination of DCC status may help clinicians select patients with stage II tumors who would benefit from adjuvant therapy.

▶ From both a clinical and a molecular biology perspective, there are 3 types of colorectal cancer: (1) the type associated with familial adenomatous polyposis, which accounts for about 1% of the cases of colon cancer in the Western world; (2) a hereditary nonpolyposis form of colorectal cancer, which accounts for about 10% of cases in the West; and (3) the "sporadic" type, which accounts for the bulk of the cases of colon cancer. Genetic abnormalities predisposing to types 1 and 2 colon cancer have been identified within the past 6 years.

The APC gene responsible for the familial adenomatous polyposis form of carcinoma of the colon was identified in 1991. This gene is located on the long arm of chromosome 5. A variety of germline mutations in the APC gene result in inactivation and loss of its gene product.

Another gene on the short arm of chromosome 2 is frequently altered in hereditary nonpolyposis colorectal cancer. It is a gene that is involved in repair of mistakes that occur in DNA replication or with DNA damage. This disorder is one the most common inherited cancers of man and may affect one in 200 individuals. It has been hypothesized that affected individuals are born with one abnormal gene. When a mutation occurs in the corresponding normal allele, mutations rapidly accumulate and cancer develops.

Other genes are known to be involved in the pathogenesis of sporadic colon cancer. It is known than alterations of one of the *ras* genes may be an early event in carcinogenesis and that loss and mutation of the p53 gene is a late event. It is also known that loss of a gene on the long arm of chromosome 18 is frequent in colon cancer. This gene is known as DCC (deleted in colorectal cancer).

For several years now, I have (somewhat pompously) been predicting that this progress in molecular carcinogenesis will lead to better tests and better treatment for cancers. This is now a reality. Lack of the DCC protein is associated with more aggressive tumor behavior.

M.J. Cline, M.D.

Hereditary Cancer Risk Notification and Testing: How Interested Is the General Population?

Andrykowski MA, Lightner R, Studts JL, et al (Univ of Kentucky, Lexington)
J Clin Oncol 15:2139–2148, 1997   14–8

Background.—The interest of the general public in hereditary cancer risk testing and notification needs to be assessed. A statewide telephone survey of adults' interest in these issues was reported.

Methods and Findings.—Six hundred fifty-four residents of Kentucky were asked about their attitudes toward hereditary cancer-risk testing and notification as part of an annual telephone survey. Eighty-two percent expressed interest in testing and 87% in notification. Logistic regression analyses showed that lack of interest in notification was associated with female sex, the practice of fewer health protective behaviors, and better perceptions of personal health. Lack of interest in testing was correlated with those factors, as well as with older age, less concern over cancer development, and a more extensive history of cancer in first-degree relatives.

Conclusion.—Hereditary-risk testing programs may have problems attracting the interest of persons at greatest risk for carrier status. By contrast, many persons at low risk for positive carrier status may seek testing, possibly for reassurance.

▶ A large number of cancer susceptibility genes have now been defined. These are related to a variety of hereditary cancer syndromes including familial breast cancer, ovarian cancer, colon cancer, retinoblastoma, familial adenomatous polyposis, multiple endocrine neoplasia, and others. In some cases, as for example in the case of the *BRCA1* gene, laboratory tests are available to identify individuals at risk of cancer development. Although the benefits of testing for cancer susceptibility have not yet been established, the technology for testing for cancer susceptibility genes is apt to increase dramatically in the next few years.

This article examines whether people are (at present) interested in such testing. The results of this telephone survey indicate that most people— more than 80 percent—are interested in testing for risks of cancer susceptibility and in notification of risk. However, those with a family history of cancer and those least interested in good preventive medicine practices are least interested in testing for cancer susceptibility. This may not be unreasonable until such time as physicians can do something effective about preventing or curing a cancer in those individuals in whom a positive test is found. How far off is that? Years? Decades?

If you are interested in this subject, you should consult this article. It has a good bibliography. Another recent article discusses the process of informed consent for cancer susceptibility testing.[1]

M.J. Cline, M.D.

Reference

1. Geller G, Botkin JR, Green MJ, et al: Genetic testing for susceptibility to adult-onset cancer. *JAMA* 277:1467, 1997.

Embryonic Lethality and Radiation Hypersensitivity Medicated by Rad51 in Mice Lacking *Brca2*
Sharan AK, Morimatsu M, Albrecht U, et al (Baylor College of Medicine, Houston)
Nature 386:804–810, 1997   14–9

Background.—Inherited mutations in the *BRCA2* gene are associated with a dominant predisposition to cancer, suggesting that this gene is a tumor suppressor. The *BRCA2* gene encodes a protein with no significant homology to any known protein. To understand the function of this gene, investigators created mice that were missing the murine homologue of the *BRCA2* gene.

Methods/Results.—Brca2-deficient embryos were normal throughout early development, but arrested at the time of detectable *BRCA2* expression after 6.5 days of gestation. Embryonic expression of *BRCA2* was associated with tissue proliferation. The yeast 2-hybrid assay was utilized to detect an interaction between a conserved region of Brca2 and MmRad51. This result was confirmed in mammalian cells. Both Brca2 and Rad51 were co-expressed in the mouse embryo. Brca2-deficient embryos were hypersensitive to γ-radiation.

Conclusions.—The association of the DNA repair enzyme Rad51 with Brca2 and the sensitivity of Brca2-deficient cells to radiation may explain the high penetrance of early-onset cancer phenotypes associated with mutations in this gene. In mammary epithelial cells that lack Brca2 function, Rad51-mediated DNA repair is presumably compromised, which would destabilize the genome and lead to malignancy. This explains the tumor-suppressor phenotype of Brca2.

▶ Mutations in either the *BRCA1* or *BRCA2* gene confer a dominant predisposition to cancer of the breast and ovary or cancer of the breast alone. They are associated with hereditary predisposition to these cancers in certain families. Screening of many breast cancers has found that mutations in *BRCA2* are very rare in sporadic nonfamilial breast cancer.

Molecular and cytogenetic evidence have suggested that *BRCA1* and *BRCA2* are *tumor suppressor* genes, but their precise roles in metabolism have not been defined, in part because the *BRCA2* protein has no homology with any other known protein. The data presented in this report are evidence for a role for the *BRCA2* gene in a complex system involved in the repair of double-stranded breaks in DNA. This is quite similar to the story of *BRCA1* and its association with a DNA repair system and also to gene defects in predisposition to hereditary nonpolyposis colorectal cancer.

As this article points out, there are still many unknowns. However, with observations such as these, we are quickly beginning to fill in the pieces of the puzzle of genes and predisposition to cancer.

M.J. Cline, M.D.

Total Synthesis of the Potential Anticancer Vaccine KH-1 Adenocarcinoma Antigen
Deshpande PP, Danishefsky SJ (Mem Sloan-Kettering Cancer Ctr, New York)
Nature 387:164–166, 1997   14–10

Background.—Human tumors can be marked by the expression of unusual carbohydrate moieties, such as surface-bound glycolipids or glycoproteins, which may have anticancer vaccine potential. Research in this field has been limited by the inability to isolate sufficient quantities of these compounds from natural sources. This report presents the successful total synthesis of an adenocarcinoma glycoplipid antigen, KH-1.

Methods.—A hexasaccaride was built, which allowed the unveiling of 3 free hydroxyls as α-fucosylation acceptor sites.

Results.—The final product structures were verified by mass spectroscopy and self-consistent NMR analysis.

Conclusions.—These successful results demonstrate the capability of oligosaccharide synthesis for the reconstruction of carbohydrate antigens. The ability to synthesize these antigens in quantity will enable research on the use of these molecules as antitumor vaccines to proceed.

▶ To the best of my knowledge, this is one of the first reports of the total synthesis of a tumor-associated carbohydrate antigen. Let us hope that it does indeed open up a new field of tumor vaccines.

M.J. Cline, M.D.

Patient Preferences Concerning the Trade-Off Between the Risks and Benefits of Routine Radiation Therapy After Conservative Surgery for Early-Stage Breast Cancer
Hayman JA, Fairclough DL, Harris JR, et al (Dana-Farber Cancer Inst, Boston; Harvard Med School, Boston)
J Clin Oncol 15:1252–1260, 1997   14–11

Introduction.—Reports vary regarding the need for radiation therapy after conservative surgery for early-stage invasive breast cancer. An important issue in deciding use of radiation therapy is how women feel about the trade-off between the fear and consequences of local recurrence vs. toxicity and inconvenience of treatment. Use of utilities (measures of patient preference) can help determine the strength of a woman's preferences for particular states of health in times of uncertainty. Preferences regarding the trade-off between the risks and benefits of routine radiation therapy and conservative surgery for early-stage breast cancer were analyzed using utilities in 97 women.

Methods.—Ninety-seven patients and 20 female oncology nurses (for comparison) participated in a 45-minute interview that included a rating scale exercise, a standard gamble exercise using a chance board, and a brief questionnaire.

Results.—Patients varied significantly in health states' utilities. Utilities scores were highest for treatment with conservative surgery and radiation therapy without a local recurrence; intermediate for treatment with conservative surgery alone, followed either by no local recurrence or by a local recurrence salvaged by conservative surgery and radiation; and lowest for treatment with or without radiation, followed by local recurrence salvaged by mastectomy and reconstructive surgery. No sociodemographic or clinical factors evaluated explained more than 5% of variability in patients' or nurses' utilities or their differences.

Conclusion.—Patients with early-stage breast cancer who valued breast preservation believed the benefits of radiation therapy outweigh the risks. This treatment should be offered to women, even though there is no proof that radiation will be beneficial to them. Patients placed significant value on local control of their cancer in terms of overall quality of life.

▶ Four published randomized trials show no statistically significant survival advantage when radiation therapy is added to conservative surgery in early-stage breast cancer. On the other hand, the addition of radiation therapy clearly reduces the risks of local recurrence of disease. In this interesting study of a relatively small group of 97 patients and 20 medical oncology nurses, it is clear that the fear of local recurrence and its consequences is sufficiently strong that most prefer the risks and inconvenience of adjuvant radiation therapy. Treating physicians and surgeons must take this preference into account in structuring therapeutic programs for early-stage breast cancer.

M.J. Cline, M.D.

Measuring the Accuracy of Prognostic Judgments in Oncology
Mackillop WJ, Quirt CF (Queen's Univ, Kingston, Ont, Canada; Kingston Gen Hosp, Ont, Canada)
J Clin Epidemiol 50:21–29, 1997   14–12

Introduction.—Accuracy of prognosis in oncology is important because treatment strategies are different for patients with expected long-term survival vs. short-term survival. The accuracy of prognostic judgments in the day-to-day practice of cancer medicine was evaluated.

Methods.—A total of 116 patients undergoing outpatient cancer treatment were interviewed regarding perception of illness, treatment, and prognosis. Physicians completed corresponding questionnaires for 98 patients regarding illness, treatment, and prognosis. Doctors were asked to estimate probability of cure and duration of survival for each patient. Patients' charts were reviewed at 5-year follow-up to determine disease outcome. Data from patients' charts were compared with estimates of probability of cure and duration of survival.

Results.—The ability of the oncologists to discriminate between curable and incurable disease compared favorably with the discrimination of prognostic judgments in acute care medicine. The estimates of duration of survival in patients with incurable disease were well calibrated. Individual predictions were not precise. There was only fair discrimination between patients who would survive for 3 months and those who would not live that long. The discrimination was very poor between patients who would survive for 1 year and those who would not survive that long.

Conclusion.—Oncologists were quite accurate in estimates of probability of cure, but were less accurate in estimates of duration of survival of patients who had incurable disease.

▶ Oncologists' predictions of probability of cure are surprisingly accurate. In fact, we are better than the weatherman!

M.J. Cline, M.D.

Physician Desire for Euthanasia and Assisted Suicide: Would Physicians Practice What They Preach?
Howard OM, Fairclough DL, Daniels ER, et al (Dana-Farber Cancer Inst, Boston; Harvard Med School, Boston)
J Clin Oncol 15:428–432, 1997   14–13

Background.—Debate regarding euthanasia and physician-assisted suicide continues to increase. A survey of oncologists determined how many could imagine a situation in which they would desire euthanasia and whether these physicians viewed euthanasia or assisted suicide acceptable for their patients.

Methods and Findings.—Three hundred fifty-five oncologists were randomly selected and interviewed. Forty-eight percent said they could imagine a situation in which they might wish for euthanasia or assisted suicide for themselves. Oncologists who were Catholic and more religious were significantly less likely to desire such an intervention for themselves. Of oncologists who could imagine a situation in which they might desire euthanasia or assisted suicide, 85.8% believed that such interventions were acceptable for their patients. Of those who could not imagine a situation in which they would want euthanasia or assisted suicide for themselves, 41.7% still viewed such interventions as ethical for their patients. Only 6.8% of oncologists viewed these interventions as acceptable for themselves but not for their patients.

Conclusion.—Most oncologists would "practice what they preach" about euthanasia and assisted suicide. Oncologists who are inconsistent in their views overwhelmingly respect patient autonomy rather than imposing their own views on their patients.

▶ This interesting article describes interviews with 355 randomly selected oncologists regarding attitudes toward euthanasia. Some 48% said that they could imagine circumstances in which they might desire euthanasia or assisted suicide for themselves. Most of these physicians also found it acceptable for their patients under some "appropriate" circumstances. Interestingly, of those physicians who could not accept the idea of euthanasia or assisted suicide for themselves, 42% still thought it might be ethically acceptable for their patients. Only 7% of oncologists could imagine circumstances in which they might desire euthanasia or assisted suicide for themselves but found it unacceptable for their patients. Although, for the moment, these weighty ethical issues have been pre-empted by legal decisions, I do not think that they will go away.

M.J. Cline, M.D.

THE HEART AND CARDIOVASCULAR DISEASE

WILLIAM H. FRISHMAN, M.D.

Introduction

Many excellent basic and clinical research studies were published last year on the prevention, diagnosis, and treatment of cardiovascular diseases. The 48 articles selected for the cardiovascular disease section of the 1998 YEAR BOOK OF MEDICINE were selected from more than 4,000 articles reviewed. Each article is followed by editorial comments and, when necessary, additional reference citations. Articles on the pathophysiology and epidemiology of cardiovascular disease are also included, as well as articles dealing with clinically relevant issues.

Chapter 26 presents articles dealing with etiologic factors in the pathophysiology of atherosclerosis. Moderate alcohol consumption appears to protect against the development of angina pectoris and myocardial infarction in men without known atherosclerotic disease. Elevated LDL-cholesterol remains a risk factor for coronary heart disease in elderly subjects. In men with known atherosclerotic disease, an elevated serum cholesterol is predictive of an unfavorable prognosis, suggesting the need for aggressive lipid lowering in these individuals. More and more evidence is appearing that psychological factors, such as depression, predict the occurrence of myocardial infarction. Studies are being conducted to determine if antidepressant medications can alter clinical outcomes in patients with known coronary artery disease.

There has been much interest in the inflammation of infectious and non-infectious etiologies as causative factors of coronary heart disease and its complications. Subjects with high C-reactive protein levels, a marker for inflammation, appear to have a higher risk for coronary events, and agents such as aspirin may provide protection against coronary events as anti-inflammatory agents, rather than as anti-thrombotic drugs.

Chapter 27 deals with acute coronary syndromes. Low-molecular-weight heparins are now being investigated as treatments for unstable angina, as alternatives to unfractionated heparin. Low-molecular-weight heparin appears to be as effective as heparin in preventing myocardial infarctions, but the former treatment is easier to administer and monitor and may be less toxic. Thrombolysis is still a mainstay treatment for acute myocardial infarction, and marked elevations in blood pressure to not appear to put patients at an increased risk of mortality; however, the risk of stroke is greater. Carvedilol, a β-adrenergic blocker, is now an approved treatment for patients with congestive heart failure. The drug also appears to be useful in the treatment of acute myocardial infarction with similar benefits as beta-adrenergic blockers.

The risk of death in patients who have survived an acute myocardial infarction complicated by ventricular fibrillation is a controversial subject. It appears that patients are at increased risk for the first 50 days postinfarction; however, after 50 days there is no greater mortality risk observed. Delayed hospital presentation increases the risk of mortality from myocardial infarction, and various factors such as patient age and female gender are associated with delay in treatment. In the managed care era, it appears that specialist care provides better clinical outcomes in patients with acute myocardial infarction than that provided by primary care physicians, albeit with increased cost.

Chapter 28 discusses chronic coronary artery disease. One study shows that exercise-induced ECG evidence of myocardial ischemia without chest pain is of less clinical significance than ischemia associated with pain. A high-carbohydrate meal appears to provoke an earlier onset of anginal symptoms than a high-fat meal.

One of the more exciting therapeutic questions is whether lipid-lowering therapy itself can reduce myocardial ischemia, allegedly due to a favorable action on endothelial function in blood vessel walls. It is suggested that lipid-lowering treatment with lovastatin can reduce the number of ischemic episodes detected by the ambulatory ECG. Lipid-lowering treatment with apheresis and concomitant drug therapy may have similar benefit in patients with ischemic vascular disease. Aggressive lipid-lowering therapy in an attempt to reduce the LDL-cholesterol below 100 mg/dl has been shown to slow the progression of atherosclerosis in coronary bypass grafts. Anti-coagulation therapy with warfarin conferred no such benefit.

Innovative treatments for chronic coronary artery disease include α-tocopherol and β-carotene. However, in male smokers, these treatments appear to increase the risk of mortality. A promising treatment is clopidogrel, a new anti-platelet drug recently approved by the FDA to reduce the risk of stroke and vascular death.

Chapter 29 contains a study demonstrating again that outcomes with coronary angioplasty procedures are more favorable if performed by experienced operators. In another study, the use of the platelet glycoprotein IIb/IIIa antagonists appears to reduce the rate of thrombotic complications in patients undergoing percutaneous transluminal coronary angioplasty who have refractory unstable angina.

Intracornary stenting is becoming utilized more commonly and data now accumulating show that in symptomatic patients with isolated stenoses of the proximal left anterior descending coronary artery, primary stent implantation provides better outcomes than percutaneous transluminal coronary angioplasty alone.

Chapter 29 concludes with a study showing that estrogen replacement therapy can improve the long-term survival of female patients undergoing coronary artery bypass grafting.

Chapter 30 is extensive. Heart failure is becoming more prevalent than in previous years. In the failing heart there appears to be an acceleration of programmed cell death (apoptosis). Heart failure is often caused by hypertensive heart disease, and antihypertensive therapy can have a significant impact on the development of heart failure in older subjects.

New drug therapies for heart failure include the α-β-adrenergic blocker carvedilol which appears to favorably alter the course of patients with nonischemic and ischemic ventricular dysfunction. The angiotension II receptor blocker losartan, was also shown to be an effective treatment in a study of older subjects. The calcium blocker, felodipine, was shown to be safe when used in patients with congestive heart failure; however, it has limited benefit on morbidity and mortality. Digoxin was shown to be an important part of an anticongestive heart failure regimen, as well as an anticoagulation regimen.

Heart transplant remains an important palliative treatment in heart failure, and there is evidence that older subjects may accrue the same benefit as younger individuals who undergo the procedure. In Chapter 31, a study gives a pathophysiologic explanation for the occurrence of angina pectoris in patients with aortic stenosis who do not have coronary artery disease. In an epidemiologic study, calcific aortic valve disease was shown not to be an inevitable result of aging, but, rather, a condition associated with male gender, hypertension, smoking, and hyperlipidemia. Balloon mitral commissurotomy has become a common procedure for treating mitral stenosis without an intraoperative approach. A study reviewed in this chapter reveals that the long-term event-free survival rate is quite favorable in patients after this procedure.

Noninvasive procedures have provided important diagnostic approaches for assessing left ventricular function after coronary revascularization procedures. In Chapter 32, data are provided to show that thallium imaging and dobutamine echocardiography provide information that is comparable in evaluating the success of coronary revascularization on ventricular functioning.

Arbutamine is a new catecholamine analogue that has been approved for use as a provocative agent in patients undergoing stress echocardiography. Both arbutamine and exercise are of comparable benefit in inducing echocardiographic ischemia.

Echocardiographic assessment of commissural calcium can be used to predict the success of a balloon mitral valvotomy. Those subjects having commissural calcium have a worse outcome following the valvotomy procedure.

Chapter 33 includes information on atrial tachyarrhythmias and an approach to managing the complications of thromboembolism. Atrial flutter may be associated with an increased risk of thromboembolism, as is atrial fibrillation. Early conversion of atrial fibrillation to sinus rhythm does not require anticoagulation or pre-screening by transesophageal echocardiography. In patients having atrial fibrillation greater than 2 days, transesophageal echocardiography may eliminate the need for patients to undergo preconversion anticoagulation if the study reveals no thrombus. Four weeks of anticoagulation would still be required postconversion. In patients with atrial fibrillation whose ventricular rate cannot be slowed down, radio frequency atrioventricular node modification provides an appropriate therapeutic option.

Regarding ventricular tachyarrhythmias, in one study nonsustained ventricular tachycardia was an independent predictor of increased mortality in patients with heart failure, and in another study, the routine use of amiodarone therapy was not found to be beneficial. Implantable defibrillators may provide a benefit in these high-risk individuals, as suggested by the findings of improved survival in patients having coronary artery disease, left ventricular dysfunction, and nonsustained ventricular tachycardia who undergo implantation.

In the last chapter of this section, an important case for cerebral thromboemboli is the finding of protruding plaque and plaque-related mobile masses on transesophageal echo exam. In another report, the diagnosis and treatment of systemic infection related to endocarditis on pacemaker leads is described.

A proper approach to anticoagulation with warfarin is provided in a dose comparative study. The use of atenolol to reduce morbidity and mortality in patients undergoing noncardiac surgery is also described.

Finally, two studies related to pacemakers are provided. In the first, the phenomenon of pacemaker interference by cellular telephones is decribed. In the second, the controversial use of dual-chamber pacing for treatment of obstructive hypertrophic cardiomyopathy is assessed in a double-blind trial.

William H. Frishman, M.D.

15 Risk Factors for Coronary Artery Disease

Moderate Alcohol Consumption and Risk for Angina Pectoris or Myocardial Infarction in U.S. Male Physicians
Camargo CA Jr, Stampfer MJ, Glynn RJ, et al (Harvard Med School, Boston; Harvard School of Public Health, Boston)
Ann Intern Med 126:372–375, 1997   15–1

Background.—Previous research has shown that moderate alcohol intake reduces the risk for myocardial infarction. However, many clinicians question the validity of this finding. Also, the relationship of moderate drinking to the risk for other events, such as angina pectoris, has not been established.

Methods.—A cohort of 22,071 apparently healthy male physicians, ages 40 to 84 years between 1981 and 1984, was studied prospectively. Annual questionnaires were sent to the participants.

Findings.—Between study enrollment and 1994, 1,368 cases of new-onset angina and 690 of myocardial infarction occurred. According to multivariate analyses controlling for several potential confounding variables, alcohol consumption was strongly, inversely correlated with the risk for each event. Compared with participants drinking less than 1 drink per week, those drinking one per day had relative risks of 0.69 and 0.65 for angina and myocardial infarction, respectively. These associations persisted when nondrinkers or occasional drinkers were used as the reference group.

Conclusions.—In this cohort of apparently healthy men, moderate alcohol drinking reduced the risk for angina pectoris and myocardial infarction. The benefits of moderate drinking must, of course, be weighed against the potential hazards of alcohol consumption.

▶ This report from the Physician's Health Study demonstrates that moderate alcohol consumption (two or more drinks daily) in men can lower the risk of angina pectoris by 53% and myocardial infarction by 44%, compared with men consuming less than 1 drink per week. This observation has been made previously.[1]

Although cardiovascular benefits in this study were with lower alcohol consumptions than the limits suggested by the 1995 US Dietary Guidelines[2] of two or fewer drinks daily for men, they must be weighed against the potential hazards of moderate alcohol consumption (alcoholism). It is suggested that life-long abstainers not be encouraged to start drinking and that occasional drinkers not be encouraged to increase their consumption. However, patients at risk for coronary artery disease should discuss their current drinking habits with their primary care physician for an individual clinical recommendation.

The mechanisms by which moderate intake of alcohol might protect against myocardial infarction include an antiplatelet effect and possibly favorable effects on HDL-cholesterol.[3]

W.H. Frishman, M.D.

References

1. Steinberg D, Pearson TA, Kuller LH: Alcohol and atherosclerosis. *Ann Intern Med* 113:967–976, 1991.
2. Dietary Guidelines Advisory Committee: Nutrition and your health: *Dietary Guidelines for Americans, 4th ed.* Washington, DC, U.S. Dept. Of Agriculture & Dept. Of Health & Human Services, 1995.
3. DelVecchio A, Frishman WH, Fadel A, Ismail A: Cardiovascular manifestations of substance abuse. In, Frishman WH, Sonnenblick EH: *Cardiovascular Pharmacotherapeutics.* New York: McGraw Hill Inc., 1997: 1115.

Serum Lipids and Incidence of Coronary Heart Disease: Findings From the Systolic Hypertension in the Elderly Program (SHEP)
Frost PH, for the Systolic Hypertension in the Elderly Research Group (Univ of California, San Francisco; et al)
Circulation 94:2381–2388, 1996   15–2

Objective.—The risk of coronary heart disease (CHD) in middle-aged individuals is directly related to total and low-density lipoprotein (LDL) cholesterol level and inversely related to high-density lipoprotein (HDL) cholesterol level. There is less information about CHD risk factors in individuals 60 years of age or older even though most CHD incidents occur in men older than 60 years and women older than 70 years. Findings of the Systolic Hypertension in the Elderly Program (SHEP), a randomized, placebo-controlled, double-blind, multicenter clinical trial, show that CHD is associated with serum total cholesterol, non-HDL cholesterol, and LDL cholesterol levels in men and women.

Methods.—Blood pressure values, cholesterol levels, and triglyceride levels were measured in 4,736 individuals (14% black, 43% men) 60 years of age or older, with elevated blood pressure. Patients were randomly allocated to therapy or placebo groups. Outcomes were decrease in occurrence of fatal and nonfatal stroke and monitoring of major coronary heart disease incidents.

Results.—Mean systolic and diastolic blood pressures were 170 and 77 mm Hg; mean total cholesterol, HDL cholesterol, and non-HDL cholesterol levels were 236 mg/dL, 54 mg/dL, and 182 mg/dL; fasting triglyceride values were 144 mg/dL. Patients were studied up for an average of 4.5 years. Patients had 245 nonfatal myocardial infarctions or fatal CHD during the study. Multivariate analysis established a relationship between myocardial infarction and CHD events and total cholesterol; LDL and non-HDL cholesterol; ratios of the 3 cholesterol measures to HDL; and triglycerides.

Conclusion.—High-density lipoprotein cholesterol was not a risk factor for CHD in this population. Non-HDL cholesterol appears to be a CHD risk factor indicator in older individuals. Controlling non-HDL cholesterol levels could reduce the incidence of CHD by 23% to 30%. The patients in this study were healthy volunteers and therefore may not be representative of the older population. Whether reducing the risk factors will result in a clinical benefit to this cohort is not known.

▶ In another report from SHEP,[1] it was shown that elevated LDL cholesterol was a predictor of subsequent CHD events in patients with isolated systolic hypertension. An increased ratio of LDL cholesterol to HDL cholesterol was also shown to be predictive, not a reduced HDL cholesterol alone. Preliminary data would suggest that elderly subjects can have changes in morbidity and mortality with drug treatment designed to reduce the level of LDL cholesterol.[2] Drug treatment can be given safely to the elderly, and more definitive clinical trials are now in progress examining the effects of cholesterol-lowering regimens on clinical outcomes in older subjects.

W.H. Frishman, M.D.

References

1. SHEP Cooperative Research Group: Prevention of stroke by antihypertensive drug treatment in older persons with isolated systolic hypertension. *JAMA* 265:3255–3264, 1991.
2. Scandinavian Simvastatin Survival Study Group: Randomized trial of cholesterol lowering in 4444 patients with coronary heart disease: the Scandinavian Simvastatin Survival Study (4S). *Lancet* 344:1383–1389, 1991.

Serum Cholesterol and Long-term Prognosis in Middle-aged Men With Myocardial Infarction and Angina Pectoris: A 16-Year Follow-up of the Primary Prevention Study in Göteborg, Sweden

Rosengren A, Hagman M, Wedel H, et al (Östra Univ Hosp, Göteborg, Sweden)

Eur Heart J 18:754–761, 1997   15–3

Background.—Previous studies have shown that drug treatment to lower serum cholesterol can reduce mortality in research subjects with coronary disease and those with no history of myocardial infarction. However, these studies were performed in selected populations. The outcomes in the placebo groups of such studies do not necessarily reflect the prognosis in an untreated population. The effects of serum cholesterol on long-term prognosis were assessed in various groups of men: those with a history of myocardial infarction, those with clinical angina without myocardial infarction, and those without clinical coronary disease.

Methods.—The study included 7,100 men participating in the second scheduled screening of a multifactor primary prevention trial conducted in Göteborg, Sweden. All men were 51–59 years old when studied at baseline in 1974–1977. This screening identified 314 men with clinical angina but no myocardial infarction and 195 men who had survived a median of 3 years after myocardial infarction. All research subjects were followed up through 1993, which yielded a mean of 16 years. The outcomes among the various groups were analyzed in terms of baseline serum cholesterol.

Results.—Among men without clinical coronary disease at baseline, the rate of death from coronary disease was 2.7 per 1,000 observation years in those with a cholesterol level of 5.2 mmol/L vs. 8.5 per 1,000 for those with a cholesterol level of 7.2 mmol/L or greater. For men with angina, coronary mortality was 5.5 per 1,000 observation years in those with a cholesterol level of 5.2 mmol/L vs. 31.0 per 1,000 observation years in those with a cholesterol level of 7.2 mmol/L. For those with a history of myocardial infarction, coronary mortality was 19.8 per 1,000 observation years in those with a cholesterol level of 5.2 mmol/L vs. 58.3 per 1,000 observation years in those with a cholesterol level of 7.2 mmol/L. The relative risk of coronary death for subjects at the higher level of serum cholesterol—after adjustment for age, smoking, systolic blood pressure, body mass index, and diabetes—was 2.42 for healthy men, 4.82 for men with angina, 2.70 for survivors of myocardial infarction, and 4.07 for men with either angina or previous infarctions.

Cholesterol had its greatest impact on mortality during the first half of follow-up, during which time the adjusted relative risk of death among men with pre-existing coronary disease and high serum cholesterol was 8.08. There was little variation in the risk of death according to baseline serum cholesterol or coronary disease status. By the end of follow-up in the healthy men, 76% of those with low cholesterol and 65% of those with high cholesterol were still alive. Of the men with previous myocardial infarctions, 50% of those with low cholesterol vs. 21% of those with high cholesterol were still alive.

Conclusions.—In men with pre-existing coronary disease, elevated serum cholesterol carries a very high long-term absolute risk of death. Such patients must receive lipid-lowering treatments of proven effectiveness. The findings in this population-based cohort suggest that studies in selected populations may underestimate the true risks of high serum cholesterol in men with coronary disease.

▶ This epidemiologic study from Sweden in men reiterates the dangers of serum cholesterol elevation in individuals with angina pectoris or a history of myocardial infarction or both.

It is of great clinical importance to reduce the cholesterol level with dietary changes and/or lipid-lowering therapy in these high-risk individuals.[1] There is also growing evidence to suggest that cholesterol-lowering therapy is a cost-effective primary prevention approach against first myocardial infarctions, at least in high-risk men.[2, 3]

W.H. Frishman, M.D.

References

1. Scandinavian Simvastatin Survival Study: Randomised trial of cholesterol lowering in 4444 patients with coronary heart disease: the Scandinavian Simvastatin Survival Study (4S). *Lancet* 344:1383–1389, 1994.
2. Shepherd J, Cobbe SM, Ford I, et al: Prevention of coronary heart disease with pravastatin in men with hypercholesterolemia. *N Engl J Med* 333:1301–1307, 1995.
3. Pharoah PD, Hollingworth W: Cost effectiveness of lowering cholesterol concentration with statins on patients with and without pre-existing coronary heart disease: life table method applied to health authority population. *BMJ* 312:1443–1448, 1996.

Depression, Psychotropic Medication, and Risk of Myocardial Infarction: Prospective Data From the Baltimore ECA Follow-up
Pratt LA, Ford DE, Crum RM, et al (Johns Hopkins School of Hygiene and Public Health, Baltimore, Md)
Circulation 94:3123–3129, 1996   15–4

Introduction.—Several studies have suggested that depression is associated with an increased risk of myocardial infarction (MI). To date, however, no prospective study has used a measure of depression that reflects clinical diagnostic criteria. It is possible that psychotropic medications could contribute to increased risk of MI in depressed patients. As part of the Baltimore Epidemiologic Catchment Area (ECA) Follow-up Study, depression was studied prospectively as a risk factor for nonfatal MI.

Methods.—The study used follow-up data from the Baltimore cohort of the ECA, a survey of psychiatric disorders in the general population. When the area probability sample was selected in 1981, 3,481 individuals were interviewed and evaluated for history of a major depressive episode; dysphoria, defined as 2 weeks of sadness; and use of psychotropic medication. In 1994, they were asked about the occurrence of MI. The data were examined to see if a major depressive episode increased the risk of MI and whether psychotropic medication played any role.

Results.—Of 1,551 subjects who were free of heart trouble in 1981, 64 reported experiencing an MI. Research subjects with a history of dysphoria had a 2.07 odds ratio (OR) for MI, compared with those who had no history of dysphoria (95% confidence interval [CI] 1.16–3.71). For subjects with a history of major depressive episode, the OR was 4.54 (95% CI 1.65–12.44). These relationships were independent of coronary risk factors. The following drugs were associated with an increased risk of MI in multivariate models, barbiturates, meprobamates, phenothiazines, and lithium. However, tricyclic antidepressants and benzodiazepines were not associated with an increased risk of MI. The only factor significantly associated with MI among subjects with no history of dysphoria was lithium use.

Conclusions.—Patients with a history of dysphoria or a major depressive episode appear to be at increased risk of MI. Previous reports of a link between psychotropic medication use and MI probably reflect an underlying primary relationship between depression and MI. Other studies provide some evidence that treatment depression might help to lower the risk of MI.

▶ Risk factors for MI include cigarette smoking, elevated cholesterol, diabetes and hypertension. There is growing evidence that a history of major psychiatric depression is also a primary risk factor for MI.[1] Already there is already evidence that depression can increase the risk of a second MI, following the initial event.[2]

Studies searching for biological factors associated with depression that may increase the risk for MI need to be done. Clinical trials examining the efficacy and safety of antidepressant pharmacotherapy in relation to risk of MI also need to be conducted.

W.H. Frishman, M.D.

References

1. Anda R, Williamson D, Jones D, et al: Depressed affect, hopelessness, and the risk of ischemic heart disease in a cohort of U.S. adults. *Epidemiology* 4:285–294, 1993.
2. Frasure-Smith N, Lesperance F, Talajic M: Depression and 18-month prognosis after myocardial infarction. *Circulation* 91:999–1005, 1995.

Inflammation, Aspirin, and the Risk of Cardiovascular Disease in Apparently Healthy Men

Ridker PM, Cushman M, Stampfer MJ, et al (Brigham and Women's Hosp, Boston; Univ of Vermont, Burlington)
N Engl J Med 336:973–979, 1997   15–5

Background.—Both laboratory and pathologic data have suggested that inflammation plays a role in the initiation and progression of atherosclerosis, but little information is available on the role of inflammation in first myocardial infarction, stroke, or venous thrombosis. C-reactive protein is a marker of systemic inflammation. Baseline plasma C-reactive protein concentration was assessed in 1,086 healthy men, who participated in the Physicians' Health Study, to examine the association between inflammation and the risk of a first cardiovascular event.

Methods.—The Physicians' Health Study was a randomized, double-blind, placebo-controlled 2 × 2 factorial trial of aspirin and beta carotene in the primary prevention of cardiovascular disease and cancer. Before randomization, participants were asked to provide baseline blood samples. Each participant who provided an adequate baseline blood sample and had a confirmed myocardial infarction, stroke, or venous thrombosis during the at least 8 years of follow-up was matched with 1 control who provided an adequate blood sample and reported no cardiovascular disease. Patients and controls were matched for age, smoking status, and length of time since randomization.

Results.—Cardiovascular disease developed in 543 participants during the course of this study, and these were matched with 543 controls. Baseline plasma C-reactive protein levels were higher among men who developed a myocardial infarction or ischemic stroke than they were among men without cardiovascular events or men who developed venous thrombosis. The men in the highest C-reactive protein quartile had 3 times the risk of myocardial infarction and 2 times the risk of ischemic stroke than the men in the lowest quartile. This risk was stable over long periods and was independent of smoking; body mass index; blood pressure; and plasma levels of total or HDL cholesterol, triglyceride, Lp(a) lipoprotein, t-PA antigen, D-dimer, fibrinogen, or homocysteine. Aspirin intake was associated with significant reductions in the risk of myocardial infarction among men in the highest quartile, but was not associated with significant risk reductions among men in the lowest quartile (Fig 2).

Conclusions.—This study indicates that the baseline plasma concentration of C-reactive protein (a marker for inflammation) in healthy men can be used to predict the risk of first myocardial and ischemic stroke but not the risk of venous thromboembolism, suggesting that the effect of inflammation on vascular risk may be limited to arterial circulation. The benefits of aspirin in reducing the risk of a first cardiovascular event were directly related to the level of C-reactive protein. This result not only implicates aspirin's anti-inflammatory, as well as its antiplatelet, activity in cardio-

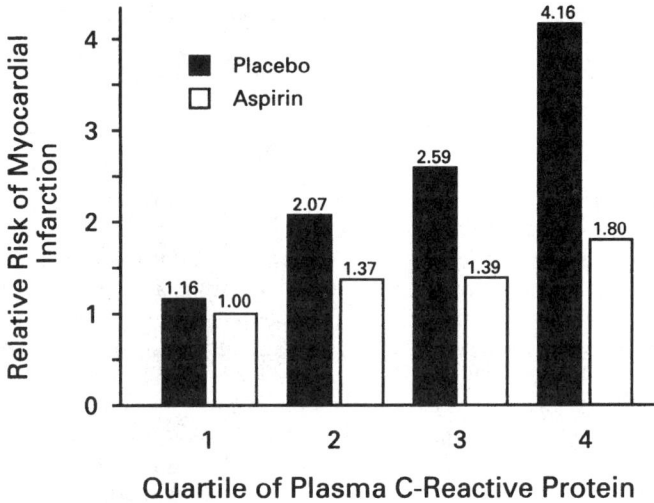

Quartile of Plasma C-Reactive Protein

FIGURE 2.—Relative risk of a first myocardial infarction associated with baseline plasma concentrations of C-reactive protein, stratified according to randomized assignment to aspirin or placebo therapy. (Reprinted by permission of *The New England Journal of Medicine*, from Ridker P, Cushman M, Stampfer M, et al: Inflammation, aspirin, and the risk of cardiovascular disease in apparently healthy men: *N Engl J Med* 338:973–979, copyright 1997, Massachusetts Medical Society.)

vascular health, but also suggests that other anti-inflammatory agents could play a role in the prevention of cardiovascular disease.

▶ Recently acquired laboratory and pathologic data support the premise that inflammation has a role in both the initiation and progression of atherosclerosis.[1, 2] Few data are available to indicate whether an inflammatory process can increase the risk of first myocardial infarction or stroke or whether anti-inflammatory therapy can decrease the risk.

This study shows that the baseline plasma concentration of C-reactive protein, an acute phase reactant, which is a marker for underlying systemic inflammation, can identify patients at risk of future myocardial infarction and stroke. Anti-inflammatory agents such as aspirin and antibiotics could reduce the risk of a vascular event in individuals having evidence of an inflammatory process in the blood vessels. Clinical studies need to be done to test this hypothesis. An anti-inflammatory effect of aspirin might suggest that higher doses than those needed for an antiplatelet effect should be used for cardioprotection. An inflammatory process may be infectious or noninfectious and may precipitate plaque rupture and thrombosis.[3-7]

W.H. Frishman, M.D.

References

1. Alexander RW: Inflammation and coronary artery disease. *N Engl J Med* 331:468–469, 1994.
2. Nieminen MS, Mattila K, Valtonen V: Infection and inflammation as risk factors for myocardial infarction. *Eur Heart J* 14:12K–16K, 1993.

3. Boyle JJ: Association of coronary plaque rupture and atherosclerotic inflammation. *J Pathol* 181:93–99, 1997.
4. Van der Wal AC, Becker AE, Van der Loos CM, et al: Site of intimal rupture or erosion of thrombosed coronary atherosclerotic plaques is characterized by an inflammatory process irrespective of the dominant plaque morphology. *Circulation* 89:36–44, 1994.
5. Melnick JL, Adam E, DeBakey ME: Possible role of cytomegalovirus in atherogenesis. *JAMA* 263:2204–2207, 1990.
6. Mendall MA, Goggin PM, Molineaux N, et al: Relation of *Helicobacter pylori* infection and coronary heart disease. *Br Heart J* 7:437–439, 1994.
7. Buja LM: Does atherosclerosis have an infectious etiology? *Circulation* 94:872–873.

16 Acute Coronary Syndromes

Comparison of Low-molecular-weight Heparin With Unfractionated Heparin Acutely and With Placebo for 6 Weeks in the Management of Unstable Coronary Artery Disease: Fragmin in Unstable Coronary Artery Disease Study (FRIC)
Klein W, for the FRIC Investigators (Graz, Austria; Göttingen, Germany; Glasgow, Scotland; et al)
Circulation 96:61–68, 1997   16–1

Introduction.—Therapeutic-dose unfractionated heparin and aspirin are effective in reducing adverse ischemic outcomes for unstable coronary artery disease, such as death and myocardial infarction, and the combination of both drugs has been found to be very effective. There are pharmacologic and pharmacokinetic advantages to low-molecular weight heparin when compared to unfractionated heparin, such as high bioavailability, long plasma half-life, and a predictable pharmokinetic profile. A previous study demonstrated that the low-molecular weight heparin, dalteparin, at 120 IU/kg administered twice daily with aspirin reduced the frequency of death and new myocardial infarction in patients with acute unstable coronary artery disease. In the acute treatment of unstable angina or non–Q-wave myocardial infarction, the efficacy and safety of weight-adjusted subcutaneous dalteparin, administered twice daily, were compared with those of IV unfractionated heparin.

Methods.—The study included 1,482 patients with unstable angina or non–Q-wave myocardial infarction. In the first phase of the study, days 1–6, either dose-adjusted IV infusion of unfractionated heparin or twice-daily weight-adjusted subcutaneous injections of dalteparin (120 IU/kg) were assigned to patients. In the second phase of the study, days 6–45, placebo or dalteparin at 7,500 IU once daily was assigned to patients.

Results.—In the patients treated with unfractionated heparin, the rate of death, myocardial infarction, or recurrence of angina was 7.6% during the first 6 days, and it was 9.3% in the dalteparin-treated patients. The composite end point of death or myocardial infarction was 3.6% in the patients treated with unfractionated heparin and 3.9% in the dalteparin-treated patients. In 5.3% of patients treated with unfractionated heparin,

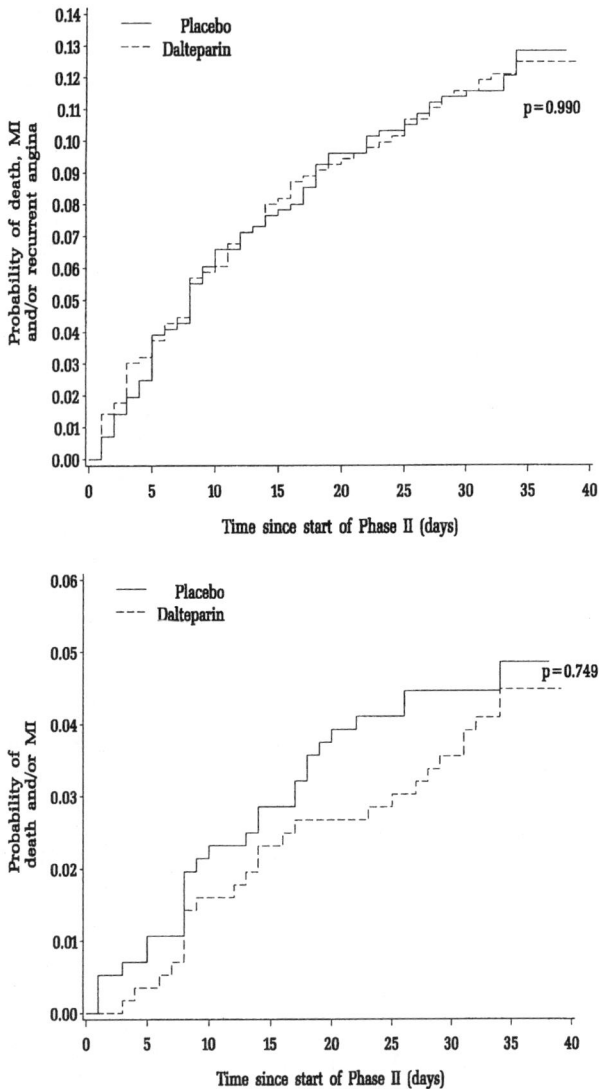

FIGURE 2.—**Top**, occurrence of the composite outcome of death, myocardial infarction, and recurrence of angina in the prolonged-treatment phase. **Bottom**, occurrence of the composite outcome of death and myocardial infarction in the prolonged-treatment phase. (Reproduced with permission from Klein W, for the FRIC Investigators: Comparison of low-molecular-weight heparin with unfractionated heparin acutely and with placebo for 6 weeks in the management of unstable coronary artery disease: Fragmin in Unstable Coronary Artery Disease Study (FRIC). *Circulation* 96:61–68, 1997. Copyright 1997, American Heart Association.)

revascularization procedures were performed, and in 4.8% of the patients in the dalteparin groups, revascularization procedures were performed. In the second phase of the study, both the placebo and dalteparin groups had a 12.3% rate of death, myocardial infarction, or recurrence of angina (Fig 2). In the placebo group, the rate of death or myocardial infarction was 4.7% and for the dalteparin group, it was 4.3%. In 14.2% of patients in the placebo group, revascularization procedures were performed, and in 14.3% of patients in the dalteparin group, revascularization was performed.

Conclusion.—An alternative to unfractionated heparin in the acute treatment of unstable angina or non–Q-wave myocardial infarction may be the low-molecular weight heparin dalteparin administered by twice-daily subcutaneous injection. No additional benefit over aspirin alone at 75–165 mg was found with prolonged treatment with dalteparin at a lower once-daily dose.

▶ In the treatment of patients with unstable angina, a therapeutic dose of unfractionated heparin and aspirin have been shown to reduce adverse outcomes, including death and myocardial infarction.[1, 2] Low-molecular-weight heparins may have pharmacologic advantages over unfractionated heparin, including a predictable pharmacokinetic profile that can result in effective and predictable anticoagulant levels after subcutaneous use, without the need for laboratory monitoring.[3, 4] Low-molecular-weight heparins have been found to be as effective or more effective than unfractionated heparin in the treatment of patients with venoembolic disease and ischemic stroke.[5, 6]

The FRIC study shows that the low-molecular-weight heparin, dalteparin, administered twice daily subcutaneously, is a safe and effective alternative to unfractionated heparin in the treatment of unstable angina, but there is no advantage to using dalteparin long term when compared to aspirin after hospital discharge. In another recent study, enoxaparin plus aspirin was shown to be more effective than unfractionated heparin plus aspirin, in reducing the incidence of ischemic events in patients with unstable angina or non–Q-wave myocardial infarction in the early phase.[7] There is growing evidence to suggest that low-molecular-weight heparin may replace unfractionated heparin in the acute management of ischemic syndromes.[8]

W.H. Frishman, M.D.

References

1. Cohen M, Adams PC, Parry G, et al: Combination antithrombotic therapy in unstable rest angina and non-Q-wave infarction in non-prior aspirin users. *Circulation* 89:81–88, 1994.
2. Theroux P, Ouimet H, McCans J, et al: Aspirin, heparin or both to treat acute unstable angina. *N Engl J Med* 319:1105–1111, 1988.
3. Frishman WH, Klein MD, Blaufarb I, et al: Antiplatelet and other antithrombotic drugs, in Frishman WH, Sonnenbick EH: *Cardiovascular Pharmacotherapeutics.* New York, McGraw Hill, 1997, pp 323–379.
4. Hirsh J, Levine MN: Low molecular weight heparin. *Blood* 79:1–17, 1992.

5. Lensing WA, Prins MH, Davidson BL, et al: Treatment of deep vein thrombosis with low molecular weight heparin: A meta-analysis. *Arch Intern Med* 155:601–607, 1995.
6. Kay R, Wong KS, Yu YL, et al: Low molecular weight heparin for the treatment of acute ischemic stroke. *N Engl J Med* 333:1588–1593, 1995.
7. Cohen M, Demers C, Gurfinkel EP, et al, for the Efficacy and Safety of Subcutaneous Enoxaparin in Non-Q-Wave Coronary Events Study Group: A comparison of low-molecular-weight heparin with unfractionated heparin for unstable coronary artery disease. *N Engl J Med* 337:447–452, 1997.
8. Armstrong PW: Heparin in acute coronary disease—requiem for a heavyweight? (editorial). *N Engl J Med* 337:492–494, 1997.

Relation of Increased Arterial Blood Pressure to Mortality and Stroke in the Context of Contemporary Thrombolytic Therapy for Acute Myocardial Infarction

Califf RM, for the GUSTO-I Investigators (Duke Univ, Durham NC)
Ann Intern Med 125:891–900, 1996   16–2

Background.—Hypertension may increase the risk for intracranial hemorrhage during thrombolysis for acute myocardial infarction. However, the precise nature of this risk has not been defined. The effects of previous hypertension and blood pressure on the outcomes of patients who had acute myocardial infarction and received thrombolysis therapy were studied.

Methods.—The randomized trial involved 1,081 hospitals in 15 countries. A total of 41,021 patients were included. All had myocardial infarction accompanied by ST-segment elevation and were brought to the hospital within 6 hours of symptom onset. The patients were treated by 1 of 4 thrombolytic regimens.

Findings.—The incidence of total stroke and intracranial bleeding increased with increasing systolic blood pressure at study entry. This incidence was especially high for systolic pressures of about 175 mm Hg or more. In patients with systolic blood pressures of 175 mm Hg or greater at study entry who received accelerated alteplase treatment, the rates of death within 30 days and of death plus disabling stroke were lower than in those receiving streptokinase, although the former had greater rates of total and hemorrhagic stroke.

Conclusions.—The risk of death is similar in patients with myocardial infarction and very elevated blood pressure undergoing thrombolysis and in those with myocardial infarction and no increases in blood pressure. However, the risk for stroke in the former group is greater. Further research is needed to determine the risk-to-benefit ratio of thrombolysis in these patients, particularly those at low risk for death resulting from cardiac causes, and whether reducing increased blood pressure before thrombolysis decreases the incidence of stroke without raising death rates.

▶ High blood pressure has always been considered a potential risk factor for stroke in patients with acute myocardial infarction undergoing thrombolysis.[1, 2] This study shows that a systolic blood pressure over 175 mm Hg greatly increases the risk of stroke with thrombolysis and might outweigh any benefit on mortality, especially in low-risk patients with myocardial infarction. In high-risk patients with infarction with hypertension, a mortality benefit is still seen with thrombolysis despite an increased rate of stroke compared to that seen in normotensive patients. It appears that the thrombolytic agent used does not impact on the risk of stroke morbidity with thrombolysis. Whether or not acute blood pressure lowering will reduce the risk of stroke in hypertensive patients receiving thrombolysis has not been determined. Although vasodilator drugs such as nitrates and calcium blockers will lower blood pressure, they can prevent vasoconstriction if bleeding occurs with thrombolysis. Vasodilator drugs themselves may have additional anticoagulant actions.

W.H. Frishman, M.D.

References

1. Gore JM, Granger CB, Simoons ML, et al: Stroke after thrombolysis. Mortality and functional outcomes in the GUSTO-1 trial. Global Use of Strategies to Open Occluded Coronary Arteries. *Circulation* 92:2811–2818, 1996.
2. A Report of the American College of Cardiology/American Heart Association Task Force on Practice Guidelines (Committee on Management of Acute Myocardial Infarction): ACC/AHA guidelines for the management of patients with acute myocardial infarction. *J Am Coll Cardiol* 28:1328–1428, 1996.

Beneficial Effects of Intravenous and Oral Carvedilol Treatment in Acute Myocardial Infarction
Basu S, Senior R, Raval U, et al (Northwick Park Hosp, Harrow, Middlesex, England)
Circulation 96:183–191, 1997

16–3

Introduction.—In reducing the mortality and ischemic events after acute myocardial infarction, early treatment with β-blockers has been shown to be beneficial with trials showing that it has reduced early mortality by 13% when used within 24 hours of chest pain. Carvedilol is a nonselective β-blocker, which is an effective antianginal and antihypertensive agent and has been shown to improve idiopathic and ischemic congestive heart failure. When added to conventional treatment for congestive heart failure, carvedilol has resulted in a 65% mortality benefit. A group of patients with myocardial infarction were treated with carvedilol and their cardiovascular outcomes were compared with those of another group receiving placebo.

Methods.—In 151 patients with acute myocardial infarction, the effects of acute, IV, and 6-month oral treatment with carvedilol were compared with placebo. Before hospital discharge and at 3 and 6 months, patients were tested with exercise ECG, ambulatory monitoring, and 2-dimensional echocardiography. Cardiovascular events were recorded during follow-up.

Results.—Compared to placebo, carvedilol was found to be safe, and it significantly reduced cardiac events: 18 cardiac events with carvedilol treatment and 31 with placebo. At study entry, there were 54 patients with heart failure and 34 received carvedilol. No excess events or adverse effects of carvedilol therapy were found in this group. Heart rate, blood pressure at rest, and rate-pressure product at peak exercise were significantly reduced with carvedilol, but there was no change in exercise capacity. Carvedilol did not alter left ventricular ejection fraction significantly, but at prehospital discharge examination, stroke volume was higher There was also improvement of diastolic filling of the left ventricle.

Conclusion.—In patients immediately after acute myocardial infarction, and in those with heart failure, carvedilol was well tolerated and safe to use. Outcome was significantly improved. There is potential to reduce ischemic events with carvedilol, but to further elucidate its beneficial effects, larger trials are required.

▶ Carvedilol is now an approved treatment for patients with New York Heart Association class II and III heart failure, who are already receiving conventional therapy with diuretics, digoxin, and angiotensin-converting enzyme inhibitor.[1] This study shows that carvedilol is a safe treatment after an acute myocardial infarction in patients with and without heart failure. There may also be a benefit on morbidity and mortality after a myocardial infarction, which is being studied now in large clinical trials. At this juncture, carvedilol is not approved for early clinical use after a myocardial infarction, unlike the beta-blockers atenolol and metoprolol.[2, 3]

W.H. Frishman, M.D.

References

1. Packer M, Bristow MR, Cohn JN, et al: The effect of carvedilol on morbidity and mortality in patients with chronic heart failure. *N Engl J Med* 334:1349–1355, 1996.
2. Yusuf S, Peto R, Lewis J, et al: Beta blockade during and after myocardial infarction: An overview of the randomised trials. *Prog Cardiovasc Dis* 17:335–371, 1985.
3. Frishman WH, Furberg CD, Friedewald WT: β-Adrenergic blockade in survivors of acute myocardial infarction. *N Engl J Med* 310:830–837, 1984.

Does In-hospital Ventricular Fibrillation Affect Prognosis After Myocardial Infarction?
Jensen GVH, Torp-Pedersen C, Hildebrandt P, et al (Glostrup Univ, Copenhagen; Gentofte Univ, Hellerup, Denmark; Frederiksberg Hosp, Denmark; et al)
Eur Heart J 18:919–924, 1997   16–4

Introduction.—In up to 15% of patients admitted to a hospital with acute myocardial infarction, ventricular fibrillation is experienced. Patients with congestive heart failure and ventricular fibrillation are known

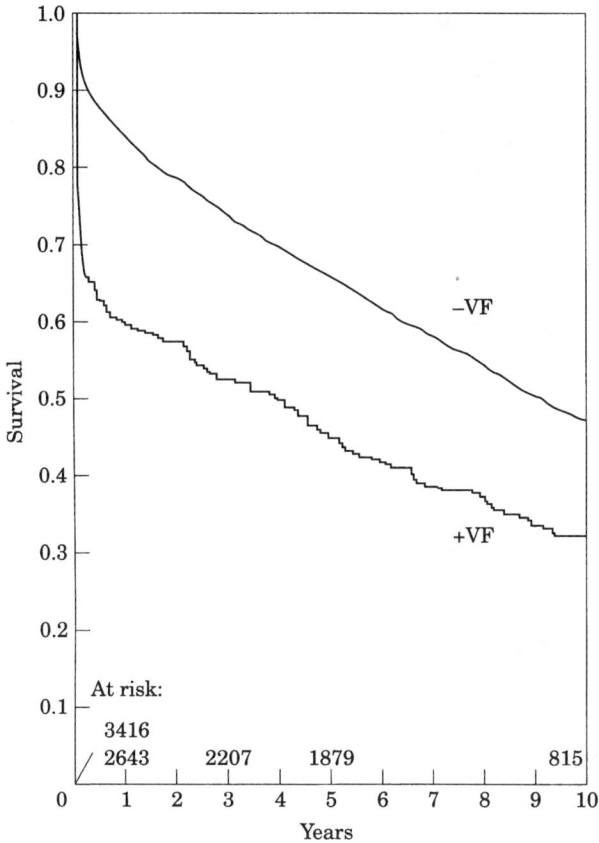

FIGURE 1.—Kaplan-Meier survival plots for 3,433 patients with myocardial infarction who survived days 0–5, grouped according to presence or absence of ventricular fibrillation. (*P* < 0.0001). *Abbreviation*: *VF*, ventricular fibrillation. (Reprinted from Jensen GVH, Torp-Pederson C, Hildebrandt P, et al: Does in-hospital ventricular fibrillation affect prognosis after myocardial infarction? *Eur Heart J* 18:919–924, 1997, by permission of the publisher WB Saunders Company Limited, London.)

to be a high-risk group. The significance of ventricular fibrillation not associated with congestive heart failure is still unknown. A population with myocardial infarction was studied to determine how ventricular fibrillation affected their outcomes.

Methods.—In a 10-year period, 4,259 patients with myocardial infarction were included in the study, and of these, 528 or 12.4% had ventricular fibrillation. To estimate their importance for 30-day and a median of 7-year prognosis, the following risk factors were included: age, gender, ventricular fibrillation, pulmonary edema, cardiogenic shock, heart failure, other cardiac arrest, and atrial fibrillation.

Results.—Patients with ventricular fibrillation had larger infarction and more signs of congestive heart failure than patients without ventricular fibrillation (Fig 1) (Fig 2). For patients with primary ventricular fibrillation and without heart failure, the odds ratio for death on days 6–30 was 6.34.

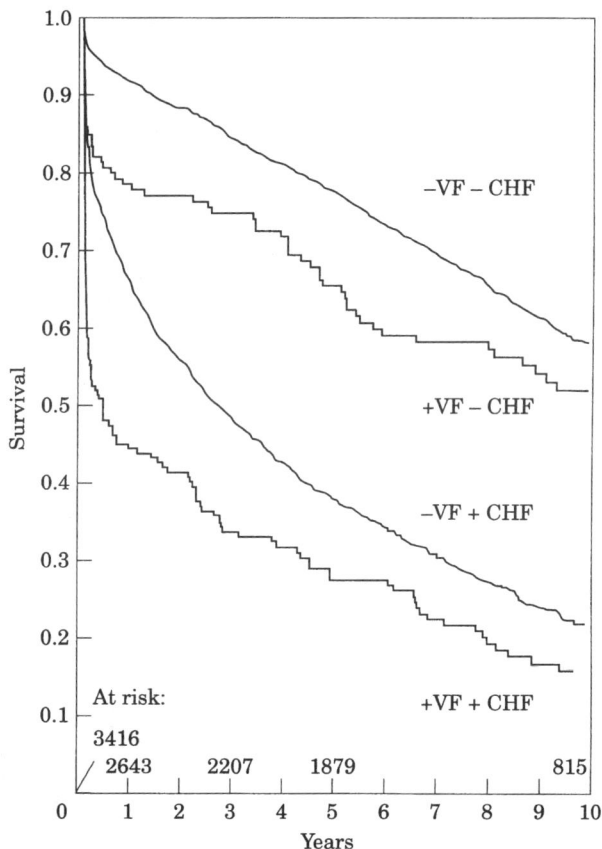

FIGURE 2.—Kaplan-Meier survival plots of 3,433 patients with myocardial infarction who survived days 0–5 grouped according to presence or absence of ventricular fibrillation and congestive heart failure. (P < 0.0001). *Abbreviations*: VF, ventricular fibrillation; CHF, congestive heart failure. (Reprinted from Jensen GVH, Torp-Pederson C, Hildebrandt P, et al: Does in-hospital ventricular fibrillation affect prognosis after myocardial infarction? *Eur Heart J* 18:919–924, 1997, by permission of the publisher WB Saunders Company Limited, London.)

For patients with ventricular fibrillation secondary to heart failure, the odds ratio for death on days 6–30 was 4.06 when compared to patients without ventricular fibrillation. In those with ventricular fibrillation, the relative risk of death for patients surviving more than 30 days was 1.11. During the initial 60 days after infarction, the importance of ventricular fibrillation for risk of death was exhausted, according to logistic regression analysis of relative risk associated with ventricular fibrillation in time intervals.

Conclusion.—Within 6–50 days after infarction, ventricular fibrillation is associated with an independent increased risk of death. The prognosis in survivors of ventricular fibrillation does not differ significantly after this period from that of patients without ventricular fibrillation.

▶ Ventricular fibrillation is seen in 10% to 15% of patients who are admitted to the hospital with acute myocardial infarction (MI). It appears that individuals who survive an episode of ventricular fibrillation are at increased risk for death up to 60 days post-MI, compared to individuals who never had an acute MI. Congestive heart failure seems to increase this risk. Beta-blockers seem to decrease this risk[1-4] and perhaps treatment of left ventricular dysfunction with early use of angiotensin-converting enzyme inhibitors may provide an additional benefit.[5]

Because the risk of ventricular fibrillation appears to be reduced beyond 60 days, this would argue against the routine use of implantable defibrillators in survivors of MI and ventricular fibrillation episodes, unless symptomatic ventricular tachyarrhythmias are present. Studies are in progress addressing this issue.

W.H. Frishman, M.D.

References

1. Ryden L, Ariniego R, Arnman K, et al: A double-blind trial of metoprolol in acute myocardial infarction. Effects on ventricular tachyarrhythmias. *N Engl J Med* 308:614–618, 1983.
2. β Blocker Heart Attack Trial Research Group: A randomized trial of propranolol in patients with acute myocardial infarction. *JAMA* 247:1707–1714, 1982.
3. The ISIS-1 Collaborative Group: Randomized trial of intravenous atenolol among 16,027 cases of suspected acute myocardial infarction: ISIS-1. *Lancet* ii:57–66, 1986.
4. Frishman WH, Furberg CD, Friedewald WT: β-Adrenergic blockade in survivors of acute myocardial infarction. *N Engl J Med* 310:830–837, 1984.
5. Ruddy MC, Kostis JB, Frishman WH: Drugs that affect the renin-angiotensin system, in Frishman WH, Sonnenblick EH: *Cardiovascular Pharmacotherapeutics*. New York, McGraw Hill Inc, 1997, pp. 131–192.

Delayed Hospital Presentation in Patients Who Have Had Acute Myocardial Infarction

Gurwitz JH, McLaughlin TJ, Willison DJ, et al (Harvard Med School, Boston; Univ of Massachusetts, Boston; McMaster Univ, Hamilton, Ont, Canada)
Ann Intern Med 126:593–599, 1997 16–5

Introduction.—In-hospital and long-term mortality have been correlated with the time from the onset of symptoms of acute myocardial infarction to hospital presentation. Delayed hospital presentation has been recognized as the largest contributor to postponed treatment of acute myocardial infarction with the advent of the thrombolytic era. A relationship between early treatment and improvement in short-term survival has been demonstrated. To develop appropriate patient-directed educational interventions to reduce delay, the identification of factors contributing to delayed hospital presentation for patients who have had acute myocardial infarction is essential. Patients with acute myocardial infarction at the time of admission to a hospital were evaluated.

Methods.—There were 2,409 patients hospitalized in 37 hospitals during a 10-month period who had a retrospective review of their charts. The main outcome measure was hospital presentation that was delayed more than 6 hours after symptoms of acute myocardial infarction became apparent. The analysis included the following factors: age, sex, marital status, living arrangement, location of residence, employment status, health insurance status, median income, presence of chest discomfort, and medical history.

Results.—Of the patients in the study, 40% were delayed for more than 6 hours for presentation to the hospital after the onset of symptoms. Advanced age and female sex were the factors associated with prolonged delay. The risk for prolonged delay was significantly reduced by the presence of chest discomfort and a history of mechanical revascularization. The risk for delay was greatest during the evening and early morning hours. Presentation was more likely to be delayed by patients with a history of hypertension. Emergency medical transport services were used by 42% of patients hospitalized with acute myocardial infarction.

Conclusion.—Hospital presentation is often delayed by patients with acute myocardial infarction. The prompt use of emergency medical transport services should be encouraged, and information targeted at elderly persons, women, and persons with cardiac risk factors should be promoted to reduce the length of delay and improve the outcome of patients with acute myocardial infarction.

▶ Studies have demonstrated repeatedly that the earlier a patient is brought to the hospital for treatment of an acute myocardial infarction, the better the outcome.[1] Consensus groups recommend early and rapid transfer to the emergency room as soon as patients have chest pain,[2] which will allow for earlier use of thrombolysis and other acute intervention procedures, thereby improving prognosis.[3]

Characteristics of patients who delay their presentation to the emergency room after onset of symptoms include advanced age and female gender. The time of day and the belief that the symptoms will disappear also influence the decision to access emergency care. A national campaign needs to be instituted to educate high-risk individuals and groups about the process of using emergency clinical services when chest pain symptoms begin.

W.H. Frishman, M.D.

References

1. Turi ZG, Stone PH, Muller JE, et al: Implications for acute intervention related to time of hospital arrival in acute myocardial infarction. *Am J Cardiol* 58:203–209, 1986.
2. ACC-AHA Guidelines for the Management of Patients with Acute Myocardial Infarction: A report of the American College of Cardiology/American Heart Assn Task Force on Practice Guidelines (Committee on Management of Acute Myocardial Infarction). *J Am Coll Cardiol* 28:1328-, 1996.

3. Fibrinolytic Therapy Trialists (FTT) Collaborative Group: Indications for fibrinolytic therapy in suspected acute myocardial infarction: Collaborative overview of early mortality and major morbidity results from all randomised trials of more than 1000 patients. *Lancet* 343:311–322, 1994.

Outcome of Acute Myocardial Infarction According to the Speciality of the Admitting Physician
Jollis JG, DeLong ER, Peterson ED, et al (Duke Univ, Durham, NC)
N Engl J Med 335:1880–1887, 1996   16–6

Background.—One strategy used by health care organizations to reduce the use of medical services and lower health care costs is to limit access to specialists. It is not known whether this practice affects the outcome of patients, especially those who are acutely ill. It has been suggested that patients with acute cardiac illnesses may have a poorer outcome when treated by a primary care physician, partially because family practitioners and internists may be less aware of life-saving drugs than cardiologists. The association between the outcome of patients with acute myocardial infarction and the type of physician who provides their care was examined.

Methods.—The medical records were reviewed of 8,241 patients from 4 states receiving Medicare who were hospitalized for acute myocardial infarction during a 7-month period in 1992. Insurance claim and survival data for all 220,535 patients receiving Medicare who were hospitalized for

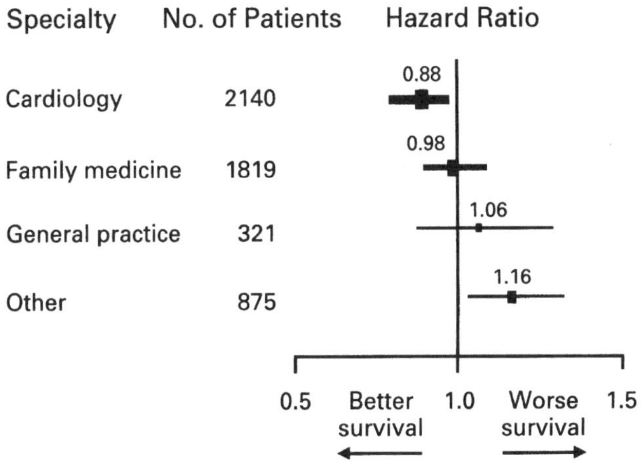

FIGURE 1.—Hazard ratios for adjusted 1-year mortality among patients with acute myocardial infarction in the Cooperative Cardiovascular Project cohort according to the specialty of the admitting physician. *Note:* The *bars* indicate the 95% confidence intervals. The hazard ratios have been adjusted for indicators of the severity of illness; the availability of facilities for coronary angiography, angioplasty, or bypass surgery at the hospital; and urban or rural hospital location. Patients admitted by physicians specializing in internal medicine served as the reference category. (Reprinted by permission of the New England Journal of Medicine, from Jollis JG, Delong ER, Peterson ED, et al: Outcome of acute myocardial infarction according to the specialty of the admitting physician. *N Engl J Med* 335:1880–1887, 1996. Copyright 1996, Massachusetts Medical Society.)

acute myocardial infarction during 1992 were also analyzed. Data were analyzed according to the specialty of the admitting physician.

Results.—Patients admitted by cardiologists were more likely to have had prior myocardial infarction, coronary bypass surgery, or anterior myocardial infarction, and to have lower blood pressure than other patients. After adjustment for patient and hospital characteristics, analysis showed that patients admitted by a cardiologist had a 12% lower risk of death within 12 months than patients admitted by a primary care physician (Fig 1). Cardiologists had the highest use rate of cardiac procedures, cardiac medications, and other medications associated with improved survival.

Discussion.—In treating elderly patients with acute myocardial infarction, cardiologists use more resources, but patients are more likely to have a better outcome than patients admitted by primary care physicians. Cardiologists were more likely to use thrombolytic agents, beta-blockers, aspirin, nitrates, and heparin than other physicians. Shifting the care of these patients to family practitioners or internists may decrease the survival of these patients. Further research should address how specialists and primary care physicians should interact in caring for these patients.

▶ To control health care costs, primary care physicians have been asked to provide more of the acute care of patients with myocardial infarction previously assigned to cardiologists.

In this retrospective Medicare database, it was shown that subspecialist care was associated with better clinical outcomes than care provided by primary care physicians. However, the cost of care was higher with the subspecialist in charge. Society cannot have it both ways regarding the care of older patients with myocardial infarction, that is, cheaper costs and better clinical outcomes. Optimal care can often be provided by individuals with the most clinical experience, and this is an issue that must be dealt with by health care economists and planners.

A similar study needs to be done in younger patients with myocardial infarction to evaluate the most cost-effective way to provide optimal medical care.

W.H. Frishman, M.D.

17 Chronic Coronary Artery Disease

Clinical Implications of Silent Versus Symptomatic Exercise-induced
Myocardial Ischemia in Patients With Stable Coronary Disease
'Narians CR, Zareba W, Moss AJ, et al (Univ of Rochester, New York;
Uniformed Services Univ, Bethesda, Md)
J Am Coll Cardiol 29:756–763, 1997   17–1

Background.—It is unclear whether painless ischemia identified during noninvasive cardiac testing is associated with a lesser extent of myocardial ischemia and/or a prognosis different from that of ischemia accompanied by angina. The functional and prognostic significance of silent ischemia compared with symptomatic ischemia was studied.

Methods.—Nine hundred thirty-six clinically stable patients were assessed 1 to 6 months after an acute coronary event (myocardial infarction or unstable angina). Ambulatory monitoring, exercise treadmill testing, and stress thallium-201 scintigraphy were performed. Mean followup was 23 months.

Findings.—Compared with the 125 patients with symptomatic ischemia during assessment, the 378 with silent ischemia showed less severe and extensive reversible defects on stress thallium scintigraphy, less functional impairment during treadmill testing (as manifested by longer exercise duration and longer time to ST segment depression), and less frequent ST segment depression during ambulatory monitoring. Patients with symptomatic ischemia had a significantly increased number of recurrent cardiac events subsequently compared with patients with silent or no ischemia, those rates being 28.8%, 18%, and 17.3%, respectively. The subgroup with symptomatic ischemia and poor exercise tolerance had an especially high number of adverse outcomes. The difference in cardiac event rates between those with silent ischemia compared with those with symptomatic ischemia persisted even after adjustment for baseline clinical characteristics (Fig 1).

Conclusions.—Myocardial ischemia was less severe and extensive in patients with stable coronary disease experiencing silent myocardial ischemia during noninvasive stress testing 1 to 6 months after a coronary event than in those with symptomatic ischemia. The presence or absence of

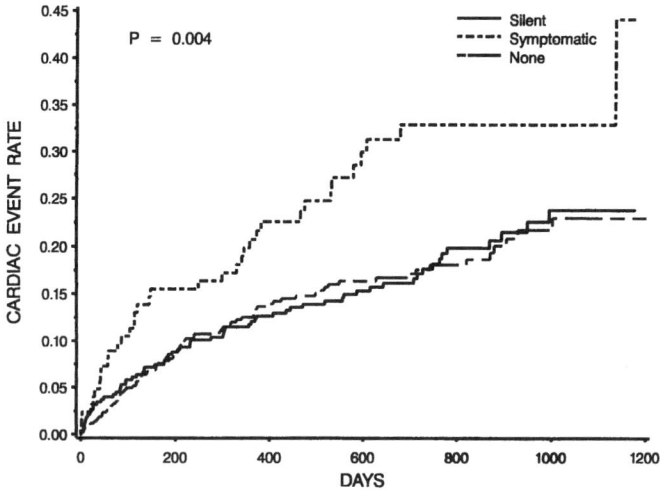

FIGURE 1.—Kaplan-Meier analysis for time to recurrent cardiac event (cardiac death, nonfatal myocardial infarction, unstable angina) according to presence and type of ischemia (symptomatic, silent, or none). (Reprinted with permission from the American College of Cardiology, 'Narians CR, Zareba W, Moss AJ, et al: Clinical implications of silent versus symptomatic exercise-induced myocardial ischemia in patients with stable coronary disease. *J Am Coll Cardiol* 29:756–763, 1997.)

angina during testing was associated with outcome in an independent fashion.

▶ The pathophysiologic implications of silent myocardial ischemia in patients with coronary disease remain unresolved.[1] This study shows that silent myocardial ischemia induced by exercise testing signifies a more favorable prognostic situation than the presence of painful ischemia. It is concluded that the presence of chest pain related to exercise-induced myocardial ischemia signifies more jeopardized myocardium and an increased risk of a subsequent adverse outcome. Patients with silent ischemia alone with exercise have less severe reversible defects with stress thallium testing.

These data would suggest that the presence of silent ischemia would argue for a conservative medical-oriented approach after a myocardial infarction rather than an invasive approach, which would be more appropriate in patients having symptomatic ischemia, in which symptoms cannot be controlled by medical therapy.

W.H. Frishman, M.D.

Reference

1. Klein J, Chao SY, Berman DS, Rozanski A: Is "silent" myocardial ischemia really as severe as symptomatic ischemia? The analytical effect of patient selection biases. *Circulation* 89:1958–1966, 1994.

William Heberden Revisited: Postprandial Angina: Interval Between Food and Exercise and Meal Composition Are Important Determinants of Time to Onset of Ischemia and Maximal Exercise Tolerance
Kearney MT, Charlesworth A, Cowley AJ, et al (Queen's Med Centre, Nottingham, England)
J Am Coll Cardiol 29:302–307, 1997   17–2

Introduction.—In patients with coronary artery disease, cardiovascular adjustments may become worse after eating a meal. Although the effects of food in healthy subjects are well established, they are not so well known in patients with coronary artery disease. In patients with angiographic evidence of coronary artery disease and normal left ventricular function, the effects of isoenergetic high-fat and high-carbohydrate meals on hemodynamic variables at rest and on the time to onset of symptom-limited maximal exercise tolerance and more than 1-mm ST-segment depression were evaluated.

Methods.—On 3 occasions, 15 patients with chronic stable angina were tested in the fasted state. While patients were standing, measurements were taken of cardiac output, heart rate, and blood pressure. Recordings were taken with the modified Bruce exercise test from time of onset of more than 1-mm ST segment depression to limiting chest pain. A high carbohydrate or 2.5 MJ high-fat meal was given to patients, with no meal given on the third occasion. Rest hemodynamic measurements and exercise tests were repeated at 30 minutes and 1 hour after eating the meals.

Results.—Exercise variables were not affected by the high-fat meal, but the high-carbohydrate meal resulted in a reduction in time to onset of ST-segment depression of 74.4±22.2 seconds during exercise at 30 minutes. Limiting chest pain occurred 50–90 seconds earlier among patients who had the high-carbohydrate meal at 30 and 50 minutes than when the patients fasted.

Conclusion.—The onset of angina during exercise occurs earlier than in the fast state 1 hour after a high-carbohydrate meal. A high-fat meal does not affect exercise time despite similar hemodynamic adjustments. The study also showed that a decrease in blood pressure occurred among patients with coronary artery disease and chronic stable angina after eating a high-fat or a high-carbohydrate meal. The effect of meals of different compositions on coronary blood flow and metabolism should be further studied.

▶ An association has been made between food intake and earlier development of angina pectoris with exertion.[1] The classic teaching is for patients with angina pectoris and coronary artery disease to avoid excessive activity after eating. After a meal is eaten, there is a decrease in splanchnic vascular resistance, which leads to a shunting of blood away from other vascular beds.[2-4] This phenomenon appears to be more marked with a high-carbohydrate meal compared to a high-fat meal. The difference between meal composition may be related to the speed of intestinal absorption of carbohydrates and lipids.

W.H. Frishman, M.D.

References

1. Goldstein RE, Redwood DR, Rosing DR, et al: Alterations in the circulatory response to exercise following a meal and their relationship to post-prandial angina pectoris. *Circulation* 44:90–100, 1971.
2. Kelback H, Munck O, Christensen NJ, et al: Central haemodynamic changes after a meal. *Br Heart J* 61:506–509, 1989.
3. Heseltine D, Potter JF, Hartley IA, et al: Blood pressure, heart rate and neuroendocrine responses to a high carbohydrate and a high fat meal in healthy young subjects. *Clin Sci* 79:517–522, 1990.
4. Sidery MB, MacDonald IA, Cowley AJ, et al: Cardiovascular responses to high-fat and high-carbohydrate meals in young subjects. *Am J Physiol* 261:H1430–H1436, 1991.

Effect of Cholesterol Reduction on Myocardial Ischemia in Patients With Coronary Disease

Andrews TC, Raby K, Barry J, et al (Harvard Med School, Boston)
Circulation 95:324–328, 1997   17–3

Introduction.—For the development of coronary artery disease and cardiac events, elevated serum cholesterol in general and serum low-density lipoprotein (LDL) cholesterol in particular are well-established risk factors. New results show improvement of characteristic cellular dysfunctions affecting atherosclerotic arteries in animals and patients with hypercholesterolemia. In patients with coronary artery disease, the effect of cholesterol lowering was determined on the scope of myocardial ischemia as measured by ST-segment depression on ambulatory ECG.

Methods.—The study included 40 patients with proved coronary artery disease, at least 1 episode of ST-segment depression on ambulatory ECG monitoring, and total serum cholesterol between 191 and 327 mg/dL. Twenty patients were randomly assigned to an American Heart Association step 1 diet plus lovastatin and the other 20 patients had the same diet with a placebo. After 4–6 months of therapy, serum cholesterol and LDL cholesterol levels and ambulatory monitoring were repeated.

Results.—At baseline, the 2 groups had comparable measurements. At the end of the study, the group receiving lovastatin had lower mean total and LDL cholesterol levels and significantly fewer episodes of ST-segment depression than the placebo group. In 13 of 20 patients receiving lovastatin (65%), ST-segment depression was completely resolved, whereas 2 of 20 (10%) in the placebo group had complete resolution (Fig). A highly significant reduction in ischemia was found in the treatment group. An independent predictor of ischemia resolution was diet and lovastatin.

Conclusion.—Over 2 years, cholesterol lowering in patients with coronary heart disease can cause physical regression of atheroma, can improve

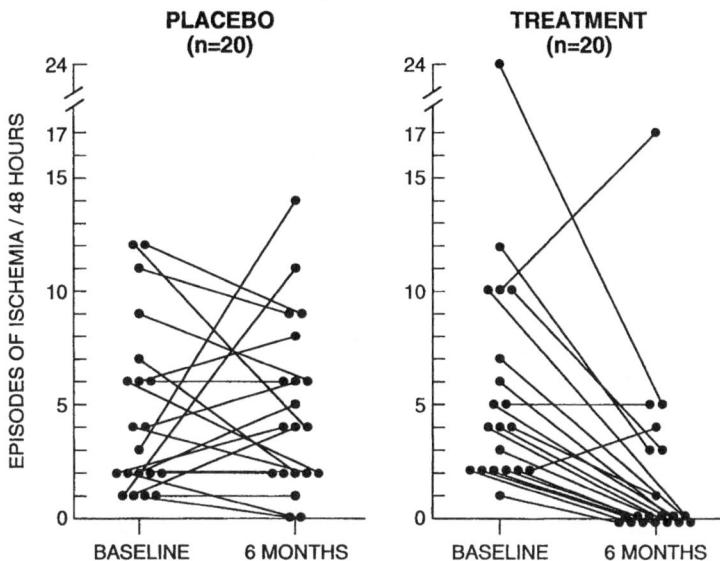

FIGURE.—Data show patient-by-patient effect of cholesterol lowering over 6 months on the number of episodes of ischemic ST-segment depression in patients with coronary disease. Two of 20 in the placebo group vs. 13 of 20 in the treatment group show resolution of ischemia. (Reproduced with permission, from Andrews TC, Raby K, Barry J, et al: Effect of cholesterol reduction on myocardial ischemia in patients with coronary disease. *Circulation* 95:324–328, 1997. Copyright 1997 American Heart Association.)

the endothelial dysfunction in atherosclerotic coronary arteries, and significantly decrease the occurrence of coronary death and myocardial infarction. An effective method to eliminate myocardial ischemia during daily life is cholesterol lowering with lovastatin in a significant proportion of patients.

▶ Aggressive lipid lowering with the 3-hydroxy-3-methylglutaryl coenzyme A reductase inhibitors has been shown to reduce morbidity and mortality from coronary artery disease[1, 2] and to modify the progression of atherosclerotic lesions of the coronary arteries.[3, 4] Elevated cholesterol levels have been associated with abnormalities of coronary vasomotion related to endothelial cell dysfunction.[5]

This study shows that another benefit of cholesterol reduction with statin drugs and diet is to reduce episodes of ST-segment depression detected by ambulatory ECG monitoring. A trial is now in progress, looking at the effects of statin-mediated cholesterol reduction on angina pectoris, with the hypothesis being improved endothelium-dependent relaxation. Similar studies are being performed in patients with peripheral vascular disease.

W.H. Frishman, M.D.

References

1. Randomized trial of cholesterol lowering in 4444 patients with coronary heart disease: The Scandinavian Simvastatin Survival Study (4S). *Lancet* 344:1383–1389, 1994.
2. Shepherd J, Cobbe SM, Ford I, et al: Prevention of coronary heart disease with pravastatin in men with hypercholesterolemia: West of Scotland Coronary Prevention Study Group. *N Engl J Med* 333:1301–1307, 1995.
3. Vos J, deFeyter PJ, Simoons ML, et al: Retardation and arrest of progression or regression of coronary artery disease: A review. *Prog Cardiovasc Dis* 35:435–454, 1993.
4. Brown BG, Zhao X-Q, Albers JJ: Lipid lowering and plaque regression: New insights into prevention of plaque disruption and clinical events in coronary disease. *Circulation* 87:1781–1791, 1993.
5. Anderson TJ, Meredith IT, Yeung AC, et al: The effect of cholesterol lowering and antioxidant therapy on endothelium-dependent coronary vasomotion. *N Engl J Med* 332:488–493, 1995.

Effect of Apheresis of Low-Density Lipoprotein on Peripheral Vascular Disease in Hypercholesterolemic Patients With Coronary Artery Disease

Kroon AA, van Asten WNJC, Stalenhoef AFH (Univ Hosp Nijmegen, The Netherlands)
Ann Intern Med 125:945–954, 1996   17–4

Background.—Hypercholesterolemic patients with coronary artery disease who are refractory to lipid-lowering medications often respond to apheresis of low-density lipoprotein (LDL). The effects of LDL apheresis plus simvastatin treatment on the progression of peripheral vascular disease was compared with that of simvastatin therapy alone.

Methods.—Forty-two men with primary hypercholesterolemia and extensive coronary atherosclerosis were enrolled in the open, randomized trial. Twenty-one received biweekly apheresis of LDL plus simvastatin, 40 mg/d (group 1), and 21 received the same dose of simvastatin alone (group 2) for 2 years.

Findings.—Mean baseline LDL cholesterol levels declined from 7.8 to 3 mmol/L in group 1 and from 7.9 to 4.1 mmol/L in group 2. Mean lipoprotein(a) levels declined from 57 to 44.5 mg/dL and from 38.4 to 44.5 mg/dL in the 2 groups, respectively. The number of group 1 patients with hemodynamically significant stenoses in the aortotibial tract declined from 9 to 7; by contrast, this number increased from 6 to 13 in group 2. Mean intima-media thickness declined by a mean 0.05 mm in group 1 and increased by 0.06 mm in group 2. A multiple regression analysis indicated that changes in apolipoprotein A, total cholesterol, and lipoprotein(a) levels accounted for changes in the aortotibial tract. Changes in the intima-media thickness of the carotid artery were explained by changes in lipoprotein(a) and apolipoprotein A1 levels (Fig 1).

Conclusions.—Aggressive lipid lowering with LDL apheresis and simvastatin reduces the intima-media thickness of the carotid artery. This

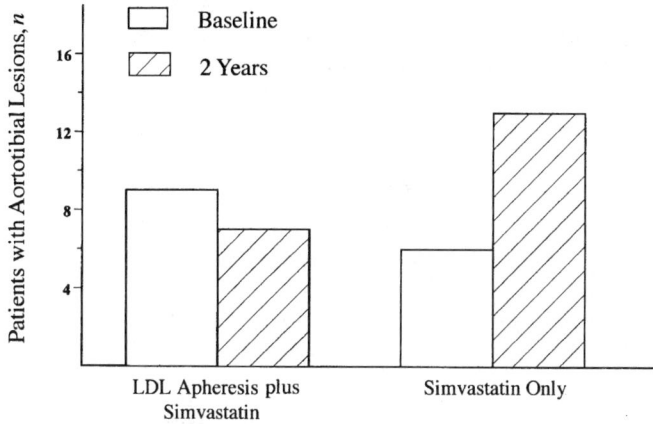

FIGURE 1.—The number of patients with hemodynamically significant stenoses in the aortotibial tract at baseline and at 2 years of treatment with low-density lipoprotein (LDL) apheresis plus simvastatin or simvastatin alone. The change in trend between both groups is statistically significant (P = 0.002). (Courtesy of Kroon AA, van Asten WNJC, Stalenhoef AFH: Effect of apheresis of low-density lipoprotein on peripheral vascular disease in hypercholesterolemic patients with coronary artery disease. *Ann Intern Med* 125:945–954, 1996.)

combination also prevents increases in the number of hemodynamically significant stenoses in the lower limbs. Treatment with simvastatin alone does not prevent carotid or aortotibial vascular disease progression.

▶ This study shows that apheresis of low-density lipoprotein (LDL) with concurrent treatment with the HMG-CoA reductase inhibitor simvastatin successfully decreased the intima-media thickness of the carotid artery while preventing progression of hemodynamically significant arterial stenoses in the lower limb. Treatment with simvastatin did not prevent progression of arterial disease in this population.

These results are from the LDL-Apheresis Atherosclerosis Regression Study (LAARS), a 2 year, open, randomized study of men with primary hypercholesterolemia and extensive coronary artery disease.[1] The study found functional improvement in exercise capacity with combined apheresis and drug treatment. There was a 63% reduction from baseline in LDL-cholesterol levels with combined apheresis and drug treatment, however, apheresis should be considered only in patients having hypercholesterolemia which is refractory to drug treatment.

W.H. Frishman, M.D.

Reference

1. Kroon AA, Aengevaeren WR, van der Werf T, et al: The LDL-Apheresis Atherosclerosis Regression Study (LAARS): Effect of aggressive versus conventional lipid lowering treatment on coronary atherosclerosis. *Circulation* 93:1826–1835, 1996.

The Effect of Aggressive Lowering of Low-Density Lipoprotein Cholesterol Levels and Low-Dose Anticoagulation on Obstructive Changes in Saphenous-Vein Coronary-Artery Bypass Grafts

The Post Coronary Artery Bypass Graft Trial Investigators (Maryland Med Research Inst, Baltimore)

N Engl J Med 336:153–162, 1997   17–5

Background.—Atherosclerosis and thrombosis often cause obstructive changes in aortocoronary saphenous-vein bypass grafts. The effect of aggressive reductions of low-density lipoprotein (LDL) cholesterol levels or low-dose anticoagulation on the progression of atherosclerosis in grafts was studied.

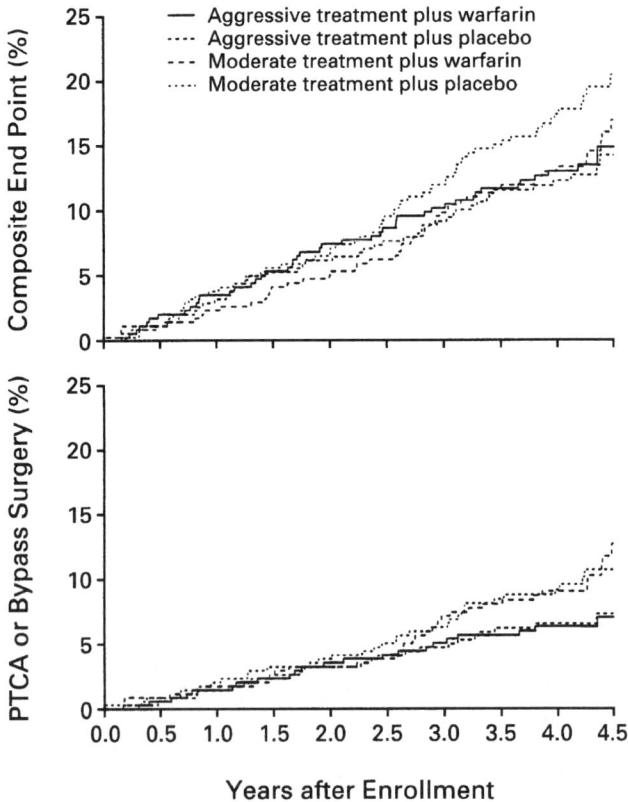

FIGURE 2.—Cumulative life-table rates of events according to study group. The composite end point was death from cardiovascular or unknown causes, nonfatal myocardial infarction, stroke, bypass surgery, or angioplasty. *Abbreviation: PTCA*, percutaneous transluminal coronary angioplasty. (Reprinted by permission of *The New England Journal of Medicine*, courtesy of The Post Coronary Artery Bypass Graft Trial Investigators: The effect of aggressive lowering of low-density lipoprotein cholesterol levels and low-dose anticoagulation on obstructive changes in saphenous-vein coronary-artery bypass grafts. *N Engl J Med* 336:153–162, copyright 1997, Massachusetts Medical Society.)

Methods.—The 1,351 patients included in the study had undergone bypass surgery 1 to 11 years before baseline angiographic study and had LDL cholesterol levels between 130 and 175 mg/dL. In addition, all had at least 1 patent vein graft on angiography. Patients were assigned to aggressive or moderate treatment with lovastatin and, if needed, cholestyramine to decrease LDL cholesterol levels and to treatment with warfarin or placebo in a 2-by-2 factorial design. Angiography was repeated at a mean of 4.3 years after the baseline study.

Findings.—The average LDL cholesterol level of patients receiving aggressive treatment ranged from 93 to 97 mg/dL, as determined annually during the study period. With moderate treatment, this range was 132 to 136 mg/dL. The mean international normalized ratios in the warfarin and placebo groups were 1.4 and 1.1, respectively. In patients with LDL cholesterol levels lowered by aggressive treatment, 27% of the grafts showed atherosclerotic progression. For those receiving moderate treatment, this value was 39%. Angiographic outcomes did not differ significantly between the warfarin and placebo groups. The revascularization rate during 4 years was 29% lower in the patients receiving aggressive treatment than in those receiving moderate treatment (Fig 2).

Conclusion.—The progression of atherosclerosis in grafts can be reduced through aggressive reduction of LDL cholesterol levels to less than 100 mg/dL. Low-dose warfarin did not decrease such atherosclerotic progression.

▶ Atherosclerosis is a common cause of chronic occlusive disease of saphenous-vein coronary bypass grafts. This prospective study demonstrates conclusively the benefit of aggressive reduction of LDL cholesterol with the hepatic hydroxymethylglutaryl coenzyme A reductase inhibitor lovastatin, and, if needed, the bile-acid resin cholestyramine in reducing the progression of atherosclerosis in grafts and the need to perform revascularization procedures. However, no effect of aggressive therapy on mortality was observed. Warfarin appeared to have no morbidity benefit in this study, but the dose used may have been inadequate (the mean international normalized ratio was 1.4). There are also no data on patients who had LDL cholesterol values before drug treatment of less than 130 mg/dL, a group for whom the benefits of lipid-lowering therapy have not been demonstrated.

Based on this study, all patients undergoing coronary artery bypass grafting who have baseline LDL cholesterol levels greater than 130 mg/dL should have their LDL cholesterol reduced below 100 mg/dL with diet and drug treatment. This reflects the guidelines of the National Cholesterol Education Program.[1] In addition, aspirin should be given, based on previous studies, and cigarette smoking behaviors should be changed. A study should be done investigating the effects of additional lipid-lowering therapies in those patients having LVL cholesterol values less than 130 mg/dL but more than 100 mg/dL.

W.H. Frishman, M.D.

Reference

1. National Cholesterol Education Program: Second report of the Expert Panel on Detection, Evaluation and Treatment of High Blood Cholesterol in Adults (Adult Treatment Panel II). *Circulation* 89:1329–1445, 1994.

Randomised Trial of α-Tocopherol and β-Carotene Supplements on Incidence of Major Coronary Events in Men With Previous Myocardial Infarction

Rapola JM, Virtamo J, Ripatti S, et al (Natl Public Health Inst, Helsinki; Natl Cancer Inst, Bethesda, Md; Univ of Helsinki)

Lancet 349:1715–1720, 1997   17–6

Objective.—Whereas data from prospective cohort studies indicate that antioxidants decrease the incidence of coronary heart disease, results of clinical trials do not support these findings. The effects of α-tocopherol and β-carotene supplements on the incidence of major coronary events among men at high risk of a coronary event because of previous myocardial infarction were investigated in the Alpha-tocopherol and Beta-carotene Cancer Prevention (ATBC) Study.

Methods.—Dietary supplements of α-tocopherol (50 mg/day), β-carotene (20 mg/day), both, or placebo were administered to 1,862 male smokers aged 50–69 years who had a previous myocardial infarction.

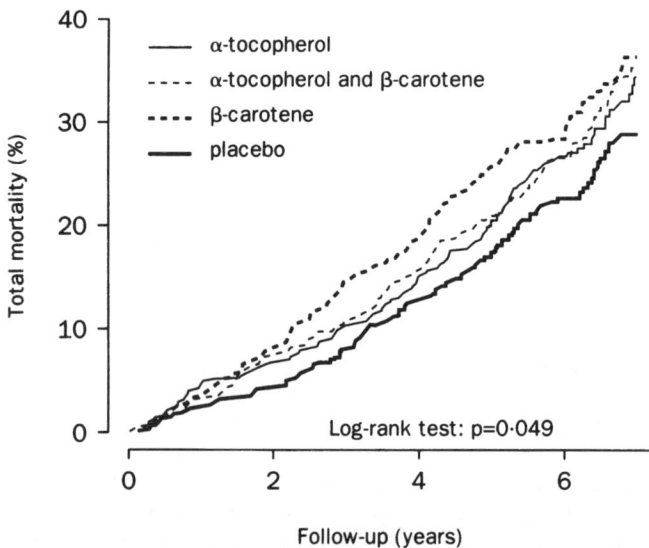

FIGURE 3.—Kaplan-Meier estimates of mortality. (Courtesy of Rapola JM, Virtamo J, Ripatti S, et al: Randomised trial of α-tocopherol and β-carotene supplements on incidence of major coronary events in men with previous myocardial infarction. *Lancet* 349:1715–1720, 1997. Copyright by the Lancet Ltd, 1997.)

Individuals completed a questionnaire about their background, smoking, and medical histories, diet, and exercise. Participants were examined 3 times a year for an average of 5.3 years. Body mass index was calculated, blood pressure was measured, and blood chemistry was performed. Serum α-tocopherol and β-carotene concentrations were determined. The end point was the first major coronary event.

Results.—Serum levels of α-tocopherol and/or β-carotene were similar among treatment groups. There were 424 major coronary events, 190 nonfatal and 234 fatal. There was no difference in the total number of coronary events among the 4 groups, although the risk of nonfatal myocardial infarction was lower in the treated groups and significantly lower in the α-tocopherol-treated group. Mortality was highest in the β-carotene group and lowest in the placebo group (Fig 3).

Conclusion.—Both α-tocopherol and β-carotene increased the risk of a fatal coronary event in male smokers with a previous myocardial infarction.

▶ This report is from the Alpha-tocopherol Beta-carotene Cancer Prevention[1] Study, a placebo-controlled longitudinal study designed to examine the cardioprotective effects of α-tocopherol, β-carotene, and their combination in male patients with a history of myocardial infarction and cigarette smoking. The study shows no benefit from either therapy on coronary events compared to placebo, and the authors (see Figure 3) discourage the use of α-tocopherol and β-carotene supplements in survivors of myocardial infarction. It has been suggested that these antioxidant drugs may interfere with the benefits of ischemic preconditioning and might also increase the risk of atherosclerotic plaque rupture.[1-3] Of concern is that many physicians take antioxidants themselves and commonly prescribe them to their patients.[4] Other prospective studies examining the clinical effects of antioxidants in coronary prone individuals are now in progress.[5, 6]

W.H. Frishman, M.D.

References

1. Sun JZ, Tang TL, Parks SW, et al: Evidence for an essential role of reactive oxygen species in the genesis of late preconditioning against myocardial stunning in conscious pigs. *J Clin Invest* 97:562–576, 1996.
2. Prince MR, LaMuraglia GM, MacNichol EF Jr: Increased preferential absorption in human atherosclerotic plaque with oral beta carotene. *Circulation* 78:338-344, 1988.
3. Mitchell DC, Prince MR, Frisoli JK, et al: Beta carotene uptake into atherosclerotic plaque: Enhanced staining and preferential ablation with the pulsed dye laser. *Lasers Surg Med* 13:149–157, 1993.
4. Mehta J: Intake of antioxidants among American cardiologists. *Am J Cardiol* 79:1558–1559, 1997.
5. Jha P, Flather M, Lonn E, et al: The antioxidant vitamins and cardiovascular disease. *Ann Intern Med* 123:860–872, 1995.

6. Vakili BA, Frishman WH, Lin TS, et al: Antioxidant vitamins and enzymatic and synthetic scavengers of oxygen-derived free radical scavengers in the prevention and treatment of cardiovascular diseases, in Frishman WH, Sonnenblick EH (eds): *Cardiovascular Pharmacotherapeutics*. New York; McGraw Hill Inc, 1997, pp 535–556.

A Randomised, Blinded Trial of Clopidogrel Versus Aspirin in Patients at Risk of Ischaemic Events (CAPRIE)

Gent M, and the CAPRIE Steering Committee (Hamilton Civic Hosps Research Centre, Ont, Canada)
Lancet 348:1329–1339, 1996   17–7

Objective.—Adverse effects and efficacy of clopidogrel and those of aspirin on the risk of ischemic stroke, myocardial infarction, and vascular death were evaluated in a randomized, comparative trial.

Background.—Various randomized trials have evaluated the effect of antiplatelet drugs on the risk of ischemic stroke, myocardial infarction, and death in patients with atherothrombotic disease or atherosclerotic peripheral arterial disease. Placebo-controlled studies have shown that aspirin and ticlopidine can reduce the risk of stroke, myocardial infarction, and vascular death, but both of these agents have serious adverse effects. Clopidogrel is a thienopyridine derivative chemically related to ticlopidine. In various animal models, it has been shown to prevent arterial and venous thrombosis and lower atherogenesis. Clopidogrel inhibits platelet aggregation induced by adenosine diphosphate.

Methods.—Clopidogrel, 75 mg/day plus placebo or aspirin, 325 mg/day, plus placebo was administered to 19,185 patients from 384 centers with

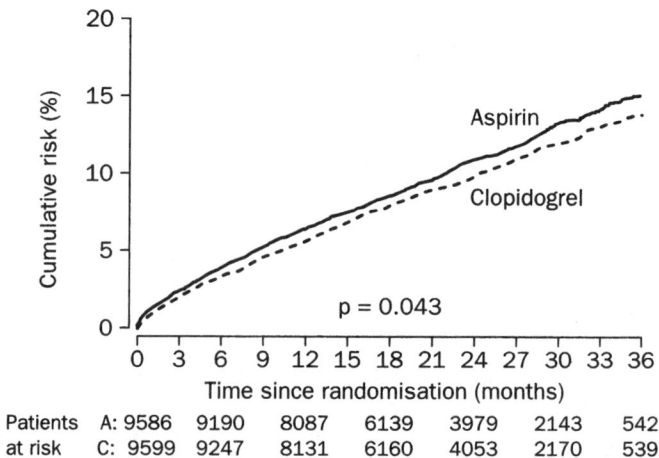

Patients							
at risk	A: 9586	9190	8087	6139	3979	2143	542
	C: 9599	9247	8131	6160	4053	2170	539

FIGURE 3.—Cumulative risk of ischemic stroke, myocardial infarction, or vascular death. *Abbreviations*: A, aspirin; C, clopidogrel. (Courtesy of Gent M, and the CAPRIE Steering Committee: A randomized, blinded, trial of clopidogrel versus aspirin in patients at risk of ischaemic events (CAPRIE). *Lancet* 348:1329–1339, 1996. Copyright 1996 by The Lancet, Ltd.)

ischemic stroke, myocardial infarction, or atherosclerotic peripheral arterial disease. Adverse effects and risk of ischemic stroke, myocardial infarction, or vascular death were calculated. Follow-up was 1–3 years.

Results.—Intention-to-treat analysis showed that the annual risk of ischemic stroke, myocardial infarction, or vascular death was 5.32% in patients treated with clopidogrel and 5.83% in patients treated with aspirin (Fig 3). The relative risk reduction was 8.7% in favor of clopidogrel, and this difference was statistically significant. On-treatment analysis showed a relative risk reduction of 9.4%. The safety of clopidogrel and aspirin was similar. Serious adverse effects in both groups included rash, diarrhea, upper gastrointestinal discomfort, intracranial hemorrhage, and gastrointestinal hemorrhage. Significant reduction in neutrophils occurred in 10 patients given clopidogrel and 16 patients given aspirin.

Conclusions.—In these patients with atherothrombotic disease, clopidogrel was more effective than aspirin in lowering risk of ischemic stroke, myocardial infarction, and vascular death. There was no evidence of excess neutropenia. Clopidogrel is safer than ticlopidine and at least as safe as medium-dose aspirin. CAPRIE was the first trial of an antiplatelet drug to include clinical subgroups of patients with ischemic cerebrovascular, cardiac, and peripheral arterial disease under a common treatment protocol.

▶ Clopidogrel is a thienopyridine antiplatelet drug in the same class as ticlopidine. Similar to ticlopidine, clopidogrel is a pro-drug that is not active in vitro but active in vivo.[1-5] It functions as an adenosine diphosphate (ADP)-selective agent whose antiaggregating properties are several times higher than those of ticlopidine and are apparently the result of the same mechanism of action, i.e., inhibition of ADP binding to its platelet receptor and triggering the release of thrombogenic factor-containing alpha granules.[4] After a single oral or IV administration, clopidogrel inhibited ADP-induced platelet aggregation for several days and potently reduced thrombus formation in various experimental animal models.[1-4]

In this study, aspirin had a slightly higher benefit than clopidogrel in preventing myocardial infarction; clopidogrel had a greater effect in preventing stroke and vascular death. On the basis of this study, clopidogrel will be marketed as an alternative antiplatelet treatment to aspirin for preventing cardiovascular events.

W.H. Frishman, M.D.

References

1. Verstraete M, Zoldhelyi P: Novel antithrombotic drugs in development. *Drugs* 49:856–884, 1995.
2. Verstraete M: New developments in antiplatelet and antithrombotic therapy. *Eur Heart J* 16 (Suppl L):16–23, 1995.
3. Schror K: Antiplatelet drugs: A comparative review. *Drugs* 50:7–28, 1995.
4. Mills DCB, Puri R, Hu CJ, et al: Clopidogrel inhibits the binding of ADP analogues to the receptor mediating inhibition of platelet adenylate cyclase. *Arterioscler Thromb* 12:430–436, 1992.

18 Coronary Interventional Procedures

Coronary Angioplasty Volume-Outcome Relationships for Hospitals and Cardiologists
Hannan EL, Racz M, Ryan TJ, et al (State Univ of New York, Albany; Boston Univ; Mid-America Heart Inst, Kansas City, Mo; et al)
JAMA 279:892–898, 1997   18–1

Objective.—Many studies have examined the association between adverse outcomes of various procedures and the volume of procedures performed by the physician or hospital. However, none of these studies have looked at the relationship between volume and outcomes for percutaneous transluminal coronary angioplasty (PTCA). In this study, outcomes of PTCA were analyzed for their relationship to various measures of provider volume.

Methods.—The study included data on 62,670 patients undergoing PTCA. All patients were discharged from New York state hospitals after PTCA from 1991 through 1994. The indicators of volume analyzed were annual hospital volume and annual cardiologist volume. The outcomes studied were in-hospital mortality and same-stay coronary artery bypass graft (CABG).

Results.—For the overall cohort, in-hospital mortality was 0.90%, and the rate of CABG during the same hospitalization was 3.43%. Risk-adjusted in-hospital mortality was 0.96% for patients undergoing PTCA at low-volume hospitals, that is, those performing less than 600 procedures per year. The risk-adjusted same-stay CABG rate for this group was 3.92%. For patients whose PTCA was performed by low-volume cardiologists—those performing less than 75 procedures per year—in-hospital mortality was 1.03%, and the same-stay CABG rate was 3.93%. The same-stay CABG rate was 2.99% for patients whose PTCA was done by a cardiologist who performed 75 to 174 procedures per year at hospitals with a volume of 600 to 999 procedures a year. For patients at these middle-volume hospitals, whose cardiologists performed 175 or more procedures per year, the same-stay CABG rate was 2.84%.

Conclusions.—The outcomes of PTCA are significantly affected by the volume of procedures performed at a given hospital and by a given cardiologist. Mortality and same-stay CABG rates are elevated for patients whose cardiologist performed less than 75 procedures per year. Mortality is significantly increased for hospitals with an annual volume of less than 600. The results suggest that minimum provider volumes for maintenance of competence should be set even higher than those recommended by the recent American College of Cardiology and American Heart Association guidelines.

▶ In recent years, studies have documented a relationship between outcomes of medical and surgical procedures, and provider volume.[1-3] From this large database in New York, it was confirmed that hospitals and cardiologists who perform more coronary angioplasty procedures have more favorable outcomes regarding mortality and the need for their patients to have same-stay CABG. There is also a need to calculate risk-adjusted outcomes. Low-risk patients may be able to travel long distances to a high-volume angioplasty center, whereas high-risk patients may go to a low-volume center closer to home.

W.H. Frishman, M.D.

References

1. Luft HS, Garnick DW, Mark DH, et al: *Hospital Volume, Physician Volume, and Patient Outcomes.* Ann Arbor, Mich, Health Administration Press, 1990.
2. Jollis JG, Peterson ED, DeLong ER, et al: The relationship between the volume of coronary angioplasty procedures at hospitals treating Medicare beneficiaries and short-term mortality. *N Engl J Med* 331:1625–1629, 1994.
3. Kimmel SE, Berlin JA, Laskey WK: The relationship between coronary angioplasty procedure volume and major complications. *JAMA* 274:1137–1142, 1995.

Immediate Coronary Angiography in Survivors of Out-of-hospital Cardiac Arrest
Spaulding CM, Joly L-M, Rosenberg A, et al (René Descartes Univ, Paris; Service d'Aide Medicale Urgente, Paris)
N Engl J Med 336:1629–1633, 1997   18–2

Purpose.—The reported incidence of acute coronary artery occlusion among patients with sudden out-of-hospital cardiac arrest varies widely. One useful treatment approach for such patients could be coronary angiography followed by angioplasty, if appropriate. A strategy of immediate coronary angiography and angioplasty was studied for use in survivors of out-of-hospital cardiac arrest.

Methods.—The experience included 84 consecutive patients with out-of-hospital cardiac arrest of no obvious cause. The patients were between

30 and 75 years old. They were brought immediately to the cardiac catheterization laboratory where they underwent immediate coronary and left ventricular angiography. If angiography showed recent coronary artery occlusion, coronary angioplasty was attempted if possible.

Results.—The patients were 70 men and 15 women (mean age, 55.5 years). Angiography revealed clinically significant coronary artery disease in 60 patients. Forty patients—48% of the total—had coronary artery occlusion. Thirty-seven underwent attempted angioplasty, which was technically successful in 28 patients. There were no clinical or ECG findings useful for predicting the presence of coronary artery occlusion. Thirty-eight percent of patients survived to hospital discharge. Successful angioplasty was a significant independent predictor of survival on multivariate logistic regression analysis (odds ratio, 5.2).

Conclusions.—Many patients who survive out-of-hospital cardiac arrest have acute coronary artery occlusion. This condition cannot be predicted by clinical and ECG findings such as chest pain or ST-segment elevation. Occlusion can be detected by immediate coronary angiography, and survival may be improved by coronary angioplasty, when appropriate. This approach may improve the long-term outcomes after out-of-hospital cardiac arrest.

▶ This study shows that many patients who survive unexpected out-of-hospital sudden cardiac death have an acute coronary thrombosis as the cause. This would suggest that out-of-hospital interventions to lyse or break up coronary clots might be better suited to improve clinical outcomes in patients with cardiac arrest because many patients will not be able to ultimately undergo coronary angiography and angioplasty because of limited resources.

W.H. Frishman, M.D.

Randomised Placebo-controlled Trial of Abciximab Before and During Coronary Intervention in Refractory Unstable Angina: The CAPTURE Study

Simoons ML, for the CAPTURE Investigators (Univ Hosp Rotterdam, The Netherlands)
Lancet 349:1429–1435, 1997   18–3

Objective.—Platelet aggregation plays a key role in the development of unstable angina, and patients undergoing percutaneous transluminal coronary angioplasty (PTCA) are at risk for thrombotic complications. By blocking the platelet glycoprotein IIb/IIIa receptor, abciximab—the Fab (fragment, antigen binding) of the chimeric antibody c7E3—can prevent platelet adhesion and aggregation. A pilot study suggested that giving abciximab before PTCA might help to prevent thrombotic complications in patients with refractory unstable angina. This intervention was studied in a multicenter, randomized, placebo-controlled trial.

Methods.—The study was scheduled to include 1,400 patients with refractory unstable angina. All had recurrent myocardial ischemia despite medical therapy, including heparin and nitrates. The patients were first evaluated by angiography, then randomized to receive either abciximab or placebo. The assigned treatment was given by infusion, starting 18-24 hours before PTCA and continuing until 1 hour afterward. The 30-day outcomes evaluated were death as a result of any cause, myocardial inrfaction, and urgent intervention for recurrent ischemia.

Results.—Recruitment into the trial was halted at a planned interim analysis; the current analysis included 1,265 patients. The incidence of 1 of the outcomes noted above was 11.3% in the abciximab group and 15.9% in the placebo group. Patients receiving abciximab had a 0.6% rate of myocardial infarction before PTCA compared with 2.1% in the placebo group. The rate of myocardial infarction during PTCA was also lower with abciximab (2.6% vs. 5.5% for the placebo group). Patients receiving abciximab were twice as likely to experience major bleeding (3.8% vs. 1.9%). By 6 months, there was no difference between groups in the rates of death, myocardial infarction, or need for repeat intervention.

Conclusions.—Abciximab treatment before PTCA significantly reduces the rate of thrombotic complications in patients with refractory unstable angina. Treatment significantly reduces the rate of myocardial infarction, before, during, and after PTCA. Beyond the first few days, abciximab has no apparent effect on myocardial infarction risk. The expense of the drug may lead some physicians to use it only to treat thrombotic complications after they have occurred; however, this use has not been tested.

▶ This study shows the short-term and long-term benefits of using abciximab in patients with unstable angina pectoris when they are undergoing angioplasty. It is not known whether infusions of abciximab for even greater time intervals after undergoing angioplasty might further improve clinical outcomes. In addition, oral agents of this class are now available and might provide long-term protection against coronary ischemic events.[1, 2]

W.H. Frishman, M.D.

References

1. Frishman WH, Klein MD, Blaufarb I, et al: Antiplatelet and other antithrombotic drugs, in Frishman WH, Sonnenblick EH (eds): *Cardiovascular Pharmacotherapeutics.* New York, McGraw Hill, 1997, p 323.
2. Frishman WH, Burns B, Atac B, et al: Novel antiplatelet therapies for treatment of patients with ischemic heart disease. Inhibitors of platelet glycoprotein IIb/IIIa integrelin receptors. *Am Heart J* 130:877–892, 1995.

A Comparison of Coronary-artery Stenting With Angioplasty for Isolated Stenosis of the Proximal Left Anterior Descending Coronary Artery

Versaci F, Gaspardone A, Tomai F, et al (Università di Roma Tor Vergata, Rome; Università Cattolica del Sacro Cuore, Rome)
N Engl J Med 336:817–822, 1997
                                                                    18–4

Background.—Recent clinical trials have suggested that primary stent implantation in large coronary arteries results in a lower rate of restenosis and less need for repeat interventions than percutaneous transluminal coronary angioplasty (PTCA) as a treatment for coronary artery disease. A prospective, randomized study was performed to compare the effectiveness of primary stent implantation with that of PTCA in the treatment of patients with symptomatic isolated stenosis of the proximal left anterior descending coronary artery.

Methods.—The study population consisted of 120 patients with typical angina pectoris and/or confirmed myocardial ischemia; a newly diagnosed, isolated stenosis of the proximal portion of the left anterior descending coronary artery; and a left ventricular ejection fraction of at least 40%. Patients were randomized to either primary stent implantation or PTCA. After discharge, patients were treated with warfarin for 3 months, and aspirin and diltiazem indefinitely. The primary clinical end points were the rate of procedural success and the rate of event-free survival, defined as freedom from death, myocardial infarction, and angina at 12 months. The amount of restenosis was assessed 12 months after the procedure.

Results.—Between March 1992 and July 1995, 105 men and 15 women were referred for isolated, symptomatic stenosis of the proximal left anterior descending coronary artery. Sixty patients were randomized to primary stent implantation and 60 to PTCA. There were no significant differences between these 2 groups in demographic, clinical, or angiographic characteristics. The rate of procedural success was similar for the 2 treatment groups. The 12-month rate of event-free survival was 87% in the stent group and 70% in the PTCA group. The rate of restenosis was 19% in the stent group and 40% in the PTCA group.

Conclusions.—These results demonstrate that in symptomatic patients with isolated stenosis of the proximal left anterior descending coronary artery, primary stent implantation was associated with both a significantly lower rate of restenosis and a better clinical outcome than PTCA.

▶ Percutaneous transluminal coronary angioplasty has been shown to be an effective alternative to medical therapy in the treatment of patients with single-vessel coronary artery disease, with no differences in mortality outcomes seen.[1, 2] In the treatment of patients with isolated stenosis of the proximal left anterior descending coronary artery who are symptomatic and considered for a catheter-based procedure, stenting has advantages over standard coronary angioplasty, with a lower rate of restenosis.[3–5] The long-term effects of stenting on the natural history of coronary artery disease still need to be determined.

W.H. Frishman, M.D.

References

1. Parisi AF, Folland ED, Hartigan P: A comparison of angioplasty with medical therapy in the treatment of single-vessel coronary artery disease. *N Engl J Med* 326:10–16, 1992.
2. Strauss WE, Fortin T, Hartigan P, et al: A comparison of quality of life scores in patients with angina pectoris after angioplasty compared with after medical therapy: outcomes of a randomized clinical trial. *Circulation* 92:1710–1719, 1995.
3. Serruys PW, deJaegere P, Kiemeneij F, et al: A comparison of balloon-expandable-stent implantation with balloon angioplasty in patients with coronary artery disease. *N Engl J Med* 331:489–495, 1994.
4. Fischman DL, Leon MB, Baim DS, et al: A randomized comparison of coronary-stent placement and balloon angioplasty in the treatment of coronary artery disease. *N Engl J Med* 331:496–501, 1994.
5. Landzberg BR, Frishman WH, Lerrick K: Pathophysiology and pharmacological approaches for prevention of coronary artery restenosis following coronary artery balloon angioplasty and related procedures. *Prog Cardiovasc Dis* 34:361–398, 1997.

Effect on Survival of Estrogen Replacement Therapy After Coronary Artery Bypass Grafting

Sullivan JM, El-Zeky F, Vander Zwaag R, et al (Univ of Tennessee, Memphis; Division of Health Services Research Baptist Mem Hosp, Memphis, Tenn)

Am J Cardiol 79:847–850, 1997   18–5

Objective.—Estrogen replacement therapy (ERT) reduces cardiovascular events in postmenopausal women. Angiographic studies have documented reduced coronary artery stenosis and mortality in women with coronary artery disease. The relationship between ERT in postmenopausal women and survival after coronary artery bypass grafting (CABG) was examined in an observational study.

Methods.—Five- and 10-year survival was compared for 92 postmenopausal women receiving ERT and 1,006 postmenopausal women not receiving ERT who underwent CABG between 1972 and 1989.

Results.—Data were obtained for at least 1 year for 861 non-ERT users and 82 ERT users. Non-ERT users were significantly older and had a higher incidence of 3-vessel disease. Non-ERT users tended to have lower cholesterol, lower ejection fractions, a higher prevalence of left main coronary stenosis, and a more frequent history of myocardial infarction. Five-year survival was significantly higher in ERT-users and also significantly higher in women who used ERT postoperatively only. When Cox's stepwise proportional hazards analysis was performed to assess the relative risks of death, the number of vessels with stenosis greater than 70% of luminal diameter (relative risk (RR) 1.43), the presence of significantly left main coronary artery stenosis (RR 1.83), the presences of diabetes mellitus (RR 1.57) significantly increased mortality, whereas only ERT significantly decreased mortality (RR 0.38).

Conclusion.—Estrogen replacement therapy significantly improves the 5- and 10-year survival of postmenopausal women undergoing CABG.

▶ Estrogen has been shown in large retrospective cohort studies in post-menopausal women to have benefits against the development of coronary artery disease and its complications.[1] The benefits of estrogen appear to be related to lipid lowering and/or vasculoprotective actions. This retrospective clinical experience, demonstrates a lower coronary event rate after coronary angioplasty in postmenopausal women receiving estrogen compared to those who were not.[2] However, the number of revascularization procedures were similar in both groups. A similar beneficial result on outcomes has been described in women who underwent CABG and who were receiving estrogen replacement.

The Womens' Health Initiative is addressing whether all postmenopausal women should receive estrogen replacement to prevent coronary artery disease, using a placebo-controlled study design, and a similar prospective, placebo-controlled study is being done in women with known coronary artery disease.[1]

Until the studies are completed, postmenopausal women with known coronary artery disease, especially those with other risk factors (e.g., diabetes, smoking), should probably receive estrogen replacement with and without progestin (depending on the presence of a uterus) unless there are contraindications to their use and only after normal findings on a mammogram and pelvic examination.

W.H. Frishman, M.D.

References

1. Gomberg-Maitland M, Frishman WH, Karch S, et al: Hormones as cardiovascular drugs: estrogens, progestins, thyroxine, growth hormone, corticosteroids and testosterone, in Frishman WH, Sonnenblick EH: *Cardiovascular Pharmacotherapeutics.* New York: McGraw Hill, 1997, pp 787–835.
2. O'Keefe JH, Kim SC, Hall RR, et al: Estrogen replacement therapy after coronary angioplasty in women. *J Am Coll Cardiol* 29:1–5, 1997.

19 Cardiomyopathy/ Heart Failure

Apoptosis in the Failing Human Heart
Olivetti G, Abbi R, Quaini F, et al (New York Med College, Valhalla; Univ of Parma, Italy; Univ of Udine, Italy; et al)
N Engl J Med 336:1131–1141, 1997   19–1

Introduction.—Patients with cardiomyopathy, whether of ischemic or nonischemic origin, have progressive loss of myocytes. Although experimental studies have demonstrated apoptosis in myocytes, it is unknown whether programmed cell death occurs in the human heart as it fails. Apoptosis of myocytes was studied in patients with intractable congestive heart failure.

Methods.—The researchers analyzed specimens of myocardial tissue from 36 patients who received heart transplants and from 3 who died soon after myocardial infarction, as well as from 11 normal hearts. Histochemical and biochemical analyses were performed, as well as a combination of histochemical analysis and confocal microscopy. The analysis also included measurement of the expression of *BCL2* and *BAX*, 2 proto-oncogenes that protect against and promote apoptosis, respectively.

Results.—The specimens from patients with heart failure had a 232-fold increase in morphologic evidence of myocyte apoptosis. On biochemical assessment, these specimens showed DNA laddering as a marker of apoptosis. Histochemically, the specimens showed DNA-strand breaks in myocyte nuclei; confocal microscopy revealed chromatin condensation and fragmentation. In failing hearts, the percentage of myocytes labeled with *BCL2* was nearly doubled; this finding was confirmed by Western blotting. There was no difference in expression of *BAX*.

Conclusions.—During failure, the human heart undergoes myocyte apoptosis. Programmed cell death occurs despite enhanced expression of *BCL2*, which protects cells from apoptosis. This suggests that the overloaded myocardium activates compensatory mechanisms in an attempt to preserve cells. Myocyte apoptosis may play a role in the progression of cardiac dysfunction.

▶ Cardiomyopathy is a growing cause of morbidity and mortality in the United States. Apoptosis is the process of programmed cell death, and this study demonstrated that heart failure itself could accelerate the apoptotic process. This additional cell loss would hasten patient decompensation and death. Ventricular dilation itself may be the apoptotic trigger in patients with congestive heart failure, which would demonstrate the need to keep ventricular volumes smaller with diuretic and vasodilating drugs.[1] Pressure loads may also be an apoptotic stimulus.[2]

Specific treatments aimed at turning on anti-apoptotic genes are now being investigated as a possible approach for the prevention and treatment of congestive heart failure.[3]

W.H. Frishman, M.D.

References

1. Vasan RS, Larson MG, Benjamin EJ, et al: Left ventricular dilatation and the risk of congestive heart failure in people without myocardial infarction. *N Engl J Med* 336:1350–1355, 1997.
2. Bing OHL: Hypothesis: Apoptosis may be the mechanism for the transition to heart failure with chronic pressure overload. *J Mol Cell Cardiol* 26:943–948, 1994.
3. Bialik S, Geenen DL, Bennett MR, et al: Cardiac myocyte apoptosis: A new therapeutic target? in Frishman WH, Sonnenblick EH (eds): *Cardiovascular Pharmacotherapeutics*. New York, McGraw Hill, 1997, pp 955–972.

Prevention of Heart Failure by Antihypertensive Drug Treatment in Older Persons With Isolated Systolic Hypertension
Kostis JB, for the SHEP Cooperative Research Group (UMDNJ, New Brunswick, NJ; Univ of Texas, Houston; Natl Heart, Lung, and Blood Inst, Bethesda, Md; et al)
JAMA 278:212–216, 1997   19–2

Introduction.—More than 2 million persons are affected by heart failure in the United States. A common antecedent is hypertension and isolated systolic hypertension. The incidence of total stroke was reduced by 36% and of major cardiovascular events by 32% in the Systolic Hypertension in the Elderly Program, in which participants aged 60 years and older had antihypertensive stepped-care drug treatment with low-dose chlorthalidone. The occurrence of heart failure in active and placebo groups in the Systolic Hypertension in the Elderly Program was studied among patients with a history of ECG evidence of prior myocardial infarction compared to the other patients..

Methods.—There were 4,736 persons aged 60 years and older with diastolic blood pressure below 90 mm Hg and systolic blood pressure between 160 and 219 mm Hg who received stepped-care antihypertensive drug therapy with the step 1 drug as chlorthalidone at 12.5–25 mg or matching placebo, and the step 2 drug as atenolol at 25–50 mg or matching placebo.

Results.—There were 55 of 2,365 patients in the active therapy group who had heart failure compared to 105 of 2,371 patients in the placebo group. A predictor of risk of fatal or hospitalized nonfatal heart failure was a history of ECG evidence of myocardial infarction at baseline. For the different heart failure end points examined, the risk reduction in the group with a history of ECG evidence of myocardial infarction at baseline ranged from 59% to 85%. A higher risk of heart failure occurred among older patients, men, and those with higher systolic blood pressure, or a history of ECG evidence of myocardial infarction.

Conclusion.—A strong protective effect was exerted in preventing heart failure among older persons with isolated systolic hypertension who received stepped-care treatment based on low-dose chlorthalidone. An 80% risk reduction was seen among patients with prior myocardial infarction.

▶ Heart failure is the most common reason for admission to the hospital for older individuals, and is increasing in prevalence in the United States. Hypertension, including isolated systolic hypertension, in the elderly[1] is a known risk factor for the development of heart failure, and the results of the SHEP study[2] show that a stepped-care treatment approach to isolated systolic hypertension in the elderly can dramatically prevent or postpone the development of heart failure in both men and women. This was most apparent in patients with a prior history of myocardial infarction.

The SHEP medical regimen included a low-dose, stepped-care treatment approach using chlorthalidone, atenolol, and reserpine.

W.H. Frishman, M.D.

References

1. SHEP Cooperative Research Group: Prevention of stroke by antihypertensive drug treatment in older persons with isolated systolic hypertension: Final results of the Systolic Hypertension in the Elderly Program (SHEP). *JAMA* 265:3255–3264, 1991.
2. Saltzberg S, Stroh JA, Frishman WH: Isolated systolic hypertension in the elderly: Pathophysiology and treatment. *Med Clin N Amer* 72:523–547, 1988.

Randomised, Placebo-controlled Trial of Carvedilol in Patients With Heart Failure Due to Ischaemic Heart Disease
Krum H, and the Australia/New Zealand Heart Failure Research Collaborative Group (Austin Hosp, Melbourne, Australia)
Lancet 349:375–380, 1997   19–3

Introduction.—Carvedilol is a β-blocker that has antioxidant and anti-ischemic properties, and has the potential to reduce morbidity and mortality in heart failure. In a previous study of 415 patients with heart failure resulting from ischemic heart disease, carvedilol was administered, and

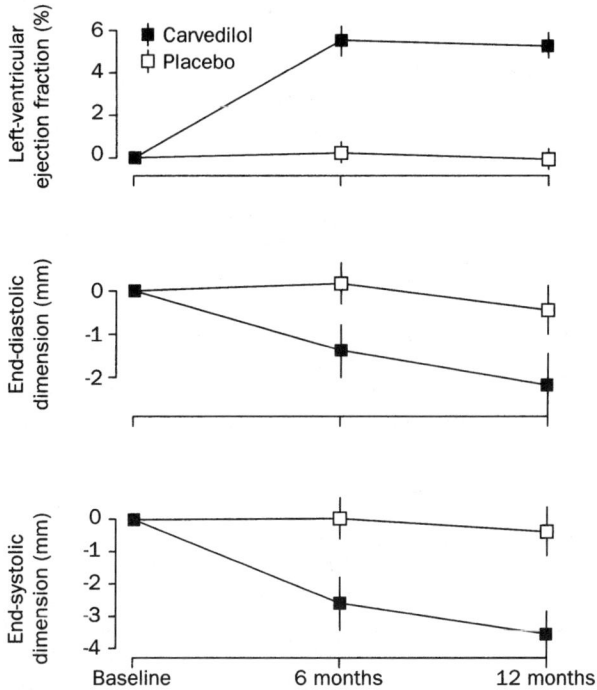

FIGURE 2.—Changes in left ventricular ejection fraction and left ventricular dimensions in carvedilol and placebo groups during 12 months of follow-up. Values at 6 and 12 months represent mean change from baseline (±SE). (Courtesy of Krum H, and the Australia/New Zealand Heart Failure Research Collaborative Group: Randomized, placebo-controlled trial of carvedilol in patients with heart failure due to ischemic heart disease. *Lancet* 349:375–380, 1997. Copyright by The Lancet Ltd, 1997.)

was shown to have improved left ventricular function. The effects of long-term treatment are still unknown; The follow-up results of these patients for an average of 19 months later were evaluated.

Methods.—There was a random assignment of treatment of 415 patients with chronic stable heart failure, with 207 receiving carvedilol and 208 receiving matching placebo. Several measurements were taken at baseline, 6 months, and 12 months, including specific activity scale score, New York Heart Association class, 6-minute walk distance, treadmill exercise duration, left ventricular dimensions, and left ventricular ejection fraction. All deaths, hospital admissions, and episodes of worsening heart failure were documented with the double-blind follow-up for an average of 19 months.

Results.—In the carvedilol group compared to the placebo group, left ventricular ejection fraction increased by 5.3% after 12 months (Fig 2), end-diastolic dimension decreased by 1.7 mm, and end-systolic dimension decreased by 3.2 mm. There were no clear changes, however, in the 6-minute walk distance, New York Heart Association class, specific activity scale, or treadmill exercise duration. The rate of death or hospital admission was lower in the carvedilol group than in the placebo group after 19 months, but the frequency of episodes of worsening heart failure was similar.

Conclusion.—For at least a year after the start of treatment, the beneficial effects of carvedilol on left ventricular function and size were maintained; however, no extra benefits were demonstrated on symptoms, exercise performance, or episodes of worsening heart failure. After a year of treatment with carvedilol, there was an overall reduction in events resulting in death or hospital admission. To show whether this drug can be recommended as first-line therapy for heart failure, together with angiotensin-converting enzyme inhibitors, trials of several thousand patients and several years must be designed to investigate the effects of carvedilol on survival.

▶ Beta-blockers have been shown to be useful in preventing morbidity and mortality in many patients with left ventricular dysfunction from both ischemic and nonischemic cardiomyopathy.[1-5] Carvedilol is the first beta-blocker approved for clinical use in congestive heart failure (CHF). The drug is usually added to stable doses of digoxin, diuretics, and angiotensin-converting enzyme inhibitors in patients who are not decompensated or who have advanced CHF. Carvedilol appears to relieve symptoms, improves left ventricular function, and can reduce mortality. The mechanism by which beta-blockers accomplish their benefit is not known. The drug must be titrated carefully, and some patients receiving carvedilol will decompensate.

A study with bucindolol in patients with advanced CHF is in progress and studies comparing carvedilol to metoprolol in patients with CHF are underway.

W.H. Frishman, M.D.

References

1. Frishman WH, Nalamati J: Carvedilol: a new alpha- and beta-adrenergic blocker for heart failure and hypertension. *N Engl J Med*, in press.
2. Packer M, Ristow MR, Cohn JN, et al: Effect of carvedilol on morbidity and mortality in chronic heart failure. *N Engl J Med* 334:1349–1355, 1996.
3. Vantrimpont P, Rouleau JL, Wun C-C, et al: Additive beneficial effects of beta blockers to angiotensin converting enzyme inhibitors in the Survival and Ventricular Enlargement (SAVE) study. *J Am Coll Cardiol* 29:229–236, 1997.
4. Colucci WS, Packer M, Bristow MR, et al: Carvedilol inhibits clinical progression in patients with mild symptoms of heart failure. *Circulation* 94:2800–2806, 1996.
5. Frishman WH: Alpha- and beta-adrenergic blocking drugs, in Frishman WH, Sonnenblick EH: *Cardiovascular Pharmacotherapeutics*. New York, McGraw Hill, 1997, pp 59–94.

Randomised Trial of Losartan Versus Captopril in Patients Over 65 With Heart Failure (Evaluation of Losartan in the Elderly Study, ELITE)

Pitt B, for ELITE Study Investigators (University Hosp, Ann Arbor, Mich)
Lancet 349:747–752, 1997   19–4

Background.—Angiotensin-converting enzyme (ACE) inhibitors are useful in the treatment of chronic heart failure and left ventricular dysfunction. However, probably because of their preservation of bradykinin, these drugs (such as captopril) are associated with significant side effects such as cough, angioedema, renal dysfunction, and hypotension. Angiotensin II type 1 receptor antagonists exert their effects without increasing bradykinin levels; thus, these drugs (such as losartan) may avoid the side effects of ACE inhibitors. This study compared the safety and efficacy of captopril and losartan were compared in the treatment of heart failure in elderly patients.

Methods.—This prospective, double-blind, randomized study involved 722 patients 65 years of age or older with New York Heart Association classes II–IV heart failure, decreased left-ventricular ejection fraction, of 40% or less, and no history of ACE inhibitor use. Patients received 48 weeks of therapy with either captopril (titrated to 50 mg 3 times daily; $n = 370$) or losartan (titrated to 50 mg once a day; $n = 352$). End points for discontinuing therapy included a persistent increase in serum creatinine levels of 0.3 mg/dL or more (indicating renal dysfunction); hospitalization for heart failure, myocardial infarction, or angina; worsening of heart failure; hypotension-related symptoms; adverse reaction to the study drugs; and death.

Findings.—The 2 groups were similar at baseline with respect to demographics, other drug therapies, and hemodynamic parameters. After treatment, both groups were also similar in the increases in serum creatinine (10.5% in each group) and symptoms related to hypotension. However, the losartan group experienced fewer all-cause deaths (4.8%) than the captopril group (8.7%), primarily as the result of fewer sudden cardiac deaths in the losartan group. Significantly more patients discontinued therapy or died while taking captopril (30%) than while taking losartan (18.5%).

Conclusion.—Neither renal dysfunction nor hospitalizations/deaths resulting from heart failure were more common with either drug. Similarly, both drugs improved cardiac function after long-term treatment. However, losartan was associated with less all-cause mortality, mainly because of fewer sudden cardiac deaths. Losartan was also associated with fewer drop-outs caused by drug intolerance. Whether the effects of losartan on reducing cardiac deaths are specific to this drug or are general to all angiotensin II type 1 receptor antagonists remains to be determined.

▶ Angiotensin-converting enzyme inhibitors have been shown to reduce mortality and morbidity in patients with congestive heart failure New York Heart Association (NYHA classes I-IV) when combined with diuretics and digoxin.[1-4] In the ELITE trial, the angiotensin II receptor blocker, losartan, was unexpectedly found to have a greater beneficial effect than the ACE inhibitor captopril on clinical outcomes in elderly patients with chronic heart failure (NYHA classes II–IV). Losartan was also tolerated better with regard to cough, and there were fewer hospitalizations with the angiotensin II receptor blocker. A larger study is now in progress comparing losartan to captopril, and studies are in progress combining ACE inhibitors with angiotensin II receptor blockers, which would allow for the potentiation of bradykinin while the effects of angiotensin on the circulation are inhibited.

W.H. Frishman, M.D.

References

1. CONSENSUS Trial Study Group: Effects of enalapril on mortality in severe congestive heart failure: Results of the Cooperative North Scandinavian Enalapril Survival Study (CONSENSUS). *N Engl J Med* 316:1429–1435, 1987.
2. SOLVD Investigators: Effect of enalapril on survival in patients with reduced left ventricular ejection fractions and congestive heart failure. *N Engl J Med* 325:293–302, 1991.
3. SOLVD Investigators: Effect of enalapril on mortality and the development of heart failure in asymptomatic patients with reduced left ventricular ejection fractions. *N Engl J Med* 327:685–691, 1992.
4. Garg R, Yusuf S: Overview of randomized trials of angiotensin converting enzyme inhibitors on the mortality and morbidity in patients with heart failure. *JAMA* 18:1450–1455, 1995.

Patients With Mild Heart Failure Worsen During Withdrawal From Digoxin Therapy

Adams KF Jr, Gheorghiade M, Uretsky BF, et al (Univ of North Carolina, Chapel Hill; Northwestern Univ, Chicago; Univ of Texas, Galveston; et al)
J Am Coll Cardiol 30:42–48, 1997   19–5

Introduction.—Digoxin therapy used in patients with heart failure is still an issue that is unresolved. The debate concerns the utility of digoxin in patients with little or no clinical evidence of classic congestive heart failure but with significant left ventricular dysfunction. The therapeutic effects of digoxin in patients with mild clinical heart failure have not been investigated either. The outcome of patients with a mild heart failure who were withdrawn from digoxin therapy was compared with that of patients with moderate heart failure who were withdrawn from digoxin and of patients who continued to receive digoxin regardless of heart failure score.

Methods.—In 3 groups of patients, potential differences in treatment failure, left ventricular ejection fraction and exercise capacity were evaluated: those with mild heart failure, with a score of 2 or less, who were withdrawn from digoxin; those with moderate heart failure with a score greater than 2 who were withdrawn from digoxin; and patients who continued receiving digoxin regardless of heart failure score.

Results.—During follow-up in the group of patients who continued receiving digoxin, heart failure score at randomization did not predict outcome during follow-up. There was an increased risk of treatment failure and deterioration of exercise capacity and left ventricular ejection fraction in the group of patients with mild heart failure who were withdrawn from digoxin compared to those who continued receiving digoxin. Treatment failure was significantly more likely to be experienced by patients with moderate heart failure score who were withdrawn from digoxin than the other 2 groups.

Conclusion.—After digoxin withdrawal, patients with systolic left ventricular dysfunction were at risk of clinical deterioration, despite mild clinical evidence of congestive heart failure.

▶ There is growing evidence that digoxin treatment can safely improve symptoms in patients with congestive heart failure who are in normal sinus rhythm, and its withdrawal will cause clinical deterioration.[1-3] Patients with even mild left ventricular dysfunction will show deterioration of exercise capacity and left ventricular ejection fraction when digoxin is withdrawn.

Digoxin should remain a standard treatment for patients with systolic heart failure, even when only a few clinical symptoms are present.

W.H. Frishman, M.D.

References

1. Uretsky BF, Young JB, Shahidi FE, et al: Randomized study assessing the effect of digoxin withdrawal in patients with mild to moderate chronic congestive heart failure: Results of the PROVED trial. *J Am Coll Cardiol* 22:955–962, 1993.
2. Packer M, Gheorghiade M, Young JB, et al, for the RADIANCE study. Withdrawal of digoxin from patients with chronic heart failure treated with angiotensin-converting enzyme inhibitors. *N Engl J Med* 329:1–7, 1993.
3. Garg R, Gorlin R, Smith T, et al, for the Digitalis Investigation Group: The effect of digoxin on mortality and morbidity in patients with heart failure. *N Engl J Med* 336:525–533, 1997.

Effect of the Calcium Antagonist Felodipine as Supplementary Vasodilator Therapy in Patients With Chronic Heart Failure Treated With Enalapril: V-HeFT III

Cohn JN, for the Vasodilator-Heart Failure Trial (V-HeFT) Study Group (Univ of Minnesota, Minneapolis)

Circulation 96:856–863, 1997   19–6

Background.—Vasodilator drugs have beneficial hemodynamic effects in congestive heart failure patients, but different categories of vasodilators appear to have different effect profiles. This suggests that adding another vasodilator to therapy with the ACE inhibitor enalapril might increase patient response. The vascular selective calcium antagonist felodipine ER was chosen, because it is easy to administer and does not have negative inotropism at clinically relevant dosages. The V-HeFT III study examined the effect of addition of felodipine to enalapril therapy on the symptoms and exercise capacity of 450 heart failure patients over a 3-month period. It also examined effects on long-term morbidity and mortality.

Methods.—This study was performed in 24 Veterans Affairs hospitals. Men over the age of 18 with histories and findings of heart failure and a reduction in exercise tolerance were included in the study group. During a 2–12 week baseline period, clinical stability was documented, and 2 consecutive valid exercise tests were performed. Radionuclide EF, echocardiography, Holter monitoring, quality of life assessment, and PNE and ANP assays were performed. Participants were then randomized in a double-blinded fashion to receive felodipine or placebo. Follow-up visits occurred at 2-week intervals for 12 weeks and then at 3-month intervals for up to 39 months.

Results.—Addition of felodipine to enalapril therapy significantly reduced blood pressure, increased injection fraction, and reduced levels of plasma atrial natriuretic peptide at 3 months, compared with placebo. Felodipine therapy had no effect on exercise tolerance, quality of life, or hospitalization. The favorable effects of felodipine therapy on ejection fraction and atrial natriuretic peptide did not persist over long-term follow-up, but felodipine therapy did prevent worsening of exercise tolerance and quality of life. Mortality and hospitalization rates were similar for both the treatment and placebo groups. A higher incidence of peripheral edema was the only side effect of felodipine therapy that was detected in this study.

Conclusions.—Although the selective calcium antagonist felodipine had a sustained vasodilator effect in heart failure patients and was well tolerated, its only long-term benefit was a trend toward better exercise tolerance and quality of life. These results do not support the use of felodipine as adjunctive therapy in patients receiving ACE inhibitors, but they do suggest that felodipine can be used safely in heart failure patients for a different indication.

▶ There is controversy regarding the efficacy and safety of using calcium channel blockers in patients with congestive heart failure.[1] There are some data suggesting that the dihydropyridine calcium channel blocker, amlodipine, a second-generation dihydropyridine, might be safe and efficacious when added to conventional therapy for patients with heart failure.[2]

This study using felodipine, another second-generation dihydropyridine, did not show that the drug could favorably augment the clinical response to ACE inhibitors in patients with heart failure. However, the findings do suggest that felodipine could be used safely in patients with heart failure if used for another indication. The study did not show an excess of cardiovascular events.

W.H. Frishman, M.D.

References

1. Frishman WH, Sonnenblick EH: β-Adrenergic blocking drugs and calcium channel blockers, in Alexander RW, Schlant RC, Fuster V: *Hurst's The Heart*, ed 9. New York: McGraw Hill Inc., pp. 1583–1618, 1998.
2. Packer M, for the Prospective Randomized Amlodipine Survival Evaluation Study Group: Effect of amlodipine on morbidity and mortality in severe chronic heart failure. *N Engl J Med* 335:1107–1114, 1996.

Effect of Antithrombotic Therapy on Risk of Sudden Coronary Death in Patients With Congestive Heart Failure
Dries DL, Domanski MJ, Waclawiw MA, et al (The Natl Heart, Lung, and Blood Inst, Bethesda, Md; Georgetown Univ, Washington, DC)
Am J Cardiol 79:909–913, 1997   19–7

Purpose.—A preponderance of evidence suggests that the pathophysiology of sudden coronary death involves acute myocardial ischemia, regardless of whether myocardial infarction is present. Lethal ventricular arrhythmias are more likely to occur when acute myocardial ischemia is superimposed on ventricles already damaged by previous infarctions. Therefore, in patients with ischemic left ventricular dysfunction, antithrombotic therapy might be expected to reduce the risk of sudden death.

A large review of patients from the Studies of Left Ventricular Dysfunction (SOLVD) prevention and treatment trials was conducted to determine the impact of regular antiplatelet and/or anticoagulant therapy on the risk of sudden cardiac death.

Methods.—The analysis included 6,797 patients: of which 4,228 from the prevention trial had asymptomatic left ventricular (LV) dysfunction, and 2,569 from the treatment trial had LV systolic dysfunction. In these 2 groups, 424 sudden deaths were classified as "probable arrhythmia with no previous worsening of heart failure." Using univariate and multivariate Cox proportional-hazards modeling, investigators studied the association between anticoagulant and antiplatelet therapy and risk for sudden cardiac death. The analysis was adjusted for the following covariates:

• Age
• Ejection fraction
• Gender
• Atrial fibrillation
• Diabetes
• History of angina
• Previous infarction
• Previous revascularization
• Regular use of β-blockers, diuretics, digoxin, antiarrhythmic agents, or enalapril.

Results.—The patients had a 2.24% incidence of sudden cardiac death per 100 patient-years of follow-up evaluation. Multivariate analysis revealed that factors independently associated with a reduced risk of sudden cardiac death included antiplatelet therapy (relative risk [RR] 0.76; 95% confidence interval [CI] 0.61–0.95) and antiplatelet monotherapy (RR risk 0.68; 95% CI 0.48–0.96). Another independent predictor was ejection fraction. A 10% reduction of this carried a 47% increase in risk of sudden coronary death. Other factors were male sex, history of angina, diabetes, use of antiarrhythmic drugs, and use of diuretics.

Conclusions.—Antiplatelet and anticoagulant therapy are both associated with a reduced risk of sudden cardiac death for patients with moderate to severe LV systolic dysfunction arising from coronary artery disease. The findings suggest that in patients with an underlying myocardial substrate for arrhythmia generation, acute myocardial events may play a key role in the occurrence of sudden death. The mechanisms of sudden coronary death among patients with heart failure and the preventive therapies remain to be defined.

▶ In a retrospective analysis of the SOLVD prevention and treatment studies,[1, 2] it was shown that research subjects receiving antithrombotic therapy, such as aspirin, warfarin or both, had a reduced rate of sudden death. These results suggest that patients with moderate to severe LV systolic dysfunction receive at least aspirin as standard treatment to prevent mortality, especially if the heart failure is associated with coronary artery disease.

W.H. Frishman, M.D.

References

1. SOLVD Investigators: Effect of enalapril on mortality and the development of heart failure in asymptomatic patients with reduced left ventricular ejection fractions. *N Engl J Med* 327:685–691, 1992.
2. SOLVD Investigators: Effect of enalapril on survival in patients with reduced left ventricular ejection fractions and congestive heart failure. *N Engl J Med* 325:293–302, 1991.

Heart Transplantation in Patients Over 54 Years of Age: Mortality, Morbidity and Quality of Life
Rickenbacher PR, Lewis NP, Valantine HA, et al (Stanford Univ, Calif)
Eur Heart J 18:870–878, 1997   19–8

Introduction.—For suitable patients with end-stage heart disease, heart transplantation is established as the treatment of choice. As survival rates of transplantation increase, age limits have expanded to include individuals who are 60 or 65 years old. In the United States, it is expected that the number of transplants will increase from 16,000 a year to 40,000 a year if individuals who are between 56 and 65 years were routinely added to the pool of heart transplants. However, there are limited donors available and

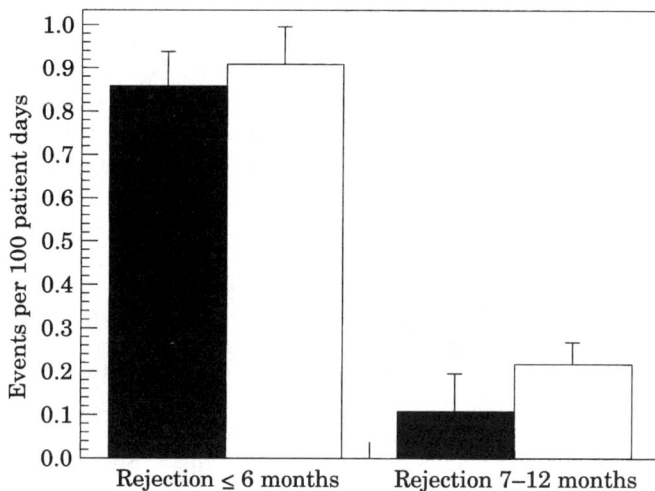

FIGURE 2.—Linearized rejection episodes during the first year posttransplant were not significantly different in patients older than 54 years (*filled bars*) and 54 years and younger (*open bars*). (Reprinted from Rickenbacher PR, Lewis NP, Valantine HA, et al: Heart transplantation in patients over 54 years of age: Mortality, morbidity and quality of life. *Eur Heart J* 18:870–878, 1997, by permission of the publisher WB Saunders Company Limited, London.)

the median wait time was more than 6 months in 1990. Thus outcomes of the elderly receiving heart transplants must be carefully monitored so that decisions can be guided on how to allocate scarce donor organs.

Methods.—In a consecutive series of patients older than 54 years at the time of transplantation with a control group of younger adult recipients, the posttransplant mortality, morbidity, and quality of life were compared. After the transplant, patients were observed for 41±27 months, and recordings were taken for the initial hospitalization, length of hospital stay, duration of intubation, hospital charges, prophylactic antilymphocytic antibody treatment, renal function, blood pressure, and dosages of immunosuppressive drugs.

Results.—In a comparison of patients older than 54 years and those younger than 54 years, the 1-year survival rate was 78±5% for the older group and 81±5% for the younger group; the 5-year survival rate was 52±7% for the older group and 66±6% for the younger group; and 46±8% for the older group and 63±6% for the younger group. Between the groups, causes of death were not significantly different. After the 6th month post transplant, patients younger than 54 years experienced significantly fewer rejection episodes (Fig 2). Between the groups, the incidence and treatment of rejection episodes and infection were comparable. In the older age group, nonlymphoid malignancies, mainly skin cancer, occurred more often in the older age group (27% vs 13%).

Conclusion.—Mortality and morbidity rates for heart transplants are comparable between carefully selected patients older than 54 years and younger than 54 years. In the older group, quality of life after the transplant seems to be even slightly better and they showed better social functioning, emotional reactions, and sleep than the younger group.

▶ Heart transplantation has become a treatment alternative for patients with advanced congestive heart failure. Advances in immunosuppression and the management of complications such as allograft rejection and accelerated atherosclerosis have improved the natural history of cardiac transplants.[1, 2]

Years ago, subjects older than 50 years were considered poor candidates for transplantation. However, this experience from Stanford, the leading transplant center in the United States, shows that carefully selected patients older than 54 years can successfully undergo transplantation with a long-term morbidity and mortality result comparable to that in younger individuals.

W.H. Frishman, M.D.

References

1. Hosenpud JD, Novick RJ, Breen TJ, et al: The Registry of the International Society of Heart and Lung Transplantation: Eleventh Official Report—1994. *J Heart Lung Transplant* 13:561–570, 1994.
2. Patel MB: Drug treatment of clinical problems related to cardiac transplantation, in Frishman WH, Sonnenblick EH: *Cardiovascular Pharmacotherapeutics.* New York, McGraw Hill, 1997, pp 1151–1164.

20 Valvular Heart Disease

Angina Pectoris in Patients With Aortic Stenosis and Normal Coronary Arteries: Mechanisms and Pathophysiological Concepts
Julius BK, Spillmann M, Vassalli G, et al (Univ Hosp, Zurich, Switzerland)
Circulation 95:892–898, 1997   20–1

Background.—Patients with severe aortic stenosis (AS) and normal coronary arteries are reported to have a high incidence (30% to 40%) of angina pectoris (AP). The pathophysiological mechanism of AP in this setting is not clear, but myocardial oxygen supply and demand may be unbalanced. The authors of a retrospective analysis of 61 patients with severe AS but without significant coronary artery disease sought to identify the various hemodynamic and angiographic determinants of myocardial perfusion.

Methods.—The patient group had a mean age of 59 years. All had undergone diagnostic catheterization at the study institution between 1977 and 1994. The patients were divided into 2 groups according to the presence or absence of AP. Thirty-two patients had a history of typical AP, and 29 did not have AP. Among those with AP, 27 had no angiographic evidence of coronary atherosclerosis, 3 had irregularities of the arterial wall, and 2 had nonsignificant coronary artery stenosis of less than 50%. Patients without AP symptoms were similarly divided: 22 had no angiographic evidence of atherosclerosis, 5 had irregularities of the arterial wall, and 2 showed nonsignificant coronary artery stenosis. A control group included 33 patients with normal coronary arteries at catheterization and atypical chest pain. Fifty-nine patients and 22 controls underwent quantitative coronary angiography. The coronary sinus thermodilution technique was used to determine coronary flow reserve in 29 patients and 7 controls.

Results.—Patients with and without AP were similar in mean age, body surface area, hemoglobin, cholesterol level, history of hypertension, and cardiothoracic ratio. The AP group had a higher New York Heart Association class and reported fewer episodes of syncope than did patients without AP. Hemodynamic data were comparable in the 2 groups, except that patients with AP had significantly increased left ventricular (LV) peak

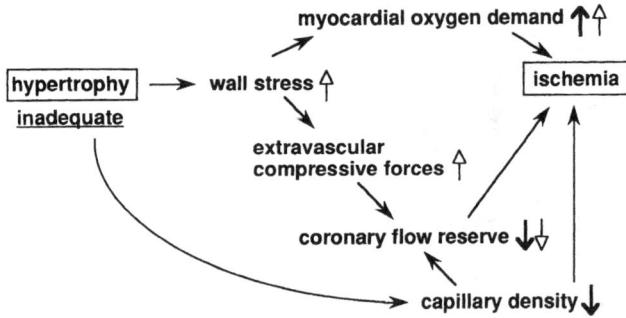

FIGURE 5.—Pathophysiology of myocardial ischemia in patients with angina pectoris (*AP*). LV hypertrophy tends to normalize (left ventricular) wall stress, but in the presence of inadequate hypertrophy, wall stress is increased. This increase leads to an increase in myocardial oxygen consumption and augmentation of extravascular compression forces. As a result, coronary flow reserve is reduced. Because of LV hypertrophy, diffusion distance is increased and capillary density decreased. Mechanisms in the presence of inadequate hypertrophy are shown by *open arrows*. (Courtesy of Julius BK, Spillmann M, Vassalli G, et al: Angina pectoris in patients with aortic stenosis and normal coronary arteries: Mechanisms and pathophysiological concepts. *Circulation* 1997; 95:892–898. Reproduced with permission [*Circulation*]. Copyright © 1997 by the American Heart Association.)

systolic pressure compared with the patients without AP. Patients with AP also had lower LV muscle mass and increased wall stress. In addition, vessels of the left coronary artery were smaller and coronary flow reserve lower in patients with AP. Only patients in the AP group showed inadequate LV hypertrophy with increased wall stress.

Conclusions.—Angina pectoris is common in patients with severe AS and appears to be associated with inadequate LV hypertrophy, high systolic and diastolic wall stresses, and reduced coronary flow reserve. Myocardial ischemia in this setting (Fig 5) may result from hypoperfusion of the myocardium under high-flow and high-demand situations.

▶ Angina pectoris of effort is a common symptom in patients with aortic valvular stenosis and is an unfavorable prognostic factor. These patients with angina and normal coronary arteries on angiography have been found to have inadequate LV hypertrophy response, increased LV wall stress, small coronary arteries, and reduced coronary flow reserve. The explanation for the inadequate hypertrophy response is not known, but in experimental studies, females may have a lesser hypertrophy response with aortic stenosis than males. The presence of angina pectoris with aortic stenosis is an important marker of the need for aortic valve surgery.

W.H. Frishman, M.D.

Clinical Factors Associated With Calcific Aortic Valve Disease

Stewart BF, Siscovick D, Lind BK, et al (Univ of Washington, Seattle; Univ of California Irvine, Orange; Georgetown Univ, Washington, DC; et al)
J Am Coll Cardiol 29:630–634, 1997   20–2

Background.—Degenerative aortic valve disease is apparently not an inevitable consequence of aging. It may be associated with specific clinical factors. The prevalence of aortic sclerosis and stenosis in the elderly was determined and the clinical factors associated with degenerative aortic valve disease identified in the current study.

Methods and Findings.—Data on 5,201 persons, ages 65 years and older enrolled in the Cardiovascular Health Study, were analyzed. Twenty-six percent had aortic valve sclerosis, and 2% had aortic valve stenosis. Sclerosis was discovered in 37% of those ages 75 years and older, and stenosis in 2.6%. Clinical factors independently correlated with degenerative aortic valve disease were age (associated with a 2-fold increase in risk for each 10-year increase in age); male sex (with a 2-fold excess risk); smoking (with a 35% increase in risk); and a history of hypertension (with a 20% increase in risk). Height and high lipoprotein(a) and low-density lipoprotein cholesterol levels were also significant variables.

Conclusions.—This study identified several clinical factors associated with degenerative aortic valve disease. A greater understanding of the cellular and molecular mechanisms involved in the pathogenesis of degenerative aortic valve disease and the risk factors for this disease may result in interventions that prevent or delay the progression of disease. Studies determining whether controlling risk factors can prevent aortic valve disease also appear to be warranted.

▶ Calcific aortic valve disease without valve commissural fusion is a common anatomic entity in older individuals. It is not an inevitable finding with aging (1), with many octogenarians showing no evidence of aortic valve calcification. This report from the Cardiovascular Health Study, a prospective, longitudinal study of older men and women, includes baseline echocardiographic data from the study cohort.

In a cross-sectional analysis, age, male gender, hypertension, smoking, level of Lp(a), and level of LDL-cholesterol are independent predictors of degenerative aortic valve disease and the association is similar for coronary artery disease risk. This finding is similar to that seen in other elderly population studies (2–4).

The study did not include quantitative Doppler data to assess valvular obstruction. The study findings suggest the possibility that calcific aortic valve disease may be preventable by specific risk factor manipulations. However, it is not certain whether the presence of aortic valve calcificiation confers any independent morbidity and mortality risk in the absence of valve obstruction.

W.H. Frishman, M.D.

References

1. Lindroos M, Kupari M, Heikkila J, Tilvis R: Prevalence of aortic valve abnormalities in the elderly: an echocardiographic study of a random population sample. *J Am Coll Cardiol* 21:1220–1225, 1993.
2. Aronow WS, Schwartz KS, Koenigsberg M: Correlation of serum lipids, calcium, and phos-phorus, diabetes mellitus and history of systemic hypertension with presence or absence of calcified or thickened aortic cusps or root in elderly patients. *Am J Cardiol* 59:998–999, 1987.
3. Gotoh T, Kuroda T, Yamasawa M, et al: Correlation between lipoprotein(a) and aortic valve sclerosis assessed by echocardiography (the JMS Cardiac Echo & Cohort Study). *Am J Cardiol* 76:928–932, 1995.
4. Lindroos M, Kupari M, Valvanne J, Strandberg T, Heikila J, Tilvis R: Factors associated with calcific aortic valve degeneration in the elderly. *Eur Heart J* 15:865–870, 1994.

Four-Year Follow-up of Patients Undergoing Percutaneous Balloon Mitral Commissurotomy: A Report From the National Heart, Lung, and Blood Institute Balloon Valvuloplasty Registry
Dean LS, Mickel M, Bonan R, et al (Univ of Alabama, Birmingham; Univ of Washington, Seattle; Univ of Montreal; et al)
J Am Coll Cardiol 28:1452–1457, 1996   20–3

Background.—Most long-term follow-up studies of patients with rheumatic mitral stenosis who have undergone percutaneous balloon commissurotomy show favorable results, but findings may have been influenced by patient selection. The authors of a multicenter study that included a wide range of patient variables examined both short- and long-term safety and efficacy of the procedure.

Methods.—All patients were enrolled in the National Heart, Lung, and Blood Institute Balloon Valvuloplasty Registry; results are reported for the 736 patients aged 18 years and older who underwent the procedure between November 1987 and October 31, 1992. Follow-up data were collected at hospital discharge, 5 weeks after percutaneous balloon mitral commissurotomy, and at 6-month intervals through October 1992. Survival and event-free survival were recorded as outcomes. Multivariate Cox regression was used to identify independent predictors of outcome.

Results.—The mean age of the patients was 54 years; 81% were women. Mean mitral valve area increased from 1.0 cm² before the procedure to 2.0 cm² after the procedure. Whereas 64% of patients were in New York Heart Association (NYHA) functional class III or IV before the procedure, 81% were in functional class I or II at 6-month follow-up. The percentage of patients in class I or II remained stable during a maximal follow-up of 5.2 years, and more than 65% of patients said they believed their overall health status had improved (Fig 1). The survival rate was 93% at 1 year, 90% at 2 years, 87% at 3 years, and 84% at 4 years. Most deaths (71%) were the result of cardiac conditions. Younger patients had better survival rates than older patients, and women had a higher rate of survival at 4

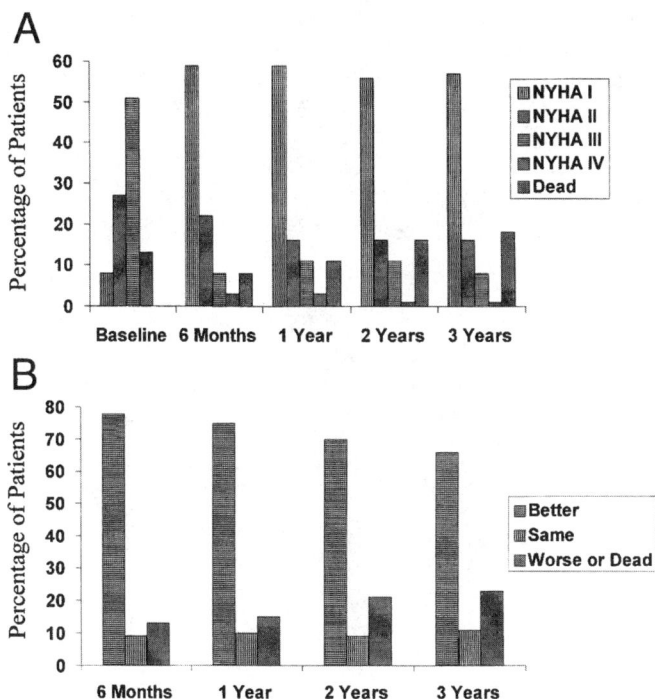

FIGURE 1.—**A**, Percentage of patients in New York Heart Association (NYHA) classes I to IV before balloon mitral commissurotomy, at 6 months and yearly thereafter to 3 years. Note that the majority of patients remain in functional class I throughout follow-up. **B**, Percentage of patients after balloon mitral commissurotomy who report their overall health status as better, the same or worse than at baseline (vs. baseline status at 6 months and then yearly thereafter to 3 years). Their impression of original overall health status closely mirrors the percentages in functional classes I and II. (Reprinted with permission from the American College of Cardiology [*J Am Coll Cardiol*] 1996; 28:1452–1457.)

years (87%) than did men (73%). Event-free survival rates (free of mitral surgery or repair balloon mitral commissurotomy) were 80% at 1 year, 71% at 2 years, 66% at 3 years, and 60% at 4 years. Multivariate predictors of death were NYHA functional class IV, higher echocardiographic score, and higher postprocedural pulmonary artery systolic and left ventricular end-diastolic pressures.

Conclusions.—This large multicenter study of percutaneous balloon mitral commissurotomy confirms the procedure's favorable effect on the hemodynamic variables of mitral stenosis. Overall survival was excellent and event-free survival quite good. With longer-term data now available, the procedure can be recommended as an alternative to surgical commissurotomy in selected patients.

▶ Percutaneous mitral balloon valvotomy is becoming a viable alternative to surgical commissurotomy in selected patients with mitral stenosis.[1] The Inoue balloon catheter (Toray, Incorporated) which was recently approved by the US Food and Drug Administration, has made the procedure less difficult and appears to have reduced the major complications of left ventricular perforation and pericardial tamponade.[2] Patients must be selected properly to ensure optimal success with the procedure. From the National Institute of Health registry report, it appears younger patients and those with echocardiographic evidence of pliable noncalcified mitral leaflets and no subvalvular fusion have better outcome after the procedure. Older patients with severe symptoms and echocardiographic evidence of immobile, calcified leaflets,[3] with concomitant subvalvular fusion, have a worse prognosis, with a palliative result at best.

W.H. Frishman, M.D.

References

1. Feldman T: Hemodynamic results, clinical outcome, and complications of Inoue balloon mitral valvotomy. *Cath Cardiovasc Diag* suppl 2:207, 1994.
2. Chen CR, Cheng TO, Chen JY, et al: Long-term results of percutaneous mitral valvuloplasty with the Inoue balloon catheter. *Am J Cardiol* 70:1445–1148, 1992.
3. Cannan CR, Nishimura RA, Reeder GS, et al: Echocardiographic assessment of commissural calcium: A simple predictor of outcome after percutaneous mitral balloon valvotomy. *J Am Coll Cardiol* 29:175–180, 1997.

21 Noninvasive Testing

Prediction of Improvement of Ventricular Function After Revascularization: ^{18}F-Fluorodeoxyglucose Single-photon Emission Computed Tomography vs Low-dose Dobutamine Echocardiography
Cornel JH, Bax JJ, Fioretti PM, et al (Univ Hosp Rotterdam-Dijkzigt; Free Univ, Amsterdam)
Eur Heart J 18:941–948, 1997   21–1

Introduction.—For the rising number of patients with left ventricular dysfunction resulting from significant coronary artery disease, assessment of myocardial viability is necessary. The most accurate method for the identification of viable myocardium is positron emission tomography of myocardial perfusion and metabolism using ^{18}F-fluorodeoxyglucose (FDG). Because this technique is of limited availability, other techniques have been proposed, including low-dose dobutamine echocardiography and imaging myocardial FDG uptake with single-photon emission CT (SPECT). To predict improvement of regional and global left ventricular function after uncomplicated coronary artery bypass grafting, thallium-201/FDG SPECT was compared with low-dose dobutamine echocardiography.

Methods.—Before surgery, low-dose dobutamine echocardiography (5 and 10 µg/kg^{-1} per min−1) and thallium-201/FDG SPECT were administered to 30 patients with regional wall motion abnormalities (mean ejection fraction 32±19%). A 13-segment model was used for comparative analysis. If there was normal perfusion or relatively increased FDG uptake in perfusion defects (mismatch) in dyssynergic segments on SPECT or if the echocardiograph showed that wall motion abnormalities were reversible during the dobutamine infusion, postoperative improvement was predicted. Ventricular function was reassessed after surgery. With the patient at rest, an echocardiogram was taken at the 3-month follow-up.

Results.—In 61 of 168 (37%) revascularized segments, regional wall motion had improved. There was a sensitivity of 89%, a specificity of 82%, a negative predictive value of 93%, and a positive predictive value of 74% for low-dose dobutamine echocardiography in predicting function outcome. For thallium-201/FDG SPECT, the sensitivity was 84%, the specificity was 86%, the positive predictive value was 78%, and the negative predictive value was 90%. There was a significant improvement in the wall motion score index, a surrogate of global ventricular function, in patients with more than 2 viable segments on either technique.

Conclusion.—Combined assessment of flow and FDG imaging is needed for the optimal prediction of functional outcome. To predict improvement of left ventricular function after surgical revascularization, thallium-201/FDG SPECT and low-dose dobutamine echocardiography appear comparable and similarly accurate.

▶ Assessment of myocardial viability is important to determine the most appropriate treatment for patients with advanced left ventricular dysfunction and coronary artery disease.[1] Many patients with ischemic cardiomyopathy could benefit from a coronary revascularization procedure if viable myocardial tissue remains.

At this juncture, positron emission tomography of myocardial perfusion and metabolism is considered to be the best modality for the identification of viable myocardium in a dysfunctional heart.[2, 3] Dobutamine echocardiography appears to be as good a methodology for predicting an improvement of regional and global ventricular function after coronary revascularization as position emission tomography,[4–6] even though they elucidate different cellular mechanisms of viability.

W.H. Frishman, M.D.

References

1. Elefteriades JA, Tolis G, Levi E, et al: Coronary artery bypass grafting in severe left ventricular dysfunction: excellent survival with improved ejection fraction and functional state. *J Am Coll Cardiol* 22:1411–1417, 1993.
2. Vom Dahl J, Eitzman DT, Al-Aouar JR, et al: Relation of regional function, perfusion and metabolism in patients with advanced coronary artery disease undergoing surgical revascularization. *Circulation* 90:2356–2366, 1994.
3. Tamaki N, Kawamoto M, Tadamura E, et al: Prediction of reversible ischemia after revascularization. Perfusion and metabolic studies with positron emission tomography. *Circulation* 91:1697–1705, 1995.
4. Arnese M, Cornel JH, Salustri A, et al: Prediction of improvement of regional left ventricular function after surgical revascularization: A comparison of low-dose dobutamine echocardiography with 201T1 single-photon emission computed tomography. *Circulation* 91:2748–2752, 1995.
5. Afridi I, Kleiman NS, Raizner AE, et al: Dobutamine echocardiography in myocardial hibernation. Optimal dose and accuracy in predicting recovery of ventricular function after coronary angioplasty. *Circulation* 91:663–670, 1995.
6. Baer FM, Voth E, Deutsch HJ, et al: Predictive value of low dose dobutamine transesophageal echocardiography and fluorine-18-flurodeoxyglucose positron emission tomography for recovery of regional left ventricular function after successful revascularization. *J Am Coll Cardiol* 28:60–69, 1996.

Comparison of Arbutamine and Exercise Echocardiography in Diagnosing Myocardial Ischemia

Cohen A, Weber H, Chauvel C, et al (Saint-Antoine Univ, Paris; Henri Mondar Univ, Paris; Broussais Univ, Paris)
Am J Cardiol 79:713–716, 1997   21–2

Background.—The new catecholamine arbutamine increases heart rate, myocardial contractility, and systolic blood pressure, thus simulating the cardiac effects of exercise. As a pharmacologic stress agent, arbutamine is given by a computerized closed-loop delivery system that controls the infusion rate in response to changes in heart rate. This allows the physician to select a desired heart rate increase and heart rate limit. The sensitivity of arbutamine was compared with that of symptom-limited exercise to induce echocardiographic signs of ischemia.

Methods.—The study included 37 patients with coronary artery disease. All stopped taking β-blockers at least 48 hours before testing. Thirty-five were tested with both arbutamine and exercise, 1 was tested with arbutamine only, and 1 was tested with exercise only. During testing, stress was stopped in case of intolerable symptoms; clinical, ECG, or echocardiographic signs of ischemia; achievement of the target heart rate of 85% of the age predicted maximum; or a plateau of heart rate response.

Results.—Thirty patients had 50% or greater narrowing of the coronary artery lumen on angiography. Both forms of stress significantly increased the rate–pressure product. The mean increase was 2,479 with arbutamine vs. 11,398 with exercise. The mean time to reach the maximal heart rate was 17 minutes with arbutamine vs. 4 minutes with exercise. The percentages of patients with interpretable echo data were 82% in the arbutamine group and 67% in the exercise group. Arbutamine was 94% sensitive in recognizing myocardial ischemia compared with 88% for exercise. Dyspnea and tremors each occurred in 5.6% of patients receiving arbutamine. Arbutamine testing had to be stopped in 2 patients, 1 because of premature atrial and ventricular beats and 1 because of premature atrial contractions and atrial fibrillation. These arrhythmias did not have any aftereffects.

Conclusions.—Arbutamine and exercise have comparable sensitivity in inducing echocardiographic signs of ischemia. The rate–pressure product of arbutamine is lower, however. Arbutamine is a well-tolerated and reliable alternative to exercise echocardiography.

▶ In practice, exercise echocardiography causes a great deal of chest wall activity and heart movement that can make interpretation of the postexercise echocardiographic study difficult. The advantage of pharmacologic echocardiographic stress testing is that it can be performed without causing major chest wall and cardiac movement so that better echocardiographic images can be obtained. There is some toxicity with drugs such as dobutamine and arbutamine, but rarely is this related to major sequelae.

Pharmacologic echocardiographic stress testing has a high predictive value in determining the presence of ischemic heart disease, and it appears to be as useful as pharmacologic testing using radionuclide methods. Pharmacologic stress testing using catecholamines should not be performed on patients receiving β-blockers because the agents can interfere with the response to catecholamine infusion.

Treadmill stress testing is still the best screening technique for detecting ischemic heart disease; pharmacologic stress testing with echocardiography or radionuclide scintigraphy is reserved for those patients who cannot exercise adequately to raise their heart rates.

W.H. Frishman, M.D.

Echocardiographic Assessment of Commissural Calcium: A Simple Predictor of Outcome After Percutaneous Mitral Balloon Valvotomy
Cannan CR, Nishimura RA, Reeder GS, et al (Mayo Clinic and Mayo Found, Rochester, Minn)
J Am Coll Cardiol 29:175–180, 1997   21–3

Introduction.—Percutaneous mitral balloon valvotomy is performed in patients with severely symptomatic mitral stenosis, but its immediate success rate and long-term outcome depend on the underlying mitral valve morphologic characteristics. A low mitral valve "score," based on leaflet thickening, calcification, mobility, and degree of subvalvular fusion (Abascal score) appears to predict immediate success and a low rate of re-stenosis. Not all patients with a low score, however, do well, and some with higher mitral valve scores have a good outcome. The predictive value of the presence or absence of calcium in mitral valve commissures by 2-dimensional echocardiography was examined in 149 patients.

Methods.—The study group consisted of consecutive patients who underwent percutaneous mitral balloon valvotomy at the Mayo Clinic between September 1987 and June 1995. They were evaluated retrospectively for mitral valve morphologic scores determined at baseline echocardiography and for calcification in each of the medial and lateral commissures. Patients were contacted by telephone every 6 months, and most were seen yearly for clinical follow-up. End points at follow-up were death, New York Heart Association functional class, repeat percutaneous mitral balloon valvotomy, and mitral valve replacement.

Results.—The average patient age was 54.6 years, and the mean follow-up period was 1.8 years. Compared with patients with an Abascal score greater than 8, there was a trend toward improved survival and freedom from repeat procedures at 36 months among patients with an Abascal score of 8 or less. There was a significant difference in outcome, however, between patients with and without commissural calcium (Fig 2). Survival at 36 months free of death, repeat valvotomy, or mitral valve replacement was 80% in those without commissural calcium vs. 40% in those with commissural calcium. In a model with Abascal score and commissural calcification and their interaction, the only significant variable was calcification.

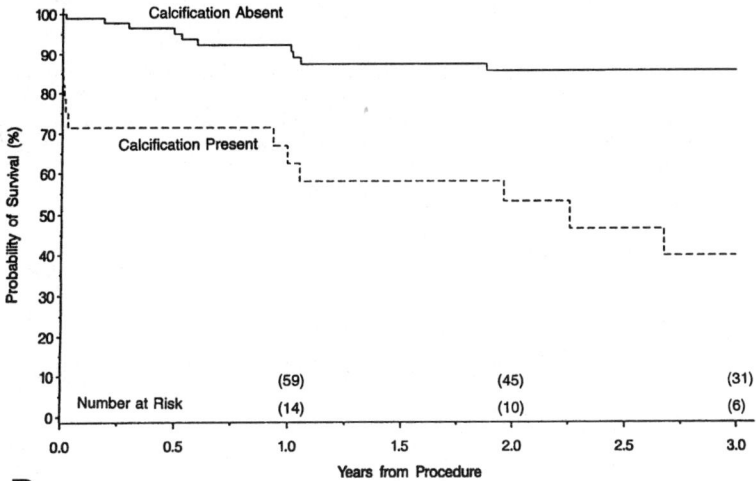

B

FIGURE 2.—B, actuarial survival curves with freedom from death, mitral valve replacement or repeat valvuloplasty for patients without commissural calcium (*solid line*) vs. those patients with calcium in a commissure (*dashed line*) (P < 0.001). (Reprinted with permission from the American College of Cardiology. Courtesy of Cannan CR, Nishimura RA, Reeder GS, et al: Echocardiographic assessment of commissural calcium: A simple predictor of outcome after percutaneous mitral balloon valvotomy. *Journal of the American College of Cardiology* 29:175–180, 1997.)

Discussion.—Commissural splitting is the dominant mechanism by which mitral valve stenosis is relieved by percutaneous mitral balloon valvotomy, and the presence of commissural calcium is a strong predictor of outcome after this procedure. This simple determination can help to identify patients who would benefit from percutaneous mitral balloon valvotomy and predict survival and the need for repeat valvotomy or mitral valve replacement after the procedure.

▶ Percutaneous mitral balloon valvotomy has become an effective and established form of treatment for selected patients with mitral valve stenosis.[1, 2] Randomized trials have demonstrated that this procedure is as effective as closed or open commissurotomy in short-term follow-up of patients with symptomatic mitral stenosis. The benefits in cost, length of hospital stay, and return to work from percutaneous mitral balloon valvotomy far outweigh surgical interventions to correct mitral stenosis.

The success rate of valvotomy is dependent on the underlying mitral valve morphologic characteristics. Those patients with pliable, noncalcified mitral leaflets and no subvalvular fusion will have a better outcome with the procedure than those patients having thickened, immobile, calcified leaflets with concomitant subvalvular fusion.

In this retrospective study, the presence of commissural calcium by 2-dimensional echocardiography was both an important and powerful predictor of an unfavorable clinical outcome with valvotomy.

W.H. Frishman, M.D.

References

1. Palacios IF, Tuzcu ME, Weyman AE, et al: Clinical follow up of patients undergoing percutaneous mitral balloon valvotomy. *Circulation* 91:671–676, 1995.
2. Reyes VP, Raju BS, Wynne J, et al: Percutaneous balloon valvotomy compared with open surgical commissurotomy for mitral stenosis. *N Engl J Med* 331:961–967, 1994.

22 Arrythmias

Risk of Thromboembolism in Chronic Atrial Flutter

Wood KA, Eisenberg SJ, Kalman JM, et al (Univ of California, San Francisco)
Am J Cardiol 79:1043–1047, 1997   22-1

Objective.—Patients with chronic atrial fibrillation are at increased risk of thromboembolus formation. Although the incidence of thromboembolus formation is not known, conventional anticoagulation therapy is generally not recommended. The frequency of, and potential risk factors for, thromboembolic events were examined in a retrospective study of patients with chronic atrial flutter referred for radiofrequency ablation treatment.

Methods.—Between May 1988 and December 1995, 86 consecutive patients (24 women), average age 60 years, without prior congenital heart surgical repair, were evaluated at the study institution, for ablation of clinical atrial flutter. Atrial flutter was classified as typical clockwise (n = 5), typical counterclockwise (n = 59), or atypical (n = 7).

Results.—Duration of flutter ranged from 2 weeks to more than 40 years. Concomitant conditions included coronary artery disease (n = 24), systemic hypertension (n = 23), ischemic or hypertrophic cardiomyopathy (n = 20), mitral valve prolapse (n = 12), and congenital heart disease (n = 5). Twelve patients (14%) had a history of embolic events. No clear risk factors could be found for thromboembolic events. In the univariate analysis, hypertension was a significant predictor of thromboembolic risk, but multivariate analysis failed to establish any significant risk factors. When patients with transient ischemic attacks or pulmonary emboli were excluded from the analysis to facilitate comparison with other atrial fibrillation studies, the overall risk was 7%, with an annual risk of 4.5 years of 1.6%.

Conclusion.—Because the risk of thromboembolus formation in patients with atrial flutter is higher than previously thought, treatment with anticoagulant therapy should be considered.

▶ Many trials have examined the incidence of thromboemboli in patients with chronic atrial fibrillation with and without valvular disease, with at least a fivefold increased incidence of stroke being seen.[1-5] In contrast, the risk of stroke in patients with chronic atrial flutter without valve disease is said to be negligible and does not require chronic anticogulation therapy. Atrial flutter is said to be associated with an increase in atrial contractile activity, which may prevent the formation of clots.

This current study suggests an increased incidence of systemic emboli in patients with chronic atrial flutter. It has been suggested that anticoagulation be considered for these patients or at least a search for atrial thrombi by echocardiographic technique. Certainly those patients with a history of an embolic event should be considered for anticoagulation therapy in the presence of chronic atrial flutter.

W.H. Frishman, M.D.

References

1. Wolf PA, Dawber TR, Thomas HE, et al: Epidemiologic assessment of chronic atrial fibrillation and risk of stroke: The Framingham Study. *Neurology* 28:973–977, 1978.
2. Petersen P, Boysen G, Godtfredsen J, et al: Placebo-controlled, randomized trial of warfarin and aspirin for prevention of thromboembolic complications in chronic atrial fibrillation: the Copenhagen AFA-SAK Study. *Lancet* 1:175–179, 1989.
3. Stroke Prevention in Atrial Fibrillation Study Group Investigators: Preliminary report of the Stroke Prevention in Atrial Fibrillation Study. *N Engl J Med* 322:863–868, 1990.
4. The Boston Area Anticoagulation Trial for Atrial Fibrillation Investigators: The effect of low dose warfarin on the risk of stroke in patients with nonrheumatic atrial fibrillation. *N Engl J Med* 323:1505–1511, 1990.
5. Atrial Fibrillation Investigators: Risk factors for stroke and efficacy of antithrombotic therapy in atrial fibrillation. Analysis of pooled data from five randomized controlled trials. *Arch Intern Med* 154:1449–1457, 1994.

Risk for Clinical Thromboembolism Associated With Conversion to Sinus Rhythm in Patients With Atrial Fibrillation Lasting Less Than 48 Hours

Weigner MJ, Caulfield TA, Danias PG, et al (Harvard Med School, Boston; Univ of Connecticut, Farmington)
Ann Intern Med 126:615–620, 1997   22–2

Background.—Patients with atrial fibrillation who undergo cardioversion to sinus rhythm may be at risk for thromboembolism if cardioversion is not preceded by several weeks of warfarin therapy. The risk for thromboembolism is believed to be quite low, however, when cardioversion is performed within 2 days or less of the onset of atrial fibrillation. To provide clinical data to support this assumption, the authors recorded the incidence of clinical thromboembolism in a large consecutive series of patients with atrial fibrillation that had lasted less than 48 hours.

Methods.—A prospective screening of 1,822 adults admitted with a diagnosis including atrial fibrillation yielded 375 patients with symptoms of less than 48 hours' duration. Patients receiving long-term warfarin treatment were excluded. Data on cardioversion and thromboembolism were obtained prospectively from hospital and outpatient records. Only clinical embolic events that occurred during the index hospitalization and within 1 month of conversion were recorded.

Results.—During the index hospitalization, 357 patients (95.2%) converted to sinus rhythm. Conversion was spontaneous in 250 (66.7%) and active in 107 (28.5%). The most common underlying systemic disorder was hypertension (41.7%); 30.4% of patients had a clinical history suggestive of coronary artery disease and 48.3% had a history of atrial fibrillation. Clinical thromboembolic events (a stroke, a transient ischemic attack, and peripheral embolus) occurred in 3 patients (0.8%), all of whom had converted spontaneously to sinus rhythm. All 3 had normal left ventricular systolic function, and none had a history of atrial fibrillation or thromboembolism.

Conclusions.—Patients admitted with atrial fibrillation of less than 48 hours' duration who underwent early cardioversion, without prolonged warfarin therapy or screening by transesophageal echocardiography, had a very low clinical rate of thromboembolism (0.8%). All 3 patients with embolic events were women older than 75 years, but the group was too small to permit identification of factors that may dispose patients to clinical thromboembolism in such populations. Data support the recommendation for early cardioversion when atrial fibrillation is known to have lasted less than 48 hours.

▶ Atrial fibrillation is the most common sustained arrhythmia and a major cause of morbidity and mortality from hemodynamic compromise and systemic emboli.[1, 2] Cardioversion of atrial fibrillation to sinus rhythm is performed in an attempt to improve cardiac function, relieve symptoms, and decrease the risk of thrombus formation. Cardioversion may be associated with clinical thromboembolism, and transesophageal echocardiography revealed the presence of left atrial thrombi in 14 patients with atrial fibrillation lasting 3 days or less. Three weeks of anticoagulation is recommended for patients with atrial fibrillation lasting 2 days or more, and the findings of this study suggest that early cardioversion may be performed in patients with atrial fibrillation lasting less than 48 hours. Patients undergoing early cardioversion should be started on heparin and anticoagulation therapy with warfarin for 3 weeks to prevent postconversion emboli.

W.H. Frishman, M.D.

References

1. Stoddard MF, Dawkins PR, Prince CR, et al: Left atrial appendage thrombus is not uncommon in patients with acute atrial fibrillation and a recent embolic event: A transesophageal echocardiographic study. *J Am Coll Cardiol* 25:452–459, 1995.
2. Pritchett EL: Management of atrial fibrillation. *N Engl J Med* 326:1264–1271, 1992.

Cardioversion Guided by Transesophageal Echocardiography: The ACUTE Pilot Study

Klein AL et al, for the ACUTE Investigators (Cleveland Clinic Found, Ohio)
Ann Intern Med 126:200–209, 1997   22–3

Background.—Successful electrical cardioversion performed for the restoration of sinus rhythm in patients with atrial fibrillation is associated with an increased risk of embolic stroke. To reduce this risk, conventional therapy involves 7 weeks of treatment with warfarin before cardioversion is undertaken. Screening for thrombi in the left atrial appendage by means of transesophageal echocardiography (TEE) may permit cardioversion to be performed earlier and more safely. A randomized, multicenter clinical trial was designed to assess the feasibility and safety of TEE-guided early cardioversion.

Methods.—The ACUTE (Assessment of Cardioversion Using Transesophageal Echocardiography) Pilot Study enrolled 126 patients from 10 hospitals in the United States, Europe, and Australia. Eligible patients had atrial fibrillation, or atrial flutter with a history of atrial fibrillation, lasting

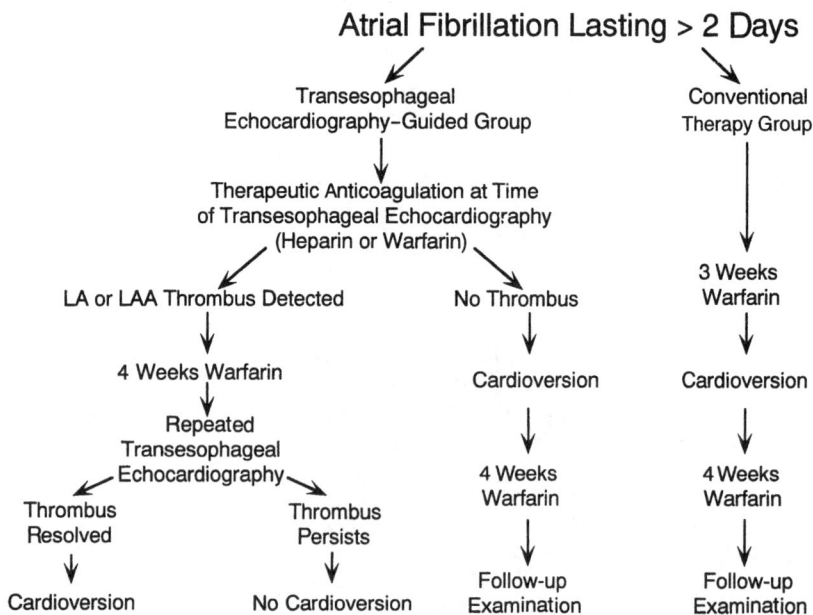

FIGURE 1.—The ACUTE (Assessment of Cardioversion Using Transesophageal Echocardiography) study protocol. Patients with atrial fibrillation were randomly assigned to undergo cardioversion with conventional therapy or cardioversion guided by transesophageal echocardiography (TEE) with brief anticoagulation therapy. The conventional-therapy group received warfarin therapy for 3 weeks before and 4 weeks after cardioversion. In the TEE group, patients were stratified according to whether a thrombus was detected in either the left atrium or the left atrial appendage. Patients in the TEE group underwent full anticoagulation therapy at the time of cardioversion and for 4 weeks after cardioversion. *Abbreviations: LA,* left atrial; *LAA,* left atrial appendage. (Courtesy of Klein AL, for the ACUTE Investigators: Cardioversion guided by transesophageal echocardiography: The ACUTE pilot study. *Ann Intern Med* 126:200–209, 1997.)

longer than 2 days and had not received anticoagulant therapy for more than 7 days. Patients were randomized to a conventional or a TEE-guided approach to cardioversion (Fig 1). Patients in the TEE group began receiving anticoagulation therapy at their initial visit; heparin was used for inpatients and warfarin for outpatients. When stable therapeutic anticoagulation was assured, TEE was scheduled, with subsequent cardioversion immediately or within 24 hours. Cardioversion was postponed and warfarin continued for 4 weeks if thrombi were detected, with TEE repeated to confirm freedom from thrombi.

Results.—Fifty-six of the 62 patients randomized to TEE-guided cardioversion underwent TEE. Cardioversion was postponed in 7 patients when atrial thrombi were detected. Thirty-eight of the 45 patients who underwent cardioversion (84%) had successful cardioversion without embolization. Of the 11 patients who underwent TEE but not cardioversion, 7 had thrombi, 3 spontaneously reverted to sinus rhythm, and 1 converted to sinus rhythm after overdrive pacing. Cardioversion was performed in 37 of the 64 patients given conventional therapy and was successful in 28 (76%). One patient had a peripheral embolism in an arm 3 days after cardioversion. Mean time to cardioversion was shorter in the TEE group (0.6 weeks) than in the conventional therapy group (4.8 weeks). The authors noted a tendency toward a greater incidence of clinical hemodynamic instability and bleeding complications in the conventional-therapy group.

Conclusions.—Preliminary findings in this pilot study of patients with atrial fibrillation suggests that TEE-guided cardioversion with short-term anticoagulation therapy is feasible and safe. Compared with conventional therapy, TEE may allow cardioversion to be performed sooner, may decrease the risk for embolism, and may be associated with less clinical instability.

▶ The ACUTE pilot study was designed to assess the optimal way of treating atrial fibrillation lasting more than 2 days. A TEE-guided cardioversion group was compared with a nonechocardiography group of patients given 3 weeks of warfarin before cardioversion. The absence of atrial thrombi on TEE permits immediate cardioversion[1,2] and reduces the time of anticoagulation from 7 to 4 weeks. Although the sample size was small, patients with low ejection fractions in the ACUTE pilot study had more atrial thrombi than those with normal ejection fractions. Patients with diminished left ventricular function and atrial fibrillation may also have left ventricular thrombi. Perhaps all patients with diminished ejection fractions and atrial fibrillation should undergo conventional treatment with 3 weeks of anticoagulation before cardioversion and those patients with normal ventricles should undergo TEE-guided anticoagulation therapy before cardioversion.

W.H. Frishman, M.D.

References

1. Manning WJ, Silverman DI, Keighley CS, et al: Cardioversion from atrial fibrillation without prolonged anticoagulation with use of transesophageal echocardiography to exclude the presence of atrial thrombi. *N Engl J Med* 328:750–755, 1993.
2. Leung DY, Grimm RA, Klein AL: Transesophageal echocardiography–guided approach to cardioversion of atrial fibrillation. *Prog Cardiovasc Dis* 39:21–32, 1996.

Long-term Follow-up After Radiofrequency Modification of the Atrioventricular Node in Patients With Atrial Fibrillation

Morady F, Hasse C, Strickberger SA, et al (Univ of Michigan, Ann Arbor)
J Am Coll Cardiol 27:113–121, 1997   22–4

Introduction.—Studies involving small numbers of patients indicate that radiofrequency energy can be used to modify atrioventricular (AV) node conduction without creating pathologic AV block in patients with atrial fibrillation and an uncontrolled ventricular rate. A study of 62 patients who underwent radiofrequency modification of the AV node was conducted to clarify several issues and describe long-term follow-up results.

Methods.—The patients, 32 men and 30 women, had a mean age of 63 years and a mean left ventricular ejection fraction of 0.44; 43 had structural heart disease. All underwent the procedure because of symptomatic, drug-refractory atrial fibrillation with an uncontrolled ventricular rate. Atrial fibrillation was chronic in 46 cases and paroxysmal in 16. During an infusion of 4 µg/min of isoproterenol, radiofrequency energy was applied to the posteroseptal or midseptal right atrium. The end point of the procedure was a ventricular rate of 120–130 beats per minute. Follow-up included ECG monitoring on an inpatient basis for at least 2 days, a treadmill test 2–4 days after the procedure, and outpatient visits at 3, 12, and 24 months. Forty-four patients have had 12 months or more of follow-up.

Results.—Fifty patients (81%) achieved short-term control of the ventricular rate without induction of pathologic AV block. In 10 patients (16%), inadvertent high-degree AV block occurred, either at the time of the procedure (6 cases) or 36–72 hours later (4 cases). Overall, 73% of patients experienced adequate rate control at rest and during exertion, without pathologic AV block. Five patients have had a symptomatic recurrence of an uncontrolled rate during atrial fibrillation. Within 1 year of the procedure, the mean left ventricular ejection fraction increased significantly among 37 patients with a successful outcome (from 0.44 to 0.51). There were 2 cases of sudden death, at 1–5 months after the procedure, in patients with idiopathic dilated cardiomyopathy.

Conclusion.—In approximately 70% of properly selected patients with atrial fibrillation and an uncontrolled ventricular rate, excellent long-term outcomes can be achieved with radiofrequency modification of the AV node. Patients experienced relief of symptoms and improved function, and some showed marked improvement in ejection fraction.

▶ Radiofrequency modification of the AV node can be performed to modify AV node conduction in patients with atrial fibrillation and rapid ventricular rates without creating pathologic AV block.[1, 2]

In 70% of properly selected patients, there is excellent long-term control of the ventricular rate observed during both rest and exercise, relief of clinical symptoms, and improvement in functional class. Compared with radiofrequency ablation of the AV node and pacemaker insertion, the principal drawbacks of the modification procedure are a recurrence rate of 10% and a facilitation of polymorphic ventricular tachycardia. In contrast, the modification procedure, if successful, will eliminate the need for a lifetime of pacemaker therapy.

Atrioventricular node ablation treatment should be used in patients prone to polymorphic ventricular tachycardia and in those who require or already have a pacemaker.

W.H. Frishman, M.D.

References

1. Williamson BD, Man KC, Daoud E, et al: Radiofrequency catheter modification of atrioventricular conduction to control the ventricular rate during atrial fibrillation. *N Engl J Med* 331:910–917, 1994.
2. Feld GK, Fleck RP, Fujimura O, et al: Control of rapid ventricular response by radiofrequency catheter modification of the atrioventricular node in patients with medically refractory atrial fibrillation. *Circulation* 90:2299–2307, 1994.

Nonsustained Ventricular Tachycardia in Severe Heart Failure: Independent Marker of Increased Mortality due to Sudden Death
Doval HC, for the GESICA-GEMA Investigators (Instituto del Corazón del Hosp Italiano, Buenos Aires, Argentina)
Circulation 94:3198–3203, 1996   22–5

Background.—Mortality remains extremely high in patients with congestive heart failure, and approximately 40% of deaths occur suddenly. Ventricular tachycardia and fibrillation appear to be frequent mechanisms of death in patients with severe heart failure. The authors studied a homogenous group of patients to determine the independent prognostic value of nonsustained ventricular tachycardia (NSVT) on total mortality and its relation to the death mechanisms.

Methods.—From December 1989 through March 1993, 516 patients were enrolled; 173 patients (33.5%) had NSVT as determined by 24-hour Holter recordings. To be included in the study, patients had to be stable and in an advanced functional capacity with adequately treated advanced chronic heart failure and marked left ventricular systolic dysfunction. None was receiving antiarrhythmic treatment, had concomitant serious

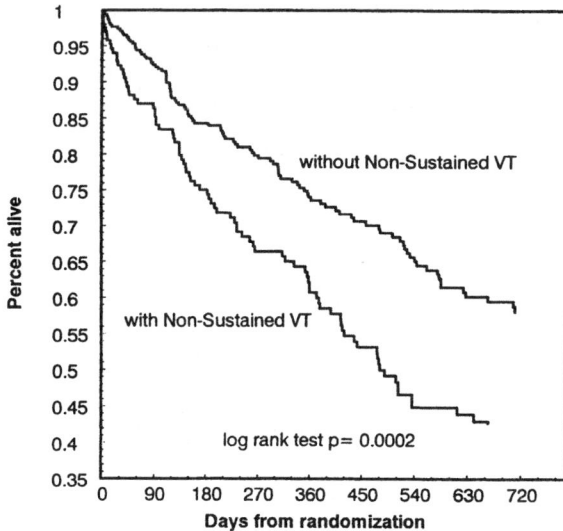

FIGURE 1.—Nonsustained ventricular tachycardia (*VT*) and total mortality. (Doval HC, for the GESICA-GEMA Investigators: Nonsustained ventricular tachycardia in severe heart failure: Independent marker of increased mortality due to sudden death. *Circulation* 1996; 94:3198–3203. Reproduced with permission [*Circulation*]. Copyright 1996 by the American Heart Association.)

associated clinical diseases, or history of sustained ventricular tachycardia or ventricular fibrillation. Follow-up continued for 2 years.

Results.—At the end of the study period, 5 patients with NSVT and 14 without NSVT were lost to follow-up; follow-up was terminated in 4 patients with and 12 without NSVT who underwent heart transplantation. With an average follow-up of 13 months, 193 of 516 patients had died (37.4%): 87 with NSVT (50.3%) and 106 without NSVT (30.9%). Independent predictors of the presence of NSVT in the 24-hour Holter monitoring were increased furosemide dose, decreased systolic blood pressure, increased serum creatinine level, faster heart rate, and Chagas' disease as the cause of heart failure. The presence of NSVT increased total mortality (Fig 1), with a relative risk (RR) of 1.69; the RR for sudden death was 2.77 with NSVT. Progressive heart failure death was also increased in the NSVT group (20.8% vs 17.5% for those without NSVT). Treatment with amiodarone did not affect mortality in the NSVT group. Quantitative analysis of 24-hour Holter monitorings showed that couplets had a similar RR to that of NSVT for both total mortality and sudden death.

Conclusions.—Nonsustained ventricular tachycardia was confirmed to be an independent marker for increased overall mortality and sudden death in patients with congestive heart failure. The absence of NSVT and ventricular repetitive beats in a 24-hour Holter monitoring may identify patients with a low probability of sudden death.

▶ Despite the recent progress in the treatment of congestive heart failure, mortality remains high. In this multicenter study[1] it was found that the presence of NSVT on a 24-hour ambulatory ECG is an independent marker for increased mortality and sudden death in patients with chronic heart failure and marked left ventricular systolic dysfunction. Antiarrhythmic therapy does not appear to reduce the incidence of total or sudden death in patients with congestive heart failure, however, if the arrhythmia spontaneously subsides, the patient will have a better prognosis.[2] This would signify that the arrhythmia is a marker for mortality rather than the cause. However, an implantable defibrillator might improve the prognosis of these patients.[3]

W.H. Frishman, M.D.

References

1. Doval H, Nul D, Grancelli, et al: Randomised trial of low dose amiodarone in severe congestive heart failure. *Lancet* 1:493–498, 1994.
2. Goldstein S, Brooks M, Ledingham R, et al: Association between ease of suppression of ventricular arrhythmia and survival. *Circulation* 91:79–83, 1995.
3. Moss AJ, Hall J, Cannom DS, et al for the Multicenter Automatic Defibrillator Implantation Trial Investigators: Improved survival with an implanted defibrillator in patients with coronary disease at high risk for ventricular arrhythmia. *N Engl J Med* 335:1933–1940, 1996.

Randomised Trial of Effect of Amiodarone on Mortality in Patients With Left-ventricular Dysfunction After Recent Myocardial Infarction: EMIAT
Julian DG, for the European Myocardial Infarct Amiodarone Trial Investigators (Netherhall Gardens, London; St George's Hosp; Sanofi Recherche, Montpellier, France; et al)
Lancet 349:667–674, 1997   22–6

Introduction.—In survivors of acute myocardial infarction, ventricular arrhythmias are one of the main causes of death. After many studies of antiarrhythmic drugs that block the sodium channel showed no efficacy in suppressing arrhythmias and preventing death in survivors of myocardial infarction, the European Myocardial Infarct Amiodarone Trial was conducted. Amiodarone and β-adrenergic blocking agents showed promise as antiarrhythmic drugs. A large trial of amiodarone in survivors of myocardial infarction at increased risk of death was conducted. The main entry criterion was the presence of depressed left-ventricular ejection fraction, which has been shown to be the single most powerful independent predictor of mortality, including sudden death.

Methods.—The effect of amiodarone on all-cause mortality, cardiac mortality, and arrhythmic death was studied in 1,486 survivors of myocardial infarction with depressed left-ventricular function of 40% or less in a randomized, placebo-controlled, double-blind trial. On-treatment and intention-to-treat analyses were conducted. Patients were divided into 2 groups with 743 in the amiodarone group and 743 in the placebo group. They were followed up for a median of 21 months.

Results.—Between the 2 groups, there was no difference in all-cause mortality with 103 deaths in the amiodarone group and 102 in the placebo

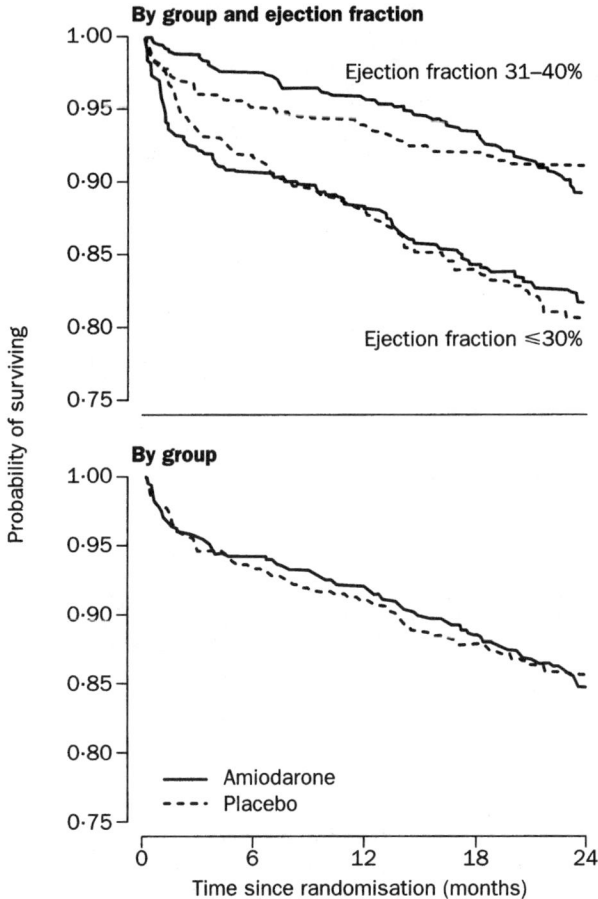

FIGURE 2.—Kaplan-Meier estimates of all-cause mortality by group and ejection fraction (Courtesy of Julian DG, for the European Myocardial Infarct Amiodarone Trial Investigators: Randomized trial of effect of amiodarone on mortality in patients with left-ventricular dysfunction after recent myocardial infarction: EMIAT. *Lancet* 349:667–674, 1997. Copyright 1997 by the Lancet Ltd.)

group (Fig 2). There was no difference in cardiac mortality in the 2 groups. There was a 35% risk reduction in arrhythmic deaths in the amiodarone group. In the amiodarone group, there were more deaths from nonarrhythmic cardiac and noncardiac causes than in the placebo group. The risk of death was significantly increased by a history of myocardial infarction.

Conclusion.—The systematic prophylactic use of amiodarone in all patients with depressed left-ventricular function after myocardial infarction was not supported by these findings. The use of amiodarone in patients for whom antiarrhythmic therapy is indicated, however, was supported by the lack of proarrhythmia and the reduction in arrhythmic death.

▶ Amiodarone, a class III antiarrhythmic agent, has been studied in multiple trials looking at the effects of drug treatment in patients at high risk of sudden cardiac death.[1-4] EMIAT showed that amiodarone is associated with an increased reduction in arrhythmic death in patients with depressed left ventricular function. However, there was no reduction in all-cause cardiac mortality. There is evidence though that amiodarone might be useful in those patients having sustained a potentially dangerous arrhythmia after myocardial infarction.

Beta-blockers remain the treatment of choice for preventing mortality and morbidity after myocardial infarction, and left-ventricular function should be treated vigorously. Implantable defibrillators may soon become the treatment of choice rather than drug therapy for the high-risk patients with ventricular arrhythmias requiring treatment.[5, 6]

W.H. Frishman, M.D.

References

1. Camm AJ, Julian DG, Janse MJ, et al: The European Myocardial Infarct Amiodarone Trial (EMIAT). *Am J Cardiol* 72:95F–98F, 1993.
2. Ceremunzynski L, Kleczar E, Krzeminska-Pakula M, et al: Effect of amiodarone on mortality after myocardial infarction: A double-blind, placebo-controlled pilot study. *J Am Coll Cardiol* 20:1056–1062, 1992.
3. Singh SN, Fletcher RD, Fisher SG, et al, for the Survival Trial of Antiarrhythmic Therapy in Congestive Heart Failure: Amiodarone in patients with congestive heart failure and asymptomatic ventricular arrhythmias. *N Engl J Med* 333:77–82, 1995.
4. Greene HL, et al, for the CASCADE Investigators: Randomized antiarrhythmic drug therapy in survivors of cardiac arrest (the CASCADE study). *Am J Cardiol* 72:280–287, 1993.
5. Moss AJ, Hall WJ, Cannom DS, et al: Improved survival with an implanted defibrillator in patients with coronary disease at high risk for ventricular arrhythmia. *N Engl J Med* 335:1933–1940, 1996.
6. Siebels J, Kuck KH, and the CASH Investigators: Implantable cardioverter-defibrillator compared with antiarrhythmic drug treatment in cardiac arrest survivors. The Cardiac Arrest Study Hamburg. *Am Heart J* 127:1139–1144, 1994.

Improved Survival With an Implanted Defibrillator in Patients With Coronary Disease at High Risk for Ventricular Arrhythmia
Moss AJ, for the Multicenter Automatic Defibrillator Implantation Trial Investigators (Univ of Rochester, NY; Good Samaritan Hosp, Los Angeles; Scripps Mem Hosp, La Jolla, Calif; et al)
N Engl J Med 335:1933–1940, 1996   22–7

Introduction.—Patients with previous myocardial infarction and left ventricular dysfunction who experience unsustained ventricular tachycardia are at increased risk of death (2-year mortality rate, approximately 30%). Although antiarrhythmic therapy has been widely used in this

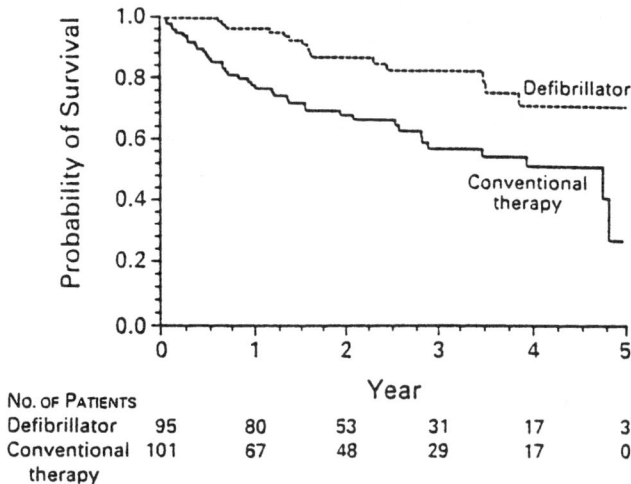

FIGURE 2.—Kaplan-Meier analysis of the probability of survival, according to assigned treatment. The difference in survival between the 2 treatment groups was significant (P = 0.009). (Reprinted by permission of The New England Journal of Medicine. Courtesy of Moss AJ, for the Multicenter Automatic Defibrillator Implantation Trial Investigators. N Engl J Med 335:1933–1940. Copyright 1996; Massachusetts Medical Society.)

high-risk group of patients, there is no evidence of improved survival. Whether an implanted cardioverter-defibrillator would improve survival was determined in a prophylactic trial.

Methods.—The trial enrolled 196 patients from 32 centers, 30 of which were in the United States and 2 of which were in Europe. Eligible patients were in New York Heart Association functional class I, II, or III with previous myocardial infarction, a left ventricular ejection fraction of 0.35 or less, a documented episode of asymptomatic unsustained ventricular tachycardia, and an inducible, nonsuppressible ventricular tachyarrhythmia on electrophysiologic study. Randomization was to conventional medical therapy in 101 patients and to an implanted defibrillator in 95. Patients were stratified according to center and to the interval between the most recent myocardial infarction and enrollment (less than 6 months or 6 months or more).

Results.—The 2 groups were similar in baseline clinical characteristics and in the proportion of patients in the transthoracic stratum or transvenous stratum groups. During follow-up (average period, 27 months), there were 15 deaths in the defibrillator group (11 from cardiac causes) and 39 in the conventional therapy group (27 from cardiac causes). The study was officially stopped when the efficacy boundary of the sequential design was crossed at 51 deaths. Three additional deaths occurred before the stopping date but were not identified until the close-out procedure. Although the implanted defibrillator significantly reduced overall mortality, antiarrhythmic therapy yielded no survival benefit (Fig 2).

Conclusion.—Use of the implanted defibrillator significantly improved survival in a narrowly defined patient population: high-risk patients with coronary heart disease and left ventricular dysfunction, spontaneous asymptomatic unsustained ventricular tachycardia, and inducible and nonsuppressible ventricular tachycardia on electrophysiologic testing.

► Nonsustained ventricular tachycardia in patients who have had a previous myocardial infarction is associated with a high mortality rate over the subsequent 2 years. This study shows that an implantable defibrillator can reduce mortality in these patients compared with medical therapy.

The implantable defibrillator provides protection against death in high-risk patients having coronary artery disease and left ventricular dysfunction, spontaneous asymptomatic unsustained ventricular tachycardia, and inducible and nonsuppressible ventricular tachyarrhythmias on electrophysiologic testing. Until the results of ongoing randomized trials of defibrillators become available[1, 2] in other populations, the device should only be used in the type of patient with myocardial infarction described in this study.

W.H. Frishman, M.D.

References

1. Bigger JT Jr: Should defibrillators be implanted in high-risk patients without a previous sustained ventricular tachyarrhythmia? in Naccarelli GV, Veltri EP (eds): *Implantable Cardioverter-Defibrillators*. Boston, Blackwell Scientific, 1993, p 284.
2. Greene HL: Antiarrhythmic drugs versus implantable defibrillators: The need for a randomized controlled study. *Am Heart J* 127:1171–1178, 1994.

23 Other Topics

Vascular Events During Follow-up in Patients With Aortic Arch Atherosclerosis
Mitusch R, Doherty C, Wucherpfennig H, et al (Univ of Lübeck, Germany; Univ of Greifswald, Germany)
Stroke 28:36–39, 1997   23–1

Background.—Although aortic arch atherosclerosis has been associated with vascular events, few follow-up data exist. Patients with moderate to severe aortic arch atherosclerosis detected by transesophageal echocardiography were studied prospectively in the current study.

Methods.—One hundred eighty-three patients were included. One hundred thirty-six had raised plaques, with a thickness of less than 5 mm, and 47 had complex plaques with thickness of 5 mm or more or plaques with mobile components. Mean follow-up was 16 months.

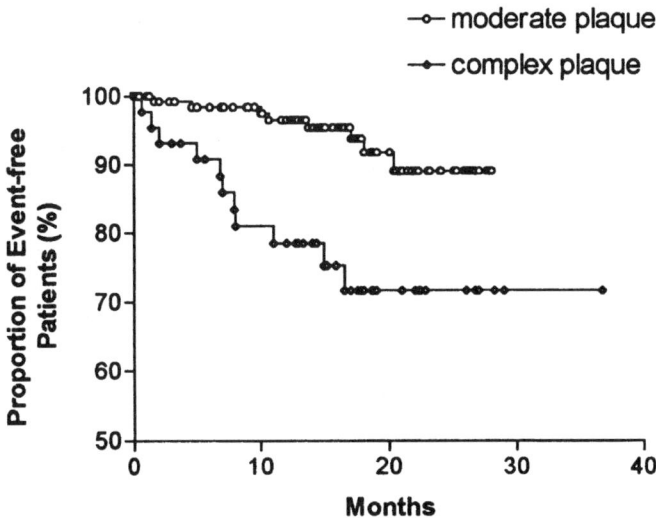

FIGURE.—Survival curves for vascular events in patients with moderate atherosclerosis (plaque thickness < 5 mm) and patients with complex atherosclerosis (plaque thickness ≥5 mm on mobile components) in the aortic arch. Kaplan-Meier analysis revealed a significant difference between the two groups of patients $P < .01$. (Courtesy of Mitusch R, Doherty C, Wucherpfennig H, et al: Vascular events during follow-up in patients with aortic arch atherosclerosis *Stroke* 28:36–39, 1997.)

Findings.—Fifteen patients experienced vascular events with a presumed embolic origin during follow-up. The incidence in patients with raised plaques and in those with complex plaques was 4.1 and 13.7 per 100 person-years, respectively. According to a Kaplan-Meier survival analysis, the rate of vascular events was significantly higher in patients with complex plaques (Fig). In a Cox proportional hazards analysis, independent predictors of vascular events were complex plaques, coronary artery disease, and a history of previous embolism.

Conclusions.—This study suggests that patients with complex aortic arch atherosclerosis are at greater risk for subsequent vascular events. Such complex disease includes protruding plaques and plaque-related mobile masses.

▶ Complex aortic arch atherosclerosis, which includes protruding plaques and plaque-related mobile thrombotic masses, is associated with an increased risk of subsequent vascular events of a presumed embolic etiology.[1-4] These lesions may also be associated with an increased risk of embolization in patients undergoing cardiac catheterization. It is recommended that transesophageal echocardiography be done in patients with unexplained embolic events to also look for protruding atherosclerotic lesions in the thoracic aorta.[5] The most important remaining question is that of treatment.[5] Surgery is technically feasible, but should be reserved for a select group of candidates with recurrent events. The role of anticoagulant drugs and pharmacologic strategies to promote atheroma regression still needs to be determined.

W.H. Frishman, M.D.

References

1. Amarenco P, Duychaerts C, Tzourio C, et al: The prevalence of ulcerated plaques in the aortic arch in patients with stroke. *N Engl J Med* 326:221–225, 1992.
2. Khatibzadeh M, Mitusch R, Stierle U, et al: Aortic atherosclerotic plaque as a source of systemic embolism. *J Am Coll Cardiol* 27:664–669, 1996.
3. Tunick PA, Rosenzweig BP, Katz ES, et al: High risk for vascular events in patients with protruding aortic atheromas: A prospective study. *J Am Coll Cardiol* 23:1085–1090, 1994.
4. Amarenco P, Cohen A, Tzourio C, et al: Atherosclerotic disease of the aortic arch and the risk of ischemic stroke. *N Engl J Med* 331:1474–1479, 1994.
5. Kronzon I, Tunick PA: Atheromatous disease of the throracic aorta: pathologic and clinical implications. *Ann Intern Med* 126:629–637, 1997.

Systemic Infection Related to Endocarditis on Pacemaker Leads: Clinical Presentation and Management

Klug D, Lacroix D, Savoye C, et al (Hôpital Cardiologique de Lille, France)
Circulation 95:2098–2107, 1997   23–2

Introduction.—Endocarditis can occur as a result of pacemaker lead infection. This is a serious complication with a reported incidence of

0.13% to 7.0% in patients with permanently implanted endocardial pacemakers. Medical treatment is not sufficient; percutaneous or surgical ablation is required. The diagnosis and management of pacemaker lead infection were studied.

Patients.—The retrospective study included 52 patients admitted during a 3-year period with suspected infection of pacemaker leads. Fourteen patients had symptoms beginning within 6 weeks after the last procedure on the pacemaker implant site. The remaining 38 patients had symptoms occurring over a longer period of time. A fever was present in 86.5% of patients. Thirty-eight percent of patients had clinical and/or radiologic signs of pulmonary involvement. Thirty-one percent had pulmonary infarcts apparent on pulmonary scintigraphy, and 52% had local complications. Ninety-six percent of patients had elevated C-reactive protein levels.

An infecting organism was identified in 88% of patients; it was *Staphylococcus* in 93.5%. Twenty-three percent of patients had vegetations detected by transthoracic echocardiography. In 94%, the pacemaker lead appeared normal on transesophageal echocardiography.

Outcomes.—Treatment was by percutaneous removal in 38 patients and by surgical removal with extracorporeal circulation in 10 patients. After the infected material was removed, all patients received antibiotics. Two patients died before the leads could be removed, and 2 died after surgical removal. In-hospital mortality was 7.6%. At a mean follow-up of 20 months, the overall mortality was 27%.

Conclusions.—Patients in whom fever, complications, or pulmonary lesions develop after pacemaker implantation should be suspected of having endocarditis related to pacemaker lead infection. Vegetations can usually be detected on transesophageal echocardiography. In most patients, the infecting organism is *Staphylococcus*. After complete removal of the endocardial system, the patients must receive 6 weeks of antibiotic therapy.

▶ Years ago, endocarditis from pacemaker lead infection was considered to be a rare occurrence worthy of case reports. However, a report of a large series demonstrates that pacemaker endocarditis is more common, and patients are often seen soon after the pacemaker implant with acute endocarditis or later with chronic endocarditis. Transesophageal echo cardiography is the best technique when looking for vegetations. Treatment consists of removal of the endocardial system by surgical or percutaneous means. Percutaneous removal seems to be safer when the vegetation size is less than 10 mm. Six weeks of continuous antibiotic therapy is also recommended.

After removal of the infected pacemaker, an abdominal pacemaker can be inserted for permanent epicardial stimulation of the ventricle for those patients who require permanent ventricular stimulation. In some patients, a new transvenous permanent pacemaker can be inserted 1–2 months after the percutaneous removal of the old system.

W.H. Frishman, M.D.

Comparison of 5-mg and 10-mg Loading Doses in Initiation of Warfarin Therapy

Harrison L, Johnston M, Massicotte MP, et al (McMaster Univ, Hamilton, Ont, Canada; Hamilton Civic Hosp Research Centre, Ont, Canada)
Ann Intern Med 126:133–136, 1997   23–3

Background.—Though loading warfarin doses greater than those used for maintenance treatment are commonly used in clinical practice, they have never been investigated prospectively. The effects of 5- and 10-mg loading doses of warfarin on laboratory markers of the anticoagulant effect of warfarin were compared.

Methods.—Forty-nine patients with a target international normalized ratio (INR) of 2 to 3 were enrolled in the randomized clinical trial. Patients were given an initial dose of 5- or 10-mg warfarin, with subsequent doses adminsitered on the basis of dosing nomograms.

Findings.—Forty-four percent of the patients in the 10-mg group had INRs exceeding 2 at 36 hours, compared with 8% of those in the 5-mg group. Factor VII levels were 27% and 54% of the 10- and 5-mg groups, respectively, at this time. Factor II levels were 74% and 82% in the 10- and 5-mg groups, respectively. At 60 hours, 36% of the 10-mg group and none of the 5-mg patients had INRs exceeding 3. At 84 hours, INRs were between 2 and 3 in 63% of the 10-mg group and in 79% of the 5-mg group. Vitamin K was needed for excessive prolongation of the INR in 4 patients in the 10-mg group and in 1 in the 5-mg group (Figure).

Conclusions.—A 5-mg loading dose of warfarin results in less excess anticoagulation than a 10-mg dose. The smaller dose also avoids the development of a potential hypercoagulable state from precipitous reductions in protein C levels in the first 36 hours of warfarin treatment.

▶ Warfarin treatment is often initiated with a 10-mg loading dose and then reduced to a dose level that maintains the international normalized ratio (INR) within the desired therapeutic range.[1] An alternative approach is to start warfarin therapy at 5 mg, which is the dose usually required to maintain the INR between 2.0–3.0.

In this study, patients who received the 10-mg loading dose achieved INRs greater than 2.0 more rapidly than patients receiving the 5-mg loading dose. However, because the change in early INR was caused by a reduction in factor VII and not factor II, an adequate anti-thrombotic effect may not be present.[2] By day 5, therapeutic INR is seen after a 10-mg and 5-mg loading dose.

The authors[2] suggest that heparin therapy be maintained for 5 days after warfarin is started, with either a 10- or 5-mg loading dose. A 5-mg loading dose may prevent a potential hypercoagulable state caused by a decline in protein C during early treatment.

W.H. Frishman, M.D.

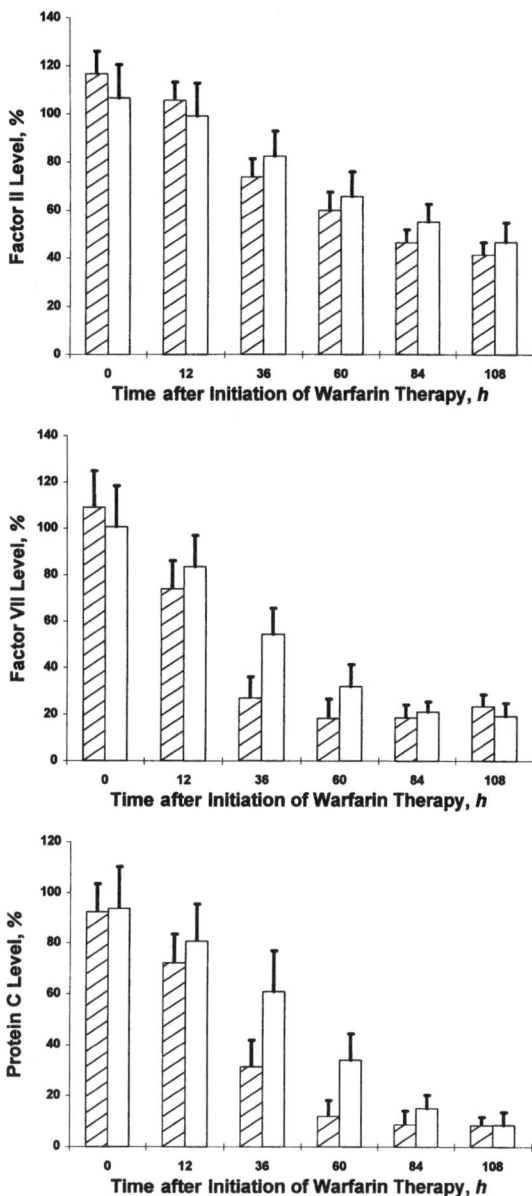

FIGURE.—Plasma levels of coagulation factors in patients receiving a 10-mg (*striped bars*) or 5-mg (*white bars*) loading dose of warfarin for each of 6 time points assessed. Levels of factor II (*top*) decreased at a similar rate in the 5- and 10-mg groups. Levels of factor VII (*middle*) and protein C (*bottom*) decreased more rapidly in the 10-mg group than in the 5-mg group. Error bars represent 95% CIs. (Courtesy of Harrison L, Johnston M, Massicotte MP, et al: Comparison of 5-mg and 10-mg loading doses in initiation of warfarin therapy. *Ann Intern Med* 126:133–136, 1997.)

References

1. Frishman WH, Klein MD, Blaufarb I, et al: Antiplatelet and antithrombotic drugs. In, Frishman WH, Sonnenblick EH (eds): *Cardiovascular Pharmacotherapeutics.* New York: McGraw Hill Inc., 1997; 323.
2. Zivelin A, Rao LV, Rapaport SI: Mechanism of the anticoagulant effect of warfarin as evaluated in rabbits by selective depression of individual procoagulant vitamin K-dependent clotting factors. *J Clin Invest* 92:2131–2140, 1993.

Effect of Atenolol on Mortality and Cardiovascular Morbidity After Noncardiac Surgery

Mangano DT, for the Multicenter Study of Perioperative Ischemia Research Group (Univ of California, San Francisco; Ischemia Research and Education Found, San Francisco)

N Engl J Med 335:1713–1720, 1996   23–4

Introduction.—Many patients undergoing noncardiac surgery have or are at risk for coronary artery disease. In this group, myocardial ischemia and nonfatal myocardial infarction occurring in the week after surgery greatly increases the risk of mortality and cardiovascular morbidity. Preoperative or intraoperative beta-blockers have yielded encouraging effects on hemodynamics and measures of myocardial ischemia; however, the effects of giving this treatment throughout the postoperative period have not been investigated. The effects of intensive beta-blocker therapy before and after noncardiac surgery in patients with or at risk for coronary artery disease were studied over a 2-year follow-up period.

Methods.—The study included 200 patients undergoing elective noncardiac surgery who either had or were at risk for coronary artery disease. They were assigned to receive either atenolol or placebo before the induction of anesthesia, immediately after surgery, and then through up to 7 days of hospitalization. Before and immediately after surgery, the study medications were given IV. Each day thereafter, if the heart rate was greater than 55 beats/min and the systolic blood pressure at least 100 mm Hg, the patients received 2 tablets of atenolol (100 mg) or placebo. Just 1 tablet was given if the heart rate was 55–65 beats/min or the systolic blood pressure was 100 mm Hg or greater. If the heart rate or blood pressure fell below these values, no treatment was given. Anesthetic and surgical management were not restricted by the study protocol. One hundred ninety-four patients survived to discharge, and outcome data were available for 192. The main outcome variable was all-cause mortality after 2 years; cardiovascular morbidity during the same period was a secondary outcome.

Results.—The overall mortality during 2 years of follow-up was 15.6%, with 21 of 30 deaths occurring in the placebo group. The overall mortality was 55% lower and cardiac mortality was 65% lower with atenolol. In the atenolol group, there was 1 noncardiac death in the first 6–8 postoperative months; during the same time, there were 10 deaths in the placebo group,

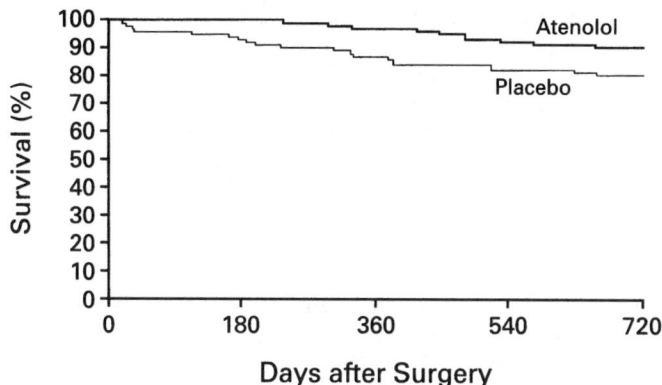

FIGURE 1.—Overall survival in the 2 years after noncardiac surgery among 192 patients in the atenolol and placebo groups who survived to hospital discharge. The rate of survival at 6 months (180 days) was 100% in the atenolol group and 92% in the placebo group ($P < 0.001$); at 1 year (360 days), the rates were 97% and 86%, respectively ($P = 0.005$); and at 2 years (720 days), 90% and 79% ($P = 0.019$). (Reprinted by permission of The New England Journal of Medicine, from Mangano DT, for the Multicenter Study of Perioperative Ischemia Research Group: Effect of atenolol on mortality and cardiovascular morbidity after noncardiac surgery. *N Engl J Med* 335:1713–1720, 1996. Copyright 1996, Massachusetts Medical Society.)

including 7 cardiac deaths. The early survival advantage with atenolol was preserved at 1 and 2 years (Fig 1).

The rate of cardiac events was lower with atenolol, with the main effect again occurring within 6–8 months. Time to the first adverse event was 6 days in the placebo group vs. 158 days in the atenolol group. On multivariate analysis, factors associated with survival at 2 years were diabetes mellitus and atenolol therapy. The risk of death was not increased for patients with diabetes treated with atenolol, compared to a 4-fold increase in patients with diabetes receiving placebo. There was no difference between groups in the use of cardiovascular medications during follow-up. Atenolol had no serious adverse effects, such as hypotension or bradycardia.

Conclusions.—Giving atenolol throughout the hospitalization period can significantly reduce the risk of mortality and cardiovascular events after noncardiac surgery in patients with or at risk for coronary artery disease. The main effect of this treatment is apparent within the first 6–8 months after surgery. Beta-blockade is a safe and well-tolerated therapy. Conservative cost estimates suggest that the overall cost per life-year saved with this therapy is $2,500.

▶ Patients at risk for the complications of coronary artery disease were shown to benefit from atenolol treatment compared to placebo when undergoing noncardiac surgery. This treatment should be started in patients preoperatively and maintained throughout the hospital stay. Patients who benefit include those having heart failure and pulmonary disease.

Patients already receiving beta-blockers before surgery should have them maintained on the morning of surgery and they should be restarted as soon as possible in the postoperative period.

Patients with suspected coronary artery disease before noncardiac surgery, who are not receiving anti-ischemic drug therapy, can be given beta-blockers rather than having to undergo an extensive preoperative evaluation to rule in or rule out coronary disease.

W.H. Frishman, M.D.

Interference With Cardiac Pacemakers by Cellular Telephones
Hayes DL, Wang PJ, Reynolds DW, et al (Mayo Clinic, Rochester, Minn; New England Med Ctr, Boston; Univ of Oklahoma, Oklahoma City; et al)
N Engl J Med 336:1473–1479, 1997   23–5

Introduction.—European studies have suggested that cellular telephones can interfere with implanted pacemakers. In the United States, in vitro studies have shown the potential for such interference. In a multicenter trial, the incidence of interference with pacemakers by cellular phones was assessed, as was the clinical risk arising from such interference.

Methods.—The prospective, cross-over, double-blind study included 980 patients with implanted cardiac pacemakers. Each patient was tested with 5 types of hand-held cellular telephones in random order, including 1 analog and 4 digital phones. In the test mode use for each phone, the phones were programmed to transmit at maximal power, thus simulating the worst-case scenario. Furthermore, 1 phone was tested during actual use. During testing, each patient underwent ECG monitoring with the phone over the ipsilateral ear and in a series of maneuvers directly over the pacemaker. When any interference occurred, it was classified as to type and clinical significance.

Results.—A total of 5,233 tests were performed, 20% of which caused any type of interference and 7.2% of which caused symptoms. Clinically significant interferences occurred in 6.6% of tests. Clinically significant interference never occurred with the phone held normally over the ear. The rate of definitely clinically significant interference was only 1.7%, and this only occurred with the phone held over the pacemaker. Dual-chamber pacemakers showed interference in 25.3% of tests compared with 6.8% for single-chamber pacemakers. The interference rate was 28.9% to 55.8% for pacemakers without feed-through filters compared to 0.4% to 0.8% for those with feed-through filters.

Conclusions.—Cellular telephones can interfere with pacemaker function. However, clinically significant interference does not occur with the phone placed over the ear, as during normal use. Cellular phones should not be placed over the pacemaker and should not be carried in a pocket close to the pacemaker when turned on.

▶ This interesting report in an era of increased cellular telephone technology shows the potential danger of cellular phone use to pacemaker function.

Future implantable pacemaker and defibrillator designs should take into consideration potential interference with these devices from electromagnetic fields close by.[1]

W.H. Frishman, M.D.

Reference

1. Carillo R, Garay O, Balzano Q, et al: Electromagnetic near field interference with implantable medical devices. Presented at the 1995 IEEE International Symposium on Electromagnetic Compatibility. Atlanta, Ga, August 14–18, 1995.

Dual-Chamber Pacing For Hypertrophic Cardiomyopathy: A Randomized, Double-Blind, Crossover Trial

Nishimura RA, Trusty JM, Hayes DL, et al (Mayo Clinic and Mayo Found, Rochester, Minn)
J Am Coll Cardiol 29:435–441, 1997   23–6

Background.—Several recent cohort studies have demonstrated that implanting a dual-chamber pacemaker in patients with severely symptomatic hypertrophic obstructive cardiomyopathy can relieve symptoms and reduce the severity of left ventricular outflow tract gradient. However, there have been no randomized, double-blind comparisons of dual-chamber pacing and standard treatment.

Methods.—Twenty-one patients with severely symptomatic hypertrophic obstructive cardiomyopathy were enrolled in the current double-blind, randomized, crossover trial after baseline studies. Minnesota quality-of-life assessment, 2-dimensional and Doppler echocardiography, and cardiopulmonary exercise testing were done. Nineteen patients completed the protocol and were randomly assigned to DDD pacing for 3 months followed by back-up AAI pacing for 3 months or to these treatments in the reverse order.

Findings.—After DDD pacing, left ventricular outflow tract gradient declined significantly to a mean 55 mm Hg, compared with the mean baseline gradient of 76 mm Hg and of 83 mm Hg after AAI pacing. Quality-of-life scores and exercise duration were improved significantly after DDD pacing compared with baseline but not compared with the back-up AAI arm. Peak oxygen consumption did not differ significantly among the 3 arms. Overall, symptomatic improvement was noted in 63% during DDD pacing and in 42% during AAI pacing. Thirty-one percent had no symptomatic change, and 5% had symptom deterioration during DDD pacing (Fig 1).

Conclusions.—Dual-chamber pacing may alleviate symptoms and reduce gradient in patients with hypertrophic obstructive cardiomyopathy. However, symptoms are unaffected or even worsen in some patients.

% pts

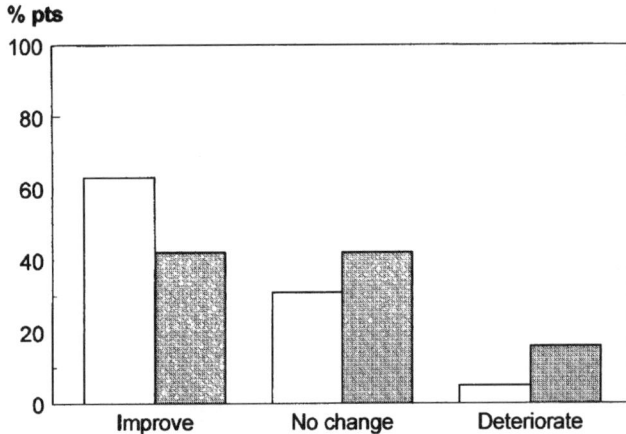

FIGURE 1.—Subjective symptomatic response after each of the 2 pacing arms. Shown are the percentages of patients (pts) who experienced improvement, no change or deterioration from the baseline state. Open columns = continuous DDD pacing; gray columns = AAI, backup mode with the atrial rate set at 30 beats/min. (Reprinted with permission from the American College of Cardiology, from Nishimura RA, Trusty JM, Hayes DL, et al: Dual-chamber pacing for hypertrophic cardiomyopathy: A randomized, double-blind, crossover trial. *J Am Coll Cardiol* 29:435–441, 1997.)

Subjective improvement may also occur after implantation of the pacemaker without the hemodynamic benefit, which suggests a placebo effect.

▶ Dual-chamber cardiac pacing has been proposed as a palliative treatment for hypertrophic cardiomyopathy in patients unresponsive to medical therapy (e.g., beta blocker, verapamil).[1] The mechanism of benefit is uncertain, but may be related to an obstructive gradient reduction related to a dyssynchronous pacing of the septum caused by right ventricular pacing and possibly ventricular remodeling.[1]

This study shows that dual-chamber pacing may relieve clinical symptoms in some patients, but has no effect in others, despite a reduction in left ventricular outflow gradient. Patients may feel subjective improvement, even in the absence of hemodynamic improvement. There is also no information regarding the impact of pacing on mortality. One cannot recommend cardiac pacing as a routine treatment for patients with severely symptomatic hypertrophic cardiomyopathy unresponsive to medical therapy, but as a possible palliative treatment perhaps in patients who cannot undergo surgical myectomy.

W.H. Frishman, M.D.

Reference

1. Fananapazir L, Epstein ND, Curiel RV, Panza JA, Tripodi D, McAreavey D: Long-term results of dual-chamber (DDD) pacing in obstructive hypertrophic cardiomyyopathy: evidence for progressive symptomatic and hemodynamic improvement and reduction of left ventricular hypertrophy. *Circulation* 1994; 90:2731–2742.

Introduction

This year I have chosen for the YEAR BOOK articles that deal predominantly with treatment. Some of the articles discuss established treatments; for example, estrogen for women with postmenopausal osteoporosis; some are new; for example, insulin lispro for diabetes; and others are promissory; for example, a drug to inhibit parathyroid hormone secretion in patients with primary hyperparathyroidism. These selections reflect the fact that more research on old treatments is being done and more new treatments are being developed. For the latter, one has only to consider diabetes mellitus, for which insulin lispro, metformin, troglitazone and acarbose have become available in recent years. Herein I comment on some of these articles, and also on other articles not included in the following chapters.

The chapter on the pituitary gland contains three articles on treatment. One describes the efficacy of a slow-release formulation of lanreotide, and analogue of somatostatin. Unlike octreotide, which must be given several times daily, lanreotide need be given only every 10 to 14 days. Although transsphenoidal surgery remains the treatment of choice for patients with acromegaly, the time may be approaching when lanreotide or a related compound will supplant surgery as primary therapy. A second article in this chapter describes the efficacy of cabergoline in patients with prolactinomas resistant to bromocriptine therapy. Cabergoline is, like bromocriptine, a dopamine agonist, but its duration of action is much longer and it seems to have fewer side effects than bromocriptine. The latter supplanted surgery as primary treatment for most patients with a prolactinoma about a decade ago, and it may soon be supplanted by cabergoline. The last article in this chapter describes the efficacy of a new synthetic vasopressin antagonist in patients with excess vasopressin secretion.

What to do about patients with adrenal incidentalomas continues to be debated. The lessons of the case study I selected on this topic for the chapter on adrenal disease—that all patients should be studied for hormonal hypersecretion and large incidentalomas should be excised—are not new, but the experience—over 200 patients studied more or less systematically—was large. To emphasize the need for study of these patients further, I also include an article describing the characteristics of patients with incidentally discovered pheochromocytomas. Several articles in the chapter on adrenal disease discuss adrenal insufficiency. One describes the presence of antibodies to 21-hydroxylase in patients with autoimmune adrenalitis. Most patients with idiopathic adrenal insufficiency have these antibodies, but it is important to remember that a positive test for them does not mean the patient has adrenal insufficiency, any more than a positive test for antithyroid peroxidase antibodies means the patient has hypothyroidism. Another article describes adrenal insufficiency in patients taking megestrol, a steroid given to women with metastatic breast carcinoma to inhibit tumor growth and to patients with wasting disorders to stimulate appetite. While the findings seem real, megestrol also causes Cushing's syndrome. Why it should cause both adrenal insufficiency and excess is unexplained. Another article in this chapter provides strong evidence that patients with Cushing's disease who are not cured by transsphenoidal surgery should be treated with radiotherapy, certainly a more appealing option than another operation.

One of the articles in the chapter on thyroid disease reminds us how variable and nonspecific the symptoms and signs of hypothyroidism are. There are several articles on thyroxine therapy. One describes a study of the bioequivalence of two brand name and two generic preparations of thyroxine. Publication of this study was originally held up by the sponsor, because the sponsor's product was not more bioavailable, though why it was expected to be escapes me. All the sponsor got for delaying publication was bad publicity and a class action suit. Another article describes the lack of efficacy of thyroxine therapy in patients with subclinical hypothyroidism. This is an important issue because so many patients have this disorder, but the new results will probably not discourage continued use of thyroxine because it *might* result in symptomatic improvement as well as prevent progression to overt hypothyroidism. Two articles concern subclinical hyperthroidism; in one it was associated with cardiovascular abnormalities (not confirmed by another study[1]) and in the other it was not associated with bone loss. The debate about the ill effects, or the lack thereof, of subclinical hyperthyroidism on the cardiovascular system and bone will no doubt continue. But, in fact, subclinical hyperthyroidism is largely avoidable anyway, because the most common cause is thyroxine therapy, and the only patients who should be given thyroxine in doses sufficient to cause subclinical hyperthyroidism are the few with carcinoma of the thyroid. Not included in the thyroid chapter, but worth mentioning, is a review of the topic of thyroid nodules detected when ultrasonography, computed tomography or magnetic resonance imaging of the neck is done for other reasons.[2] Such incidental nodules are found in up to 50% of patients having these tests, and are best managed by watchful waiting.

The chapter on the parathyroid glands and bone focuses on primary hyperparathyroidism and bone. One article on the former topic describes a decline in the frequency of hyperparathyroidism at the Mayo Clinic. The decline there has been substantial, but it has not yet, to my knowledge, been corroborated elsewhere. One of the most important fundamental advances in the area of calcium metabolism in recent years is the identification and cloning of the calcium receptor.[3] The article describing reduction of parathyroid hormone secretion in patients with primary hyperparathyroidism by a drug that binds to the receptor is surely the forerunner of many more. Among the articles on bone are two about the effects of estrogen. One indicates that the efficacy of estrogen in increasing bone density can be predicted by measuring biochemical markers of bone turnover rather soon after therapy is initiated, rather than waiting a year or more to see if bone density has increased. Routine measurements of bone markers are not necessary, but they may be worthwhile in women with severe osteoporosis. The reason is that estrogen is not effective in all women, and it is better to learn sooner rather than later that a woman with severe osteoporosis is not responding to it. The other article about estrogen suggests that its effect on the skeleton is sustained during prolonged therapy, reinforcing the view that estrogen therapy should be continued indefinitely. An article on alendronate confirms that its action to increase bone density in postmenopausal women with osteoporosis translates into a decrease in fractures; thus, gain in bone density induced by alendronate is accompanied by a gain in bone strength. Vitamin D and calcium supplementation—a simple and less expensive treatment—had similar positive effects on bone density and nonvertebral fractures in a study of older men and women included in this chapter. The final two articles deal with corticosteroid-induced osteoporosis; both vitamin D and calcium supplementation and intermittent etidronate proved effective in preventing loss of bone; a comparison of the two would be useful now.

An article in the chapter on reproduction describes the changing pattern of onset of puberty in girls—it occurs earlier than commonly believed. The practical implications of the results involve counseling anxious parents about normal pubertal development in their children and knowing when development is precocious. I include an article on a telephone survey of postmenopausal women who were asked about estrogen therapy. The results reveal, among other things, the disconnect between what physicians recommend and what women do regarding this treatment. Only one article on reproductive function in men appears in this year's volume, a case study of a group of men who had acquired, or at least late-onset, hypogonadotropic hypogonadism.

On the topic of carbohydrate metabolism and diabetes mellitus, there is an article on the high frequency of eating disorders in young women with diabetes. This finding is, perhaps, not surprising given the high frequency of eating disorders in young women in general and the stresses of parental and physician requests for controlled diets and regular food intake in young patients with diabetes. An article on insulin lispro, which is more rapid acting than regular insulin, is included. This drug will not revolutionize the treatment of patients with diabetes, but it may make life simpler for some, because they can inject their short-acting insulin and eat immediately. With respect to injection of insulin, I include an article demonstrating the safety of injecting insulin through clothing, something that I suspect all diabetic patients do, even if they don't tell us. Another article provides further evidence that administration of an angiotensin-converting enzyme inhibitor is beneficial in normotensive patients with type 1 diabetes who have microalbuminuria, but no evidence of benefit in those with no albuminuria. These data may slow the rush to treat everyone with either type 1 or type 2 diabetes with one of these drugs. On the topic of the complications of diabetes, a study is presented which demonstrates that granulocyte-colony stimulating factor is beneficial in diabetic patients with foot ulcers.

An important event in the area of diabetes last year was the recommendation of an expert committee that the classification "diabetes" be changed to an etiologic one, and the terms "insulin-dependent" and "non-insulin-dependent" be eliminated.[4] Thus, type 1 diabetes is immune-mediated or idiopathic diabetes, and everything else is type 2 diabetes (except for specific types of diabetes such as those due to genetic defects in insulin secretion or action, infection or endocrinopathies). The change in terminology is designed primarily to eliminate the confusion about insulin therapy caused by the old terminology, specifically the question of how to categorize those patients with nonautoimmune diabetes who must be treated with insulin. More important, the diagnostic criteria were changed; diabetes is now defined as symptoms of hyperglycemia plus a casual plasma glucose concentration of 200 mg/dL (11.1 mmol/L) or more, a fasting plasma glucose concentration of 126 mg/dL (7.0 mmol/L) or more, or a plasma glucose concentration of 200 mg/dL (11.1 mmol/L) or more two hours after ingestion of 75 grams of glucose. These changes reflect the awareness that slightly lower plasma glucose concentrations than previously thought are risk factors for the vascular complications of diabetes. On a more practical level, the committee came down firmly in favor of measurements of fasting plasma glucose for diagnosis, except in pregnant women. This is recognition of reality—few glucose tolerance tests are being done now, nor should they be (except in pregnant women).

Two of the three articles in the chapter on obesity concern the physiology of leptin. The key findings are that obese humans of all ages have high serum leptin concentrations, and therefore leptin resistance, but why they are leptin-resistant is unknown. There are differences in serum leptin concentrations among women and men, and among subjects of different ages. There is also a suggestion of a role in reproduction, and leptin production declines with caloric restriction. The main therapeutic question is whether serum leptin concentrations can be raised further or sensitivity to leptin increased in obese patients somehow, and, if so, whether doing so will promote weight loss. The third article describes a comparative study of the effect of estrogen-progestin and simvastatin on hypercholesterolemia in postmenopausal women; the former was effective, but not as effective as the latter. Overshadowing this area in 1997 was the recognition of valvular heart disease in obese patients taking dexfenfluramine alone or in combination with phentermine, which led to the withdrawal of fenfluramine.[5] The magnitude of the risk is not known, and may never be, nor is the pathophysiology, but, when added to the risk of pulmonary hypertension reported in patients taking these drugs,[6] the withdrawal seems eminently prudent.

The next seven chapters contain more extensive comments about these and other articles and, of course, the abstracts of the articles themselves. I hope readers find both the abstracts and the comments both useful and provocative.

Robert D. Utiger, M.D.

References

1. Shapiro LE, Sievert R, Ong L, et al: Minimal cardiac effects in asymptomatic athyreotic patients chronically treated with thyrotropin-suppressive doses of L-thyroxine. *J Clin Endocrinol Metab* 82:2592–2595, 1997.
2. Tan GH, Gharib H: Thyroid incidentalomas: Management approaches to nonpalpable nodules discovered incidentally on thyroid imaging. *Ann Intern Med* 1226:226–231, 1997.
3. Brown EM, Pollak M, Seidman CE, et al: Calcium-ion-sensing cell-surface receptors. *N Engl J Med* 333:234–239, 1995.
4. The expert committee on the diagnosis and classification of diabetes mellitus. Report of the Expert Committee of the Diagnosis and Classification of Diabetes Mellitus. *Diabetes Care* 20:1183–1197, 1997.
5. Connolly HM, Crary JL, McGoon MD, et al: Valvular heart disease associated with fenfluramine-phenteramine. *N Engl J Med* 337:581–588, 1997.
6. Mark EJ, Patalas ED, Chang HT, et al: Fatal pulmonary hypertension associated with short-term use of fenfluramine and phenteramine. *N Engl J Med* 333:602–606, 1997.

24 The Pituitary Gland

Three Year Follow-up of Acromegalic Patients Treated With Intramuscular Slow-release Lanreotide
Caron P, Morange-Ramos I, Cogne M, et al (CHU Rangueil, Toulouse, France; CHU la Timone, Marseilles, France)
J Clin Endocrinol Metab 82:18–22, 1997   24–1

Background.—An alternative to pituitary surgery and radiotherapy in acromegalic patients is treatment with somatostatin analogues. Recently, a depot long-lasting formulation of slow-release (SR) lanreotide was found to be effective in the short-term control of growth hormone (GH) hypersecretion in such patients. The long-term affects of SR lanreotide in a group of acromegalic patients was evaluated.

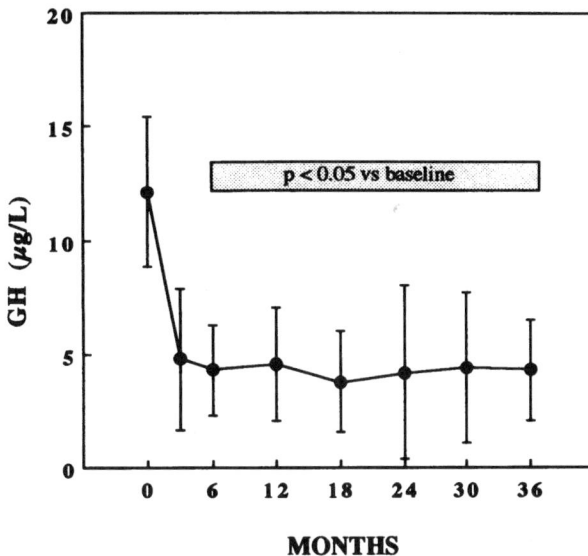

FIGURE 1.—Mean (±SE) plasma growth hormone concentrations in 22 acromegalic patients before and during long-term treatment with slow-release lanreotide. *Abbreviation: GH,* growth hormone. (Courtesy of Caron P, Morange-Ramos I, Cogne M, et al: Three year follow-up of acromegalic patients treated with intramuscular slow-release lanreotide. *J Clin Endocrinol Metab* 82:18–22, 1997; Copyright The Endocrine Society.)

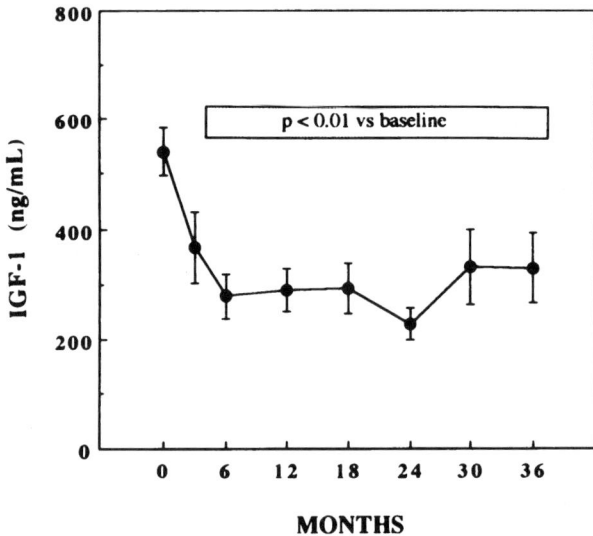

FIGURE 2.—Mean (±SE) plasma insulin-like growth factor-1 concentrations in 22 acromegalic patients before and during long-term treatment with slow-release lanreotide. *Abbreviation: IGF*-1, insulin-like growth factor-1. (Courtesy of Caron P, Morange-Ramos I, Cogne M, et al: Three year follow-up of acromegalic patients treated with intramuscular slow-release lanreotide. *J Clin Endocrinol Metab* 82:18–22, 1997; Copyright The Endocrine Society.)

Methods.—Thirteen women and 9 men, mean age 51 years, were studied. Twelve had pituitary macroadenomas; 8, microadenomas; and 2, empty sella. Seven patients had had partial surgical removal of adenomas. Twenty-one had plasma GH concentrations less than 5 µg/L during previous octreotide treatment. On the basis of plasma GH values after 3 months of twice monthly IM injections of 30 mg of SR lanreotide, SR lanreotide was given every 14 or 10 days.

Findings.—At 6 months, the plasma GH concentrations were 5 µg/L or less in 68% of the patients and 2.5 µg/L or less in 27%. These values remained unchanged during 1–3 years of continued treatment. During treatment, plasma insulin-like growth factor-1 concentrations were in the normal range in 63% of the patients (Figs 1 and 2). Thirteen percent had a significant reduction in pituitary tumor volume. Minor digestive problems within 48 hours after each injection, occurring in 13 patients, were the main side effects. Gallstones developed in 18% of patients.

Conclusions.—SR lanreotide may be of value after unsuccessful surgery and radiotherapy in acromegalic patients.

▶ The best treatment for acromegaly is surgery. The options for those who refuse surgery or those in whom it is contraindicated or is unsuccessful are radiotherapy, bromocriptine, and octreotide. Radiotherapy results in gradual clinical improvement, a gradual fall in GH production, and a lesser and more gradual fall in insulin-like growth factor-1 (IGF-1) production. Bromocriptine is effective in less than half of patients, and then only when given in large, poorly tolerated doses. Octreotide is perhaps the most effective of all treatments; it results in clinical improvement and substantial decreases in GH and IGF-1 production in up to 80% of patients, but it must be given subcutaneously 2 or 3 times daily or by continuous subcutaneous infusion (and it is very expensive).[1]

Lanreotide, like octreotide, is an octapeptide analogue of somatostatin. When formulated so as to be long-acting, 2 or 3 injections monthly effectively reduced GH and IGF-1 production in these patients for up to 3 years. Headache, paresthesias, and soft-tissue swelling decreased, but nothing more is said about the symptoms and signs of acromegaly. This treatment has the same gastrointestinal side effects as octreotide, but they occur less often because the drug is given less often. All the patients in this study received 30-mg doses of lanreotide, but more can be given if necessary.[2] A long-acting preparation of octreotide that is given once monthly has also proved effective.[3]

Cure of acromegaly is often defined as a serum GH concentration of 5 µg/mL or less, whether measured once (ideally just before the next dose in drug-treated patients) or several times during the day and night. Reduction to only slightly below 5 µg/L is inadequate, because mean 24-hour serum GH concentrations in normal adults are less than 1 µg/L. Therefore, it should be no surprise that clinical improvement is incomplete and serum IGF-1 concentrations remain near or above the upper limit of normal in many patients considered to have "normal" GH secretion. Life expectancy is decreased in treated acromegalic patients,[4] which likely means that they should be treated more vigorously. These new long-acting preparations of lanreotide or octreotide should make that much easier, and maybe in time there will be an orally active preparation.

R.D. Utiger, M.D.

References

1. Vance ML, Harris AG: Long-term treatment of 189 acromegalic patients with the somatostatin analog octreotide: Results of the International Multicenter Acromegaly Study Group. *Ann Intern Med* 151:1573–1578, 1991. (1992 YEAR BOOK OF MEDICINE, p. 457).
2. Giusti M, Gussoni G, Cuttica CM, Giordano G, and the Italian Multicenter Slow Release Lanreotide Study Group. *J Clin Endocrinol Metab* 81:2089–2097, 1996.
3. Flogstad AK, Halse J, Bakke S, et al: Sandostatin LAR in acromegalic patients: Long term treatment. *J Clin Endocrinol Metab* 82:23–28, 1997.
4. Rajasoorya C, Holdaway IM, Wrightson P, et al: Determinants of clinical outcome and survival in acromegaly. *Clin Endocrinol (Oxf)* 41:95–102, 1994.

Hyperprolactinemia in Postmenopausal Women

Maor Y, Berezin M (Tel Aviv Univ, Tel Hashomer, Israel)
Fertil Steril 67:693–696, 1997   24–2

Background.—Hyperprolactinemia, often the result of pituitary microadenoma, is a common cause of amenorrhea, galactorrhea, and infertility among young women. Much less information is available on prolactin (PRL)-secreting pituitary tumors in postmenopausal women. A group of women aged 49 to 68 years (mean 58) with hyperprolactinemia were studied.

Study Design.—All 6 women were seen at a clinic in a tertiary care hospital. A complete history was obtained and serum prolactin, luteinizing hormone, and follicle-stimulating hormone were measured, and CT of the pituitary gland was obtained. After diagnosis, bromocriptine treatment was initiated. These women were followed for 3 years.

Results.—The average serum prolactin concentration was 1,427 ng/mL in these 6 women at presentation. All had secondary amenorrhea, with an average duration of 32 years, and 5 had galactorrhea at some time. CT revealed a pituitary macroadenoma in 4 women, an enlarged sella suggesting a macroadenoma in 1, and a microadenoma in 1. After 6 months of treatment with bromocriptine, all had normal serum prolactin concentrations. Five of the 6 women then had hot flashes.

Conclusions.—In younger women, most cases of hyperprolactinemia result from microadenomas, whereas in most older women it results from a macroadenoma, reflecting the continuing growth of tumor over time. All of the older women in this series had a history that was compatible with long-standing hyperprolactinemia beginning long before the expected age of menopause.

▶ Among young women, hyperprolactinemia causes infertility, oligomenorrhea or amenorrhea, and galactorrhea; it is usually one or more of these symptoms that leads to its recognition. If the woman has a prolactinoma, it grows slowly and prolactin secretion gradually increases, so that she eventually has amenorrhea if it was not present initially. Therefore, it is not surprising that 5 of these 6 older women had a macroprolactinoma. What is surprising is that 5 had a history of galactorrhea and had received treatment—successfully—for infertility, presumably without having a determination of serum prolactin. It should be measured in any infertile woman before treatment to induce ovulation is initiated.

The course of events in these women serves as a reminder that hyperprolactinemia can cause secondary amenorrhea (premature menopause), and that prolactinomas often grow very slowly. A clinical difference between secondary amenorrhea caused by hyperprolactinemia and that caused by primary ovarian failure (whether premature or not) or gonadotropin deficiency (but no hyperprolactinemia) is that women with hyperprolactinemia do not have hot flashes.[1, 2] A biochemical difference is the finding of normal or low serum follicle-stimulating hormone (FSH) and luteinizing hormone (LH) concentrations in hyperprolactinemic women, whereas they are high in women with primary ovarian failure. The occurrence of hot flashes and a rise in serum FSH and LH concentrations during treatment with bromocriptine in 5 of the women reported here can be taken as evidence that excess prolactin has hypothalamic actions.

Were hyperprolactinemia to occur in a woman who had a normal menopause, it would of course be clinically silent until whatever was causing it caused symptoms.

R.D. Utiger, M.D.

References

1. Gambone J, Meldrum DR, Laufer L, et al: Further delineation of hypothalamic dysfunction responsible for menopausal hot flashes. *J Clin Endocrinol Metab* 59:1097–1102, 1984.
2. Soccia B, Schneider AB, Marut EL, et al: Pathological hyperprolactinemia suppresses hot flashes in menopausal women. *J Clin Endocrinol Metab* 66:868–871, 1988.

Prolactinomas Resistant to Standard Dopamine Agonists Respond to Chronic Cabergoline Treatment
Colao A, Di Sarno A, Sarnacchiaro F, et al (Univ Federico II, Naples, Italy)
J Clin Endocrinol Metab 82:876–883, 1997   24–3

Background.—Patients with prolactinomas are usually treated with dopamine agonists, such as bromocriptine and quinagolide (CV 205–502). Recently, cabergoline, a long-acting selective dopamine agonist, has been developed. The effectiveness of cabergoline in the treatment of patients with prolactinomas who had not responded to treatment with bromocriptine or quinagolide was examined.

Methods.—The study group consisted of 9 men and 18 women with an age range of 15 to 64 years. Of the 27 patients, 19 had macroprolactinomas and 8 had microprolactinomas. The patients with macroprolactinoma had undergone surgery or radiotherapy or both. All patients had previously been treated with bromocriptine and 20 had also been treated with quinagolide. Before cabergoline treatment, baseline serum prolactin concentrations were 108–3,500 ng/mL in patients with macroprolactinoma and 64–205 ng/mL in patients with microprolactinoma. All patients had gonadal failure, and symptoms of tumor expansion were present in 10 patients Cabergoline was given in a dose of 0.25 mg once weekly for the first week, 0.25 mg twice during the second week, then 0.5 mg twice weekly.

Results.—Treatment with cabergoline normalized serum prolactin concentrations in 15 of 19 patients with macroprolactinoma and all 8 patients with microprolactinoma (Fig 2). In 3 of the 4 remaining patients, it caused a significant decrease in hyperprolactinemia. Therapy was stopped in one patient at the end of 3 months of therapy because of no response. Gonadal function returned in 18 of 27 patients, galactorrhea disappeared in 5 of 6 women, and headache improved in 7 of 8 patients. Significant tumor shrinkage was detected by CT or MRI in 13 patients. Cabergoline was well tolerated by all patients, although 6 had nausea, postural hypotension, abdominal pain, dizziness, and sleepiness at the start of therapy.

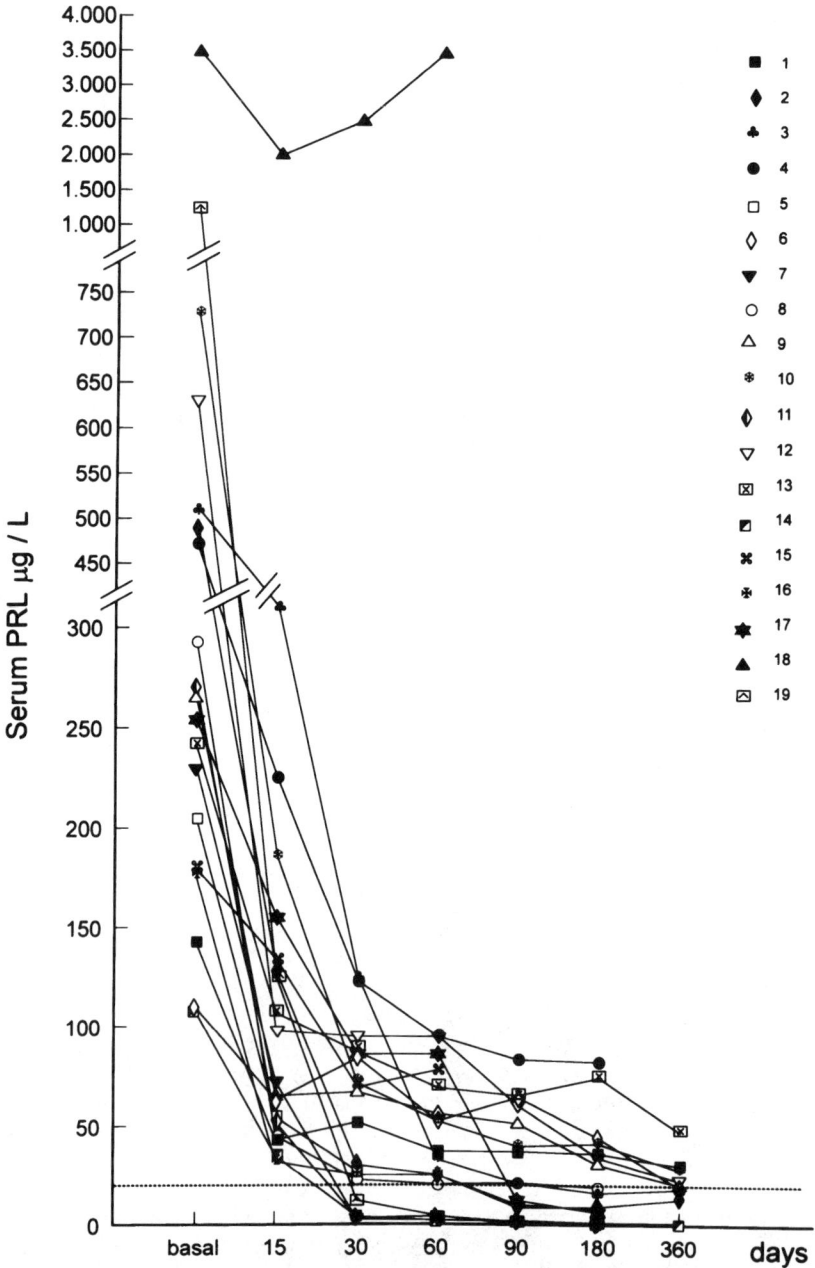

FIGURE 2.—Serum prolactin (PRL) profile before and during cabergoline therapy in 19 patients with a macroprolactinoma. The *broken line* indicates the upper limit of the normal range. (Courtesy of Colao A, Di Sarno A, Sarnacchiaro F, et al: Prolactinomas resistant to standard dopamine agonists respond to chronic cabergoline treatment. *J Clin Endocrinol Metab* 82:876–883, 1997. Copyright The Endocrine Society.)

Conclusions.—Treatment of patients with prolactinomas who were resistant to standard dopamine agonist drugs with cabergoline demonstrated that cabergoline is a safe, effective, and well-tolerated therapy. It is the only therapy available for patients with prolactinomas that do not respond to conventional dopamine agonist therapy.

▶ Standard therapy for patients with prolactin-secreting micro- or macroadenomas is bromocriptine. It is nearly always effective, reducing both tumor size and prolactin secretion, and therefore reversing hypogonadism and restoring fertility. However, a minority of patients cannot tolerate the drug, because of persistent nausea, vomiting, headache, or other side effects, or are resistant to its action (in doses that the patient can tolerate), so that prolactin secretion does not decline much or tumor size does not decrease or even increases.

This study demonstrates the efficacy of cabergoline in patients with macro- and microprolactinomas in whom bromocriptine had not reduced serum prolactin concentrations to normal. The results were particularly impressive in the 19 patients with macroprolactinomas; their mean serum prolactin concentration fell from 520 to 122 ng/mL, and the values during treatment were 20 ng/mL or lower in all but 4 patients.

Cabergoline is a dopamine agonist, like bromocriptine, and is now available in the United States. Its duration of action is much longer than that of bromocriptine; it was given twice weekly in this study, except in 2 patients who ultimately required daily therapy; and once-weekly therapy has proved effective in some patients.[1] In a direct comparison of cabergoline and bromocriptine in women with microprolactinomas or idiopathic hyperprolactinemia, about 70% of whom had not been treated previously, cabergoline given twice weekly was more effective in both restoring ovulatory menstrual cycles and reducing serum prolactin concentrations than bromocriptine given daily and had fewer side effects.[2]

Taken together, these results suggest that cabergoline, initially given once weekly, will become the treatment of choice for patients with prolactinomas.

R.D. Utiger, M.D.

References

1. Biller BMK, Molitch ME, Vance ML, et al: Treatment of prolactin-secreting macroadenomas with the once-weekly dopamine agonist cabergoline. *J Clin Endocrinol Metab* 81:2338–2343, 1996.
2. Webster J, Piscitelli G, Polli A, et al: A comparison of cabergoline and bromocriptine in the treatment of hyperprolactinemic amenorrhea. *N Engl J Med* 331:904–909, 1994.

Acute Aquaresis by the Nonpeptide Arginine Vasopressin (AVP) Antagonist OPC-31260 Improves Hyponatremia in Patients With Syndrome of Inappropriate Secretion of Antidiuretic Hormone (SIADH)

Saito T, Ishikawa S-E, Abe K, et al (Jichi Med School, Tochigi, Japan; Tohoku Univ, Sendai, Japan; Nagaoka Red Cross Hosp, Japan; et al)
J Clin Endocrinol Metab 82:1054–1057, 1997   24–4

Introduction.—Hyponatremia is the major manifestation of the syndrome of inappropriate secretion of antidiuretic hormone (SIADH). A previous study demonstrated that the non-peptide arginine vasopressin antagonist OPC-31260 had a diuretic effect in conscious rats and was therapeutically effective in rats with SIADH. In patients with SIADH, it was determined whether OPC-31260 produces water diuresis and improves hyponatremia.

Methods.—A protocol of 3 successive days was designed for 11 patients with SIADH. There were 9 men and 2 women (mean age 64). The first day served as the control day and the next 2 days the patients were given OPC-31260 intravenously. On each day, 5 blood and urine samples were collected at 1-hour intervals.

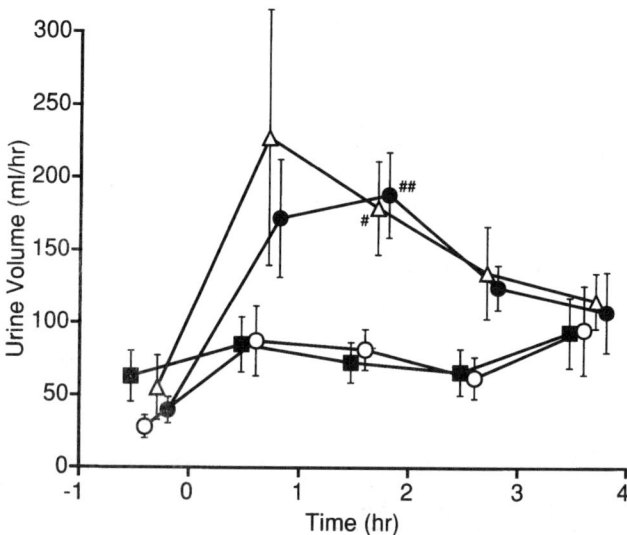

FIGURE 1.—Alteration in urine volume after iv administration of OPC-31260 in patients with SIADH. *Closed squares* show the control (n=8). *Open circles* show the 0.1 mg/kg OPC-31260 group (n=6). *Open triangles* show the group of 0.25 mg/kg OPC-31260 group (n=4). *Closed circles* show the 0.5 mg/kg OPC-31260 group (n=8). *Single hatchmark* P<0.05 and *double hatchmark* P<0.01 *vs.* the respective urine volume at the first urine collection, which was before the administration of OPC-31260. Values are means ±SE. (Courtesy of Saito T, Ishikawa S-E, Abe K, et al: Acute Aquaresis by the Nonpeptide Arginine Vasopressin (AVP) Antagonist OPC-31260 Improves Hyponatremia in Patients With Syndrome of Inappropriate Secretion of Antidiuretic Hormone (SIADH). *J Clin Endocrinol Metab* 82:1054–1057, copyright 1997, The Endocrine Society.)

Results.—The 4-hour cumulative urine volume was increased, and urinary osmolality was decreased to below 225 mOsm/kgH20 after single doses of OPC-31260 (Fig 1). Urinary solute excretion increased independently of the diuretic effect of the drug. The mean serum sodium concentration increased after administration of 0.5 mg/kg OPC-31260.

Conclusion.—OPC-31260 is an effective therapeutic agent in patients with SIADH.

▶ Mild, and sometimes not so mild, hyponatremia caused by inappropriate vasopressin secretion is a rather common problem among hospitalized patients.[1] The cardinal manifestations, in addition to hyponatremia, are high urinary osmolality (and sodium excretion) in the absence of volume depletion; if the patient is volume-depleted then the vasopressin secretion must be presumed to be appropriate. The causes of inappropriate vasopressin secretion include central nervous system disease, pulmonary disease, and vasopressin-secreting tumors—nearly always small-cell carcinomas of the lung, hypothyroidism, and secondary adrenal insufficiency. An essential component of its causation is an inappropriate increase in thirst; the normal response to vasopressin-induced water retention and increased extracellular volume is a decrease in thirst. Often, however, the syndrome is iatrogenic, the result of excessive fluid administration in a patient in whom vasopressin secretion is increased slightly as a result of pain, anesthetic. and analgesic drugs or both.

The usual treatment is water restriction, although sometimes hypertonic saline is given. Water restriction can be unpleasant in patients who are alert, because they are thirsty. Patients with chronic excess vasopressin secretion can also be treated with drugs that cause nephrogenic diabetes insipidus such as lithium or demeclocycline. These drugs inhibit vasopressin action, but neither is a specific inhibitor of vasopressin action, their efficacy is variable, and they have many side effects. Therefore, the idea of treatment with a specific inhibitor of vasopressin action, as described by Saito et al, is attractive. Theirs was only a preliminary study, but the inhibitor clearly increased urine volume and decreased urine osmolality for several hours (while not changing plasma vasopressin concentrations). Now all that is needed is a long-acting analogue of OPC-31260, and a practical alternative to water deprivation will be at hand.

R.D. Utiger, M.D.

Reference

1. Anderson RJ: Hospital-associated hyponatremia. *Kidney Int* 29:1237–1247, 1986.

25 Adrenal Glands

Incidentally Discovered Adrenal Mass (Incidentaloma): Investigation and Management of 208 Patients
Kasperlik-Zaluska AA, Roslonowska E, Slowinska-Srzednicka J, et al (Centre of Postgraduate Med Education, Warsaw)
Clin Endocrinol (Oxf) 46:29–37, 1997   25–1

Introduction.—Adrenal masses that are incidentally discovered (incidentalomas) during imaging of the abdomen require specific diagnostic and therapeutic approaches. A large group of patients with incidentalomas was reviewed for clinical and endocrine features, management, pathologic findings, and outcome.

Patients and Methods.—During a 10-year period, 220 patients with adrenal tumors incidentally detected by ultrasonography were referred to the study institution for CT. Ten were excluded because CT did not confirm the tumor, and 2 received a diagnosis of congenital adrenal hyperplasia. The remaining 208 patients, 148 women and 60 men, had a mean age of 51.8 years. Bilateral tumors were discovered in 36 patients. Tumor diameter was less than 3.0 cm in 119 patients, 3.1–4.0 cm in 38, 4.1–9.9 cm in 40, and greater than 10.0 cm in 18. Symptoms prompting the initial ultrasound examination included abdominal or lumbar pain, nephrolithiasis, and urinary tract infection. 36 patients had hypertension, 23 were obese, and 8 had diabetes mellitus. After discovery of the adrenal tumor, patients underwent urinary and plasma hormone assays, and dynamic endocrine tests.

Results.—Common findings were low plasma corticotropin (ACTH) concentrations (in 33 of 98 investigated patients) and diminished dexamethasone suppressibility and lack of ACTH response in the corticotropin-releasing hormone (CRH) test (2 of 12 patients). Cortisol hypersecretion was found in 2 patients with clinical Cushing's disease and in 6 with preclinical Cushing's syndrome. Surgery was performed in 85 patients. A recommendation for surgery was made if the mass was greater than 4.0 cm in diameter, in patients with known tumor or or suspected metastatic disease, and in patients with overproduction of catecholamines or aldosterone, or a lack of dexamethasone suppressibility. The most frequent pathological findings were adrenocortical adenoma (21), carcinoma (17), pheochromocytoma (13), metastatic masses (12), and myelolipoma (10)

TABLE 1.—Pathological Diagnosis in 85 Patients Treated by Surgery
Because of Adrenal Incidentalomas

Pathological diagnosis	Number of tumours
Adenoma	21
Carcinoma	17
Phaeochromocytoma	13
Metastatic tumour	12
Myelolipoma	10
Cyst	4
Nodular hyperplasia	3
Aldosteronoma	2
Lipoma	1
Lymphoma (bilateral)	1
Neurilemmoma	1
Haematoma	1

(Courtesy of Kasperlik-Zaluska AA, Roslonowska E, Slowinska-Srzednicka J, et al: Incidentally discovered adrenal mass [incidentaloma]: Investigation and management of 208 patients. *Clin Endocrinol [Oxf]* 46:29–37. Copyright 1996, Blackwell Science Ltd.)

(Table 1). The carcinomas ranged in size from 3.2 to 20.0 cm and the nonmalignant tumors from 1.5 to 21.0 cm.

Discussion.—Patients with an incidentally discovered adrenal mass need to be investigated for malignancy and subclinical endocrine hypersecretion. Although patients with small tumors might be followed up, those with tumors greater than 4.0 cm should be treated by surgery.

▶ Incidental adrenal masses may be detected by any current imaging procedure—ultrasonography, CT, and MRI. The latter 2 methods are more sensitive in patients suspected on clinical and biochemical grounds to have adrenal tumors, so it is likely that ultrasonography misses some incidental adrenal tumors (it can be difficult to see the left adrenal at all). The reverse seems not to be true. In this study, in which almost all the incidental tumors were detected by ultrasonography, CT confirmed the presence of all but 10 of them.

The questions posed by the incidental identification of an adrenal mass are: Is the mass secreting anything, and should it be removed, either because it is secreting something or because it may be an adrenal carcinoma? In the absence of hypertension, hypokalemia, or any clinical manifestations of cortisol or androgen excess, the probability that the mass is functioning is very small.[1] Nevertheless, there is general agreement that any patient with a mass should have studies to determine whether the mass is a pheochromocytoma, even in the absence of hypertension, because this condition is potentially life-threatening. How much more should be done is debatable, because the probability of clinically important adrenal disease is very small.[1] A search for hypokalemia—indicative of hyperaldosteronism—is appropriate in a hypertensive patient, and measuring serum cortisol or urinary cortisol excretion to look for clinically unrecognized Cushing's syndrome is reasonable in any patient (cortisol and catecholamines can be measured in the same urine sample). Others argue that some type of dexamethasone suppression testing should be done to detect subclinical Cushing's syndrome.[2] Some would also, like Kasperlik-Zaluska et al., routinely measure serum dehydroepiandrosterone sulfate or urinary 17–ketosteroid excretion as a test for adrenal carcinoma, but normal results do not exclude that diagnosis. I think these latter tests are unnecessary, preferring to rely on size (4 cm or more in diameter; as was done in this study). In addition, adrenal carcinomas tend to have regions of necrosis or hemorrhage and irregular borders detectable by imaging.[3] These carcinomas must be small at some time, but their frequency relative to that of small adrenal adenomas is so low that routine operation cannot be justified.

R.D. Utiger, M.D.

References

1. Ross NS, Aron DC: Hormonal evaluation of the patient with an incidentally discovered adrenal mass. *N Engl J Med* 323:1401–1405, 1990.
2. McLeod MK, Thompson NW, Gross MD, et al: Sub-clinical Cushing's syndrome in patients with adrenal gland incidentalomas. Pitfalls in diagnosis and management. *Am Surg* 56:398–403, 1990. (1992 YEAR BOOK OF MEDICINE, pp 463–464.)
3. Kloos RT, Gross MD, Francis IR, et al: Incidentally discovered adrenal masses. *Endocr Rev* 16:460–484, 1995.

Steroid 21-Hydroxylase Autoantibodies: Measurements With a New Immunoprecipitation Assay

Tanaka H, Perez MS, Powell M, et al (FIRS Labs, Cardiff, Wales; Univ of Padua, Italy)

J Clin Endocrinol Metab 82:1440–1446, 1997   25–2

Objective.—An important type of adrenocortical autoantibodies is antibodies to steroid 21-hydroxylase. They are a distinguishing feature of autoimmune Addison's disease and, therefore, the diagnosis of autoimmune adrenal disease would be facilitated by a convenient assay for antibodies to 21-hydroxylase. A new technique for measuring antibodies to 21-hydroxylase is described and its use in various groups of patients evaluated.

Methods.—The assay was based on the ability of serum from patients to precipitate ^{125}I-labeled recombinant human 21-hydroxylase. It was used to study serum samples from 60 patients with Addison's disease, 12 with autoimmune polyglandular syndrome type I, 27 with autoimmune polyglandular syndrome type II, and 30 who had positive tests for adrenal antibodies by immunofluorescence but no biochemical evidence of Addison's disease. Also tested were serum samples from 243 normal subjects, 150 patients with type 1 diabetes mellitus, 77 with Graves' disease, 67 with Hashimoto's thyroiditis, 9 with Addison's disease caused by tuberculosis, 32 with type 2 diabetes mellitus, 35 with myasthenia gravis, and 17 with premature ovarian failure.

Results.—The assay detected 21-hydroxylase antibodies in 72% of patients with Addison's disease, 92% of those with autoimmune polyglandular syndrome type I, 100% of those with autoimmune polyglandular syndrome type II, and 80% of those with anti-adrenal antibodies but no biochemical evidence of Addison's disease. In contrast, 21-hydroxylase antibodies were present in 3% or fewer of the normal subjects and patients with type 1 diabetes mellitus, Graves' disease or Hashimoto's thyroiditis, and in no patients in the other groups tested.

Conclusion.—The new assay for 21-hydroxylase is sufficiently simple and convenient for routine use and should facilitate assessment of the prevalence and pattern of inheritance of adrenal autoimmunity.

▶ The most common cause of Addison's disease is autoimmune adrenalitis, which has long been a diagnosis of exclusion. The reason is that the only way to confirm the diagnosis positively was by testing the patient's serum for anti-adrenal antibodies using an immunofluorescence technique, and this test was not widely available. There is now evidence that anti-adrenal antibodies include antibodies against several adrenal enzymes, especially 21–hydroxylase but also 17-hydroxylase and the P450 side-chain cleavage enzyme,[1] and perhaps other adrenal components as well. The latter 2 enzymes are found in the gonads, whereas 21-hydroxylase is found only in adrenal tissue; therefore, anti–21-hydroxylase antibodies are more specific indicators of adrenal disease.

The introduction of a simple immunoprecipitation test for anti–21-hydroxylase antibodies should make it easier to confirm autoimmune adrenalitis as the cause of Addison's disease. The vast majority of patients with Addison's disease who have anti-adrenal antibodies (and some who do not) have these antibodies. They can be detected many years after the diagnosis of Addison's disease,[2] and they are not detected in the serum of patients with tuberculous or other causes of Addison's disease. Note that both types of antibodies can sometimes be detected in patients with other autoimmune endocrine disorders who do not have Addison's disease. These patients are at risk for the development of the disease.

Some patients with anti–21-hydroxylase antibodies have persistently normal adrenal function, suggesting that the antibodies do not inhibit enzyme function in vivo.[3] These differences in adrenal function may simply reflect differences in antibody titers, but the antibodies in different patients could be directed against different regions (epitopes) of the enzyme molecule and, therefore, affect its biological activity differently.

R.D. Utiger, M.D.

References

1. Chen S, Sawicka J, Betterele C, et al: Autoantibodies to steroidogenic enzymes in autoimmune polyglandular syndrome, Addison's disease, and premature ovarian failure. *J Clin Endocrinol Metab* 81:1871–1876, 1996.
2. Soderbergh A, Winqvist O, Norheim I, et al: Adrenal autoantibodies and organ-specific autoimmunity in patients with Addison's disease. *Clin Endocrinol* 45:453–460, 1996.

3. Betterele C, Volpate M, Rees Smith B, et al: I. Adrenal cortex and steroid 21-hydroxylase autoantibodies in adult patients with organ-specific autoimmune disease: Markers of low progression to clinical Addison's disease. *J Clin Endocrinol Metab* 82:932–938, 1997.

Clinical Adrenal Insufficiency in Patients Receiving Megestrol Therapy
Subramanian S, Goker H, Kanji A, et al (Mercy Hosp and Med Ctr, Chicago; Univ of Illinois, Chicago)
Arch Intern Med 157:1008–1011, 1997   25–3

Introduction.—Megestrol acetate has been used extensively in women with metastatic breast cancer. Although primarily a progestin, secondary adrenal suppression has been reported with prolonged administration. The clinical and biochemical features of women who developed symptoms of adrenal insufficiency during megestrol acetate therapy for advanced breast cancer were described.

Methods and Results.—13 women, aged 48 to 89 years, who developed fatigue and weakness while receiving megestrol (160 mg/day) for metastatic breast cancer were studied. Each had measurements of serum cortisol and rapid corticotropin stimulation tests.

Results.—Eight women had hypotension, and 3 had nausea, anorexia, vomiting, and diarrhea. Their mean basal plasma cortisol concentration was 41 nmol/L (1.5 µg/dL), with a range of 28 to 110 nmol/L (1.0 to 4.0 µg/dL). At 30 minutes after corticotropin stimulation the mean serum cortisol concentration was 239 nmol/L (8.7 µg/dL), with a range of 94 to 447 nmol/L (3.4 to 16.2 µg/dL). The values 60 minutes after corticotropin stimulation were similar. Eleven women were treated with prednisone and improved.

Conclusion.—When profound fatigue occurs in women receiving megestrol treatment, screening for adrenal insufficiency is indicated.

▶ Megestrol acetate is a progestational steroid that also inhibits corticotropin (ACTH) secretion by the pituitary, thereby reducing endogenous cortisol secretion.[1] The result is low basal and ACTH-stimulated serum cortisol concentrations, as were found in the 13 patients of this study; serum ACTH concentrations, measured in 2 patients, were low. If megestrol acetate inhibits ACTH secretion, then almost by definition it has glucocorticoid activity. How, then, to explain the occurrence of symptoms of adrenal insufficiency—weakness, hypotension, and anorexia and other gastrointestinal symptoms? Either the glucocorticoid potency of megestrol acetate in peripheral tissues is less than that in the pituitary, or the symptoms have some other explanation.

The fact that those patients given prednisone improved supports the conclusion they had glucocorticoid deficiency, but, on the other hand, the symptoms are rather nonspecific and I know of no direct evidence that megestrol acetate has differential effects on peripheral and pituitary glucocorticoid receptors. The potency of megestrol acetate as an inhibitor of

ACTH secretion must vary because at least other patients studied by Subramanian et al. taking the same dose had no clinical or biochemical evidence of adrenal dysfunction. That megestrol acetate has glucocorticoid activity is confirmed by its ability (usually in high doses) mg/day to cause Cushing's syndrome (with low serum ACTH and cortisol concentrations).[2, 3]

As a practical matter, the possibility of adrenal insufficiency should be kept in mind in any patient receiving moderate doses of megestrol acetate who becomes weak or hypotensive. These problems are even more likely to occur if the patient has an acute illness or after withdrawal of megestrol acetate, because of inability to increase endogenous ACTH and cortisol secretion promptly.[1] Keep in mind, too, that megestrol acetate is given not only to patients with breast and other cancers as antitumor therapy, but also to patients with AIDS to stimulate appetite and weight gain as well as hypogonadal patients to relieve hot flashes—so many different patients are at risk.

R.D. Utiger, M.D.

References

1. Leinung MC, Liporace R, Miller CM: Induction of adrenal suppression by megestrol acetate in patients with AIDS. *Ann Intern Med* 122:843–845, 1995.
2. Steer KA, Kurtz AB, Honour JW: Megestrol-induced Cushing's syndrome. *Clin Endocrinol* 42:91–93, 1995.
3. Mann M, Koller E, Murgo A, et al: Glucocorticoidlike activity of megestrol: A summary of Food and Drug Administration experience and a review of the literature. *Arch Intern Med* 157:165101656, 1997.

An Assessment of Optimal Hydrocortisone Replacement Therapy
Howlett TA (Leicester Royal Infirmary, England)
Clin Endocrinol (Oxf) 46:263–268, 1997   25–4

Background.—Although hydrocortisone is now the standard form of glucocorticoid replacement in patients with primary and secondary adrenal insufficiency, there is still no agreement on the appropriate dose, timing, or monitoring of such therapy. The use of hydrocortisone replacement therapy at 1 center was reviewed.

Methods.—The case notes of 210 patients who had been treated with hydrocortisone were reviewed. One hundred thirty patients, whose records contained the findings of at least 1 valid hydrocortisone day curve (consisting of measurements of serum cortisol at 0900, 1230, and 1730 hours and 24-hour urinary cortisol execretion while receiving usual therapy) were identified. Data on 174-day curves were, therefore, analyzed. A quality score was calculated by giving 1 point for each of the following: normal urinary cortisol execretion, 0900 hours serum cortisol value, 1230 hours serum cortisol >50 nmol/L (1.8 µg/dL), and 1730 hours serum cortisol >100 nmol/L (3.6 µg/dL).

TABLE 1.—Proportion of Patients Receiving Different Dose Regimens Who Achieved Target Cortisol Levels for Hydrocortisone Replacement

Hydrocortisone regimen	n	Urine free cortisol* 50–220 nmol/24 h	Percentage of day curves achieving …			
			0900 h cortisol† 100– 700 nmol/l	1230 h cortisol‡ >50 nmol/l (>100 nmol/l)	1730 h cortisol§ >50 nmol/l (>100 nmol/l)	All 4 criteria‖ using 50 nmol/l (100 nmol/l)
All thrice daily regimens	109	68%	87%	95% (77%)	98% (85%)	60% (41%)
All twice daily regimens	65	65%	63%	97% (86%)	48% (23%)	15% (8%)
10 mg/5 mg AM/noon/PM	53	77%	92%	94% (74%)	98% (85%)	66% (47%)
10 mg/10 mg/5 mg AM/noon/Pm	28	57%	79%	96% (86%)	100% (86%)	50% (32%)
10 mg/–/5 mg AM/noon/PM	18	78%	83%	94% (83%)	72% (33%)	39% (22%)
20 mg/–/10 mg AM/noon/PM	29	55%	48%	100% (97%)	45% (21%)	10% (3%)

*Differences not significant by χ^2, except 10/5/5 vs. 20/–/10: $P = 0.036$.
†Twice vs. thrice daily and 10/5/5 vs. 20/–/10: $P \leq 0.001$ by χ^2.
‡Differences not significant by χ^2, except 10/5/5 vs. 20/–/10 using 100 nmol/L: $P = 0.01$.
§Twice vs. thrice daily and 10/5/5 vs. 20/–/10: $P \leq 0.001$ by χ^2.
‖Twice vs. thrice daily and 10/5/5 vs. 20/–/10: $P \leq 0.001$; 10/5/5 vs. 20/–/10: $P \leq 0.01$; 10/5/5 vs. 10/10/5: $P \geq 0.1$ by χ^2.
(Courtesy of Howlett TA: An assessment of optimal hydrocortisone replacement therapy. *Clin Endocrinol* 46:263–268, 1997. Blackwell Science Ltd.)

Findings.—Optimal replacement was achieved in only 15% of the patients receiving twice-daily hydrocortisone therapy, as compared with 60% receiving thrice-daily therapy (Table 1). The mean overall "quality score" for the twice-daily regimen was 2.7, and the quality score for the thrice-daily regimen was 3.5. In 66% of the patients, a regimen of 10 mg/5 mg/5 mg (on rising, at lunch, and in the evening) provided optimal replacement. The mean quality score in these patients was 3.6. By contrast, a regimen of 10 mg/10 mg/5 mg provided optimal replacement in 50% and had a corresponding quality score of 3.3; a regimen of 20mg/10mg provided optimal replacement in 10% and resulted in a corresponding quality score of 2.5.

Conclusions.—Optimal replacement is achieved with thrice-daily hydrocortisone regimens. An appropriate starting dose is 10 mg/5 mg/5 mg, and subsequent individual adjustments should be based on hydrocortisone day curves.

▶ The standard glucocorticoid replacement regimen for patients with adrenal insufficiency has long been 15–20 mg hydrocortisone (cortisol) in the morning and 5–10 mg in the late afternoon. These doses were based on subjective responses to therapy, the diurnal rhythm of serum cortisol, and evidence that normal subjects secreted about 20 mg cortisol daily. There has been concern that the doses are excessive because some patients treated with them have low bone density,[1] because peak serum cortisol concentrations often exceed those in normal subjects,[2] and because of a recent estimate that normal subjects secrete about 10 mg cortisol daily.[3] (I have never understood why we use the term *hydrocortisone* in reference to pills and therapy, but *cortisol* in reference to endogenous hormone secretion.)

Reasoning from these considerations, the author established what I think are reasonable biochemical criteria for optimal replacement therapy. Based on these criteria, a dose of 30 mg hydrocortisone daily is too much for most patients, and it ought to be given 3 times rather than twice daily. The authors of another, similar study of glucocorticoid replacement therapy published at the same time reached the same conclusion, and, in addition, they found that a 30% reduction in the daily dose of hydrocortisone resulted in a significant increase in serum osteocalcin, indicative of an increased rate of bone formation.[4]

I am convinced that 20 mg hydrocortisone daily is adequate therapy for most patients with either primary of secondary adrenal insufficiency, and that a 3–dose regimen (10 mg in the morning, 5 mg at noon, and 5 mg in the late afternoon) provides more physiologic replacement than a 2-dose regimen. Someone should carefully assess clinical well-being and the like in patients with adrenal insufficiency treated with multiple regimens, but a study of that type would be difficult and is not likely to be done. Biochemical monitoring is rarely performed in these patients, but both Howlett and Peacey et al.[4] present persuasive evidence that it can provide useful guidance. It is easier to measure cortisol in a 24-hour urine sample than to measure serum cortisol 3 times during a day, but either can provide useful information, especially when overtreatment is suspected.

R.D. Utiger, M.D.

References

1. Zelissen PMJ, Croughs RJM, van Rijk PP, et al: Effect of glucocorticoid replacement therapy on bone mineral density in patients with Addison's disease. *Ann Intern Med* 120:207–210, 1994 (1995 YEAR BOOK OF MEDICINE, pp 596–597).
2. Kehlet H, Binder C, Blichert-Toft M: Glucocorticoid maintenance therapy following adrenalectomy: Assessment of dosage and preparation. *Clin Endocrinol* 5:37–41, 1976.
3. Esteban NV, Loughlin T, Yergey AL, et al: Daily cortisol production rate in man determined by stable isotope dilution/mass spectrometry. *J Clin Endocrinol Metab* 71:39–45, 1991.
4. Peacey SR, Guo C-Y, Robinson AM, et al: Glucocorticoid replacement therapy: Are patients overtreated and does it matter? *Clin Endocrinol* 46:255–261, 1997.

A Double-blind Study of Perioperative Steroid Requirements in Secondary Adrenal Insufficiency

Glowniak JV, Loriaux DL (Oregon Health Sciences Univ, Portland)
Surgery 121:123–129, 1997   25–5

Introduction.—The adrenal glands secrete increased amounts of cortisol during acute stress such as a major operation. To maintain hemodynamic stability under these circumstances, increased cortisol is thought to be necessary, but the amount needed is not known. How much glucocorticoid is necessary to prevent hypotension was studied in patients having elective operations who had been treated with glucocorticoids.

Methods.—All patients took 7.5 mg of prednisone daily for at least 2 months and had secondary adrenal insufficiency, as defined by corticotropin stimulation testing. There were 2 groups of patients, with 6 patients receiving saline solution and cortisol perioperatively and 12 patients receiving saline solution alone. The usual daily prednisone dose (7.5–20 mg in most patients) was administered to all patients throughout the study.

Results.—The operations were joint replacements, abdominal operations, and other procedures. During surgery, one patient from each group had hypotension, which resolved with volume replacement. During the perioperative period, the average pulse rates and blood pressures in the two groups were similar. Three patients in the placebo group had postoperative complications, none of which were serious; they included transient ileus, pneumonia and fever.

Conclusion.—When given only their daily dose of prednisone during surgical procedures, patients with secondary adrenal insufficiency do not have hypotension or tachycardia indicative of glucocorticoid deficiency.

Therefore, additional glucocorticoid is not required to prevent hemodynamic compromise in the perioperative period.

▶ There is no doubt that endogenous corticotropin (ACTH) and cortisol secretion is decreased in a dose-dependent manner in patients taking prednisone or other glucocorticoids for any reason. There also is no doubt that acute illness and injury (generically called stress) call forth a transient increase in ACTH and cortisol secretion, and that the increase in cortisol secretion plays an important role in maintaining hemodynamic stability during stress. These two facts, plus a few reports many years ago of vascular collapse during stress in patients taking glucocorticoid, have led to the practice of giving all glucocorticoid-treated patients supplemental glucocorticoid when they are sick or injured. The usual practice has been to give large doses, based mostly on the notion that 'if some is good, more is better.'

The findings of this study challenge the idea that glucocorticoid-treated patients need supplemental glucocorticoid therapy when stressed, in this case by elective surgery. Most of the patients were taking 10 or 15 mg of prednisone daily, not a large dose, and some had small rises in serum cortisol in response to administration of a large dose of ACTH, indicating they did not have severe adrenal atrophy. But whether they could—when stressed—make more ACTH and cortisol was unfortunately not tested. The fact remains that the patients who got only their regular dose of prednisone had no more perioperative or postoperative hypotension or other difficulties than those who received additional glucocorticoid. The regular dose, however, was not trivial, so the results do not mean that patients need no glucocorticoid when stressed, but simply no extra glucocorticoid, only what they were already getting. In another study, patients taking 5–10 mg of prednisone daily needed no supplemental glucocorticoid perioperatively,[1] and in adrenalectomized monkeys a replacement dose of glucocorticoid was no less effective than 10 times more in preventing hypotension and death during and after cholecystectomy.[2]

The conclusion seems clear—glucocorticoid-treated patients do not need additional large doses of glucocorticoid when stressed. Those patients taking low doses, for example, 5–7.5 mg of prednisone daily, can make additional cortisol if need be, and those receiving larger doses have enough exogenous glucocorticoid to meet their needs. However, the tradition of giving supplemental glucocorticoid to anyone taking exogenous glucocorticoid who is stressed is so ingrained in medical lore that it is not likely to change soon. Still, the practice ought to be questioned more, and if a supplement is to be given, the dose need not be large (for example, 75–100 mg, not 300 mg, of hydrocortisone on day 1, half that on day 2, and none on day 3).

R.D. Utiger, M.D.

References

1. Bromberg JS, Alfrey EJ, Barker CF, et al: Adrenal suppression and steroid supplementation in renal transplant recipients. *Transplantation* 51:385–390, 1991.

2. Udelsman R, Ramp J, Gallucci, WT, et al: Adaptation during surgical stress: A reevaluation of the role of glucocorticoids. *J Clin Invest* 77:1377–1381, 1986.

The Long-term Outcome of Pituitary Irradiation After Unsuccessful Transsphenoidal Surgery in Cushing's Disease

Estrada J, Boronat M, Mielgo M, et al (Universidad Autónoma, Madrid)
N Engl J Med 336:172–177, 1997   25–6

Background.—When transsphenoidal surgery is unsuccessful in patients with Cushing's disease, irradiation of the pituitary is generally considered the most appropriate treatment. However, the long-term efficacy of this treatment is not well established.

Methods.—Thirty adults with persistent or recurrent Cushing's disease underwent external pituitary radiation after unsuccessful transsphenoidal surgery. The mean radiation dose was 50 Gy. Median follow-up was 42 months after therapy.

Findings.—Eighty-three percent of the patients had remissions during follow-up, beginning 6–60 months after radiation therapy. In most patients, remissions occurred in the first 2 years (Fig 1). None of the 25 patients achieving remission had a relapse of Cushing's disease. The response to radiotherapy was unassociated with sex, age, urinary cortisol excretion before radiotherapy, the interval between surgery and radiotherapy, the finding of a pituitary adenoma on pathologic assessment, or tumor size at surgery earlier. In 17 patients, growth hormone deficiency was noted after radiotherapy. In addition, 10 patients developed gonadotropin deficiency, 4 thyrotropin deficiency, and 1 corticotropin deficiency.

Conclusions.—Although other treatments are available, radiotherapy is often recommended for patients with Cushing's disease after noncurative pituitary surgery. The current findings confirm that this treatment is effective and well tolerated.

▶ Most patients with Cushing's syndrome have Cushing's disease, usually caused by a corticotropin-secreting tumor of the pituitary. The treatment of choice is transsphenoidal surgery, but the operation is successful in only about 75% of patients.[1, 2] Either the tumor is incompletely resected, it proves to be an unrelated non-secreting tumor, or no tumor is found. Partial or even complete hypophysectomy is sometimes done when no tumor is found, but even these steps may not be curative, and partial or complete hypopituitarism is likely.

The most appropriate management of those patients who are not cured by transsphenoidal surgery has been a matter of some controversy. The first step must be to reconfirm that the patient has excess corticotropin secretion of pituitary origin. That having been done, the options are another pituitary operation, pituitary irradiation, and total adrenalectomy. This study by Estrada et al. provides strong evidence for the value of pituitary irradiation. Most of the patients had a remission, and none has yet relapsed. One very

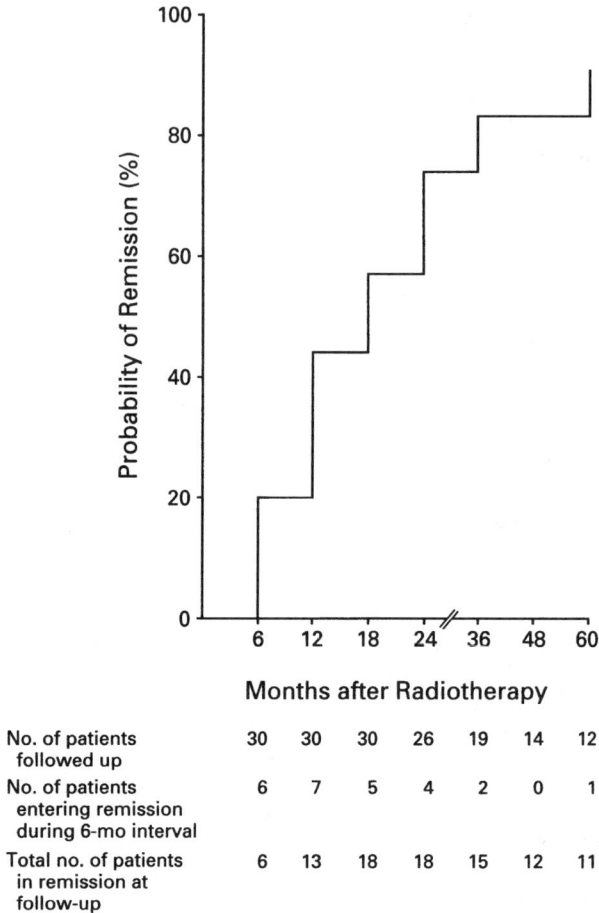

	6	12	18	24	36	48	60
No. of patients followed up	30	30	30	26	19	14	12
No. of patients entering remission during 6-mo interval	6	7	5	4	2	0	1
Total no. of patients in remission at follow-up	6	13	18	18	15	12	11

FIGURE 1.—Probability of remission of Cushing's disease in 30 patients treated with pituitary irradiation after unsuccessful transsphenoidal surgery. (Reprinted by permission of the *New England Journal of Medicine*, from Estrada J, Boronat M, Mielgo M, et al: The long-term outcome of pituitary irradiation after unsuccessful transsphenoidal surgery in Cushing's disease. *N Engl J Med* 336:172–177, 1997. Copyright 1997, Massachusetts Medical Society.)

important aspect of the treatment program was the use of ketoconazole to control adrenal hypersecretion while awaiting the effects of the radiotherapy. Pituitary radiation has not been widely used in the past in patients with Cushing's syndrome as either primary or secondary therapy because its effects are slow, as shown in Figure 1 of the article, and because no one has been comfortable allowing the ravages of cortisol excess—muscle weakness, osteoporosis, psychiatric disturbances, hyperglycemia, etc.,—to continue while awaiting the effects of radiotherapy. Ketoconazole, by reducing cortisol secretion, changes all that, and, of course, if it is not effective or cannot be tolerated, then one can always undertake total adrenalectomy.

I think this study should rekindle interest in pituitary radiation in patients with Cushing's disease who are not cured by transsphenoidal surgery, and I am sufficiently persuaded by the results to view it as the treatment of choice for these patients.[3]

R.D. Utiger, M.D.

References

1. Bochicchio D, Losa M, Buchfelder M, et al: Factors influencing the immediate and late outcome of Cushing's disease treated by transsphenoidal surgery: A retrospective study by the European Cushing's Disease Survey Gropup. *J Clin Endocrinol Metab* 80:3114–3120, 1995. (1997 YEAR BOOK OF MEDICINE, p 482).
2. Sonino N, Zielezny M, Fava GA, et al: Risk factors and long-term outcome in pituitary-dependent Cushing's disease. *J Clin Endocrinol Metab* 81:2647–2652, 1996. (1997 YEAR BOOK OF MEDICINE, p 484).
3. Utiger RD: Treatment, and retreatment, of Cushing's disease. *N Engl J Med* 1997:215–217, 1997.

Inhaled Beclomethasone Dipropionate Suppresses the Hypothalamo-Pituitary-Adrenal Axis in a Dose Dependent Manner

Grebe SKG, Feek CM, Durham JA, et al (Wellington School of Medicine, New Zealand; Wellington Hosp, New Zealand)
Clin Endocrinol (Oxf) 47:297–304, 1997   25–7

Background.—The dose-response relationship of the effects of inhaled beclomethasone dipropionate on hypothalamo-pituitary-adrenal function is unclear. The dose-response relationship of inhaled beclomethasone dipropionate on the hypothalamo-pituitary-adrenal axis was investigated in a general practice patient population.

Methods.—Twenty-one patients receiving inhaled beclomethasone were recruited to participate in a controlled observational study. The patients had minimal past and no present exposure to other glucocorticoids. Twenty-one age- and sex-matched normal subjects were also studied. Measurements obtained included 24-hour urinary cortisol excretion, serum cortisol before and 30 minutes after injection of 1 µg and 250 µg of tetracosactrin, serum insulin-like factor (IGF)-1, and serum osteocalcin. The use of beclomethasone was estimated by inhaler weighing and prescription counts.

Findings.—Patients receiving inhaled beclomethasone had significantly lower 24-hour urinary cortisol excretion, and increase in serum cortisol after 250 µg tetracosactrin, as compared with the normal subjects (Fig 4). Measures of hypothalmo-pituitary-adrenal function were inversely associated with the dose of beclomethasone as estimated by inhaler weighing. Serum IGF-1 and osteocalcin concentrations were comparable in the two groups.

Conclusion.—Hypothalamo-pituitary-adrenal axis suppression occurs in asthmatic patients receiving moderate-to-large doses of inhaled beclomethasone. When accurate measurements of inhaled glucocorticoid dose are

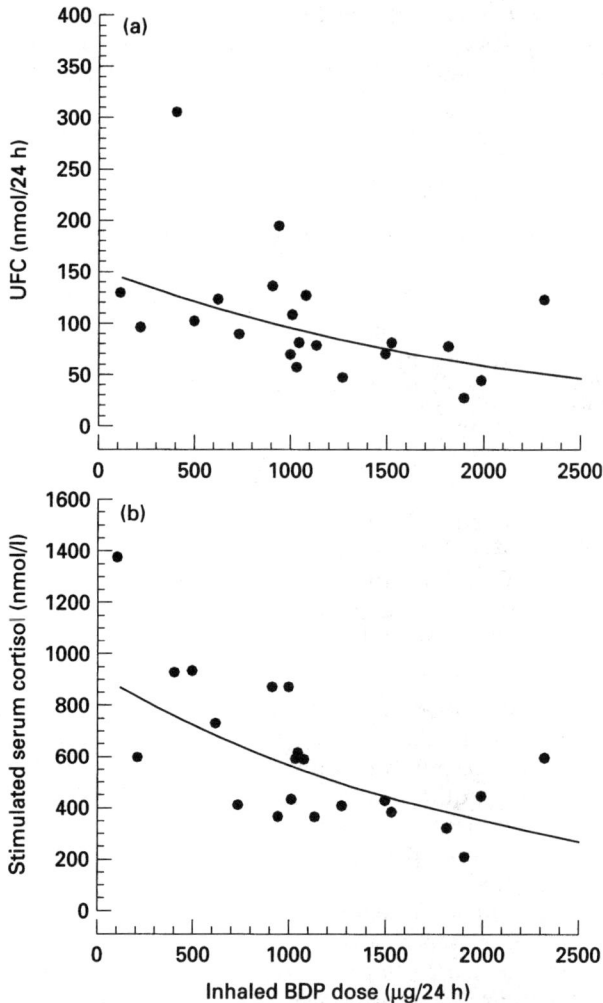

FIGURE 4.—*A*, 24-hour urinary cortisol excretion (nmol/24 hr), *B*, Serum cortisol concentrations (nmol/L) 30 minutes after IM injection of 250 μg tetracosactrin in 21 patients receiving inhaled beclomethasone dipropionate plotted against daily inhaled beclomethasone dipropionate dose, as estimated by inhaler weighing. There was a significant negative exponential relationship ($P < 0.03$) between dose of beclomethasone, and both 24-hour urinary cortisol excretion and tetracosactrin-stimulated serum cortisol concentrations. All other measurements of hypothalamo-pituitary-adrenal function (data not shown), except serum cortisol concentrations 30 minutes after IM injection of 1 μg tetracosactrin, were also significantly inversely correlated with inhaled dose of beclomethasone. (Courtesy of Grebe SKG, Feek CM, Durham JA, et al: Inhaled beclomethasone dipropionate suppresses the hypothalamo-pituitary-adrenal axis in a dose dependent manner. *Clin Endocrinol (Oxf)* 47:297–304, 1997. Reprinted by permission of Blackwell Science Ltd.)

used, an exponential relationship between dose and hypothalamo-pituitary-adrenal function is evident.

▶ Inhaled glucocorticoids have many fewer systemic effects than do oral glucocorticoids. Nevertheless, some inhaled glucocorticoid does reach the systemic circulation and can, therefore, inhibit endogenous hypothalamic-pituitary-adrenal function. Indeed, measuring the extent of inhibition is the best way to determine just how much inhaled glucocorticoid is being absorbed into the systemic circulation, whether via the lungs or after being swallowed.

Previous studies suggested that 800 μg of inhaled beclomethasone or budesonide was equivalent to 4 to 6 mg of oral prednisone, but most of these were acute studies done in normal subjects.[1] In contrast, this study was done in patients with asthma who had been treated with inhaled beclomethasone for years. Although the overall effects of inhaled beclomethasone (mean daily dose, 1,120 μg), in terms of inhibition of hypothalamic-pituitary-adrenal function, were very small, the figure shows clearly that high doses did have an inhibitory action. The changes seem roughly comparable to those in normal subjects, suggesting that neither chronic therapy nor asthma affect the absorption of inhaled beclomethasone.

Thus, high doses of inhaled beclomethasone can cause any of the clinical manifestations of Cushing's syndrome, including, of course, osteoporosis. With respect to that problem, the mean serum osteocalcin concentrations were similar in the patients with asthma and the normal subjects. Nevertheless, the patients receiving higher doses of beclomethasone would be expected to have lower values, indicating a lower rate of bone formation and, perhaps, lower bone density. In another study, asthmatic patients receiving 1,000 μg beclomethasone daily had low bone density, but all had received systemic glucocorticoid therapy in the past.[2]

Patients receiving 1,000 μg (or perhaps 800 μg) or more of inhaled beclomethasone daily should be considered at risk for glucocorticoid side effects. They should be managed accordingly, including measures to protect the skeleton.

R.D. Utiger, M.D.

References

1. Jenning BH, Andersson K-E, Johansson SA: Assessment of systemic effects of inhaled glucocorticosteroids: Comparison of the effects of inhaled budesonide and oral prednisolone on adrenal function and bone turnover. *Eur J Clin Pharmacol* 40:77–82, 1991.
2. Packe GE, Robb O, Robins SP, et al: Bone density in asthmatic patients taking inhaled corticosteroids: Comparison of budesonide and beclomethasone dipropionate. *J R Coll Physicians London* 30:128–132, 1996.

Clinical Experience With Incidentally Discovered Pheochromocytoma
Miyajima A, Nakashima J, Baba S, et al (Keio Univ, Tokyo)
J Urol 157:1566–1568, 1997   25–8

Background.—The rate of incidentally discovered adrenal tumors, including pheochromocytoma, has increased significantly because of advances in diagnostic imaging. It is important to identify incidental pheochromocytomas among hormonally active tumors so that appropriate perioperative treatment can be given. The characteristics of incidentally discovered pheochromocytoma are not well known.

Methods.—The medical records of 17 patients with resected pheochromocytomas were reviewed; 7 patients had symptomatic tumors and 10 had unsuspected or incidentally discovered tumors. Patient characteristics were compared and features of incidentally discovered lesions were examined; these included tumor localization, detection methods, imaging findings, urinary catecholamine excretion, treatment at operation, and tumor size.

Results.—All patients with symptomatic tumors had typical hypertension-related symptoms. Six of the 10 patients with incidentally discovered tumors had hypertension; 3 of these 6 patients had low grade fever without typical symptoms, and 1 percent was asymptomatic. Seven patients with symptomatic tumors and 8 patients with incidentally discovered tumors had increased urinary norepinephrine excretion, but the values in the latter group were considerably lower. The difference in urinary epinephrine and vanillylmandelic acid values between the 2 groups was not significant. The average diameter of the incidentally discovered tumors was significantly larger than the diameter of the symptomatic tumors.

Discussion.—Patients with incidentally discovered pheochromocytomas may, in fact, have symptoms of catecholamine excess. Their tumors tend to secrete lesser amounts of catecholamines but are larger than the tumors in patients with symptomatic tumors.

▶ It is no surprise that patients with incidentally discovered pheochromocytomas are less likely to have either hypertension or elevated urinary norepinephrine and dopamine excretion than those with symptomatic pheochromocytomas. Given these differences, I am not sure why urinary vanillylmandelic acid excretion was similar in the 2 groups in this study, but it is the least specific of the tests used to evaluate patients suspected to have a pheochromocytoma. Urinary metanephrine excretion—a widely used test in the United States—was not measured, but if a patient had, for example, only a small increase in urinary norepinephrine excretion, both urinary metanephrine and vanillylmandelic acid excretion might be normal. The pattern of results described in the patients studied by Miyajima et al. indicates that individual catecholamines should be measured to identify those incidentally discovered adrenal masses that are pheochromocytomas.

Whatever other evaluation is done in patients with an incidentally discovered adrenal mass, the important thing is not to miss a pheochromocytoma. When the hypertension is mild or the biochemical results nearly normal, magnetic resonance imaging (many pheochromocytomas have high signal intensity on T2-weighted images) or radionuclide imaging with ^{131}I-meta-iodobenzylguanidine (MIBG) or ^{111}In-pentetreotide (each of which are taken up by about 85% of pheochromocytomas[1]) is indicated.

R.D. Utiger, M.D.

Reference

1. Kloos RT, Gross MD, Francis IR, et al.: Incidentally discovered adrenal masses. *Endocrine Rev* 16:460–484, 1995.

26 The Thyroid Gland

Estimation of Tissue Hypothyroidism by a New Clinical Score: Evaluation of Patients With Various Grades of Hypothyroidism and Controls
Zulewski H, Müller B, Exer P, et al (Univ Hosp of Basel, Switzerland)
J Clin Endocrinol Metab 82:771–776, 1997   26-1

Background.—The development of modern assays for thyroid hormones has made confirming a diagnosis of obvious thyroid dysfunction easy. Subclinical hypothyroidism, on the other hand, is usually identified only by testing, and treatment of it is often based on the physician's subjective assessment of clinical severity. It would be useful to have a symptom-rating scale to evaluate clinical status and treatment outcome. Possible symptoms and signs of hypothyroidism were re-examined in an attempt to develop a convenient new clinical score for evaluation of the severity of subclinical hypothyroidism.

Study Design.—The study group consisted of 332 women studied in a prospective fashion at the Endocrine Outpatient Clinic of the University Hospital of Basel. Fourteen symptoms and signs of hypothyroidism were evaluated in a blinded manner in 50 women with overt hypothyroidism and 80 euthyroid women to derive the new clinical score. The score was validated by assessment in 93 women with subclinical hypothroidism, 109 euthyroid women, and 67 women with hypothyroidism who had become euthyroid after 3 months of treatment.

Results.—The most frequent findings in women with overt hypothyroidism were prolonged ankle reflex relaxation time and dry skin (Fig 1). Among the euthyroid women, those aged 55 years and older had more hypothyroid symptoms, especially constipation and dry skin, than younger women. To adjust for this, 1 point was added to the score of women younger than 55 years. The clinical score was defined as: hypothyroid, more than 5 (of 14) points; intermediate, 3–5 points; and euthyroid, 0–2 points. These ranges were set to achieve positive and negative predictive values of more than 90% for the diagnosis or exclusion of hypothyroidism. This score classified 62% of all women with overt hypothyroidism as clinically hypothyroid and 61% of euthyroid women as clinically euthyroid. Of the women with subclinical hypothyroidism, 24% were designated hypothyroid, 29% euthyroid, and 47% intermediate. Among women with overt hypothyroidism, the new score had excellent correla-

Frequency of hypothyroid symptoms and signs (in %) in patients (n=50) and controls (n=80)

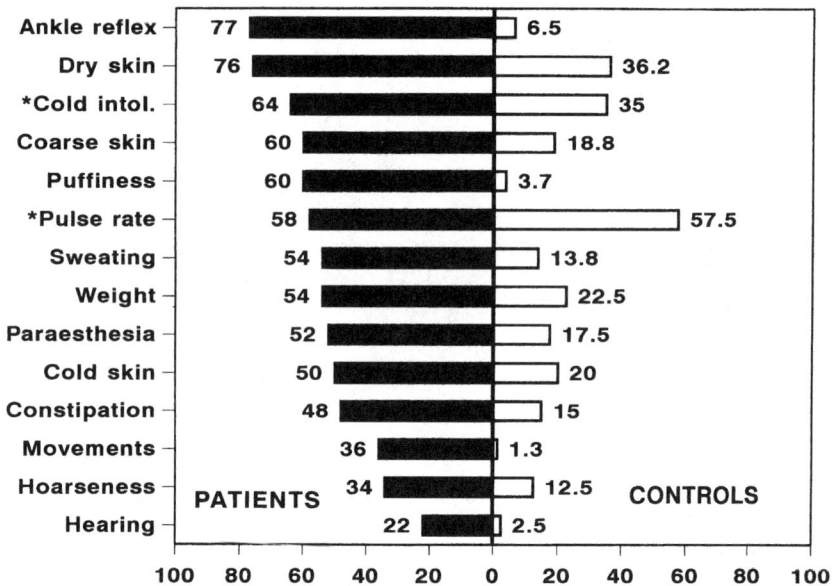

	PATIENTS	CONTROLS
Ankle reflex	77	6.5
Dry skin	76	36.2
*Cold intol.	64	35
Coarse skin	60	18.8
Puffiness	60	3.7
*Pulse rate	58	57.5
Sweating	54	13.8
Weight	54	22.5
Paraesthesia	52	17.5
Cold skin	50	20
Constipation	48	15
Movements	36	1.3
Hoarseness	34	12.5
Hearing	22	2.5

FIGURE 1.—Frequency of hypothyroid symptoms and signs (percentage) in 50 women with overt hypothyroidism and 80 euthyroid women. Two symptoms (pulse rate and cold intolerance) showed positive and negative predictive values of less than 70% and were, therefore, excluded from the new score. (Courtesy of Zulewski H, Müller B, Exer P, et al: Estimation of tissue hypothyroidism by a new clinical score: Evaluation of patients with various grades of hypothyroidism and controls. *J Clin Endocrinol Metab* 82:771–776, 1997. Copyright The Endocrine Society.)

tion with tests of peripheral hormone action, but not with serum thyrotropin (TSH) concentrations. In subclinical hypothyroidism, the best correlation was between the new score and serum TSH or free thyroxine concentrations.

Conclusions.—The clinical findings in overt and subclinical hypothyroidism are quite variable. Therefore, the new clinical score cannot be recommended to establish a diagnosis; it must be based on standard thyroid function testing. This score may be useful to evaluate the severity of hypothyroidism, assess patients with inconsistent laboratory results, and monitor the effectiveness of treatment.

▶ It is not easy to make a clinical diagnosis of overt hypothyroidism (low serum thyroxine [T_4] and triiodothyronine [T_3] and high serum thyrotropin [TSH] concentrations), which is, of course, why so much testing of thyroid function is done. None of the symptoms or signs is specific for hypothyroidism, and many normal subjects have a few of them. Determining a clinical score or index by combining the symptoms and signs is a reasonable enough approach, and indeed this was done almost 40 years ago by Billewicz et al.[1] I found that score difficult to work with because some symptoms were given positive scores if present and negative ones if absent, and they were weighted unevenly. This new system described by Zulewski et al. is simpler to use, because symptoms are scored simply as present (1) or not present (0). There is still the problem of having to make yes-no decisions about symptoms that may be mild and inconstant, especially if the patient cannot remember when they began, and signs like slow ankle reflexes also may be inconstant. Using the new scheme devised, 62% of the overtly hypothyroid patients in the derivation group had a hypothyroid score, 36% were intermediate, and 2% were euthyroid. All these patients were seen in an endocrine clinic, so someone else may have thought the patient had thyroid disease, and the scores would likely be lower in a less-selected group. Nevertheless, there are patients with overt hypothyroidism in the community. My favorite case is that of a woman who was traveling through the United States by bus and answered an advertisement seeking healthy women aged 60 or more years for a short thyroid study. She had no symptoms or signs of anything, but proved to have a very low serum T_4 concentration and a serum TSH concentration of about 150 µU/mL.

In this study, only 29% of the patients with subclinical hypothyroidism (normal serum T_4 and T_3 and high serum TSH concentrations) were classified as being euthyroid. This percentage seems low; for example, in a study of 272 patients attending a primary care geriatric clinic, the frequency of dry skin, cold skin, puffiness, and weight gain were similar in the patients with subclinical hypothyroidism and those who were euthyroid.[2] These results suggest that the presence of symptoms in a patient with subclinical hypothyroidism could be coincidental. One might assume that the question of whether symptoms are caused by thyroid deficiency or are coincidental could be resolved by giving T_4 or a placebo. That has been done, with conflicting results, and a new study of the question with extensive evaluation of quality of life and cognitive function is described in Abstract 26–3.

R.D. Utiger, M.D.

References

1. Billewicz WZ, Chapman RS, Crooks J, et al: Statistical methods applied to the diagnosis of hypothyroidism. *Quart J Med* 38:255–266, 1969.
2. Bemben DA, Hamm RM, Morgan L, et al: Thyroid disease in the elderly: Part 2. Predictability of subclinical hypothyroidism. *J Fam Pract* 38:583–588, 1994.

Bioequivalence of Generic and Brand-name Levothyroxine Products in the Treatment of Hypothyroidism
Dong BJ, Hauck WW, Gambertoglio JG, et al (Univ of California, San Francisco)
JAMA 277:1205–1213, 1997   26–2

Introduction.—Some 8 million Americans are estimated to be taking thyroid hormone therapy, mostly levothyroxine. Because of concern about the therapeutic equivalency of less costly generic products, brand-name products are often recommended as the levothyroxine preparations of choice. Whether different brands of levothyroxine are therapeutically interchangeable and bioequivalent is controversial. The relative bioavailability of Synthroid, Levoxine (now called Levoxyl), and 2 generic levothyroxine preparations was compared.

Methods.—For 6-week periods, 22 women with hypothyroidism who were clinically and chemically euthyroid while receiving levothyroxine sodium (0.1 or 0.15 mg), took each of the 4 levothyroxine products in sequence, with no intervening washout periods. The order of the different products was randomly determined. For all 4 products, measurements were taken of time to peak serum concentrations, area under the serum concentration curves, serum free thyroxine index values, and serum concentrations of thyroxine and triiodothyronine after levothyroxine ingestion at the end each 6-week period.

Results.—There were no significant differences among the 4 products in peak serum thyroxine or triiodothyronine concentrations or area under their serum concentration curves. Serum triiodothyronine concentrations increased transiently after Synthroid and decreased slightly after the other products; however, the differences were not statistically significant. For all four products, the United States Food and Drug Administration criterion for relative bioequivalence within 90% confidence intervals was met. There was considerable variability among the 4 products in the rate of absorption, but these differences also were not statistically significant.

Conclusion.—For patients receiving thyroxine replacement therapy, the 4 levothyroxine preparations are bioequivalent by current Food and Drug Administration criteria and are interchangeable.

▶ Are there any differences among the 4 brand-name and 3 generic preparations of thyroxine (official name, levothyroxine sodium) available in the United States?[1] No one will ever study all of them, but the 2 brand-name preparations and 2 generic preparations (neither now marketed in the United States, according to reference.[1]) given to the 22 women with hypothyroidism in this crossover study had quite similar effects. Ingestion of each was followed by transient 15% increases in serum free thyroxine index values and transient 30% to 50% reductions in serum thyrotropin (TSH) concentrations.

One curious (although not statistically significant) difference was that serum triiodothyronine concentrations increased transiently by about 10% for a few hours after ingestion of Synthroid, but decreased transiently by about 5% after the other 3 preparations. The simple explanation is that there were a few micrograms of triiodothyronine in the Synthroid tablets; in this regard, chromatographic analyses revealed the appropriate amount of thyroxine in all brands, but their triiodothyronine content was not measured.

The women were not allowed to eat for at least 8 hours before or for 4 hours after thyroxine administration. I suspect there would be less fluctuation in serum thyroxine concentrations and, therefore, in serum TSH concentrations if food was eaten soon after the thyroxine was taken. I (and probably most everyone else) pay little attention either to when patients last took their daily dose or when they last ate when I order serum TSH or thyroxine determinations, and I do not propose that we now standardize ordering of these tests. Nevertheless, we should ask patients when they took their dose and keep the answer in mind when we interpret the results. For serum TSH measurements, this means that a slightly low value several hours after levothyroxine administration does not mean the dose is too high, nor does a slightly high value 18 to 24 hours after the dose mean that the dose is too low.

Publication of this article was delayed for several years because the sponsor (the manufacturer of Synthroid) did not agree with the authors' conclusion that all 4 preparations were bioequivalent (and the authors' institution did not vigorously support the authors' right to publish). Two of the sponsors' criticisms of the study were that the causes of hypothyroidism varied and some patients had residual thyroid function.[2] The causes did vary and some patients may have had residual thyroid function, but the fact that each patient received all 4 preparations—and had similar serum thyroid hormone and TSH concentrations after doing so—is far more important. There is no reason not to write prescriptions for plain levothyroxine.

R.D. Utiger, M.D.

References

1. *Physicians Desk Reference*, ed 51. Medical Economics Inc, Montvale, NJ, p 125.
2. Spigelman M: Bioequivalence of levothyroxine preparations for treatment of hypothyroidism. *JAMA* 277:1199, 1997.

Does Treatment With L-Thyroxine Influence Health Status in Middle-aged and Older Adults With Subclinical Hypothyroidism?
Jaeschke R, Guyatt G, Gerstein H, et al (McMaster Univ, Hamilton, Ont, Canada)
J Gen Intern Med 11:744–749, 1996   26–3

Introduction.—Thyroid replacement therapy in patients with subclinical hypothyroidism is controversial. Thirty-seven patients (28 women, 9 men) aged 56 years and older were evaluated to determine whether L-thyroxine (T_4) replacement therapy improved health-related quality of life.

Methods.—Patients were randomly assigned to receive T_4 in a dose sufficient to reduce serum thyrotropin (TSH) concentrations to normal or placebo for 6 to 10 months. The mean daily dose was 68 µg. The patients completed thyroid-specific and general health-related quality of life questionnaires, and had a battery of cognitive function tests periodically during the study.

Results.—In the treatment group, the mean serum TSH concentration decreased by 8.6 mIU/L and the mean serum T_4 concentration increased by 27.9 nmol/L (2.2 µg/dL). There was a significant improvement in memory score in the T_4-treatment group, but no change in the placebo group. There were no between-group differences in any of the other tests of cognitive function. The results of the health-related quality of life questionnaires indicated no clinically important trends in favor of treatment.

Conclusion.—Treatment of patients with subclinical hypothyroidism results in little change in measures of quality of life or cognitive function.

▶ Subclinical hypothyroidism is common, affecting 5% to 10% of women aged 60 years or older and 3% to 5% of younger women. Although individual patients may have some symptoms of hypothyroidism, such as lethargy and constipation, as a group they cannot be distinguished from patients who have normal thyroid function.[1] They do tend to have slightly increased serum total cholesterol (and low-density lipoprotein cholesterol concentrations.[2]

Whether patients with subclinical hypothyroidism should be treated has been debated since assays for serum TSH were introduced and the disorder was identified. There are several arguments for treatment: the patient may feel better; lowering serum cholesterol may be beneficial; and the risk of overt hypothyroidism is substantial, so why not treat now. The counter-arguments are: there was little symptomatic benefit in 3 placebo-controlled trials of T_4 therapy (2 previous ones[3, 4] and this new one); serum cholesterol concentrations may not fall during therapy (they didn't in this study either), and besides there is no evidence that patients with subclinical hypothyroidism have accelerated vascular disease; and the risk of overt hypothyroidism is low (2.6% per year in patients with high serum TSH concentrations, rising to 4.1% per year in patients with high serum TSH values and a positive test for antithyroid peroxidase antibodies).[5]

I conclude that either choice–T_4 therapy or no T_4 therapy—can be defended, but in recent years I have tended to advise therapy if the patient has any symptoms possibly attributable to hypothyroidism (T_4 is a rather inexpensive placebo anyway) and has a positive test for antithyroid antibodies.

R.D. Utiger, M.D.

References

1. Bemben DA, Hamm RM, Morgan L, et al: Thyroid disease in the elderly: Part 2. Predictability of subclinical hypothyroidism. *J Fam Pract* 38:583–588, 1994.
2. Tanis BC, Westendorp RGJ, Smelt AHM, et al: Effect of thyroid substitution on hypercholesterolemia in patients with subclinical hypothyroidism. *Clin Endocrinol* 44:643–649, 1996.
3. Cooper DS, Halperin R, Wood LC, et al: L-Thyroxine in subclinical hypothyroidism: A double-blind, placebo-controlled trial. *Ann Intern Med* 101:18–24, 1984.
4. Nystrom E, Caidahl K, Fager G, et al: A double-blind cross-over 12-month study of L-thyroxine treatment of women with 'subclinical' hypothyroidism. *Clin Endocrinol* 29:63–76, 1988.
5. Vanderpump MPJ, Tunbridge WMG, French JM, et al: The incidence of thyroid disorders in the community: A twenty-year follow-up of the Whickham survey. *Clin Endocrinol* 43:55–68, 1995.

Impaired Cardiac Reserve and Exercise Capacity in Patients Receiving Long-term Thyrotropin Suppressive Therapy With Levothyroxine

Biondi B, Fazio S, Cuocolo A, et al (Univ Federico II, Naples, Italy)
J Clin Endocrinol Metab 81:4224–4228, 1996   26–4

Background.—Levothyroxine (T_4) is widely used to suppress thyrotropin (TSH) secretion in patients with nontoxic goiter and after surgery for differentiated thyroid carcinoma. Although usually considered safe, chronic T_4 administration may cause some cardiovascular manifestations of hyperthyroidism. Cardiac function and exercise tolerance were assessed in patients receiving long-term TSH-suppressive treatment with T_4.

Methods.—Ten patients who had been taking T_4 for 5–9 years and 10 matched normal subjects were studied. Maximal exercise capacity was studied using a bicycle ergometer. Left ventricular function at rest and during physical exercise was assessed by radionuclide angiography. After administration of T_4 and the selective β-adrenergic antagonist bisoprolol for 4 months, the patients were assessed again.

Findings.—At rest, the T_4-treated patients had impaired left ventricular diastolic filling. Systolic function was unaffected. Left ventricular ejection fraction increased in the normal subjects during submaximal physical exercise, whereas it dropped from 63% to 53% in the patients, primarily because of increased end-systolic left ventricular volume. The patients also had decreased exercise capacity as demonstrated by peak workload and exercise duration. β-Adrenergic blockade prevented the decline in ejection fraction and the increase in end-systolic volume during exercise and increased exercise tolerance.

Conclusions.—Long-term T_4-suppressive treatment with may decrease cardiac functional reserve and exercise capacity, and the effects of T_4 are ameliorated by β-adrenergic antagonist drug therapy.

▶ This study provides further evidence that subclinical hyperthyroidism (low serum TSH and normal serum thyroid hormone concentrations) causes cardiac dysfunction. These investigators had previously demonstrated that patients with this condition had a more rapid pulse rate, more frequent atrial premature contractions, poorer diastolic function, and increased left ventricular systolic function and mass, as compared with age- and sex-matched normal subjects.[1, 2] In this new study, they found that patients with subclinical hyperthyroidism had decreases in left ventricular function and exercise capacity. These results support the view that subclinical hyperthyroidism has deleterious cardiovascular effects. These various changes have not been equated with major clinical disability, other than an increased risk of atrial fibrillation,[3] but they can hardly be deemed beneficial. (I should note here that, in another recent study, patients with subclinical hyperthyroidism had few cardiac abnormalities.[4])

The patients in this and the other studies conducted by these investigators had subclinical hyperthyroidism as a result of administration of T_4 for nontoxic goiter or thyroid carcinoma, but, of course, equal suppression of TSH secretion from endogenous thyroid excess would have similar effects. Overtreatment with T_4 should be avoided unless there is a very good reason to do so (i.e., high-risk patients with thyroid carcinoma) and T_4 should not be given at all to patients with either solitary thyroid nodules or nontoxic multinodular goiters, in whom it has little, if any, efficacy. The fact that at least some of the cardiovascular effects of subclinical hyperthyroidism can be partially ameliorated with a β-adrenergic antagonist drug may make T_4 administration safer, but doesn't make it any more effective.

R.D. Utiger, M.D.

References

1. Biondi B, Fazio S, Carella C, et al: Cardiac effects of long term thyrotropin-suppressive therapy with levothyroxine. *J Clin Endocrinol Metab* 77:334–338, 1993.
2. Fazio S, Biondi B, Carella C, et al: Diastolic dysfunction in patients on thyroid-stimulating hormone suppressive therapy with levothyroxine: Beneficial effect of β-blockade. *J Clin Endocrinol Metab* 80:2222–2226, 1995.
3. Sawin CT, Geller A, Wolf PA, et al: Low serum thyrotropin: A risk factor for atrial fibrillation in older persons. *N Engl J Med* 331:1249–1252, 1994.
4. Shapiro LE, Sievert R, Ong L, et al: Minimal cardiac effects in asymptomatic athyreotic patients chronically treated with thyrotropin-suppressive doses of L-thyroxine. *J Clin Endocrinol Metab* 82:2592–2595, 1997.

Low Thyrotropin Levels Are Not Associated With Bone Loss in Older Women: A Prospective Study
Bauer DC, Nevitt MC, Ettinger B, et al (Univ of Calif, San Francisco; Kaiser Permanente Med Care Program, Oakland, Calif)
J Clin Endocrinol Metab 82:2931–2936, 1997   26–5

Background.—The relationship of excess thyroid hormone to bone loss is debated. Whether low serum thyrotropin (TSH) concentrations, indicating excessive thyroid hormone, are associated with low bone mass or accelerated bone loss in older women was investigated.

Methods.—A cohort of 458 women aged 65 years or older was studied prospectively. At the first visit, medical history, medication use, and calcaneal bone mineral density were recorded. Serum samples were obtained and stored at −190°C for measurement of TSH. About 2 years later, hip and spinal bone density were measured. Follow-up measurements of calcaneal and hip density were obtained a mean 5.7 and 3.5 years later, respectively.

Findings.—After adjustment for age, weight, previous hyperthyroidism, and estrogen therapy, bone loss during 4–6 years was similar in women with low, normal, and high baseline serum TSH concentrations (Fig 1). The initial bone density of the calcaneus, spine, and femoral neck or

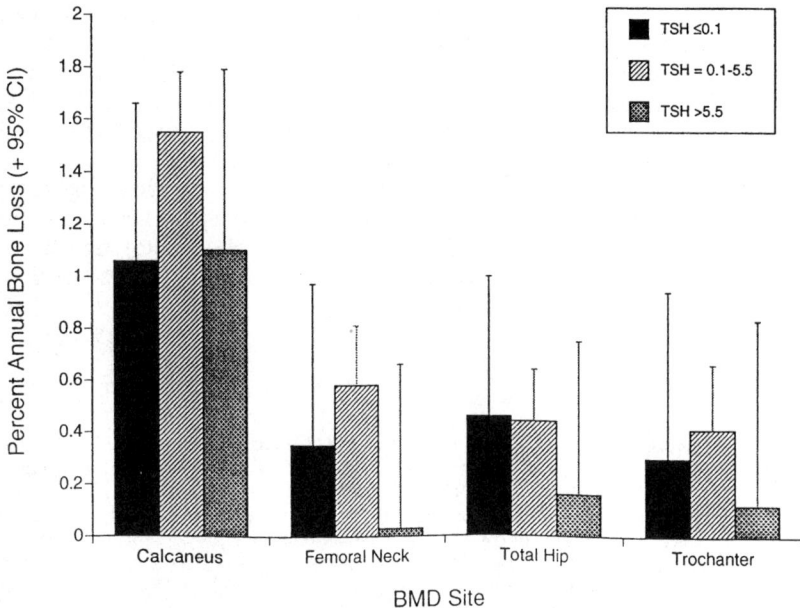

FIGURE 1.—Annual bone loss among women not taking oral estrogen as a function of serum thyrotropin (TSH) concentration at the baseline visit. The data shown are based on 266 paired calcaneal measurements and 239 paired hip measurements, adjusted for age, weight, previous hyperthyroidism, and clinic. (Courtesy of Bauer DC, Nevitt MC, Ettinger B, et al: Low thyrotropin levels are not associated with bone loss in older women: A prospective study. *J Clin Endocrinol Metab* 82:2931–2936, 1997. Copyright The Endocrine Society.)

trochanteric hip subregions did not differ significantly among the three serum TSH groups. The initial total hip density was 6% lower in the women in the low serum TSH group. The findings were similar in analyses of women not taking estrogen.

Conclusions.—Low serum TSH concentrations were not associated with low bone density or accelerated bone loss in older ambulatory women.

▶ This study provides more evidence that women treated with thyroxine who have low serum TSH concentrations do not lose bone at an excessive rate. Among the women with low serum TSH concentrations, the mean duration of treatment was more than 20 years and the mean thyroxine dose was 0.15 mg daily, so it is likely that most, if not all, of them had normal serum thyroid hormone concentrations, or nearly so; they can be said to have subclinical hyperthyroidism. Why they were taking thyroxine is not stated, but 40% had a history of hyperthyroidism and most likely had iatrogenic hypothyroidism, and, therefore, were not being intentionally over-treated.

It seems clear now that bone loss is not excessive not only in women receiving slightly overzealous thyroxine replacement therapy, but also in most of those with nodular goiter or thyroid carcinoma receiving suppressive therapy.[1, 2] Still, the results of 2 meta-analyses, 1 in 1994 and another in 1996,[3, 4] based on studies of varying design and quality, suggest increased loss at some skeletal sites in postmenopausal women. I think the way to view all these results is to consider subclinical hyperthyroidism a risk factor for bone loss in the same way as smoking or low physical activity. Like the latter, it should be avoided whenever possible. That often is not hard to do, because overtreatment with thyroxine is the most common cause of subclinical hyperthyroidism.

R.D. Utiger, M.D.

References

1. Marcocci C, Golia F, Bruno-Rosso G, et al: Carefully monitored levothyroxine suppressive therapy is not associated with bone loss in premenopausal women. *J Clin Endocrinol Metab* 78:818–823, 1994.
2. Muller CG, Bayley A, Harrison JE, et al: Possible limited bone loss with suppressive thyroxine therapy is unlikely to have clinical relevance. *Thyroid* 5:81–87, 1995.
3. Faber J, Galloe AM: Changes in bone mass during prolonged subclinical hyperthyroidism due to L-thyroxine treatment: A meta-analysis. *Eur J Endocrinol* 130:350–356, 1994 (1995 YEAR BOOK OF MEDICINE, p. 610.)
4. Uzzan B, Campos J, Cucherat M, et al: Effects on bone mass of long term treatment with thyroid hormones: A meta-analysis. *J Clin Endcrinol Metab* 81:4278–4289, 1996.

Interest of Routine Measurement of Serum Calcitonin: Study in a Large Series of Thyroidectomized Patients
Niccoli P, Wion-Barbot N, Caron P, et al (CHU la Timone, Marseille, France; CHU Angers, France; CHU Rangueil, Toulouse, France; et al)
J Clin Endocrinol Metab 82:338–341, 1997   26–6

Background.—There are 2 forms of medullary carcinoma of the thyroid—familial and sporadic. Familial medullary carcinoma can be detected by genetic or biochemical screening, enabling early diagnosis and treatment, which result in a high cure rate. However, sporadic medullary carcinoma is usually diagnosed at the stage of nodal involvement, precluding complete resection in most patients. The prevalence of sporadic medullary carcinoma in patients with thyroid nodular disease, and the value of measurements of basal and pentagastrin-stimulated serum calcitonin to improve the preoperative diagnosis of medullary carcinoma, were investigated.

Methods and Findings.—Basal serum calcitonin was determined in 1,167 patients with thyroid nodular disease before surgery. A pentagastrin stimulation test was performed in 121 patients with normal basal serum calcitonin concentrations. Histopathologic assessment of surgical specimens revealed medullary carcinoma in 16 patients (1.4%). Fourteen

(41.1%) of these tumors were found in the 34 patients with abnormal serum calcitonin values, and 2 were in the 1,133 patients (0.2%) with normal basal serum calcitonin values.

Conclusions.—Measurement of serum calcitonin to detect medullary carcinoma of the thyroid should be a routine part of the diagnostic assessment of patients with thyroid nodular diseases.

▶ Most, if not all, medullary carcinomas of the thyroid gland secrete calcitonin, like their parent C cells. Furthermore, we know from studies of families with multiple endocrine neoplasia (MEN) type 2 that serum calcitonin concentrations are high in patients with very small medullary carcinomas. Thus, measuring serum calcitonin in patients with thyroid nodular disease might be a simple way to identify those patients whose nodule is a medullary carcinoma. That can also be done by fine needle aspiration biopsy, because the cytologic appearance of medullary carcinoma differs from that of carcinomas of thyroid follicular cells and immunostaining reveals calcitonin only in the former.

The problem with measurements of serum calcitonin for differential diagnosis in patients with thyroid nodules is that medullary carcinomas account for only about 3% of all thyroid cancers,[1] and thyroid cancers account for only about 5% of all thyroid nodules. So, elevated serum calcitonin values in even a few patients who did not have medullary carcinoma would seriously compromise the value of the test. In this study of 1,167 patients with thyroid nodular disease, the majority of whom had nontoxic multinodular goiters and all of whom underwent surgery, 14 of the 34 patients with elevated serum calcitonin values had medullary carcinomas, and 2 patients with normal values had medullary carcinomas, albeit microscopic ones. However, the values in the patients with false positive elevations were, in general, only minimally elevated, whereas half the patients with medullary carcinoma had values more than 10 times the upper limit of normal. There were fewer false positive results in another study of patients with thyroid nodular disease,[2] in that all the patients who had elevated values had medullary carcinoma, but not all the patients were operated on.

In the United States, most patients with solitary thyroid nodules or a multinodular goiter with 1 or 2 dominant nodules undergo fine needle aspiration biopsy, and in most of the few patients who have medullary carcinoma, the carcinoma will be detected by cytologic examination. On the basis of the calcitonin screening studies, a few patients with thyroid nodular disease have small medullary carcinomas that cannot be detected by fine needle aspiration biopsy but can be by measurement of serum calcitonin. Of course, that doesn't mean that their survival is increased. On the other hand, some patients operated on because their serum calcitonin value is high will not have medullary carcinoma. I conclude serum calcitonin should not be measured in all patients with thyroid nodular disease, or even in all patients with solitary thyroid nodules.

R.D. Utiger, M.D.

References

1. Gilliland FD, Hunt WC, Morris DM, et al: Prognostic factors for thyroid carcinoma: A population-based study of 15,698 cases from the Surveillance, Epidemiology, and End Results (SEER) Program 1973–1991. *Cancer* 79:564–573, 1997.
2. Pacini F, Fontanelli M, Fugazzola L, et al: Routine measurement of serum calcitonin in nodular thyroid disease allows the preoperative diagnosis of unsuspected sporadic medullary thyroid carcinoma. *J Clin Endocrinol Metab* 78:826–829, 1994.

27 The Parathyroid Glands and Bone

The Rise and Fall of Primary Hyperparathyroidism: A Population-based Study in Rochester, Minnesota, 1965–1992
Wermers RA, Khosla S, Atkinson EJ, et al (Mayo Clinic and Mayo Found, Rochester, Minn)
Ann Intern Med 126:433–440, 1997
27–1

Background.—When routine measurement of serum calcium by automated technology was begun in the early 1970s, the number of identified cases of primary hyperparathyroidism increased dramatically. Trends in the incidence of this condition since the mid-1970s were studied.

Methods and Findings.—All residents of Rochester, Minnesota, receiving an initial diagnosis of primary hyperparathyroidism between 1965 and 1992 were identified through the Rochester Epidemiology Project medical records linkage system. In the prescreening era, from 1965 to 1974, the age- and sex-adjusted incidence of primary hyperparathyroidism was 15 cases per 100,000 person-years. After the introduction of automated screening in 1974, the incidence increased to 77 per 100,000 person-years, and it was 112 per 100,000 person years in 1975. After some fluctuation in the next 5 years, the incidence has declined progressively, despite improved case ascertainment, and was only 4 per 100,000 person-years in 1992. Survival was not compromised in the pre- or postscreening period. The maximum serum calcium concentrations were similar during the different time periods (Table 1).

Conclusions.—The incidence of primary hyperparathyroidism has been declining progressively since 1975. This unexpected finding suggests a change in the epidemiology of this disease.

▶ No one disputes that the introduction of widespread biochemical testing in the 1970s led to a substantial increase in the diagnosis of primary hyperparathyroidism. And, because we now know the disorder is usually very mild and rarely progressive, and that only a small minority of patients with the disorder will have kidney stones or bone disease,[1, 2] there is little doubt that most of the patients would never have been recognized.

How can we explain the fall in frequency of the disorder found by this study? The fall has continued too long to be ascribed to sudden recognition

TABLE 1.—Clinical and Demographic Characteristics of Residents of Rochester, Minnesota, Who Received a Diagnosis of Definite or Possible Primary Hyperparathyroidism From 1965 to 1992

Characteristic	Time Period		
	1965–June 1974 ($n = 63$)	July 1974–1982 ($n = 289$)	1983–1992 ($n = 123$)
Mode of diagnosis, n (%)			
Histologic evidence	23 (36.5)	78 (27.0)	21 (17.1)
Inappropriately elevated immunoreactive parathyroid hormone level	25 (39.7)	135 (46.7)	49 (39.8)
By exclusion	13 (20.6)	60 (20.8)	31 (25.2)
Possible primary hyperparathyroidism	2 (3.2)	16 (5.5)	22 (17.9)
Sex, n (%)			
Female	48 (76.2)	222 (76.8)	89 (72.4)
Male	15 (23.8)	67 (23.2)	34 (27.6)
Age, y			
Mean	53.7	57.2	52.4
Median (range)	56.5 (20.3–86.3)	58.7 (15.8–87.8)	53.0 (19.2–89.4)
Presentation, n (%)			
Symptom or complication of primary hyperparathyroidism	14 (22.2)	23 (8.0)	2 (1.6)
Abnormal serum calcium level	47 (74.6)	264 (91.4)	119 (96.8)
Other biochemical abnormality	1 (1.6)	0 (0)	2 (1.6)
Autopsy finding	0 (0)	2 (0.7)	0 (0)
Uncertain	1 (1.6)	0 (0)	0 (0)
Maximum serum calcium level, *mmol/L*			
Mean	2.72	2.72	2.67
Median (range)	2.69 (2.54–3.04)	2.69 (2.54–3.99)	2.64 (2.54–3.07)
Initial management, n (%)			
Surgery ≤6 months after diagnosis	18 (28.6)	63 (21.8)	16 (13.0)
Surgery recommended but refused	6 (9.5)	10 (3.5)	3 (2.4)
Surgery recommended but patient too ill	2 (3.2)	13 (4.5)	0 (0)
Decision to observe	35 (55.6)	203 (70.2)	104 (84.6)
Uncertain	2 (3.2)	0 (0)	0 (0)

(Courtesy of Wermers RA, Khosla S, Atkinson EJ, et al: The rise and fall of primary hyperparathroidism: A population-based study in Rochester, Minnesota, 1965–1992. *Ann Intern Med* 126:433–440, 1997.)

of the disease in patients in whom it would have been recognized in the next decade or so. The known risk factors for primary hyperparathyroidism are the multiple endocrine neoplasia syndrome, familial primary hyperparathyroidism, and head and neck irradiation in infancy and childhood, but none of these factors has been present in appreciable numbers of patients in any study of the disease.

A more attractive possibility is an increase in dietary intake of calcium, vitamin D, or both (perhaps coupled with more sunlight exposure). Increases in either would tend to raise serum calcium and, hence, inhibit parathyroid secretion and cellular growth, and, hence, possibly formation of parathyroid adenomas. We now know that patients with secondary hyperparathyroidism caused by renal insufficiency can have parathyroid nodules that are mono-clonal,[3] so I see no reason why the same couldn't happen in patients with secondary hyperparathyroidism, even very mild secondary hyperparathyroidism, of other causes. Increases in dietary calcium and vitamin D intake could also contribute to the lack of progression of primary hyperparathyroidism after it does occur and the patient becomes mildly hypercalcemic.

R.D. Utiger, M.D.

References

1. Scholz DA, Purnell DC: Asymptomatic primary hyperparathyroidism: 10 year prospective study. *Mayo Clin Proc* 56:473–478, 1981.
2. Silverberg SJ, Gartenberg F, Jacobs TP, et al: Longitudinal bone density measurements in untreated primary hyperparathyroidism. *J Clin Endocrinol Metab* 80:723–728, 1995. (1996 YEAR BOOK OF MEDICINE, p 544.)
3. Arnold A, Brown MF, Urena P, et al: Monoclonality of parathyroid tumors in chronic renal failure and in primary parathyroid hyperplasia. *J Clin Invest* 95:2047–2053, 1995.

Optimal Dietary Calcium Intake in Primary Hyperparathyroidism

Locker FG, Silverberg SJ, Bilezikian JP (Columbia Univ, New York)
Am J Med 102:543–550, 1997   27–2

Introduction.—Many patients with primary hyperparathyroidism are treated conservatively rather than by surgery. The usual recommendation is to restrict dietary intake of calcium in hope of preventing further elevation of the serum calcium concentration and renal stone formation. There is concern, however, that a low calcium intake may stimulate further increases in parathyroid hormone secretion and worsen bone disease. To determine what advice should be given regarding dietary calcium intake, 71 patients enrolled in a study of the natural history of primary hyperparathyroidism were studied.

Methods.—All the patients had undergone an evaluation that included a complete blood count; chemistry profile; measurements of serum parathyroid hormone, 25-hydroxyvitamin D, 1,25-dihydroxyvitamin D, and magnesium; and repeated measurements of 24-hour urinary excretion of calcium, creatinine, and phosphorus. Bone density was measured, and baseline food intake records were obtained. Calcium intake was defined as very low (less than 300 mg/day), low (300 to 800 mg/day), and adequate (more than 800 mg/day). No patient took medication that would affect bone and mineral metabolism.

Results.—The baseline biochemical values in all 3 groups were typical of patients with mild primary hyperparathyroidism (Table 1). All the patients had mild hypercalcemia, and low normal serum phosphorus, elevated parathyroid hormone and high-normal 1,25-dihydroxyvitamin D concentrations and high-normal urinary calcium excretion. Their mean dietary protein intake was 69 g/day, and their mean dietary sodium intake was 1,831 mEq/day; both increased with increasing calcium intake. There was no relationship between dietary protein or sodium intake and urinary calcium excretion. The level of calcium intake was not related to the bone density of the lumbar spine, femoral neck, or distal radius. Serum 1,25-dihydroxyvitamin D concentrations were elevated in 37 patients, and these patients had higher serum parathyroid hormone concentrations and higher urinary calcium values.

Conclusion.—The findings of this study suggest that dietary calcium intake up to 1,000 mg is safe and desirable for with primary hyperpara-

TABLE 1.—Baseline Indices in Patients with Primary Hyperparathyroidism by Dietary Calcium Group

	All Patients n = 71	Very Low n = 17	Low n = 46	US RDA n = 8
Dietary intake				
Calcium (mg/day)	506 ± 32	199 ± 14*	529 ± 21*	1023 ± 73*
Serum index				
Calcium (mmol/L)	2.79 ± 0.02	2.79 ± 0.05	2.77 ± 0.02	2.82 ± 0.05
Phosphorus (mmol/L)	0.90 ± 0.03	0.90 ± 0.03	0.90 ± 0.03	0.94 ± 0.03
Creatinine (μmol/L)	90 ± 3	100 ± 7	80 ± 3†	80 ± 4
Alk. phos. (μkat/L)	1.8 ± 0.1	2.0 ± 0.2	1.7 ± 0.1	1.8 ± 0.2
Magnesium (mmol/L)	0.82 ± 0.01	0.82 ± 0.04	0.82 ± 0.01	0.86 ± 0.04
MM-PTH (pg/mL)	764 ± 69	865 ± 206	751 ± 78	655 ± 92
IRMA-PTH (pg/mL)	118 ± 8	112 ± 11	123 ± 11	107 ± 10
25(OH)D (ng/mL)	21 ± 1	22 ± 4	20 ± 1	26 ± 3
1,25(OH)2D (pg/mL)	60 ± 3	56 ± 7	62 ± 3	64 ± 7
Urine index				
Calcium (mmol/d)	6.3 ± 0.4	6.2 ± 0.9	6.3 ± 0.42	69 ± 1.2
Phosphorus (mmol/d)	25 ± 1	21 ± 2	25 ± 1	29 ± 5
Calcium/mmol CR	0.70 ± 0.03	0.59 ± 0.07	0.72 ± 0.04	0.80 ± 0.13

*Different from other 2 groups at P<0.0001.
†Different from very low Ca diet at P<0.05.
Abbreviations: Alk. phos., alkaline phosphatase; *MM-PTH,* parathyroid hormone by mid-molecule assay; *IRMA-PTH,* parathyroid hormone by immunoradiometric assay; *25(OH)D,* 25-hydroxyvitamin D; *1,25(OH)2D,* 1,25-dihydroxyvitamin D; *CR,* creatinine.
(Reprinted by permission of the publisher from Locker FG, Silverberg SJ, Bilezikian JP: Optimal dietary calcium intake in primary hyperparathyroidism. *Am J Med* 102:543–550, copyright 1997 by Excerpta Medica, Inc.)

thyroidism who do not have high serum 1,25-dihydroxyvitamin D concentrations. Those with elevated serum 1,25-dihydroxyvitamin D values should restrict dietary calcium intake to prevent hypercalciuria and reduce their risk of kidney stones.

▶ Most patients with primary hyperparathyroidism are asymptomatic and have only modest hypercalcemia, which changes little with time. Similarly, although these patients may have low bone density at the time of diagnosis, it, too, changes little thereafter.[1] As a result, many patients are followed with no treatment. The question then arises, What should their intake of calcium be? Might a low calcium intake result in more bone disease or a high intake result in increased urinary calcium excretion and, therefore, a greater risk of hypercalciuria and formation of renal calculi?

These questions are not likely to be studied prospectively, but this study provides some clues as to what the results might be. Keeping in mind that the patients in this study were not considered candidates for surgery because they had mild hypercalcemia (and no renal calculi), there was no relationship between estimated dietary calcium intake and serum or urinary calcium values, serum parathyroid hormone concentrations, or bone density. Parathyroid hormone stimulates real hydroxylation of 25-hydroxyvitamin D to form 1,25-dihydroxyvitamin D, and some patients with hyperparathyroidism have high serum 1,25-dihydroxyvitamin D concentrations. The latter patients did excrete more calcium in the urine, independent of calcium intake, and could possibly be at risk for renal calculi.

There is no reason to restrict calcium intake in patients with primary hyperparathyroidism. In fact, based on the assumption that all the other factors which affect bone density in aging are operative in these patients, they should probably take in at least 1,000 mg of calcium daily. The authors recommend measuring serum 1,25-dihydroxyvitamin D and advising the patient to take in less calcium if it is high; a more direct approach would be to measure urinary calcium, and advise the patients to take in less calcium if it is high.

R.D. Utiger, M.D.

Reference

1. Silverberg SJ, Gartenberg FR, Jacobs TP, et al: Longitudinal measurements of bone density and biochemical indices in untreated primary hyperparathyroidism. *J Clin Endocrinol Metal* 80:723–728, 1995.

Short-term Inhibition of Parathyroid Hormone Secretion by a Calcium-receptor Agonist in Patients With Primary Hyperparathyroidism

Silverberg SJ, Bone HG III, Marriott TB, et al (Columbia Univ, New York; Henry Ford Hosp, Detroit; NPS Pharmaceuticals, Salt Lake City; et al)
N Engl J Med 337:1506–1510, 1997   27–3

Background.—The usual treatment for primary hyperparathyroidism is surgery. The efficacy of a calcimimetic drug that inhibits parathyroid hormone secretion in vitro in reducing serum parathyroid hormone and calcium concentrations in patients with this disorder was determined.

Methods.—Twenty postmenopausal women with mild primary hyperparathyroidism were enrolled in this randomized, placebo-controlled study. Eight women received placebo followed by 2 different single oral doses of 4, 10, or 20 mg of R-568 in ascending order, and 12 received placebo and 2 different doses of 20, 80, or 160 mg in ascending order. Their mean serum calcium concentration at baseline was 10.7 mg/dL (2.7 mmol/L). Serum parathyroid hormone and calcium were measured repeatedly after each dose.

Findings.—The administration of R-568 was associated with dose-dependent inhibition of parathyroid hormone secretion. The mean serum parathyroid hormone concentration declined by 26% after 20 mg of R-568, by 42% after 80 mg, and by 51% after 160 mg. Serum ionized calcium concentrations declined only after the 160-mg dose, the decline closely following the decline in serum parathyroid hormone concentrations (Fig 1).

Conclusions.—A calcimimetic drug can inhibit parathyroid hormone secretion in patients with primary hyperparathyroidism. Thus, medical therapy for primary hyperparathyroidim is a feasible goal.

▶ Nonsurgical therapy for patients with primary hyperparathyroidism usually consists of watchful waiting, except in postmenopausal women, in whom estrogen decreases bone turnover and increases bone density (as it

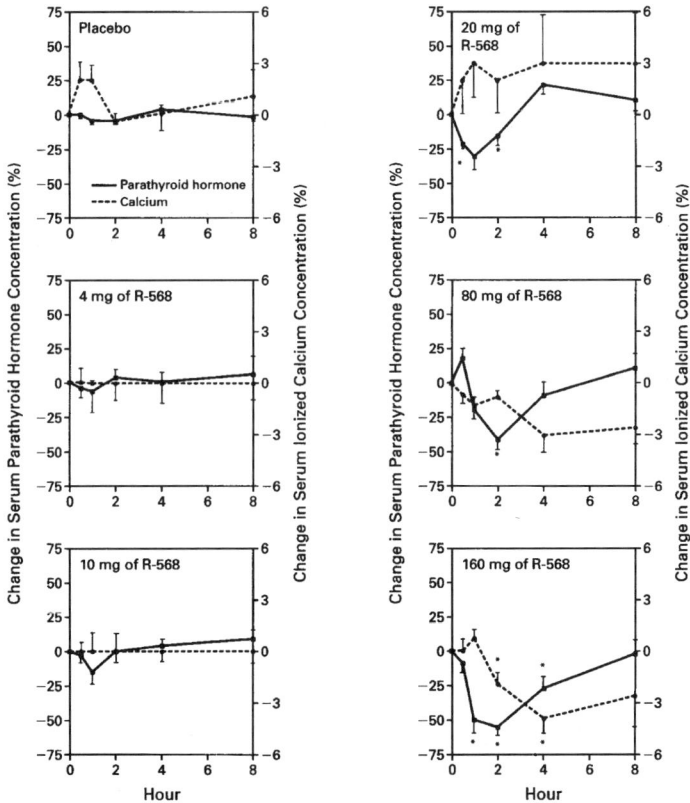

FIGURE 1.—Mean (± SE) changes in serum parathyroid hormone and ionized calcium concentrations after the administration of the calcimimetic drug R-568 in postmenopausal women with primary hyperparathyroidism. Eighteen women received placebo, 4 received the 4-mg dose of R-568, 6 received the 10-mg dose, 13 received the 20-mg dose, 8 received the 80-mg dose, and 8 received the 160-mg dose. The *asterisks* indicate P < 0.05 for the comparison with placebo. (Reprinted by permission of the *New England Journal of Medicine*, from Silverberg SJ, Bone HG III, Marriott TB, et al: Short-term inhibition of parathyroid hormone secretion by a calcium-receptor agonist in patients with primary hyperparathyroidism. N Engl J Med 337:1506–1510 copyright 1997, Massachusetts Medical Society.)

does in normal postmenopausal women).[1] Watchful waiting is a perfectly satisfactory "treatment" for asymptomatic patients with mild hyperparathyroidism, because the disease rarely worsens.[2] Nevertheless, a medical therapy suitable for men and women of all ages, not just postmenopausal women, would be useful, for example, for patients who are poor candidates for surgery, those in whom surgery is unsuccessful, and those with severe secondary hyperparathyroidism.

R-568 is the first pharmacologic fall-out of the recognition that calcium regulates parathyroid hormone secretion via a calcium-sensing receptor on the membrane of parathyroid cells.[3] The drug acts by activating the receptor; in other words, it mimics the action of calcium. Its activity in patients who have parathyroid adenomas means these tumors do not have loss-of-function mutations in the calcium-receptor gene, and it probably inhibits adenoma growth as well as parathyroid hormone secretion. It is far too short-acting to be useful clinically, and of course nothing is known about long-term safety. Nevertheless, it is proof-of-principle (e.g., that calcium receptors are physiologically important) and it opens the door to true antiparathyroid therapy.

R.D. Utiger, M.D.

References

1. Grey AB, Stapleton JP, Evans MC, et al: Effect of hormone replacement therapy on bone mineral density in postmenopausal women with mild primary hyperparathyroidism: A randomized, controlled trial. *Ann Intern Med* 125:360–368, 1996. (1997 YEAR BOOK OF MEDICINE, p 513.)
2. Silverberg SJ, Greenberg F, Jacobs TP, et al: Longitudinal measurements of bone density and biochemical indices in untreated primary hyperparathyroidism. *J Clin Endocrinol Metab* 80:723–728, 1995. (1996 YEAR BOOK OF MEDICINE, p 544.)
3. Brown EM, Pollak M, Seidman CE, et al: Calcium-ion–sensing cell-surface receptors. *N Engl J Med* 333:2334–240, 1995.

Broadband Ultrasound Attenuation Predicts Fractures Strongly and Independently of Densitometry in Older Women
Bauer DC, for the Study of Osteoporotic Fractures Research Group (Univ of California, San Francisco)
Arch Intern Med 157:629–634, 1997   27–4

Background.—Quantitative ultrasonography of bone is a new, radiation-free test that is useful for determining bone mass and, possibly, bone quality. Low attenuation of ultrasound by the calcaneus appears to be associated with an increased risk for hip and other fractures in older women. The value of quantitative calcaneal ultrasonography of bone for predicting fractures was determined and the results were compared with those obtained by bone densitometry.

Methods.—This prospective cohort study was done within the Study of Osteoporotic Fractures. A total of 6,189 postmenopausal women older than 65 years seen at 4 U.S. centers were included. Bone mineral density of the calcaneus and hip were measured, along with broadband ultrasound attenuation, a measure of the differential attenuation of sound waves transmitted through the calcaneus. The occurrence of hip and other non-spine fractures was recorded during a mean follow-up period of 2 years.

Findings.—Each standard deviation decrease in calcaneal broadband ultrasound attenuation was associated with a doubling of the risk for hip fractures after adjustment for age and clinic. The relationship was similar for bone mineral density of the calceneus and femoral neck. Decreased broadband ultrasound attenuation was associated with an increased risk for hip fracture. A low broadband ultrasound attenuation value was particularly strongly correlated with intertrochanteric fractures.

Conclusion.—Decreased broadband ultrasound attenuation predicts the occurrence of fracture in elderly women. It is also a useful diagnostic test for osteoporosis.

▶ Based on the results of this and a similar study done in Europe,[1] measurements of ultrasound transmission through bone provide information about bone strength comparable to that of measurements of bone density by absorptiometry or computed tomography. The procedure is simple and fast, involves no radiation, and may be even more useful if it can be done at sites at which fractures are likely to occur, such as the hip, spine, and radius. All of these measurements have clinical value because they identify patients at risk for fracture and, therefore, those in whom some intervention is indicated, even it is only an increase in calcium intake.

A more difficult question is who should have these measurements—all postmenopausal women or only those with risk factors for osteoporosis such as smoking, immobility, low body weight, and previous therapy with glucocorticoids? The presence of risk factors correlates poorly with low bone density[2, 3] and, therefore, cannot be substituted for measurements of bone density. Nevertheless, I have been unable to bring myself to recommend that all elderly people—or even all postmenopausal women—have a measurement of bone density. That may change because this technique should be much less expensive than the other methods. The machine and technique were recently approved by the Food and Drug Administration, and more data regarding the efficacy of the procedure should be available soon.

R.D. Utiger, M.D.

References

1. Hans D, DargentMolina P, Schott PM, et al: Ultrasonographic heel measurements to predict hip fracture in elderly women: The EPIDOS prospective study. *Lancet* 348:511–514, 1996.
2. Slemenda CW, Hui SL, Johnston CC Jr, et al: Predictors of bone mass in postmenopausal women: A prospective study of clinical data using photon absorptiometry. *Ann Intern Med* 112:96–101, 1990.
3. 1993 YEAR BOOK OF MEDICINE, pp 550–552.

Hormone Replacement Therapy in Postmenopausal Women: Urinary N-telopeptide of Type I Collagen Monitors Therapeutic Effect and Predicts Response of Bone Mineral Density
Chesnut CH III, Bell NH, Clark GS, et al (Univ of Washington, Seattle; Med Univ of South Carolina, Charleston; Osteoporosis Ctr of Santa Barbara, Calif; et al)
Am J Med 102:29–37, 1997   27–5

Introduction.—Postmenopausal women have increased bone resorption, a decline in bone mass, and subsequent increased risk for osteoporosis and fracture. Bone mass is increased and the incidence of fractures is

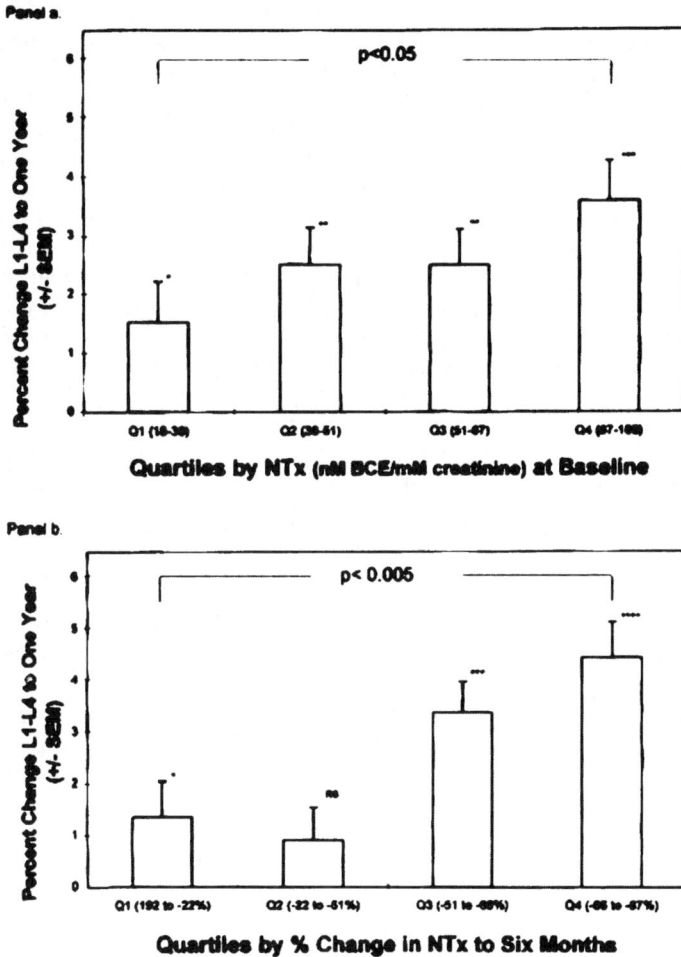

FIGURE 3.—Response to estrogen and progesterone replacement therapy at the spine by quartiles of urinary excretion of N-telepeptide of type I collage ([Ntx]; baseline, percent change to 6 months). *Ns* indicates not significantly different from baseline bone mineral density. *Asterisk* indicates significantly different (P<0.05) from baseline. *Double asterisk* indicates significantly different (P<0.001) from baseline. *Triple asterisk* indicates significantly different (P<0.0001) from baseline. *Quadruple asterisk* indicates significantly different (P<0.00001) from baseline. (Reprinted by permission of the publisher, courtesy of Chesnut CH III, Bell NH, Clark GS, et al: Hormone replacement therapy in postmenopausal women: Urinary N-telopeptide of type I collagen monitors therapeutic effect and predicts response of bone mineral density. *Am J Med* 102:29–37, copyright 1997 by Excerpta Medica, Inc.)

reduced with estrogen therapy. To monitor treatment, bone mineral density is measured, usually by dual energy x-ray absorptiometry; however, bone density increases slowly, and may not be evident for up to 2 years. Bone markers are dynamic indicators of bone remodeling, including bone resorption and formation. To monitor therapeutic response, the clinical utility of urinary excretion of the N-telopeptide of type I collagen was assessed.

Methods.—A total of 236 women who were 1 to 3 years postmenopausal participated in this 2-year randomized, controlled study. The women were divided into 2 groups, with 1 group receiving estrogen and progesterone plus calcium and the other group receiving calcium alone.

Results.—Urinary N-telopeptide excretion significantly decreased, and spine and hip bone mineral density significantly increased in the women receiving estrogen-progestin therapy plus calcium. Bone mineral density decreased significantly, but the bone marker did not change in the group of women receiving calcium alone. The greatest gain in bone mineral density in response to estrogen-progestin therapy was in the women in the two highest quartiles for baseline urinary N-telopeptide excretion and those in whom excretion decreased the most during the first 6 months (Fig 3). The odds of gain in bone mineral density in response to estrogen-progestin plus calcium therapy increased by a factor of 5.0 for every increase of 30 units in baseline urinary N-telopeptide excretion.

Conclusion.—Measurements of urinary N-telopeptide excretion may be useful to predict the antiresorptive effect of estrogen-progestin therapy in postmenopausal women.

▶ Not all women with postmenopausal osteoporosis have an increase in bone density during antiresorptive treatment such as estrogen-progestin, alendronate, or calcium–vitamin D, but even in responsive patients changes in bone density occur slowly. This means that measurements of bone density may change little for many months; measurements after less than 6 months of treatment are not useful, and even at that time may be misleading. So what is needed is a biochemical test that can be done either before treatment, or soon after treatment is begun, that indicates that the treatment will slow bone resorption and, therefore, increase bone density.

The number of substances released during bone resorption that can be measured has increased substantially in recent years. They are all fragments of collagen, either the molecules that hold the collagen chains together (pyridinoline and deoxypyridinoline) or collagen peptides, (cross-linked N-terminal peptides [telopeptides], or cross-linked C-terminal peptides.)[1] They are usually measured in urine, and diet need not be restricted before sample collection. Among them, urinary N-telopeptide excretion seems to be elevated the most in postmenopausal women and fall the most when they are given antiresorptive therapy.[2]

In this study of postmenopausal women, urinary N-telopeptide excretion decreased 23%, 39%, and 52% after 3, 6, and 12 months of treatment, respectively, in the estrogen-progestin plus calcium group, as compared with no change in the calcium group. More important, among women with low baseline urinary N-telopeptide excretion, bone density increased little during estrogen-progestin therapy, and among women with higher urinary N-telopeptide excretion at baseline, the values decreased more during estrogen-progestin plus calcium therapy in those who ultimately had the greatest increase in bone density. These results can probably be extrapolated to other treatments such as alendronate and calcium–vitamin D, allowing either efficacy to be predicted before treatment or lack of efficacy to be detected and change made within 6 months after treatment is begun.

R.D. Utiger, M.D.

References

1. Eriksen EF, Brixen K, Charles P: New markers of bone metabolism: Clinical use in metabolic bone disease. *Eur J Endocrinol* 132:251–263, 1995.
2. Garnero P, Sornay-Rendu E, Chapuy M-C, et al: Increased bone turnover in late postmenopausal women is a major determinant of osteoporosis. *J Bone Miner Res* 11:337–349, 1996.

Effects on Bone Mass After Eight Years of Hormonal Replacement Therapy
Eiken P, Nielsen SP, Kolthoff N (Hillerød Sygehus, Denmark)
Br J Obstet Gynaecol 104:702–707, 1997   27–6

Background.—Osteoporosis is an age-related disease that causes morbidity for millions of women. Estrogen deficiency is an important cause of osteoporosis, and estrogen therapy can slow or reverse it. However, the long-term effects of estrogen have not been thoroughly assessed. The long-term effects of therapy with estrogen—continuous, combined, and sequential—were analyzed in a double-blind, placebo-controlled, prospective 2-year study. This was followed by an open study.

Study Design.—From March 1984 to July 1985, 151 women who had their last vaginal bleeding more than 6 months and less than 24 months earlier and had no signs of osteoporosis entered this study. These women were randomly assigned into group 1, 50 women who received continuous estrogen and progesterone therapy; group 2, 50 women who received sequential estrogen and progesterone therapy; and group 3, 51 women who received placebo. After 24 months, the women were invited to continue participating in an open study. The lumbar spine bone mineral density and forearm bone mineral content were measured initially and at 8 years.

Results.—Only the 73 women who completed the entire trial were included in the analysis. The women who received estrogen therapy had significantly higher mean lumbar spine bone mineral density after 8 years than those who received placebo (1.084 g/cm² vs 0.944 g/cm²). There was no significant difference between those who received sequential or continuous estrogen therapy. The mean forearm bone mineral content was also significantly higher in the treated than in the untreated women at the end of the 8-year period. Femoral bone density, measured only after 8 years, was higher in the area of Ward's triangle, but not the femoral neck, trochanteric region or intertrochanteric region, in the estrogen-treated women.

Conclusions.—In these women who began estrogen soon after menopause, 8 years of therapy was associated with a sustained increase in bone mineral density, as compared with women who did not receive estrogen.

▶ This is the longest prospective study, albeit small in numbers, of the effect of estrogen on bone density in postmenopausal women that I am aware of. The women were unselected in terms of their bone density, and they began therapy within 2 years after the menopause, at a time when bone loss is more rapid and the effect of estrogen is less, as compared with 10 or more years after the menopause.[1] The therapeutic regimens of continuous or sequential administration of estradiol and norethisterone are rarely, if ever, used in the United States. Nevertheless, the dose of estradiol is comparable to 0.625 mg of conjugated equine estrogen, and the dose of norethisterone is comparable to 5 mg of medroxyprogesterone, the usual estrogen and progestin preparations and doses prescribed in the United States. The results are, therefore, probably applicable to early postmenopausal women here.

The increase in lumbar spine bone density of 12.1% above baseline in the estrogen-treated women was about 3 times that in a 3-year U.S. study.[1] The pattern of changes in the density of the distal radius was different—no change in the estrogen-treated women and a decrease in the untreated women. However, the differences between the 2 groups at both sites at 8 years (12% to 14%) were comparable. So, although the balance between bone resorption and formation at each site varied, the ability of estrogen to alter it continues. On the other hand, the effect on the bone density of the hip—the site of the most devastating fractures—was disappointingly small.

In other words, prolonged estrogen therapy leads to continued—indeed, increasing—benefit. This supports the results of studies of much older women, which revealed higher bone density at several sites only in those women who had taken estrogen for at least 7 years.[2] In sum, postmenopausal estrogen therapy must be given for prolonged periods if it is to have a large effect on fracture rates in women in their 60s and beyond.

R.D. Utiger, M.D.

References

1. Mebane-Sims I, for the Writing Group of the PEPI Trial: Effects of hormone therapy on bone mineral density: Results from the Postmenopausal Estrogen/Progestin Interventions (PEPI) trial. *JAMA* 276:1389–1396, 1996. (1997 YEAR BOOK OF MEDICINE, p 518.)
2. Felson DT, Zhang Y, Harmon MT, et al: The effect of postmenopausal estrogen therapy on bone density in elderly women. *N Engl J Med* 329:1141–1146, 1993. (1995 YEAR BOOK OF MEDICINE, p 651.)

Effect of Calcium and Vitamin D Supplementation on Bone Density in Men and Women 65 Years of Age or Older

Dawson-Hughes B, Harris SS, Krall EA, et al (Tufts Univ, Boston)
N Engl J Med 337:670–676, 1997   27–7

Objective.—Inadequate intake of calcium and vitamin D may increase the risk of bone loss in older subjects. The effect of combined calcium and vitamin D supplements on bone loss, biochemical measures of bone metabolism, and incidence of nonvertebral fractures was studied in community-living men and women aged 65 years and older.

Methods.—Three hundred eighty nine healthy subjects (176 men and 213 women) were enrolled in the 3-year, double-blind, placebo-controlled trial. They received either placebo or 500 mg of calcium and 700 IU of vitamin D₃ daily. Blood urine studies were done and bone mineral density was measured by dual-energy x-ray absorptiometry every 6 months, and fractures were recorded.

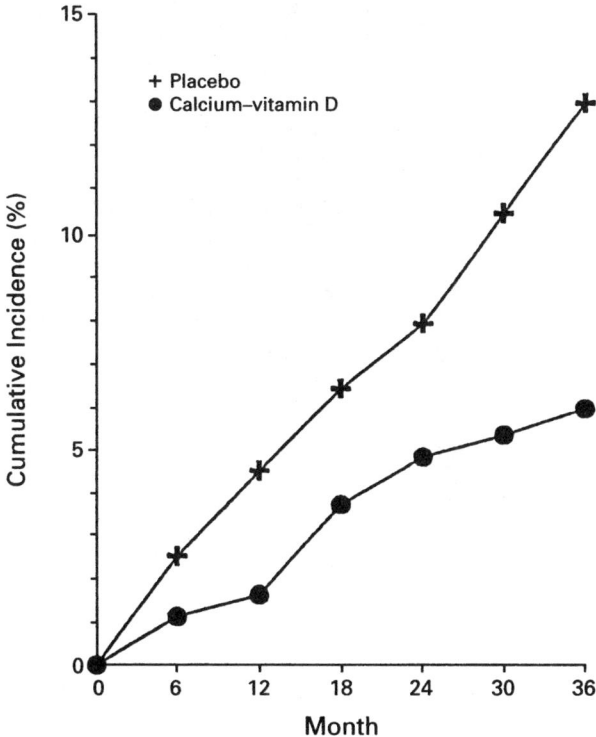

FIGURE 1.—Cumulative percentage of all 389 subjects with a first nonvertebral fracture, according to study group. By 36 months, 26 of 202 subjects in the placebo group and 11 of 187 subjects in the calcium-vitamin D group had had a fracture (P = 0.02). (Reprinted by permission of *The New England Journal of Medicine.* Courtesy of Dawson-Hughes B, Harris SS, Krall EA, et al: Effect of calcium and vitamin D supplementation on bone density in men and women 65 years of age of older. *N Engl J Med* 337:670–676. Copyright 1997, Massachusetts Medical Society.)

Results.—At 3 years, bone mineral density increased at all sites in the supplemented group and increased less or decreased in the placebo group: femoral neck, +0.50% versus −0.70%; spine, +2.12% vs. + 1.22%; total body +0.06% versus −1.09%. Thirty-seven nonvertebral fractures (fractures after severe trauma) were reported, 5 in men and 32 in women (Fig 1). There was a significantly higher incidence of fractures in the placebo group than in the supplemented group at 3 years (12.9 versus 5.9%). Twenty-eight subjects had osteoporotic fractures (fractures after moderate-to minor trauma). The 3-year incidence of osteoporotic fractures was significantly lower in the supplemented group than in the placebo group. In the supplement group, serum calcium values did not change, but serum 25-hydroxy vitamin D concentrations and urine calcium excretion increased. There were no biochemical changes in the placebo group.

Conclusion.—Vitamin D and calcium supplementation reduced bone loss and the incidence of nonvertebral fractures in a 3-year study in community-dwelling subjects aged 65 and older.

▶ The men and women in this study had baseline dietary intakes of calcium and vitamin D averaging about 717 mg and 190 IU daily, respectively, well below the recommended intakes of 1500 mg[1] and 400 IU. In this regard, they were probably representative of most Americans aged 65 and older. Undoubtedly, some had biochemical evidence of vitamin D deficiency (low serum 25–hydroxyvitamin D and high serum parathyroid hormone concentrations), but we are not told how many. Among those with vitamin D deficiency, the resulting bone disease may be either osteoporosis or osteomalacia,[2] but from a practical perspective the distinction is unimportant.

This is at least the second study to demonstrate that calcium and vitamin D supplementation can increase bone density and lower the rate of fracture.[3] In another study, vitamin D supplementation increased bone density but did not reduce the fracture rate, perhaps because the study subjects received no calcium supplements.[4, 5] Vitamin D increases calcium absorption no matter what the calcium intake, but it will be less effective if the calcium intake is low and, therefore, there isn't much calcium to be absorbed.

The evidence that vitamin D and calcium supplementation are beneficial in older persons is so extensive that it is hard to escape the conclusion that higher intakes of both throughout life would go far toward minimizing osteoporosis (and fractures) in older men and women.

R.D. Utiger, M.D.

References

1. NIH Consensus Panel on Optimal Calcium Intake: Optimal calcium intake. *JAMA* 272:1942–1948, 1994.
2. Compston JE: The role of vitamin D and calcium supplementation in the prevention of osteoporotic fractures in the elderly. *Clin Endocrinol* 43:393–405, 1995.
3. Chapuy MC, Arlot ME, Duboeuf F, et al: Vitamin D and calcium to prevent hip fractures in elderly women. *N Engl J Med* 327:1637–1642, 1992. (1994 YEAR BOOK OF MEDICINE, pp. 607–609.)

4. Ooms ME, Roos JC, Bezemer PD, et al: Prevention of bone loss by vitamin D supplementation in elderly women: A randomized, double-blind trial. *J Clin Endocrinol Metab* 80:1052–1057, 1995. (1996 YEAR BOOK OF MEDICINE, pp. 551–553.)

5. Lips P, Graafmans WC, Ooms ME, et al: Vitamin D supplementation and fracture incidence in elderly persons. *Ann Intern Med* 124:400–406, 1996.

Prevention of Nonvertebral Fractures by Alendronate: A Meta-Analysis

Karpf DB, for the Alendronate Osteoporosis Treatment Study Groups (Merck Research Labs, Rahway, NJ)

JAMA 277:1159–1164, 1997   27–8

Introduction.—Osteoporosis, results in 1.5 million fractures in the United States each year. Most of the morbidity, mortality, and cost associated with the disease is caused by nonvertebral fractures, particularly those involving the hip. The effect of treatment with alendronate, a potent aminobisphosphonate, on the incidence of nonvertebral fractures in postmenopausal women was studied.

Methods.—Data from 5 prospective, placebo-controlled, randomized trials of alendronate of at least 2 years' duration were analyzed. The study subjects were women with osteoporosis who had been postmenopausal for at least 4 years; and their lumbar spine bone mineral density was at least 2.0 SD below the mean for young adult women, as measured by dual-energy x-ray absorptiometry. The women were randomly assigned to treatment with alendronate at a dose higher than 1 mg per day or to placebo.

Results.—Sixty women in the placebo group of 590 women had nonvertebral fractures during 1,347 patient-years at of follow-up. The overall rate in this group was 4.45 women with fractures per 100 patient-years at risk. Seventy-three of 1,102 women in the alendronate group had nonvertebral fractures during 2,240 patient-years at risk. Their overall rate was 3.26 women with fractures per 100 patient-years at risk. In the placebo group, after 3 years, the estimated cumulative incidence of nonvertebral fractures was 12.6%, whereas, in the alendronate group, it was 9%. The reduction of risk was consistent at each major site of osteoporotic fracture, including the hip and wrist, and across each of the studies.

Conclusion.—Treatment with alendronate reduces the risk of nonvertebral fractures for at least 3 years in postmenopausal women with osteoporosis.

▶ While all the women in these studies had osteoporosis, as it is now defined (lumbar spine bone density at least 2 standard deviations below the peak bone density for young women), the daily doses of alendronate varied from 2 to 40 mg/day, and the duration of treatment with a particular dose varied from as little as 3 months to 3 years. The average age of the women in the different studies ranged from 59 to 71 years, and the average time since menopause ranged from 11 to 23 years. Alendronate decreased the nonvertebral fracture rate by 18% in women aged less than 65 years of age and by 35% in those aged 65 years or older. The benefit in terms of fracture reduction increased during the 3-year study, presumably because bone density increased progressively.[1] This drug also decreases vertebral fractures.[1]

The usual dose of alendronate is 10 mg daily because that is the dose that increases bone density at multiple sites. That dose might also be expected to result in a larger decrease in fractures. The duration of therapy is probably more important than the dose, and it is likely that bone loss will resume and fracture rate increase after alendronate is discontinued, as is the case after estrogen is discontinued. Perhaps a regimen of 10 mg daily for several years and then 2 or 5 mg daily indefinitely would prove optimal for increasing and then maintaining bone density.

I know of no study in which alendronate was compared with estrogen-progestin in postmenopausal women with osteoporosis. The 2 treatments cause about the same increase in bone density and, presumably, have the same benefit in terms of fracture reduction. Alendronate is clearly the treatment of choice for women with osteoporosis who cannot or will not take estrogen-progestin, and there is no reason to doubt that it will increase bone density in postmenopausal women who do not have osteoporosis.

R.D. Utiger, M.D.

Reference

1. Liberman UA, Weiss SR, Broll J, et al: Effect of oral alendronate on bone mineral density and the incidence of fractures in postmenopausal osteoporosis. *N Engl J Med* 333:1437–1443, 1995.

Intermittent Etidronate Therapy to Prevent Corticosteroid-induced Osteoporosis
Adachi JD, Bensen WG, Brown J, et al (McMaster Univ, Hamilton, Ont, Canada; Centre Hospitalier de l'Université Laval, Ste-Foy, Quebec; Univ of Calgary, Alta, Canada; et al)
N Engl J Med 337:382–387, 1997   27–9

Background.—Corticosteroid treatment commonly causes osteoporosis, suggesting the need for preventive therapy for patients who will be taking corticosteroids for more than a few weeks. There is some evidence that intermittent cyclic therapy with etidronate can prevent corticosteroid-induced osteoporosis. The ability of etidronate to prevent corticosteroid-induced osteoporosis was assessed in a randomized, controlled trial.

Methods.—The study included 141 adult patients who had started high-dose corticosteroid therapy within the previous 100 days. All were expected to receive at least 1 year of treatment with prednisone or its equivalent, at a mean daily dose of 7.5 mg for 90 days followed by a mean daily dose of 2.5 mg or greater. The patients were randomly assigned to receive cycles of etidronate, 400 mg/day for 14 days, or placebo. Both

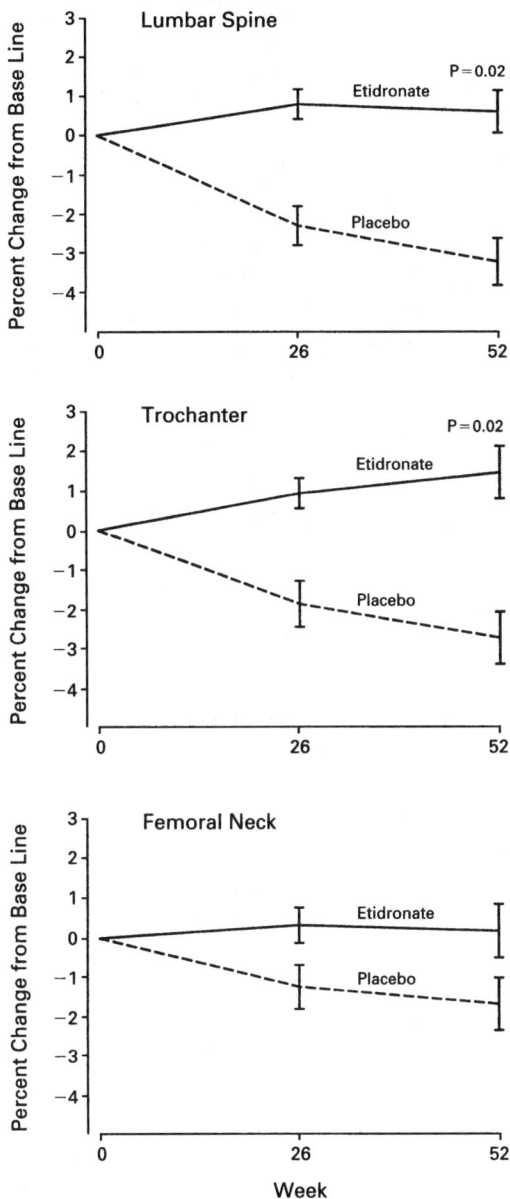

FIGURE 1.—Mean (±SE) change in the bone density of the lumbar spine (top panel), trochanter (middle panel), and femoral neck (bottom panel) between base line (week 0) and weeks 36 and 52 in the etidronate and placebo groups. The P values indicate significant differences between treatment groups. (Reprinted by permission of *The New England Journal of Medicine*. Courtesy of Adachi JD, Bensen WG, Brown J, et al: Intermittent etidronate therapy to prevent corticosteroid-induced osteoporosis. *N Engl J Med* 337:382–387, copyright 1997, Massachusetts Medical Society.)

treatments were followed by 76 days of treatment with calcium carbonate, 500 mg daily. During the 1-year treatment period, the cycle was repeated 3 times. The main outcome measure was the mean percent change in lumbar spine bone density at one year. Bone density was measured in other sites as well, and the incidence of vertebral fractures was compared.

Results.—One hundred seventeen patients completed the study. The 2 groups had comparable mean daily prednisone doses throughout the study: 14 mg/day in the placebo group and 13 mg/day in the etidronate group at 26 weeks, and 11 mg/day in both groups at 52 weeks. The cumulative corticosteroid doses were 4,119 mg and 3,911 mg, respectively. One-way analysis of variance revealed no significant changes in lumbar spine and trochanter density in the etidronate group, but a decline in the placebo group (Fig 1). The difference in mean percentage change from baseline was 3.72% in the lumbar spine, 4.14% in the trochanter, and 1.88 in the femoral neck. Etidronate was associated with a smaller decrease in lumbar spine density in men than in premenopausal and postmenopausal women; the mean one-year differences between groups were 2.50%, 4.47%, and 4.56%, respectively. A response to treatment—the slope of the bone density of the spine greater than zero, as determined by linear regression analysis—was present in 59% of the etidronate group versus 23% of the placebo group.

Vertebral fractures occurred in 15% of the placebo group versus 9% of the etidronate group, for a relative risk of 0.6. For postmenopausal women, etidronate treatment reduced vertebral fractures by 85%. At 26 weeks, serum bone-specific alkaline phosphatase was reduced by 18% in the etidronate group. At 52 weeks, the values were similar in the two groups.

Conclusions.—Intermittent etidronate therapy prevents bone loss and vertebral fractures in patients receiving long-term corticosteroid therapy.

▶ Here is another way to prevent corticosteroid-induced osteoporosis. It is only slightly more complicated than the vitamin D-calcium regimen given by Buckley et al. (Abstract 40–1),[1] and is equally safe. The 2 studies differ in several respects, the most important being that Adachi et al. started their anti-osteoporosis treatment at about the same time as corticosteroid treatment was started, whereas, the patients treated by Buckley et al. had received corticosteroids for a while (duration not stated, but the cumulative prednisone dose at baseline was greater than 5,000 mg) before being given vitamin D and calcium. The yearly changes in bone density were rather similar in the treatment and placebo groups in the 2 studies, but since more bone is lost in the first few months after corticosteroid therapy is begun than later, the etidronate-calcium regimen may well be more effective than the vitamin D-calcium regimen. It is likely that the more potent bisphosphonates alendronate and tiludronate will prove as effective as etidronate for this purpose.

As I noted in my comments about the study by Buckley et al., I think that everyone about to be treated with corticosteroids for more than a few weeks should take supplemental calcium and vitamin D. I am not certain that more aggressive therapy is indicated routinely, but one way to decide is to measure bone density. If it is already low, then more aggressive antiresorptive therapy with etidronate or another bisphosphonate (or estrogen in a woman who is amenorrheic or postmenopausal) is indicated.

R.D. Utiger, M.D.

Reference

1. Buckley LM, Leib ES, Cartularo KS, et al: Calcium and vitamin D3 supplementation prevents bone loss in the spine secondary to low-dose cotricosteroids in patients with rheumatoid arthritis. *Ann Intern Med* 125:961–968, 1996.

28 The Reproductive System

Secondary Sexual Characteristics and Menses in Young Girls Seen in Office Practice: A Study From the Pediatric Research in Office Settings Network

Herman-Giddens ME, Slora EJ, Wasserman RC, et al (Univ of North Carolina, Chapel Hill; American Academy of Pediatrics, Elk Grove Village, Ill; Univ of Vermont, Burlington; et al)

Pediatrics 99:505–512, 1997   28–1

Background.—The lack of nationally representative pubertal data for girls in the United States has necessitated reliance on Marshall and Tanner's classic 1969 studies on variations of pubertal changes in girls in the United Kingdom. The presence of secondary sexual characteristics and menses in U.S. girls aged 3 to 12 years was established in the current study to provide pubertal data pertinent to girls currently seen in pediatric office practices.

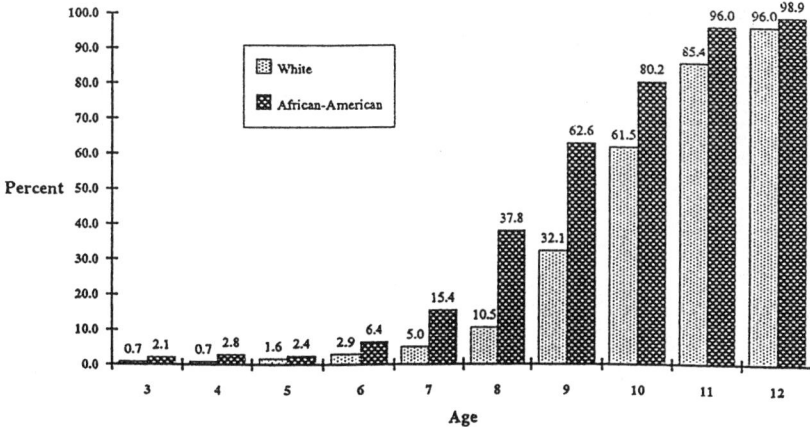

FIGURE 1.—Prevalance of breast development at Tanner stage 2 or greater by age and race (Cochran-Mantel-Haenszel ^{2} = 168.6, df = 1, P<0.001; Breslow-Day ^{2} = 10.7, df = 9, P=0.300). (Reproduced by permission of *Pediatrics*. Courtesy of Herman-Giddebs ME, Slora EJ, Wasserman RC, et al: Secondary sexual characteristics and menses in young girls seen in office practice: A study from the pediatric research in office settings network. *Pediatrics* 99:505–512, 1997.)

Methods and Findings.—Two hundred twenty-five clinicians in a practice-based research network conducted the cross-sectional study. After standardized training in the evaluation of pubertal maturation, the clinicians rated the level of sexual maturation of 17,077 girls, aged 3 through 12 years. Nine and a half percent were black and the rest were white. At 3 years of age, 3% of black girls and 1% of white girls had breast or pubic hair development. These proportions increased to 27.2% and 6.7%, respectively, at 7 years of age and 48.3% and 14.7%, respectively, at 8 years of age (Fig 1). The mean age of onset of breast development was 8.9 years for the black girls and 10.0 years for the white girls. The mean age for pubic hair development was 8.8 and 10.5 years, respectively. Menses occurred at 12.2 and 12.9 years of age among the black and white girls, respectively.

Conclusions.—Pubertal characteristics are developing in girls at younger ages than currently used norms indicate. Criteria for referring girls with precocious puberty may need to be revised, with attention given to racial differences.

▶ The age of onset of puberty may not be a subject of concern to the patients of most internists, but those same patients may have questions about the pubertal development of their children. Sexual development is usually considered precocious when it occurs before age 8 years in girls (and 9 years in boys),[1] based on studies done several decades ago. Based on this large, contemporary study, some pubertal development at age 8 years in girls should be considered normal, and the threshold age should be lowered to at least 7 years, especially in black girls. The fall in the age of onset of pubertal development is usually attributed to better nutrition and more rapid growth, but no one really knows the explanation.

This is not to say that precocious puberty is a problem of the past, but only that, for example, 7- or even 6-year-old girls with some breast development or pubic hair growth do not need extensive evaluation for ovarian, adrenal, and intracranial disease or hypothyroidism (which usually includes measurements of serum gonadotropins, estradiol, dehydroepiandrosterone sulfate, and thyrotropin, and cranial or ovarian imaging studies). This is particularly true when there is no evidence of accelerated growth, the girl's bone age is not advanced, she has not had any vaginal bleeding, and she is otherwise healthy. All these findings suggest that there is no large increase in sex steroid secretion and, therefore, the girl is very unlikely to have an identifiable cause of her precocious development. These girls should be monitored closely, with particular attention being given to acceleration in growth and bone age, but most will develop normally.

R.D. Utiger, M.D.

Reference

1. Kasa-Vubu JZ, Kelch RP: Precocious and delayed puberty: Diagnosis and treatment. In DeGroot LJ, ed. *Endocrinology*, 3rd ed. WB Saunders Co., Philadelphia 1995, pp. 1953–1977.

Prostate-specific Antigen in Female Serum, a Potential New Marker of Androgen Excess

Melegos DN, Yu H, Ashok M, et al (Univ of Toronto; Univ of Southern California, Los Angeles)

J Clin Endocrinol Metab 82:777–780, 1997   28–2

Introduction.—Prostate-specific antigen (PSA) was believed to be absent from female tissues until it was recently detected in female breast tissue. The production of PSA by steroid hormone receptor-positive breast cancer cells is regulated by steroid hormones via action of steroid hormone receptors. Since there is a relationship between androgen and PSA production in men, PSA may be a marker of androgen action in women.

Methods.—Serum PSA was measured in 22 women with hirsutism (Ferriman-Gallwey score higher than 8) and 50 normal women. Serum 3α-androstanediol glucuronide (3α-AG) was measured in all women as a marker of tissue dihydrotestosterone metabolism.

Results.—Serum, PSA concentrations were higher in the women with hirsutism than in the normal women (mean 43 vs. 3 pg/mL). There wasa positive correlation between the serum PSA and 3α-AG concentrations, and a negative correlation between serum PSA and 3α-AG concentrations and age. The serum 3α-AG value was a slightly better marker of androgen excess than the serum PSA value.

Conclusion.—Serum PSA concentrations are significantly higher in women with hirsutism than in normal women. There is a significant positive correlation between serum PSA and 3α-AG concentrations and a negative correlation with age. Serum PSA may be considered a biochemical marker of androgen action in women.

▶ What we call prostate-specific antigen is a serine protease whose function in the prostate (or anywhere else) is not known. That it is present in the prostate gland and serum and that its production is androgen dependent in men are well known. That it is present in breast, ovarian, and endometrial tissue and, in very small amounts, in serum of women, are much less well known.[1] What is perhaps more surprising is that, if Melegos et al. are correct, it is androgen dependent in women as well.

The mean serum prostate-specific antigen concentration in the normal women was 3 pg/mL, about 0.1% of the concentration in normal men. Many of the hirsute women had anovulatory cycles, but they were not otherwise characterized; their serum PSA concentrations ranged from < 1 to 579 pg/mL (median 4, mean 43). Hormonally, the authors focused on serum 3α-androstanediol glucuronide because it is produced in androgen-sensitive tissues from dihydrotestosterone and is, therefore, thought to be a good indicator of androgen action in tissues. However, not all the hirsute women studied had high serum 3α-androstanediol glucuronide concentrations.

Measurements of serum prostate-specific antigen are not a good test for androgen excess in women, because the range of values is so great. Furthermore, the source of the excess prostate-specific antigen in those hirsute women with elevated value is anyone's guess; it could be the hair follicles, the ovaries, or any other tissue that has androgen receptors (bone, muscle, breast). What can be said is that the name is a misnomer. It is not prostate specific, and, of course, it is not really an antigen.

R.D. Utiger, M.D.

Reference

1. Diamandis EP, Yu H: New biological actions of prostate-specific antigen? *J Clin Endocrinol Metab* 80:1515–1517, 1995.

Women's Beliefs and Decisions About Hormone Replacement Therapy
Newton KM, LaCroix AZ, Leveille SG, et al (Group Health Cooperative of Puget Sound, Seattle; Natl Inst on Aging, Gaithersberg, Md; Natl Ctr for Chronic Disease Prevention and Health Promotion, Atlanta, Ga)
J Women's Health 6:459–465, 1997   28–3

Background.—The reasons why United States women initiate, maintain, or stop estrogen replacement therapy have not been clearly defined. Decision making regarding this therapy was explored among women at a large Health Maintenance Organization in Washington state.

Methods.—Computer-assisted telephone interviews were conducted with 1,082 women aged 50 to 80 years. The response rate was 80.3%. Based on data from the interviews, 42.5% of the women were classified as current estrogen users, 20.9% as past users, and 36.6% as never users.

Findings.—The most common reasons for initiating estrogen therapy were menopausal symptoms, reported by 47.3%; prevention of osteoporosis, 32.4%; and physician advice, 30.3%. The most common reasons for quitting therapy were adverse effects, reported by 26.6%; physician's advice, 22.9%; fear of cancer, 15.4%; and not wanting menstrual periods or bleeding, 15.2%. Fifty-four percent of past users stopped estrogen therapy on their own. The most commonly given reasons for never initiating estrogen therapy were that it was not needed, cited by 49.9%, and that menopause is a natural event, cited by 17.9%. Thirty-three percent of never users said they had considered estrogen therapy. Only 46.6% of never users had discussed estrogen therapy with their physician, and 5% had been given a prescription for estrogen which they did not fill.

Conclusion.—Many postmenopausal women apparently make decisions about estrogen therapy independent of their physicians. The development of more effective counseling strategies depends on a better understanding of the beliefs and decisions that affect women's choices to use or not to use take estrogen therapy.

▶ More and more postmenopausal women are taking estrogen (always in combination with a progestin unless they have had a hysterectomy), whether for treatment of menopausal symptoms or prevention of coronary heart disease or osteoporosis. Because menopausal symptoms tend to subside with time, treatment need not be prolonged, whereas, it must be continued to obtain the other benefits. In the latter circumstance, the question of side effects—particularly vaginal bleeding—becomes more important, as does the question of whether long-term estrogen therapy increases the risk of breast cancer. Vaginal bleeding may be minimized by changes in regimen, for example, by switching from an intermittent to a continuous estrogen-progestin regimen. Even if the cardiovascular (and skeletal) benefits of estrogen considerably outweigh the risk of breast cancer (and the latter is still rather hotly debated), many women are much more fearful of breast cancer than of cardiovascular disease.

Based on the results of this and other questionnaire studies,[1] it is clear that there are many reasons why women either do not begin or discontinue estrogen therapy. Advice from friends or the media was not often a determinant of behavior, but I suspect that such advice contributed strongly to the other responses, for example, fear of cancer. There is much public information regarding the benefits and risks of estrogen therapy, and, no doubt, much of it is biased in 1 way or another. It also seems clear that physicians are not involved in the majority of these decisions, particularly those relating to the decision to stop treatment, although, again, a physician's views may have contributed to other responses.

The premise of these studies seems to be that every postmenopausal woman should be taking estrogen. But some women have no menopausal symptoms and in others they are very mild, so there is no immediate benefit of treatment.[2] Others probably have a low risk of cardiovascular disease or osteoporosis. The problem is that we do not know how to identify the low-risk women, and, therefore, we do not know how to lower the number needed to treat to obtain benefit. That is why all women should be considered candidates for estrogen therapy. But, we must accept that many will refuse for sensible reasons.

R.D. Utiger, M.D.

References

1. Salamone LM, Pressman AR, Seeley DG, et al: Estrogen replacement therapy: A survey of older women's attitudes. *Arch Intern Med* 156:1293–1297, 1996.
2. Porter M, Penney GC, Russell D, et al: A population-based survey of women's experience of the menopause. *Br J Obstet Gynaecol* 103:1025–1028, 1996.

Ovarian Hyperthecosis, Diabetes, and Hirsuties in Post-menopausal Women

Barth JH, Jenkins M, Belchetz PE (Leeds Gen Infirmary, London)
Clin Endocrinol (Oxf) 46:123–128, 1997   28–4

Introduction.—Hirsutism in postmenopausal women is an uncommon problem, and the diagnostic protocols for hirsutism used in premenopausal women do not apply to postmenopausal women. Body hair growth may be a useful marker of pathologic hirsutism in this age group. Four cases of ovarian hyperthecosis in postmenopausal women, marked by generalized hirsutism, are described.

Patients.—The 4 women all had substantial hair growth on the chest, upper back, and shoulders. The diagnosis of ovarian hyperthecosis was made by histologic study in 3 of the women, whereas the fourth was found to have large ovaries on ultrasonography. All the women had risk factors for vascular disease, including hypertension, hyperlipidemia, and glucose intolerance, and three had symptomatic vascular disease. Their serum testosterone concentrations ranged from 3.3 to 8.9 nmol/L (95 to 257 ng/dL).

Outcomes.—All the women were treated with gonadotropin-releasing hormone agonist (goserelin)—3.6-mg implants were placed in the abdominal wall approximately every 8 weeks for 6 months. The treatment produced a substantial reduction in serum testosterone and in hirsutism; however, hyperlipidemia was unaffected.

Conclusions.—In postmenopausal women, androgen excess is manifested by hirsutism, marked growth of hair across the upper trunk, and it can be caused by ovarian hyperthecosis.

▶ Postmenopausal women tend to have an increase in facial hair growth and loss of scalp hair, perhaps because serum testosterone concentrations fall less during menopause than do those of estradiol. Therefore, a pathologic increase in androgen production may result in a more striking increase in hair growth on the chest, back, and shoulders than on the face. Nevertheless, facial hair growth would be expected to increase, and, indeed, the women reported by Barth et al. had high scores for hair growth on the upper lip and chin. Were that not so, one would have to postulate that there were regional changes in the sensitivity of hair follicles to androgen after the menopause, for which there is no evidence. Recall also that hirsutism is likely to be the only manifestation of moderate androgen excess in postmenopausal women, until the excess is sufficiently great to cause virilization, with deepening of the voice, clitoral hypertrophy, or changes in body habitus.

Hyperthecosis of the ovaries may be viewed as a severe form of the polycystic ovary syndrome, in which there are not only multiple follicular cysts lined by increased numbers of luteinized theca cells but also severe stromal hyperplasia with or without clusters of luteinized theca cells within the hyperplastic stroma (in postmenopausal women, the follicles are absent). In premenopausal women, the polycystic ovary syndrome tends to persist but not worsen; after menopause, their serum testosterone concentrations are slightly higher than those in normal postmenopausal women, and many have hyperinsulinemia, obesity, diabetes mellitus, and hypertension.[1] Three of the 4 postmenopausal women reported here had the onset of hirsutism after menopause, and did not have the polycystic ovary syndrome as usually defined (hyperandrogenism and menstrual irregularity). All were obese (duration not stated) and likely had hyperinsulinemia. The improvement during gonadotropin-releasing hormone agonist therapy indicates that their hyperandrogenism was dependent on luteinizing hormone, but hyper-insulinemia undoubtedly contributed to it as well.[2]

Androgen excess can begin after the menopause, and its major effect is to cause hirsutism. In addition to hyperthecosis, it can be caused by ovarian and adrenal tumors, so appropriate evaluation of a postmenopausal woman with hirsutism should include not only measurement of serum testosterone and ovarian ultrasonography but also measurement of serum dehydro-epiandrosterone sulfate and, if it is abnormal, adrenal imaging to look for an adrenal carcinoma.[3]

R.D. Utiger, M.D.

References

1. Dahlgren E, Janson PO, Johansson S, et al: Women with polycystic ovary syndrome wedge resected in 1956 to 1965: A long-term follow-up focusing on natural history and circulating hormones. *Fertil Steril* 57:505–513, 1992.
2. Nestler JE, Jakubowicz DJ: Decreases in ovarian cytochrome P450c17α activity and serum free testosterone after reduction of insulin secretion in polycystic ovary syndrome. *N Engl J Med* 335:617–623, 1996.
3. Derksen J, Nagesser SK, Meinders AE, et al: Identification of virilizing adrenal tumors in hirsute women. *N Engl J Med* 331:968–973, 1994.

Adult-onset Idiopathic Hypogonadotropic Hypogonadism: A Treatable Form of Male Infertility

Nachtigall LB, Boepple PA, Pralong FP, et al (Massachusetts Gen Hosp, Boston; Centre Hospitalier Universitaire Vaudois, Lausanne, Switzerland)

N Engl J Med 336:410–415, 1997   28–5

Background.—Pubertal development is typically absent in men with isolated deficiency of gonadotropin-releasing hormone (GnRH). An adult-onset form of idiopathic hypogonadotropic hypogonadism developing after puberty was described.

Methods.—Ten men aged 27–57 years were studied. All had normal sexual maturation, idiopathic infertility, sexual dysfunction, low serum testosterone concentrations, and apulsatile secretion of luteinizing hormone on frequent blood sampling. Anterior pituitary hormone secretion and sellar anatomy were otherwise normal. The results of semen analysis and measurements of testicular volume and serum testosterone, inhibin B, and gonadotropins in these men were compared with the results in 24 men with classic GnRH deficiency before and during GnRH replacement treatment and with those of 29 normal men of comparable age.

Findings.—Serum gonadotropin concentrations in the men with adult-onset GnRH deficiency were comparable with those in men with classic GnRH deficiency before and during pulsatile GnRH administration. Compared with men with classic GnRH deficiency, those with adult-onset hypogonadotropic hypogonadism had higher mean testicular volumes and serum testosterone and inhibin B concentrations. In the 5 men undergoing long-term treatment, GnRH reversed the hypogonadism and restored fertility.

Conclusions.—Adult-onset hypogonadotropic hypogonadism is a unique form of isolated hypogonadotropic hypogonadism occurring in sexually mature men. Recognizing this syndrome clinically is important because it is one of the few treatable forms of male infertility.

▶ The first step in the evaluation of any man with onset of symptoms of testosterone deficiency or infertility after puberty is to confirm the presence of testosterone deficiency. If it is confirmed, the next step is to determine whether the hypogonadism is primary or secondary by measuring serum follicle-stimulating hormone (FSH) and luteinizing hormone (LH). Among men with acquired postpubertal hypogonadotropic hypogonadism, the most common causes are pituitary tumors (before or after treatment) and infiltrative diseases of the hypothalamus and pituitary, such as hemochromatosis, sarcoidosis, histiocytosis, and hyperprolactinemia. Further evaluation should include looking for other pituitary hormone deficiencies, MR imaging of the hypothalamus and pituitary, and tests for causative disorders such as measurements of serum prolactin, ferritin, and angiotensin-converting enzyme.

Having identified none of these disorders, one is left with acquired idiopathic hypogonadotropic hypogonadism, like the men studied by Nachtigall et al. These men differed from men with prepubertal hypogonadotropic hypogonadism mostly in having less severe hypogonadism, but, like the latter, most had no pulses of LH secretion, indicating that the fundamental problem was GnRH deficiency. Determining whether LH secretion is pulsatile or not is difficult in practice, and, besides, LH secretion may be apulsatile in patients with very few or no pituitary gonadotropic cells and it may be pulsatile in men presumed to have GnRH deficiency.[1] Determination of the serum LH response to a single dose of GnRH also is not helpful, because gonadotropic cells long deprived of GnRH may not respond unless repeatedly stimulated. The only solution if the man desires fertility is a trial of pulsatile GnRH administration; otherwise, testosterone should be given,

Biochemically, this syndrome seems to be the male counterpart of so-called hypothalamic amenorrhea, that is, decreased GnRH secretion in the absence of structural hypothalamic-pituitary disease, usually in women who have psychological problems or those who exercise excessively or who have lost weight.[2] The men studied by Nachtigall et al. were not exercising excessively nor had they lost weight. Perhaps more important, a small decrease in GnRH secretion undoubtedly has more obvious clinical consequences in women—loss of cyclic pituitary-gonadal function and amenorrhea—than in men—a modest fall in serum testosterone.

R.D. Utiger, M.D.

References

1. Spratt DI, Carr DB, Merriam GR, et al: The spectrum of abnormal patterns of gonadotropin-releasing hormone secretion in men with idiopathic hypogonadotropic hypogonadism: Clinical and laboratory correlations. *J Clin Endocrinol Metab* 64:283–291, 1987.
2. Yen SSC: Female hypogonadotropic hypogonadism: Hypothalamic amenorrhea syndrome. *Endocrinol Metab Clin North Am* 22:29–58, 1993.

29 Carbohydrate Metabolism and Diabetes Mellitus

Disordered Eating Behavior and Microvascular Complications in Young Women With Insulin-dependent Diabetes Mellitus
Rydall AC, Rodin GM, Olmsted MP, et al (Toronto Hosp; Hosp for Sick Children, Toronto; Univ of Toronto)
N Engl J Med 336:1849–1854, 1997   29–1

Background.—Insulin-dependent (type 1) diabetes mellitus is a common chronic illness of childhood and adolescence in North America. Many young women with type 1 diabetes may also have eating disturbances, which could affect diabetes management. The natural history of disordered eating behavior was studied in young women with type 1 diabetes.

TABLE 2.—Prevalence and Persistence of Disordered Eating Behavior in Young Women With Insulin-dependent Diabetes Mellitus

BEHAVIOR*	BASE LINE	FOLLOW-UP	BOTH TIMES	P VALUE FOR PREVALENCE†	P VALUE FOR PERSISTENCE‡
		number (percent)			
Binge eating (n = 87)	39 (45)	48 (55)	31 (36)	0.11	<0.001
Omission on underdosing of insulin for weight loss (n = 88)	12 (14)	30 (34)	5 (6)	0.003	0.53
Self-induced vomiting (n = 89)	7 (8)	15 (17)	4 (4)	0.06	0.01
Laxative use (n = 88)	2 (2)	7 (8)	1 (1)	0.13	0.15
Dieting for weight loss (n = 90)	34 (38)	49 (54)	26 (29)	0.01	0.002

*Only patients who responded to each item on both the baseline and follow-up questionnaires were included in each analysis.
†The P values are for comparison of the prevalence of each form of behavior between baseline and follow-up, by McNemar's test.
‡The P values are for the persistence of disordered eating behavior, by Fisher's exact test.
(Reprinted by permission of *The New England Journal of Medicine*, from Rydall AC, Rodin GM, Olmstead MP, et al: Disordered eating behavior and microvascular complications in young women with insulin-dependent diabetes mellitus. *N Engl J Med* 336:1849–1854, 1997. Copyright 1997, Massachusetts Medical Society.)

Study Design.—From June to December 1988, 121 female patients aged 12–18 years with type 1 diabetes were recruited to participate in a self-reported survey of eating attitudes and behaviors. Of those participants, 91 were recontacted 4–5 years later for follow-up.

Results.—At baseline assessment, 29% of the 91 women in the study group had highly or moderately disordered eating behavior, which persisted in 18% and improved in 11%. Of those women with normal eating behavior at baseline, 15% had disordered eating at follow-up (Table 2). Omission or underdosing of insulin to lose weight was reported by 14% at baseline and 34% at follow-up. At baseline, average hemoglobin A_{lc} values were higher in the group with highly disordered eating habits than in the other groups. Disordered eating behavior at baseline was significantly associated with retinopathy at 4-year follow-up.

Conclusions.—Disordered eating behavior is common and persistent in young women with type 1 diabetes. It is associated with decreased metabolic control and increased risk of diabetic retinopathy. Routine screening for eating disturbances may be indicated for young women with type 1 diabetes and intervention undertaken if necessary to prevent later complications.

▶ It should be no surprise that young women with type 1 diabetes who have eating disorders, particularly those disorders characterized by marked variations in food intake, are likely to have difficulty controlling their diabetes and, therefore, an increased risk of the complications of the disease. Constancy of food intake is obviously important in patients taking insulin if major fluctuations in blood glucose concentrations are to be avoided, unless the patients are prepared to measure blood glucose and vary their insulin dosage constantly.

It is also probably no surprise that the frequency of eating disorders is high among young women with diabetes. To all the social and psychological factors that affect how adolescent girls and young women view their body image, and, therefore, alter their eating behavior, must be added the stresses imposed by advice from physicians and parents to maintain constant food intake and not to gain weight, plus the tendency of insulin to stimulate weight gain. Psychiatric problems in addition to eating disorders are common among older children and adolescents with diabetes; for example, in a recent study, 42% of 92 patients (49 girls) aged 8–14 years at the time of diagnosis of diabetes had a psychiatric disorder (including 6% with eating disorders) at some time during a 10-year follow-up period.[1]

Young women with diabetes who have eating disorders might be expected to have very unstable ("brittle") diabetes, with multiple episodes of diabetic ketoacidosis and hypoglycemia.[2] Rydall et al. did not systematically collect data on this point, but 6 of the women had 1–3 episodes of ketoacidosis and 14 had 1–4 episodes (and 1 had 20 episodes) of hypoglycemia during follow-up; the number of episodes of hypoglycemia is surely an underestimate.

Thus, although women with eating disorders may not often have brittle diabetes, their glycemic control is clearly not good. Those caring for young patients—especially young women—with diabetes must be alert to the presence of eating disorders and other psychiatric disturbances, or, better yet, try to anticipate them, for the sake of the patient's physical and mental health.

R.D. Utiger, M.D.

References

1. Kovacs M, Obrosky DS, Goldston D, et al: Psychiatric disorders in youths with IDDM: Rates and risk factors. *Diabetes Care* 20:36–44, 1997.
2. Kent LA, Gell GV, Williams G: Mortality and outcome of patients with brittle diabetes and recurrent ketoacidosis. *Lancet* 344:778–781, 1994.

Distinct Genetic and Immunological Features in Patients With Onset of IDDM Before and After Age 40
Lohmann T, Rotger J, Seissler J, et al (Univ of Leipzig, Germany; Diabetes Specialty Practice, Leipzig, Germany)
Diabetes 20:524–529, 1997
29–2

Background.—Although insulin-dependent diabetes mellitus (IDDM) is usually diagnosed in childhood or young adulthood, the disease occurs after age 40 years in a subgroup of patients. In this subgroup, residual β-cell function tends to be preserved and the frequencies of insulin autoantibodies and HLA-DR3/4 heterozygosity are lower, as compared with young patients with IDDM. A consecutive series of patients with IDDM was examined to define the genetic and immunologic features of IDDM with onset before and after age 40 years.

Methods.—Twenty-three patients (IDDM group 1) were diagnosed at a young age and 24 had disease onset after age 40 years (IDDM group 2). Children younger than age 12 years and patients with pancreatitis or who were receiving glucocorticoid therapy were excluded. The duration of diabetes was less than two years and most patients were moderately well controlled. Insulin treatment was started at diagnosis or within the first year after diagnosis. A control group included 12 normal subjects. Blood samples were obtained for measurements of islet-cell and other antibodies, T-cell responses to glutamic acid decarboxylase (GAD) peptides, and HLA class II isotypes. Islet-cell antibodies were measured by indirect immunofluorescence, and anti-GAD and anti-tyrosine phosphatase (IA 2) antibodies were measured by immunoprecipitation. five-day proliferation assays were used to test T-cell responses against GAD peptides. HLA class II alleles were typed by polymerase chain reaction.

Results.—The 2 IDDM groups did not differ significantly in duration of diabetes or frequency of ketonuria. Islet cell and GAD antibodies were present in most diabetic patients, but no normal subject. Antibodies to IA2 were present only in the group 1 patients and the other antibodies were more often present in this group than in group 2. T-cell responses to GAD peptides were detected in 67% of the group 1 patients and 71% of those in group 2. Compared with the group 2 patients, those in group 1 were more frequently HLA-DR4+/DQ8+ and less frequently HLA-DR2+/DQ0602+.

Conclusion.—Both groups of patients with IDDM had evidence of autoimmunity, such as islet-related antibodies. Patients with late-onset disease, however, differed from those with earlier onset disease with respect to antibody profiles. These findings may help clinicians recognize latent autoimmune IDDM in adults and to identify those patients who may need early insulin therapy.

▶ Type 1 (autoimmune) diabetes is not exclusively a disease of children and young adults. The peak incidence is at the time of puberty, but there is a second small peak in incidence in the fifth decade of life.[1] As compared with patients less than 20 years of age, the duration of symptoms before diagnosis is longer in older patients and their islet function, as measured by basal and stimulated serum C-peptide concentrations, is reduced less.[2] The frequency of positive tests for islet-cell antibodies—the most widely available and sensitive test for autoimmune diabetes—has varied, being similar in younger and older patients in some studies but higher in young patients in other studies, including this one.[2, 3] The frequency of positive tests for anti–glutamic acid decarboxylase (GAD) and anti–tyrosine phosphatase (IA2) antibodies has also tended to be higher in young patients, but not greatly so. Anti–islet cell antibodies seem to have cytotoxic actions, but whether the other antibodies do anything to islets is not known.

As a practical matter, the important question is not whether there are immunologic differences between younger and older patients with autoimmune diabetes, but whether the older patients can be distinguished from those who have nonautoimmune diabetes (e.g., non–insulin-dependent diabetes, especially those who are not obese). This distinction may be important in deciding whether to try an oral hypoglycemic drug—particularly one of those such as glipizide or glyburide that act mostly by stimulating insulin secretion—or just give insulin. The simple pragmatic approach is to try a drug and see what happens. Measuring serum C-peptide or possibly other antibodies can also provide information to help make the choice between the 2 treatments.

R.D. Utiger, M.D.

References

1. Krolewski AS, Warram JH, Rand LLI, et al: Epidemiologic approach to the etiology of type 1 diabetes mellitus and its complications. *N Engl J Med* 317:1390–1398, 1987.
2. Karjalainen J, Salmela P, Ilonen J, et al: A comparison of childhood and adult type 1 diabetes mellitus. *N Engl J Med* 220:881–886, 1989.
3. Vandewalle CL, Falomi A, Svanholm S, et al: High diagnostic sensitivity of glutamate decarboxylase autoantibodies in insulin-dependent diabetes mellitus with clinical onset between age 20 and 40 years. *J Clin Endocrinol Metab* 80:846–851, 1995.

Reduction of Postprandial Hyperglycemia and Frequency of Hypoglycemia in IDDM Patients on Insulin-Analog Treatment

Anderson JH Jr, Brunelle RL, Koivisto VA, et al (Helsinki Univ, Finland)
Diabetes 46:265–270, 1997   29–3

Background.—Insulin lispro is a recently developed insulin analogue that acts rapidly and has a short duration of action. The effects of insulin lispro for pre-meal therapy of patients with type 1 diabetes mellitus was studied.

Methods.—This multinational, multicenter, open-label crossover trial included 1,008 patients. For 6 months, injections of insulin lispro were

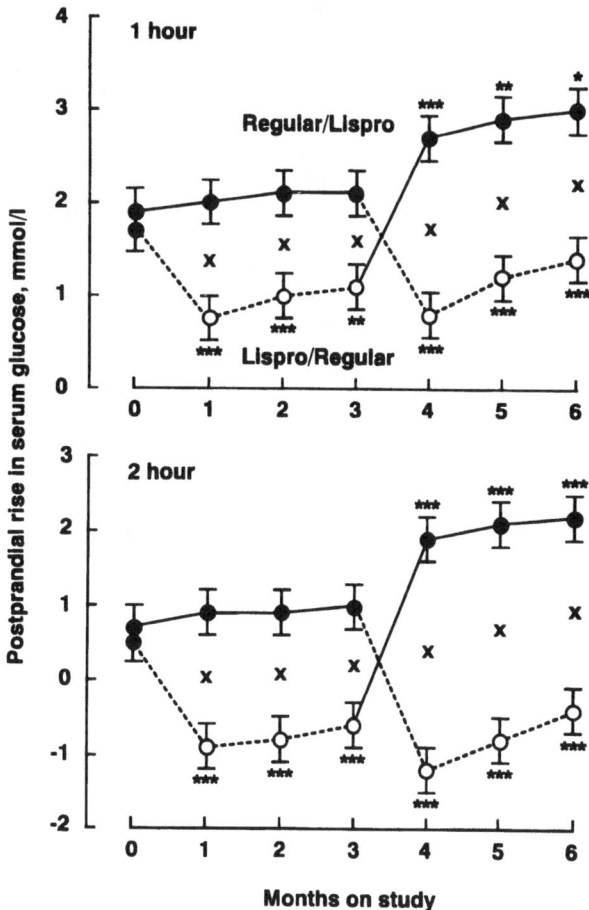

FIGURE 1.—The 1- and 2-h postprandial serum glucose excursion at each visit during the study. Pre-meal injections were either regular human insulin (●) or insulin lispro (○). *$P<0.05$; **$P<0.01$; ***P <0.001, compared with baseline; *$P<0.001$ between regular human insulin and insulin lispro. (Courtesy of Anderson JH Jr, Brunelle RL, Koivisto VA, et al: Reduction of postprandial hyperglycemia and frequency of hypoglycemia in IDDM patients on insulin-analog treatment. *Diabetes* 46:265–270, 1997.)

given immediately before meals, and injections of regular human insulin were given 30–45 minutes before meals.

Findings.—The postprandial increase in serum glucose was significantly lower during insulin lispro treatment throughout the study. At 6 months, the postprandial increase in serum glucose was reduced at 1 hour by 1.3 mmol/L (23 mg/dL) and at 2 hours by 2 mmol/L (36 mg/dL) in patients receiving insulin lispro. In addition, the rate of hypoglycemia during insulin lispro therapy was 12% lower than during regular insulin therapy, independent of the basal insulin regimen or HbA_{1c} values (Fig 1). An analysis of the total number of episodes of hypoglycemia for each patient according to time of occurrence revealed that fewer episodes occurred with insulin lispro than with regular human insulin therapy in 3 of the 4 quarters of the day. The greatest relative improvement was at night.

Conclusions.—Compared with regular human insulin, insulin lispro improves postprandial control in patients with type 1 diabetes mellitus. It also reduces the frequency of hypoglycemic episodes.

▶ Regular insulin has traditionally been considered short-acting, but serum insulin concentrations are highest about 60–120 minutes after its subcutaneous injection. In contrast, serum insulin concentrations are highest about 30 minutes after a meal in normal subjects. Therefore, to minimize postmeal excursions in serum glucose in diabetic patients, regular insulin should be given about 30 minutes before the meal, and the closer the injection to the meal, the greater the risk of hypoglycemia several hours after the meal.

Insulin lispro is insulin in which the sequence of lysine and proline residues in the B chain of the 2-chain insulin molecule has been reversed. As a result, the insulin molecules aggregate much less at injection sites, and the insulin is more rapidly absorbed into the circulation and acts more rapidly. Therefore, the insulin can be given nearer meal time and is less likely to cause hypoglycemia several hours later. This study by Anderson et al. nicely demonstrates the ability of insulin lispro to reduce postmeal rises in serum glucose concentrations and reduce the frequency of hypoglycemia several hours after the meal, even if overall glycemic regulation, as determined by HbA_{1c} values, was similar in the 2 groups. Mixing insulin lispro with intermediate- or long-acting insulin attenuates its action, as it attenuates the action of regular insulin, but the differences between insulin lispro and regular insulin persist.

Insulin lispro is the first of a series of insulin analogues, both short- and long-acting, to become available.[1] Its rapid onset and dissipation of action should provide diabetic patients treated with premeal short-acting insulin one or more times daily with more flexibility and safety, and consideration should be given to using it in patients—usually those with type 1 diabetes—who are to be managed with 1 daily injection of long-acting insulin plus pre-meal doses of rapid-acting insulin.

R.D. Utiger, M.D.

Reference

1. Barnett AH, Owens DR: Insulin analogues. *Lancet* 349:47–51, 1997.

The Safety of Injecting Insulin Through Clothing

Fleming DR, Fitzgerald JT, Jacober SJ, et al (Wayne State Univ, Detroit; Univ of Michigan, Ann Arbor)
Diabetes Care 20:244–247, 1997   29–4

Objective.—Typial antiseptic practices for injecting insulin are time-consuming and complicated. Although many patients inject the drug through their clothing, there have been no studies on the safety of this practice. Results of a 20-week, single-blinded, prospective, cross-over trial comparing the safety and perceived benefits of injecting insulin through clothing vs. conventional subcutaneous injection practice were evaluated.

Methods.—At enrollment and at 10 weeks and 20 weeks of the study, blood analyses were performed on 50 patients randomly allocated to the conventional thigh injection technique or the through-clothing thigh injection technique and crossed over at 10 weeks. White blood cell counts, differential counts, and glycosylated hemoglobin (HbA_{1c}) values were compared for the 2 groups. Patients were to record problems, perceived benefits, and other comments in log books.

Results.—Forty-two patients (21 women), aged 23–63 years, who completed the study. The average duration of diabetes was 14 years. A total of 7,275 injections through clothing were made. There were no significant differences in white blood cell or neutrophil counts or HbA_{1c} values between groups at any time point. Perceived benefits according to log entries were convenience of injecting through clothing, particularly when away from home, and less constraint in rotating injection sites. Difficulty in injecting through thick clothing and small blood stains on clothing were listed as disadvantages.

Conclusion.—Injecting insulin through clothing does not pose a safety risk.

▶ The results of this study provide support for what many patients have long been doing, probably often unknown to their doctors. As evidence, the authors describe a retrospective survey of 21 diabetic patients who had been injecting insulin (an estimated 66,807 injections) through clothing for years with not a single infection. The results of the prospective study certainly confirm the safety and benefits of through-clothing injection; the danger seems to be greater to the clothing than to the patient. The study patients were asked to inject insulin only into the thighs during both phases of the study, but injection through clothing into the abdomen—assuming not too many undergarments—or arms should be equally innocuous and convenient.

As the benefits of close control of hyperglycemia have become more evident, patients are being advised to take insulin more often. Any way to simplify therapy is, therefore, welcome, and telling patients they can safely inject insulin through clothing should be especially welcome because so many now eat away from home.

R.D. Utiger, M.D.

Acarbose in the Treatment of Type I Diabetes

Hollander P, Pi-Sunyer X, Coniff RF (Park Nicollet Clinic, St Louis Park, Minn; St Luke's/Roosevelt Ctr, New York; Bayer Corp, West Haven, Conn)
Diabetes Care 20:248–253, 1997   29–5

Introduction.—Acarbose, a complex oligosaccharide that inhibits intestinal glucosidoses, represents a novel therapeutic approach for the treatment of hyperglycemia in diabetic patients. This study was done to determine the long-term safety and efficacy of acarbose with diet and insulin therapy in patients with insulin-dependent (type I) diabetes.

Methods.—Two hundred thirty six patients age 18 years and older participated in the 24-week study, 122 patients in the placebo group and 114 in the acarbose group. The acarbose was given by means of a forced titration protocol in dosages ranging from 50 to 300 mg 3 times a day. The patients were followed up every 6 weeks with a full-meal tolerance test in which plasma glucose was measured before the meal and 60, 90, and 120 minutes after it.

Results.—The mean plasma glucose concentration 60 minutes after the test meal was 59 mg/dl (3.3 mmol/L) lower and the mean glycohemoglobin (Hb A_{1c}) value was 0.48% lower in the acarbose group than in the placebo group at the end of the study. There was no difference in the incidence of hypoglycemia between the treatment groups. The acarbose-treated patients had more gastrointestinal symptoms, including flatulence, diarrhea, and abdominal pain.

Conclusion.—For the treatment of type I diabetes, acarbose was found to be safe and effective agent when given in combination with diet and insulin therapy. With acarbose, postprandial plasma glucose and HbA_{1c} values were significantly decreased, with no increase in the incidence of hypoglycemia.

▶ Acarbose inhibits intestinal glucosidase activity, so that complex dietary carbohydrates are not broken down to form glucose and other monosaccharides. Most studies of acarbose have been done in patients with non-insulin-dependent (Type II) diabetes mellitus; in these patients, the drug reduces postprandial blood glucose concentrations sufficiently to lower HbA_{1c} values by about 0.8%.[1]

The effect of acarbose on HbA_{1c} values in this study of patients with insulin-dependent diabetes was smaller, but, nevertheless, it reduced the postprandial rises in plasma glucose concentrations after the 600-calorie test meal by about 60 mg/dL (3.3 mmol/L) without increasing the frequency of hypoglycemia. The final dose of acarbose was 300 mg 3 times daily, and the fall in HbA_{1c} averaged about 0.3% at the end of the treatment periods with 50 mg, 100 mg, and 200 mg before each meal. Looked at in terms of individual patients, however, the results do not seem as good. Only 19% of the acarbose-treated patients had a fall in HbA_{1c} of 1% or more, as compared with 8% in the placebo group. Acarbose often causes abdominal pain, bloating, or diarrhea, and in this study, 18% of the patients stopped taking it for these reasons.

Does acarbose have a role for patients with Type I diabetes? It may be a safer way to reduce postprandial rises in plasma glucose concentrations than by giving more pre-meal regular insulin (or lispro insulin; see Abstract 29–3). If the results of this study are correct, only a minority of patients will benefit appreciably from acarbose, but it still may be worth trying.

R.D. Utiger, M.D.

Reference

1. 1996 YEAR BOOK OF MEDICINE, pp 576–578.

Islet Transplantation in IDDM Patients
Secchi A, Socci C, Maffi P, et al (Univ of Milan, Italy; Istituto Nazionale dei Tumori, Milan, Italy)
Diabetologia 40:225–231, 1997   29–6

Background.—Several studies have demonstrated that intrahepatic transplantation of purified islets can replace pancreatic endocrine function in diabetic patients without major side effects. However, data from the International Islet Transplant Registry are not encouraging: only 16% of 180 patients treated between 1989 and 1994 were able to maintain insulin independence for more than 1 week. Factors correlating with success after islet allotransplantation in patients with type 1 diabetes mellitus at 1 center were investigated.

Methods and Findings.—After or along with kidney transplantation, 21 intrahepatic transplantations of fresh cadaver islets were done in 20 patients. One patient, who died from cardiac arrest several hours after islet transplantation, was not included in the final analysis. Acute, irreversible, early failure of islet function, presumed to be rejection, occurred in 15% of the patients. Forty-five percent of the patients had complete insulin independence or a more than 50% decrease in exogenous insulin requirements for from 1 to 40 months. Liver biopsy performed 3 years after transplantation in 1 patient revealed normal islets in the hepatic parenchyma. Forty percent of the patients had no benefit from islet transplantation. Metabolic studies in patients with successful results demonstrated an early phase of insulin release after arginine, mild postprandial hyperglycemia and normal HbA_{1c} values. Successful islet transplantation correlated positively with the number of islets that were transplanted.

Conclusions.—Islet transplantation is a safe procedure, with a 45% success rate as defined by transient insulin independence or substantial reduction of exogenous insulin requirement.

▶ Transplantation of pancreatic islets would seem the ideal treatment for patients with type 1 diabetes mellitus. Islets can easily be injected into the portal vein so they end up in the liver, the site that insulin and other islet hormones normally reach and act upon first, and islet transplantation would avoid the drainage and inflammatory problems that accompany pancreatic transplantation. Unfortunately, islet transplantation has not often been successful. A lot of islets are needed, and sometimes the minimum number needed—about 6,000 per kg, according to Secchi et al.—cannot be obtained from a single pancreas. What is worse, of course, is the poor success rate.

I include this article because patients ask about transplantation of insulin-producing tissue. What they must be told is that, at present, it can be done only by pancreatic transplantation, and that is nearly always done only when the patient also has end-stage renal disease and needs renal transplantation. This policy is easy to justify; substituting the necessary immunosuppressive therapy for insulin injections is not an even trade-off in terms of safety, cost, or efficacy, even if tissue availability was not a problem. Among patients receiving cadaver pancreas-kidney transplants, about 70% do not need insulin 1 year later,[1] and 3% to 5% have graft failure and must resume insulin therapy each year thereafter. These results are obviously better that those after islet transplantation, but it seems clear that any form of transplantation therapy for diabetes will be widely feasible only when ways can be found to grow insulin-secreting cells in vitro and problems of graft failure can be overcome.

R.D. Utiger, M.D.

Reference

1. Gruessner AC, Sutherland DERC: Pancreas transplant registry, United Network for Organ Sharing and International Data Report, in Terasaki PI, Cecka JM (eds): *Clinical Transplants—1994.* Los Angeles, UCLA Tissue Typing Laboratory, 1995, pp 47–69.

Randomised Placebo-controlled Trial of Lisinopril in Normotensive Patients With Insulin-dependent Diabetes and Normoalbuminuria or Microalbuminuria
Chaturvedi N, and the EUCLID Study Group (Univ College, London)
Lancet 349:1787–1792, 1997   29-7

Background.—People with insulin-dependent (type 1) diabetes mellitus have higher rates of morbidity and mortality than the general population. Some of this increased risk is the result of renal and cardiovascular com-

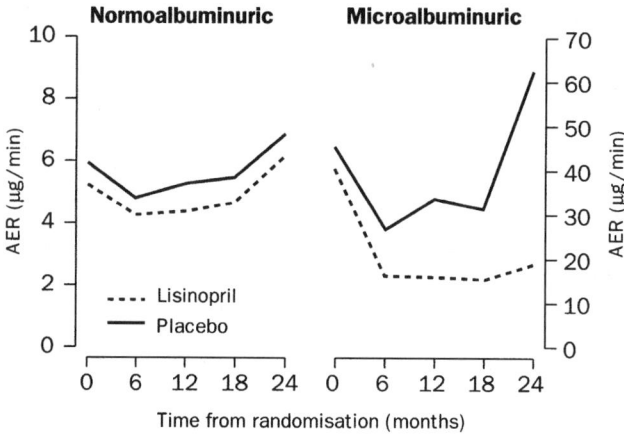

FIGURE 4.—Albumin excretion rate (AER) over time in EUCLID by initial microalbuminuric status. (Courtesy of Chaturvedi N and the EUCLID Study Group: Randomised placebo-controlled trial of lisinopril in normotensive Patients with insulin-dependent diabetes mellitus and normoalbuminuria or microalbuminuria. *Lancet* 349:1787–1792, 1997. Copyright 1997 by the Lancet Ltd.)

plications of diabetes. A prognostic factor for these complications is the appearance of protein, mostly albumin, in the urine. Elevated blood pressure is a modifiable risk factor for progression of renal disease. Inhibitors of angiotensin-converting enzyme (ACE) appear to be especially effective in controlling renal-disease progression in patients with type 1 diabetes and macroalbuminuria. To determine its effect in patients with type 1 diabetes with microalbuminuria or normoalbuminuria, a 2-year, randomized, placebo-controlled, clinical trial with the ACE-inhibitor lisinopril was performed.

Study Design.—The EURODIAB controlled trial of lisinopril in type 1 diabetes (EUCLID) was a double-blind, randomized, parallel-design clinical trial of lisinopril and placebo conducted at 18 European centers. Men and women aged 20–59 years with type 1 diabetes were recruited for this study if their resting blood pressure was at least 75 and no more than 90 mm Hg diastolic and no more than 155 mm Hg systolic. At their initial visit, participants had blood pressure readings to determine eligibility and were issued 1 month's supply of placebo to determine compliance. One month later, at the randomization visit, blood pressure was reassessed. 530 Patients were enrolled stratified by center and extent of albuminuria. Patients were re-examined at 1, 3, 6, 12, 18, and 24 months.

Results.—There were no significant differences in baseline characteristics of the patients by treatment group. Intention-to-treat analysis at 2 years demonstrated that albumin excretion rate was 2.2 μg/min lower in the treatment group than in the placebo group. This was equivalent to an 18.8% difference between the albuminuria groups. Among the patients with microalbuminuria, in albumin excretion rate difference was 34.2

µg/min. For those who completed the full 2 years of this trial, the difference was 38.5 µg/min in those with microalbuminuria and 0.23 µg/min in those with normoalbuminuria at baseline (Fig 4). There was no difference in hypoglycemic events or in metabolic control between the 2 treatment groups.

Conclusions.—The ACE-inhibitor lisinopril was of clinical benefit to a large group of patients with type 1 diabetes with early signs of renal disease, but without hypertension. The effect was greater in patients with microalbuminuria than in patients with normoalbuminuria, but the exact threshold where therapy should begin could not be determined. Long-term follow-up is required to determine the full impact of lisinopril therapy on outcome.

▶ No one questions now that microalbuminuria (urinary albumin excretion of 20–200 µg/min [30–300 mg/day]) is a risk factor for not only macroalbuminuria, but also renal insufficiency in patients with type 1 diabetes mellitus. And it is clear that treatment with an ACE inhibitor slows the increase in urinary albumin excretion and the decline in renal function in normotensive and hypertensive patients with either type 1 or type 2 diabetes.[1-3] In fact, treatment with an ACE inhibitor has become standard practice in diabetic patients with microalbuminuria.

The EUCLID study group consisted of patients with type 1 diabetes with both microalbuminuria (15%) and normoalbuminuria (85%). The results in the former group provide further evidence that ACE-inhibitor therapy slows the increase in urinary albumin excretion in patients with microalbuminuria. The more important finding is the lack of effect of ACE-inhibitor therapy in the much larger group of patients with normoalbuminuria. In this context, however, it should be remembered that only about 30% of patients with type 1 diabetes ever have overt diabetic nephropathy (renal failure and end-stage renal disease), and that, among them, microalbuminuria usually appears after they have had diabetes for about 10 years. The mean duration of diabetes in the patients in this study was 13 years, and all had had diabetes for at least 8 years, so many of those with normoalbuminuria may well be among the fortunate 70% not destined to have diabetic nephropathy.

This reasoning leads to the conclusion that ACE-inhibitor therapy is not indicated in normotensive patients with normoalbuminuria, at least those who have had diabetes for about a decade. What is needed now is a study of ACE inhibition limited to patients with normoalbuminuria who have had diabetes for less time.

R.D. Utiger, M.D.

References

1. Viberti GC, Mogensen CE, Groop LC, et al: Effect of captopril on progression to clinical proteinuria in patients with insulin-dependent diabetes mellitus and microalbuminuria. *JAMA* 271:274–279, 1994. (1995 YEAR BOOK OF MEDICINE, p 675.)
2. Lewis EJ, Hunsicker LG, Bain RP, et al: The effect of angiotensin-converting enzyme inhibition on diabetic nephropathy. *N Engl J Med* 329:1456–1462, 1993.

3. Ravid M, Lang R, Rachmani R, et al: Long-term effect of angiotensin-converting enzyme inhibition in non-insulin-dependent diabetes mellitus: A 7-year follow-up study. *Arch Intern Med* 156:286–289, 1996. (1997 YEAR BOOK OF MEDICINE, p 561.)

Estrogen Replacement Therapy Decreases Hyperandrogenicity and Improves Glucose Homeostasis and Plasma Lipids in Postmenopausal Women With Noninsulin-dependent Diabetes Mellitus
Andersson B, Mattsson L-Å, Hahn L, et al (Sahlgren's Hosp, Göteborg, Sweden; Univ of Göteborg, Sweden)
J Clin Endocrinol Metab 82:638–643, 1997   29–8

Introduction.—There is a close correlation between hyperandrogenicity (as indicated by low serum concentrations of sex hormone–binding globulin (SHBG)) and insulin resistance in women. A low serum SHBG concentration is a strong and independent risk factor for type 2 diabetes mellitus serum in women. Women who were postmenopausal, had diabetes, and had low serum SHBG concentrations were treated with estradiol to determine its effect on hyperandrogenicity and insulin resistance.

Methods.—Twenty-five women with diabetes who were naturally or surgically postmenopausal (21 vs. 4 women) and had serum SHBG concentrations less than 60 nmol/L received 2 mg 17-β-estradiol for 30 days with 1 mg norethisterone acetate for 10 days in a double-blind, cross-over, placebo-controlled trial. At baseline and after 2 cycles of active or placebo treatment, samples were obtained for measurements of blood glucose, glycosylated hemoglobin, and serum insulin, C-peptide, lipoproteins, sex steroid hormones, growth hormone, and insulin-like growth factor I (IGF-I) concentrations. The euglycemic hyperinsulinemic clamp method was used to determine insulin sensitivity.

Results.—There was a marked increase in serum SHBG concentrations and a decrease in serum-free testosterone concentrations during the estradiol treatment period, as compared with the placebo period. There also was a significant decrease in blood glucose, glycosylated hemoglobin, and serum C-peptide, total cholesterol, low-density lipoprotein cholesterol, and IGF-I concentrations, and a significant increase in serum high-density lipoprotein cholesterol concentrations during estradiol treatment.

Conclusion.—Estrogen replacement therapy decreased hyperandrogenism, decreased hyperglycemia, and improved serum lipids in postmenopausal women with diabetes.

▶ In normal, postmenopausal women, estrogen replacement therapy has little effect on glucose homeostasis. It does, however, increase insulin sensitivity, and insulin secretion declines slightly.[1] This decline probably contributes to the beneficial effect of estrogen on coronary heart disease morbidity and mortality in postmenopausal women, because insulin may act on endothelial cells as a growth factor. (It is generally accepted that the ability of estrogen to lower serum low-density lipoprotein (LDL) cholesterol concentrations and raise serum high-density lipoprotein (HDL) cholesterol concentrations[1] in these women does not account for all the benefit, and that estrogen has some more direct vascular actions.)

Does estrogen have similar effects in postmenopausal women with type 2 diabetes mellitus? According to Andersson et al., it does, at least in women with diabetes who are receiving diet or oral hypoglycemic drug therapy (hemoglobin A1c values of 7.0% or higher) and have mild androgen excess (as defined by a serum SHBG concentration of less than 60 nmol/L). We are not told the normal range for serum SHBG (or serum total or free testosterone) in the authors' laboratory, or how many women with NIDDM had to be screened to find women who met these criteria. These unknowns obviously affect the generalizability of the results. Nevertheless, estrogen had the expected effects on serum LDL and HDL cholesterol concentrations; it increased insulin sensitivity, as measured by the increase in glucose disappearance rate, and it decreased hyperandrogenism.

The extent to which these changes were caused by the decrease in hyperandrogenism, whatever its extent, is uncertain. Estrogen raises serum SHBG concentrations and, therefore, lowers serum-free testosterone concentrations in all women. Lowering insulin secretion has the same effect in women with insulin resistance and hyperinsulinemia.[2] With respect to the estrogen-induced changes in serum LDL and HDL cholesterol concentrations, the action of estrogen in improving insulin sensitivity is likely to be more important than its action to lower serum-free testosterone concentrations.

Whatever the details of the interactions among estrogen, androgen, insulin, and cholesterol, I see these results as more evidence that increasing insulin sensitivity is beneficial in ways that extend beyond reducing hyperglycemia. Estrogen therapy may be even more strongly indicated in women with diabetes than in nondiabetic women.

R.D. Utiger, M.D.

References

1. Nabulsi AA, Folsom AR, White A, et al: Association of hormone-replacement therapy with various cardiovascular risk factors in postmenopausal women. *N Engl J Med* 328:1069–1075, 1993.
2. Dunaif A, Scott D, Finegood D, et al: The insulin-sensitizing agent troglitazone improves metabolic and reproductive abnormalities in the polycystic ovary syndrome. *J Clin Endocrinol Metab* 81:3299–3306, 1996.

Subscribe to the related journal in your field!

Yes! Begin my one-year subscription to *Disease-a-Month®* (12 issues).

Name _____

Institution _____

Address _____

City _____ State _____

ZIP/PC _____ Country _____

Specialty _____
(Students/residents, please list Institution)

Subscription prices (through 9/30/98)

		USA	Canada*	Int'l
Individuals	❏	$88.00	$110.21	$103.00
Institutions	❏	136.00	161.57	151.00
Students, residents	❏	49.00	68.48	64.00

Method of payment

Enclose payment (check or credit card number) and we'll send an extra issue FREE!

❏ Check (in U.S. dollars, drawn on a U.S. bank, and payable to *Disease-a-Month®*)

❏ VISA ❏ MasterCard ❏ Discover
❏ AmEx ❏ Bill me Exp. date_____

Card #_____

Signature _____

*Includes Canadian GST

Individual/student subscriptions must be in the name of, billed to, and paid for by the individual.

Airmail rates available upon request.
Prices subject to change without notice.

J062983YC

Reservation Card for the Year Book

Yes! I would like my own copy of *Year Book of Medicine®* at the price of **$75.00** plus sales tax, postage, and handling. Please begin my subscription with the current edition according to the terms described below.* I understand that I will have 30 days to examine each annual edition.

Name _____

Address _____

City _____ State _____ ZIP_____

Method of Payment

Check (in U.S. dollars, drawn on a U.S. bank, payable to *Year Book of Medicine®*)

❏ VISA   ❏ MasterCard   ❏ Discover   ❏ AmEx   ❏ Bill me

Card number _____ Exp. date: _____

Signature _____

Prices are subject to change without notice.   PMC-018

Your Year Book service guarantee:

When you subscribe to the *Year Book*, you will receive advance notice of future annual volumes about two months before publication. To receive the new edition, you need do nothing—we'll send you the new volume as soon as it is available. If you want to discontinue, the advance notice allows you time to notify us of your decision. If you are not completely satisfied, you have 30 days to return any *Year Book*.

BUSINESS REPLY MAIL
FIRST-CLASS MAIL   PERMIT NO 135   ST LOUIS MO

POSTAGE WILL BE PAID BY ADDRESSEE

SUBSCRIPTION SERVICES
MOSBY–YEAR BOOK, INC.
11830 WESTLINE INDUSTRIAL DRIVE
ST. LOUIS   MO 63146-9988

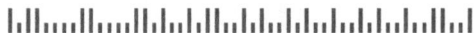

BUSINESS REPLY MAIL
FIRST-CLASS MAIL   PERMIT NO 135   ST LOUIS MO

POSTAGE WILL BE PAID BY ADDRESSEE

M Mosby

PAT NEWMAN
11830 WESTLINE INDUSTRIAL DRIVE
PO BOX 46908
ST. LOUIS   MO 63146-9934

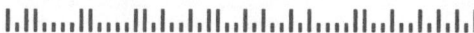

Want to speed up the process?

**To order the *Year Book*,
you also may call 1-800-426-4545**

**To subscribe to the journal today,
call toll-free in the U.S.:
1-800-453-4351
or fax 314-432-1158
Outside the U.S., call: 314-453-4351**

Visit us at:
www.mosby.com/Mosby/Periodicals

Mosby–Year Book, Inc.
Subscription Services
11830 Westline Industrial Drive
St. Louis, MO   63146   U.S.A.

M Mosby

Randomised Placebo-controlled Trial of Granulocyte-colony Stimulating Factor in Diabetic Foot Infection

Gough A, Clapperton M, Rolando N, et al (King's College School of Medicine and Dentistry, London)

Lancet 350:855–859, 1997   29-9

Background.—Diabetic patients have impaired neutrophil superoxide generation, which is an essential part of neutrophil bactericidal activity. Granulocyte colony stimulating factor (G-CSF) increases neutrophil release from the bone marrow and improves neutrophil function. The value of G-CSF as adjuvant therapy for the treatment of foot infections in diabetic patients was investigated.

Methods.—Forty diabetic patients with foot infections participated in the double-blind, placebo-controlled trial. The patients were randomly assigned to treatment with G-CSF (filgrastim) or placebo for 7 days. Both groups received similar antibiotic and insulin therapy. Neutrophils from peripheral blood obtained from the patients and from normal subjects were stimulated with opsonized zymosan. and Superoxide production was measured by spectrophotometric assay.

Findings.—Treatment with G-CSF was associated with earlier eradication of pathogens from the infected ulcer, faster resolution of cellulitis, briefer hospitalization, and a shorter duration of intravenous antibiotic therapy. None of the patients given G-CSF needed surgery, as compared

TABLE 2.—Clinical Outcome and Metabolic Control

	G-CSF	Placebo	p
Median (range) time in days			
To hospital discharge	10 (7–31)	17·5 (9–100)	0·02
To resolution of cellulitis	7 (5–20)	12 (5–93)	0·03
To withdrawal of intravenous antibiotics	8·5 (5–30)	14·5 (8–63)	0·02
To negative swab culture*	4 (2–10)	8 (2–79)	0·02
Foot temperature difference (°C)			
Baseline	4·3 (1·4–11·2)	3·1 (0–9·1)	0·033
Day 7	1·1 (0·1–2·8)	2·1 (0·1–5·8)	0·011
Number of patients			
Surgery†	0	4 (20%)	0·114
Cellulitis resolved at day 7	11 (55%)	4 (20%)	0·05
Ulcer healed at day 7‡	4 (21%)	0	0·09
Glucose (mmol/L)	12·4 (3·0–27·2)	11·5 (2·7–24·4)	0·42
Insulin dose (U/kg daily)	0·58 (0·11–1·12)	0·48 (0·15–1·01)	0·38
Angiography			
Total	4	7	0·5
Percutaneous transluminal balloon angioplasty	2	3	
Vascular surgery	1	3	
No intervention	1	1	

*Time for positive wound swabs to become sterile (granulocyte colony-stimulating factor [G-CSF] N=16, placebo N=15).

†Débridement under general anesthesia and/or ray amputation.

‡1 G-CSF patient cellulitis alone.

(Courtesy of Gough A, Clapperton M, Rolando N, et al: Randomised placebo-controlled trial of granulocyte-colony stimulating factor in diabetic foot infection. *Lancet* 350:855–859, 1997. Copyright by The Lancet Ltd.)

with 4 patients in the placebo group. Two of the latter needed toe amputation and 2 required extensive débridement under anesthesia (Table 2). After treatment for 7 days, neutrophil superoxide production was significantly greater in the G-CSF group than in the placebo group. Treatment with G-CSF was generally well tolerated.

Conclusion.—Treatment with G-CSF improved the clinical outcomes of foot infection in diabetic patients. Increased neutrophil superoxide production may be responsible for this improvement.

▶ Foot infections can be a terrible problem in diabetic patients because of vascular and neurologic disease abetted by poor neutrophil function.[1] The standard treatment is hospitalization, débridement, and intravenous antibiotic therapy, although débridement and prolonged oral antibiotic therapy may be equally effective.[2] If Gough et al. are right, the addition of G-CSF will be very beneficial, resulting in less surgery and shorter hospitalizations.

With respect to some details that may have affected the results, most of the patients had ulcers for less than 6 weeks, 60% had osteomyelitis, pathogenic organisms were recovered in 78%, and the severity of hyperglycemia was similar in the 2 groups, both before and during hospitalization. The patients given G-CSF had threefold to fourfold increases in neutrophil counts during the week of treatment, whereas the counts decreased slightly in the placebo group. Therefore, the benefits of G-CSF might have been the result of its effects on neutrophil number, neutrophil function, or both. No matter, the benefit seems real, and, although G-CSF is expensive, it is not as expensive as a hospital day or an amputation.

R.D. Utiger, M.D.

References

1. Caputo GM, Cavanagh PR, Ulbrecht JS, et al: Assessment and management of foot disease in diabetic patients. *N Engl J Med* 331:854–860, 1994.
2. Eckman MH, Greenfield S, Mackey WC, et al: Foot infections in diabetic patients: Decision and cost-effectiveness analysis. *JAMA* 273:712–720, 1995.

30 Obesity and Lipid Metabolism

The Metabolic Significance of Leptin in Humans: Gender-based Differences in Relationship to Adiposity, Insulin Sensitivity, and Energy Expenditure
Kennedy A, Gettys TW, Watson P, et al (Med Univ of South Carolina, Charleston; Charleston Veterans Affairs Med Ctr, SC)
J Clin Endocrinol Metab 82:1293–1300, 1997   30–1

Background.—Leptin, an adipocyte-derived hormone, regulates body weight by interacting with putative receptors in the hypothalamus. The relationship between leptin and the metabolic abnormalities associated with obesity and the hormonal and substrate regulation of leptin were studied.

Methods.—One hundred sixteen men and women with a body mass index (BMI) ranging from 17 to 54 kg/m² were studied. Body composition, glucose intolerance, insulin sensitivity, energy expenditure, substrate utilization, and blood pressure were assessed. Glucose tolerance was normal in 85 subjects, and 31 (19 women and 12 men) type 2 had (non–insulin-dependent) diabetes mellitus.

Findings.—In both sexes, fasting serum leptin concentrations were strongly associated with BMI and percent body fat. Men had lower serum leptin concentrations than women at any given measure of obesity. Serum leptin concentrations increased 3.4 times faster as a function of BMI and 3.2 times faster as a function of body fat in women than in men (Fig 1). Hyperleptinemia was correlated with insulin resistance and a high waist-to-hip ratio in men only. However, during hyperinsulinemic euglycemic clamp studies, serum leptin concentrations increased only in women. Fasting leptin concentrations were not associated with resting energy expenditure and insulin-induced thermogenesis. Serum leptin concentrations were similar in the diabetic and non-diabetic subjects (Fig 1).

Conclusions.—Important sex differences exist in the regulation of leptin in humans. Although serum leptin concentrations rise with progressive obesity in both women and men, serum leptin concentrations are higher in women than men for any given measure of obesity, consistent with a state of relative leptin resistance. The lack of correlation between serum leptin

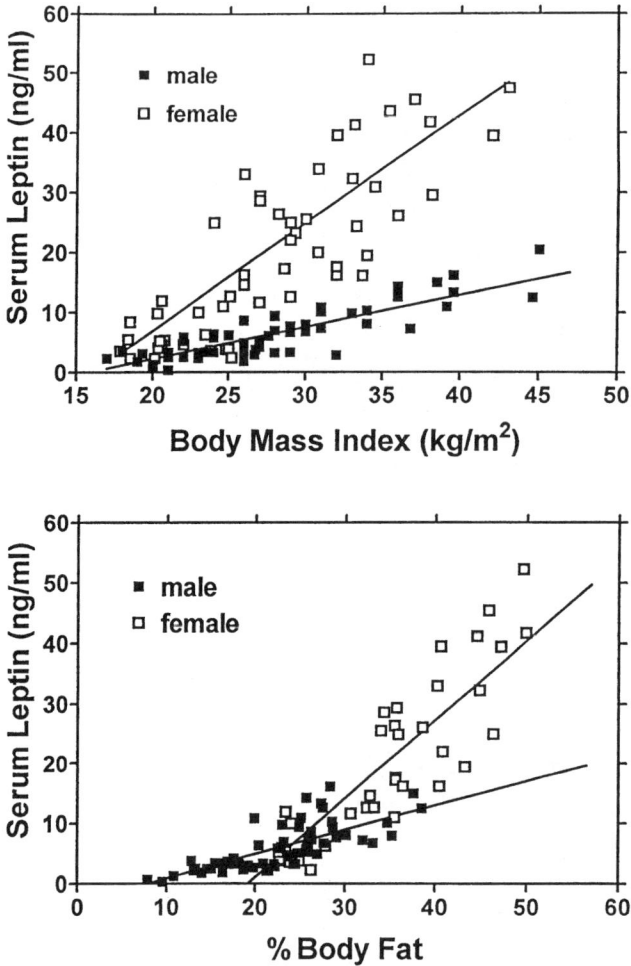

FIGURE 1.—Relationship between serum leptin and obesity in men and women. Serum leptin concentrations were measured in 116 subjects (62 men and 54 women) over a wide range of body mass indexes (17–54 kg/m^2) and percent body fat (7% to 50%). In individual men (*filled squares*) and women (*open squares*), values for body mass index (**upper panel**) and percent body fat (**lower panel**) were correlated with serum leptin concentrations. (Courtesy of Kennedy A, Gettys TW, Watson P, et al: The metabolic significance of leptin in humans: Gender-based differences in relationship to adoposity, insulin sensitivity, and energy expenditure. *J Clin Endocrinol Metab* 82:1293–1300, 1997. Copyright The Endocrine Society.)

and energy expenditure rates suggests that leptin regulates body fat mainly by changing eating behavior rather than calorigenesis.

Sexual Dimorphism in Plasma Leptin Concentration

Saad MF, Damani S, Gingerich RL, et al (Univ of Southern California, Los Angeles; Linco Research Inc, St Louis)

J Clin Endocrinol Metab 82:579–584, 1997   30–2

Background.—Leptin is the product of the *obese (ob)* gene. It appears to be a lipostatic hormone that affects the regulation of body weight by modulating feeding behavior or energy expenditure or both. The determinants of plasma leptin were assessed in subjects with normal glucose tolerance, impaired glucose tolerance, and type 2–non-insulin-dependent-diabetes.

Methods and Findings.—The subjects were 140 female and 127 male Asian Indians living in Los Angeles. Glucose tolerance was normal in 106 subjects and impaired in 102, and 59 type 2 had diabetes. Fasting plasma leptin concentrations ranged from 1.8 to 79.6 ng/mL. The concentrations were higher in obese subjects and were unaffected by changes in glucose tolerance (Fig 2). Also, the concentrations were about 40% greater in women than in men at any level of adiposity. After adjustment for body fat, postmenopausal women had higher plasma leptin concentrations than men of comparable age, but not different from those in younger women. In a multiple regression analysis, adiposity, sex, and fasting plasma insulin

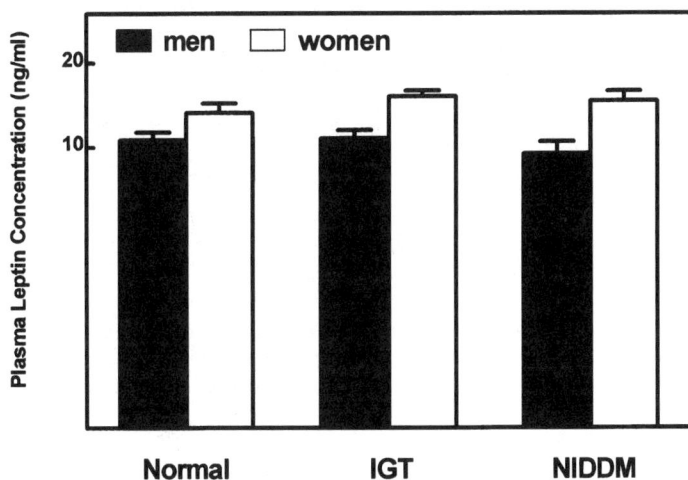

FIGURE 2.—Fasting plasma leptin concentrations, adjusted for percent body fat, in men and women in the three glucose tolerance categories. By 2-way analysis of variance: $P = 0.18$ for glucose tolerance status, and $P < 0.001$ for gender. *Abbreviations: IGT,* impaired glucose tolerance; *NIDDM,* non–insulin-dependent diabetes mellitus. (Courtesy of Saad MF, Damani S, Gingerich RL, et al: Sexual dimorphism in plasma leptin concentration. *J Clin Endocrinol Metab* 82:579–584, 1997. Copyright The Endocrine Society.)

concentrations were significant determinants of the plasma leptin concentration, accounting for 42%, 28%, and 2% of the respective variance. Plasma leptin was not significantly associated with age or waist/hip ratio.

Conclusions.—Sex is a major determinant of plasma leptin concentrations. This difference is apparently not a result of sex hormones or body fat distribution. The sexual dimorphism of leptin suggests that women may be resistant to its putative lipostatic actions and that it may have a function in reproduction.

▶ Leptin (from *leptos*, the Greek word for thin) inhibits food intake. It is the product of the *ob* gene, and is produced primarily and perhaps only by adipose tissue. As reported in these articles, serum leptin concentrations are more highly correlated with measures of adipose tissue mass, such as percent body fat, than weight or body mass index. These interrelationships hold true for both normal-weight and obese subjects; thus, in most humans, obesity is characterized by leptin resistance rather than deficiency (assuming the leptin that is produced has normal biological activity).

Serum leptin concentrations are higher in women than in men at any given level of adiposity, higher in girls than in boys,[1] and, at least among girls, higher concentrations (and more adiposity) are associated with earlier puberty.[2] In this regard, injections of leptin accelerate pubertal development in mice. Among subjects of similar adiposity, they are not different in diabetic and nondiabetic subjects, despite widely varying serum insulin concentrations, or among different races.[3] Both prolonged infusions of insulin (with glucose to maintain normal serum glucose concentrations) or glucose (which raises endogenous insulin secretion) raise serum leptin concentrations slightly.[4] The concentrations decline slightly in obese subjects who fasted for several days, but rise quickly when they are re-fed.[5] Among subjects with eating disorders, the concentrations are correlated with lack of adiposity, but not diagnosis (anorexia nervosa, bulimia, other).[6] Similarly, thyroxine and cortisol excess have little effect on serum leptin concentrations independent of adiposity.

It seems, therefore, that leptin production is little affected by either short-term metabolic perturbations, except alterations in caloric intake, or many disorders, except insofar as they affect adiopsity. Although high serum leptin concentrations do not seem to decrease food intake, they may somehow stimulate maturation of pituitary-gonadal function, thus being the signal leading to earlier sexual development in overweight children and later sexual development in very thin ones. Thus, it appears that obese humans are resistant to the appetite-suppressant actions of leptin but not its effects on reproduction.

R.D. Utiger, M.D.

References

1. Nagy TR, Gower BA, Trowbridge CA, et al: Effects of gender, ethnicity, body composition, and fat distribution on serum leptin concentrations in children. *J Clin Endocrinol Metab* 82:2148–2152, 1997.
2. Matkovic V, Ilich JK, Skugor M, et al: Leptin is inversely related to age at menarche in human females. *J Clin Endocrinol Metab* 82:3239–3245, 1997.
3. Widjaja A, Stratton IM, Horn R, et al: UKPDS 20: Plasma leptin, obesity, and plasma insulin in type 2 diabetic subjects. *J Clin Endocrinol Metab* 82:654–657, 1997.
4. Boden G, Chen X, Kolaczynski JW, et al: Effects of prolonged hyperinsulinemia on serum leptin in normal subjects. *J Clin Invest* 100:1107–1113, 1997.
5. Wiegle DS, Duell PB, Connor WE, et al: Effect of fasting, re-feeding, and dietary fat restriction on plasma leptin levels. *J Clin Endocrinol Metab* 82:561–565, 1997.
6. Ferron F, Considine RV, Peino R, et al: Serum leptin concentrations in patients with anorexia nervosa: Bulimia and non-specific eating disorders correlate with the body mass index but are independent of the respective disease. *Clin Endocrinol (Oxf)* 46:289–293, 1997.

Estrogen and Progestin Compared With Simvastatin for Hypercholesterolemia in Postmenopausal Women

Darling GM, Johns JA, McCloud PI, et al (Jean Hailes Found, Melbourne, Australia; Austin and Repatriation Med Centre, Melbourne, Australia; Monash Univ, Melbourne, Australia)
N Engl J Med 337:595–601, 1997   30–3

Background.—Both estrogen and lipid-lowering drugs improve serum lipid concentrations and may reduce cardiovascular mortality in postmenopausal women. A randomized, crossover trial compared the effects of estrogen and progestin with those of simvastatin in postmenopausal women with hypercholesterolemia.

Methods.—Postmenopausal women eligible for the study had a fasting serum total cholesterol value of more than 250 mg/dL (6.5 mmol/L), a serum follicle-stimulating hormone value of more than 20 IU/L, and normal mammography within the last 2 years. All were given dietary advice at enrollment, then entered into two 8-week treatment periods separated by an 8-week washout period. Simvastatin (10 mg daily) was given during 1 treatment period and conjugated estrogens (1.25 mg daily) and medroxyprogesterone acetate, (5 mg daily) were given during the other treatment period. Blood was sampled at weeks 4, 8, 16, 20, and 24 to measure serum lipids and lipoproteins.

Results.—The mean baseline serum total cholesterol was 305 mg/dL [7.9 mmol/L] high density lipoprotein cholesterol was 62 mg/dL (1.6 mmol/L) and low density lipoprotein cholesterol was 217 mg/dL (5.6 mmol/L). Estrogen-progestin therapy resulted in a mean 14% decrease in serum total cholesterol vs. a mean 26% decrease with simvastatin. For serum LDL cholesterol, the mean decreases were 24% with estrogen-progestin and 36% with simvastatin. The 2 treatments had a similar effect on serum HDL cholesterol concentrations, increasing the values by 7%.

Serum triglyceride concentrations increased during estrogen-progestin (mean, 29%), but decreased during simvastatin (mean, 14%). Only estrogen-progestin therapy led to a decrease in serum Lp(a) lipoprotein (mean decrease, 27%).

Conclusion.—Estrogen plus progestin therapy has beneficial effects in postmenopausal women with hypercholesterolemia. Simvastatin resulted in greater reductions in both serum total and LDL cholesterol concentrations, but the clinical importance of this difference is unclear.

▶ Estrogen therapy reduces cardiovascular disease mortality in postmenopausal women in part by lowering serum LDL cholesterol and raising serum HDL cholesterol concentrations[1, 2] It had similar effects on the serum cholesterol concentrations in these postmenopausal women with hypercholesterolemia, although the increase in serum HDL cholesterol was somewhat less than that reported in unselected women. Therefore, to the extent that changes in serum LDL and HDL cholesterol induced by estrogen account for the reduction in cardiovascular disease mortality, the benefit of estrogen should be of roughly similar magnitude in normocholesterolemic and hypercholesterolemic women.

The greater fall in serum LDL cholesterol in the women treated with simvastatin (36% vs. 24%) might be expected to confer greater benefit in terms of reduction in cardiovascular mortality. However, if lipid-lowering therapy is indicated in a postmenopausal woman, estrogen should be the first choice because of its other beneficial effects—on menopausal symptoms and bone density, for example—and its lower cost. (Remember that estrogen can raise serum triglyceride concentrations, sometimes dramatically.)

R.D. Utiger, M.D.

References

1. Lobo RA: Effects of hormonal replacement on lipids and lipoproteins in postmenopausal women. *J Clin Endocrinol Metab* 73:925–930, 1991.
2. Walsh BW, Schiff I, Rosner B, et al: Effects of postmenopausal estrogen replacement on the concentrations and metabolism of plasma lipoproteins. *N Engl J Med* 325:1196–1204, 1991.

KIDNEY, WATER, AND ELECTROLYTES

SAULO KLAHR, M.D.

Introduction

The section on glomerular disease includes a study performed by Radford et al. at the Mayo Clinic that examines the histopathologic and clinical features predicting an adverse outcome in patients with IgA nephropathy. These include an elevated serum creatinine, and the presence of hypertension and proteinuria. The overall 10-year survival in this group of patients with IgA nephropathy was 67%, a figure that is below the percentage reported in large cohort studies from Australia, Europe, and Japan.

Systemic lupus erythematosus (SLE) is an autoimmune disorder affecting several organs, including the central nervous system, the joints, serosal membranes, the skin, and the kidneys. In a mouse model of lupus nephritis, it was found that anti-DNA antibodies can cause renal disease. Since anti-DNA antibodies bind directly to renal tissue, it may be possible to prevent renal disease of this etiology by targeting non-tissue–bound antigens to anti-DNA antibodies. Gaynor et al. report on the development of antigens that can be used for this purpose. This may represent a novel therapy for lupus nephritis. Obviously, additional studies are needed before such strategies can be applied to humans.

Mak et al. from the Manchester Royal Hospital in the United Kingdom report on the long-term outcome of adult-onset minimal change nephropathy. At presentation, about half of the patients had an elevated serum creatinine and hypertension. The mean follow-up of these 51 patients was 14.1 years (range 0.5 to 38.9 years). Partial or complete remission of the nephrotic syndrome occurred in 46, 72, and 92% of patients within 4, 8, and 21 weeks of therapy with corticosteroids. In this group, 4 patients, or 8%, were steroid-resistant. Patients who had multiple relapses were treated with cyclophosphamide. This study indicates that adults with minimal change nephropathy have a good long-term outcome.

The chapter on other diseases of the kidney includes a study of the incidence of end-stage renal disease (ESRD) among silica exposed gold miners. The cohort included 2,412 male gold miners. The authors suggest that exposure to silica is associated with an increased risk for ESRD, particularly ESRD associated with glomerulonephritis. Previous studies from the United Kingdom, in patients exposed to silica, suggested that tubular dysfunction appears initially and is followed by glomerular injury.

Approximately half a million individuals in the United States carry a mutant gene for autosomal dominant polycystic kidney disease (ADPKD). Autosomal dominant polycystic kidney disease affects several organs and systems. There is a 10- to 20-fold increased risk of subarachnoid hemorrhage in patients with ADPKD, compared with the general population, and an increased risk of subarachnoid hemorrhage in patients with ADPKD compared to the general population, and an increased risk for a variety of vascular pathological conditions. In their report, Griffin et al. described the detection of polycystin within the smooth muscle cells of arteries of normal adults. Polycystin is a large protein encoded by the

PKD1 gene, the mutations of which have been implicated in the development of ADPKD. The presence of polycystin in arterial walls indicates that the vascular disorders seen in patients with ADPKD could be genetic manifestations of the disease rather than secondary events. Additional studies are required to understand the mechanisms by which polycystin impairs the normal biology of the arterial wall.

Acute renal failure (ARF) is characterized by a marked decrease in glomerular filtration rate over a period of hours or days. Non-steroidal anti-inflammatory drugs (NSAIDs) are known to cause acute renal failure. In addition, NSAID administration can cause interstitial nephritis, the nephrotic syndrome, hyperkalemia, and salt and water retention. All NSAIDs are administered orally. In the recent past, ketorolac tromethamine was approved in the United States for parenteral use as an analgesic. This retrospective study investigates the risk for ARF associated with ketorolac. The incidence of ARF was low in a group of patients receiving keterolac in the hospital. As a matter of fact, the incidence of ARF was not different from that of patients receiving opioids for analgesia. However, the authors suggest that parenteral ketorolac administration might be associated with a greater risk for ARF when therapy is prolonged beyond 5 days. The results of this study should be interpreted with caution, since this was not a prospective randomized clinical trial.

The administration of radiocontrast agents into the bloodstream for diagnostic purposes is associated with vasoconstriction of the renal ascular tree and, in some instances, with the development of ARF. Clark et al. examined the effect of administration of radiocontrast on the levels of endothelin (a powerful vasconstrictor) and atrial peptide (a vasodilator). The authors found an increase in the levels of both compounds in the circulation after administration of radiocontrast. Patients with underlying disease or diabetes had higher basal levels of both vasoactive substances and a greater tendency to develop increased endothelin levels after administration of radiocontrast. Although endothelin may contribute to renal vasoconstriction after radiocontrast administration, the simultaneous rise in the levels of atrial natriuretic peptide may offset the effect of endothelin and protect renal function in most cases.

The chapter on chronic renal failure describes the potential role of homocysteinemia in the vascular disease of patients with end-stage renal failure. Several studies indicate that an elevated level of homocysteine is an important risk factor for atherosclerotic vascular disease. The mean value for homocysteine (a sulfur containing amino acid formed during the metabolism of methionine) is 10 µmol/L and the level for the 95th percentile is about 16 µmol/L. In patients with ESRD or on dialysis, the plasma levels of homocysteine averaged 26.6 ± 1.5 µmol/L. Several reports indicate that elevated plasma levels of homocysteine are an independent risk factor for vascular disease in patients with ESRD. Chronic renal failure and absolute or relative deficiencies of folate, vitamin B_{12}, or vitamin B_6 are the major causes of increased plasma levels of homocysteine.

Giatras et al. utilized a meta-analysis of the effect of angiotensin-converting enzyme (ACE) inhibitors on the progression of renal disease, excluding patients with diabetic nephropathy. Patients receiving ACE inhibitors (806) were compared with those given other antihypertensive medications (788). The study concludes that ACE inhibitors are more effective than other antihypertensive agents in reducing the development of ESRD in non-diabetic patients. Mortality was comparable between the groups receiving ACE inhibitors and those receiving other antihypertensive medications: 2.1% in those taking ACE, as compared with 1.5% in those receiving other drugs.

The chapter on hypertension includes a report by Fogo et al. regarding the accuracy of the diagnosis of nephrosclerosis in blacks. It has been reported that the occurrence of ESRD is four times greater in blacks than in whites. In addition, blacks account for 41% of new patients admitted to ESRD programs with the diagnosis of hypertensive nephrosclerosis. This diagnosis is usually made on clinical grounds. The present study utilizes renal biopsies in an effort to substantiate the accuracy of the diagnosis of nephrosclerosis in blacks. Of 46 biopsies attempted, 39 were adequate for histological studies. Thirty-eight cases had arteriolar sclerosis or arteriosclerosis. Arteriolar thickening was present and hyaline deposits were observed in arterioles and arteries. These observations indicate that the diagnosis of hypertensive nephrosclerosis made on clinical and laboratory grounds is highly accurate in blacks.

Aperloo et al. from Holland examine, prospectively, the renal hemodynamic response in 40 nondiabetic patients with varying degrees of renal functional impairment before antihypertensive treatment and after withdrawal of that treatment. Patients were given an ACE inhibitor (enalapril) or a β blocker (atenolol) for a 4-year period. An initial fall in glomerular filtration rate after the onset of antihypertensive treatment in these patients, with mild-to-moderate loss of renal function, was associated with a slower loss of renal function over time. The initial fall in glomerular filtration rate is reversible after discontinuation of antihypertensive therapy of long duration.

Other articles in this section examined: the vascular effects of L-arginine and the role of endogenous insulin (Gugliano et al.); the effect of lazaroid therapy on the altered nitric oxide metabolism and increased oxygen-free radical activity in lead-induced hypertension (Vaziri et al.); and the potential role of the AT2 angiotensin receptor in mediating the renal production of nitric oxide (Sirugy et al.).

In the transplantation section, Jordan et al. report on their 5-year experience with the use of tacrolimus as rescue therapy for renal allograft rejection. Although the molecular structure of tacrolimus is dissimilar from that of cyclosporine, the two drugs share similar targets and inhibit similar interleukin gene products. One hundred sixty-nine patients who experienced failing cyclosporine immunosuppression with ongoing rejection were switched to tacrolimus at an average of 4.3 ± 2.6 months following transplantation. At the time of the report, 159 of the 169 patients (94%) were alive and 125 of the 169 (79%) were considered to have achieved graft rescue. Based on this experience, the authors recommend that tacrolimus be used as an alternative to the conventional agents used for rejection episodes in patients with a kidney graft.

The article by Koning et al. of the University of Wisconsin calls attention to delayed function of the transplant kidney as an important complication. In this multicenter study, delayed graft function resulted in a 10% higher rate of graft failure.

In the chapter on dialysis, Held et al. report on the relationship of the hemodialysis "dose" to patient mortality. This study supports the generalization and reports on the impact of "skipped" dialysis treatments on patient survival. The authors suggest that even one "skipped" treatment per month correlates with higher mortality. Other reports in this section discuss the effects of recombinant human growth hormone on muscle protein turnover in malnourished patients on hemodialysis; the fact that the levels of leptin (a protein secreted by fat cells that has been shown to control appetite in rodents) are elevated in the plasma of patients on hemodialysis. Suh et al. report on the depletion of L-arginine in patients on continuous ambulatory peritoneal dialysis when they develop acute peritonitis. L-arginine is the precursor for the synthesis of nitric oxide (NO). Defective production of NO may lead to persistence of bacterial infections. In this study, the majority of the patients with acute bacterial peritonitis had increased NO production. However, there was a smaller subset of patients that had low levels of nitrite (a marker of NO production).

In the chapter on water, electrolytes and acid-base, Takito et al. describe a new protein (hensin), which is localized in the collecting duct and appears to have a role in the secretion of H^+ or bicarbonate by intercalated cells of this segment of the nephron. Xu et al. report on the upregulation of the aquaporin-2 water channel in rats with chronic heart failure, providing evidence that antidiuretic hormone is responsible for the upregulation of aquaporin water channels and water retention in this setting. It should be remembered that hyponatremia is a common finding in patients with congestive heart failure, due to water retention.

The chapter on calcium, phosphorus, and bone contains an article by Kronmal et al., titled "Vasectomy is associated with an increased risk for urolithiasis." Although the mechanisms by which vasectomy increases the risk of urolithiasis have not been elucidated, the association between vasectomy and renal stone formation is in itself an important finding. Men contemplating vasectomy for contraception should be informed of the potential of urolithiasis. In another article, Curhan et al. report on a comparison of dietary calcium and other nutrients as factors affecting the risk for kidney stones in women.

Saulo Klahr, M.D.

31 Glomerular Disease

Predicting Renal Outcome in IgA Nephropathy
Radford MG Jr, Donadio JV Jr, Bergstralh EJ, et al (Mayo Clinic and Found, Rochester, Minn)
J Am Soc Nephrol 8:199–207, 1997   31–1

Objective.—Although IgA nephropathy (IgAN) has a variable clinical course. many patients exhibit a slowly progressive disease that ultimately results in end-stage renal disease (ESRD). Finding clinical, laboratory, and histologic features predictive of outcome in individual patients is difficult. Clinical and histologic features, including Mib-1 immunostaining, that might be predictive of progressive renal disease in patients with IgAN were evaluated.

Methods.—A retrospective review was conducted at the Mayo Clinic of medical records of 148 patients (41 females), average age 39 years, with primary IgAN who underwent renal biopsy between January 1973 and December 1994. Data compared and analyzed included assessments of 6 glomerular, 8 interstitial, and 6 vascular histopathologic features of the disease including results of Mib-1 immunostaining. Survival from date of biopsy to death or renal failure was estimated by the Kaplan-Meier method. Survival free of renal failure and life-table survival were determined. Univariate and multivariate analyses were performed.

Results.—Overall survival estimate was 97% at 5 years and 89% at 10 years. Mean time to renal failure was 6.3 years. There were 39 patients who progressed to ESRD for an estimated survival free of renal failure of 79% at 5 years and 67% at 10 years. Total glomerular and interstitial Mib-1 scores, vascular scores, total and individual histopathologic scores, and hypertension (Fig 1) were significantly associated with outcome. Glomerular component scores, including matrix increase, capillary narrowing or disruption, and fibrous adhesions were highly predictive of renal failure. Histopathologic scores of 11 or higher, tubulointerstitial scores of 8 or higher, and total vascular scores of 5 or higher were significantly associated with a higher risk of progression to ESRD. Multivariate analysis showed that higher glomerular score, increased serum creatinine, and younger age were significant independent predictors of renal failure, but Mib-1 scores were not.

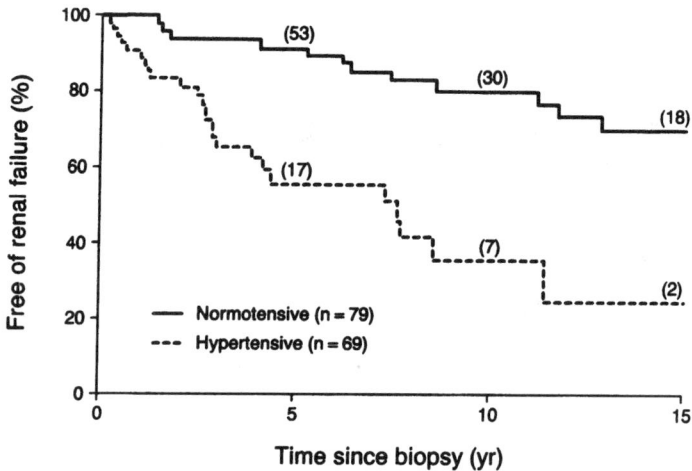

FIGURE 1.—Hypertension present at the time of renal biopsy was associated with decreased survival free of renal failure ($P < 0.001$; N = 148 patients). Numbers in parentheses indicate the number of patients at risk at 5, 10, and 15 years. (Courtesy of Radford MG Jr, Donadio JV Jr, Bergstralh EJ, et al: Predicting renal outcome in IgA nephropathy. *J Am Soc Nephrol* 8:199–207, 1997).

Conclusion.—Although this study was small, it demonstrates that histopathologic scores are significant indicators of risk of progression to ESRD in patients with primary IgAN.

▶ Immunoglobulin A nephropathy (IgAN) is a common disorder, although its incidence varies widely in different geographic areas. It is very common in Southern Europe, Asia, and Australia. IgA nephropathy accounts for 20% to 25% of all primary glomerular diseases in Southern Europe and Australia and for 30% to 40% of primary glomerular diseases in Japan. The pathogenesis of IgAN has not been completely elucidated. It is likely an immune complex glomerulonephritis caused by mesangial deposition of IgA immune complexes. The clinical course of the disease is highly variable. Some patients have rapidly progressive renal insufficiency, whereas others retain adequate renal function for decades. Approximately 30% to 50% of patients with IgAN have ESRD over a period of about 20 years after diagnosis. The most characteristic and common abnormality in renal biopsies of patients with IgAN is mesangial expansion. The increased amount of mesangial matrix is often more prominent than the mesangial proliferation.

Immunoglobulin A nephropathy has been considered a relatively uncommon entity in the United States. This report from the Mayo Clinic examines the histopathologic and clinical features that predict an adverse outcome in 148 individuals with IgAN who had a renal biopsy at that institution between 1973 and 1995. A number of clinicopathologic findings were associated with adverse outcomes. These included the presence of an elevated creatinine, hypertension (see Fig 1), and proteinuria. Histologic and immunohistologic features of renal biopsies that indicate a less favorable outcome include: diffuse and severe mesangial proliferation, lesions of the glomerular capillary wall, advanced glomerular sclerosis, pronounced interstitial infiltration or fibrosis, the presence of arteriolar hyalinosis, and clear evidence of extra-capillary proliferation. The overall 10-year survival in this group of patients with IgAN seen at the Mayo Clinic was 67%, a percentage that is below the percentage reported in large cohort studies undertaken in Australia, Japan, and Europe.[1-4]

S. Klahr, M.D.

References

1. Alamartine E, Sabatier JC, Guerin C, et al. Prognostic factors in mesangial IgA glomerulonephritis: An extensive study with univariate and multivariate analyses. *Am J Kidney Dis* 18:12–19, 1991.
2. Johnston PA, Brown JS, Braumholtz DA, et al: Clinicopathological correlations and long-term follow-up of 253 United Kingdom patients with IgA nephropathy: A report from the MRC glomerulonephritis registry. *Q J Med* 84:619–627, 1992.
3. Katafuchi R, Oh Y, Hori K, et al: An important role of glomerular segmental lesions on progression of IgA nephropathy: A multivariate analysis. *Clin Nephrol* 41:191–198, 1994.
4. Ibels LS, Gyory AG: IgA nephropathy: Analysis of the natural history, important factors in the progression of renal disease, and a review of the literature. *Medicine* 73:79–102, 1994.

Peptide Inhibition of Glomerular Deposition of an Anti-DNA Antibody
Gaynor B, Putterman C, Valadon P, et al (Albert Einstein College of Medicine, Bronx, NY)
Proc Natl Acad Sci U S A 94:1955–1960, 1997   31–2

Background.—Antibodies to double-stranded DNA are pathognomonic of systemic lupus erythematosus (SLE). These antibodies deposit in the kidney and cause glomerulonephritis. Recent research indicates that a significant percentage of anti-DNA antibodies may cross-react with renal antigens and, consequently, may be sequestered in the kidney. If this is true, then antigenic competition for pathogenic antibodies may prevent deposition of them in the kidney as well as the ensuing tissue damage. In the current study, surrogate antigens were generated for this use.

Methods and Findings.—Peptide display phage libraries were used to identify peptides that would react with R4A, a pathogenic mouse mono-clonal anti-DNA antibody, which deposits in glomeruli. The peptides were observed to bind in or near the double-stranded DNA binding site. Also, the peptides were bound preferentially by the R4A antibody, compared with 2 closely associated antibodies derived from it, one depositing in renal tubules and the other showing no renal pathogenicity. Administering 1 of these peptides in a soluble form in vivo protected mice from R4A anti-DNA antibody deposition in the kidney.

Conclusions.—The observation that peptide can greatly inhibit deposition of R4A in glomeruli in vivo suggests a new therapeutic approach to

SLE, in which target organs would be protected from antibody-mediated injury. Further research is now needed.

▶ Systemic lupus erythematosus is an autoimmune disorder characterized by multiple derangements of the immune system, including B-cell hyperactivity and excessive immune complex formation. The central nervous system, joints, serosal surfaces, skin, and kidneys are most commonly involved.

The pathogenesis of lupus nephritis is incompletely understood. The chronic deposition of preformed immune complexes and the in situ formation of immune complexes may have a significant role in changes in glomerular mesangial cells. Such complexes may be deposited in subendothelial locations, as well as in vascular and tubulointerstitial areas. Immune complexes then may activate complement and attract inflammatory cells, which, in turn, may release cytokines and other mediators of inflammation. Anti–double-stranded DNA antibodies are diagnostic of SLE, and serum titers of these antibodies correlate with disease activity in humans. In a mouse model, it has been shown that anti-DNA antibodies can cause renal disease. Since anti-DNA antibodies bind directly to renal tissue, it may be possible to prevent this type of renal disease by targeting nontissue–bound antigens to anti-DNA antibodies. The authors of this study describe the development of antigens that can be used for this purpose. They focused on peptides that react with R4A, a pathogenic mouse monoclonal anti-DNA antibody, which is deposited in glomeruli. These peptides apparently bind in or near the double-stranded DNA binding site. The administration of one of these peptides protected mice from the deposition of the R4A anti-DNA in the kidney in vivo. This may represent a novel therapy for lupus nephritis. Obviously, additional studies are needed to explore this possibility.

S. Klahr, M.D.

Long-term Outcome of Adult-onset Minimal-change Nephropathy
Mak SK, Short CD, Mallick NP (Manchester Royal Infirmary, England)
Nephrol Dial Transplant 11:2192–2201, 1996   31–3

Objective.—In children, minimal-change nephropathy (MCN) is associated with a consistent response to corticosteroid therapy and a good prognosis, with low risk of chronic renal failure. In adults, MCN is slower to respond to corticosteroids and may have a worse prognosis. There are few data on the long-term outcomes of adults with MCN. A long-term follow-up study of adult-onset MCN was conducted.

Patients.—The retrospective study included 51 patients with adult-onset MCN. All were treated in a single renal unit between 1950 and 1993. The patients were 30 women and 21 men, mean age 37 years. They were studied for an average of 14 years. One third of the patients had comorbidity, most commonly, allergy, and recent upper respiratory tract infection. All patients had nephrotic syndrome with a mean proteinuria of 16 g/24 hr. Serum creatinine was elevated in 55% of patients, but almost

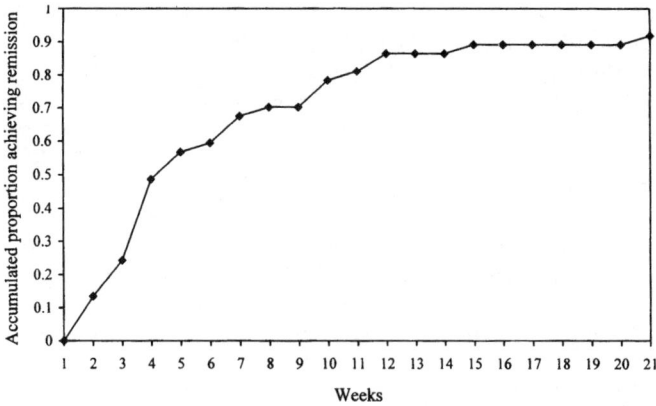

FIGURE 1.—Rate of first remission with corticosteroid treatment. (From Mak SK, Short CD, Mallick NP: Long-term outcome of adult-onset minimal-change nephropathy. *Nephrol Dial Transplant* 11:2192–2201, 1996. Reprinted by permission of Oxford University Press.)

always normalized when the patient went into remission. When first receiving a diagnosis of MCN, 47% of patients had hypertension, 33% had microscopic hematuria, 96% had hypercholesterolemia and hypertriglyceridemia, and 42% had hyperuricemia.

Outcomes.—Ninety-two percent of the patients went into remission within 21 weeks of steroid treatment (Fig 1). (The remission rate was 46% at 4 weeks and 70% at 8 weeks.) The remaining 8% of patients were steroid-resistant. With advancing age and rising initial albumin level, the time to remission increased. Time to remission was negatively correlated with number of relapses. A spontaneous remission occurred in one third of the patients. When multiple relapses occurred, cyclophosphamide was given. Sixty-three percent of the patients treated in this way were still in remission after 5 years. One fourth of the patients had hypertension after an average interval of 11 years. All but 3 patients were in complete remission at their last evaluation, and only 3 had an elevated serum creatinine level.

Conclusions.—As in children, MCN has a good long-term prognosis in adults. Patients with adult-onset MCN achieve sustained remission and long-term maintenance of renal function. There are some differences from childhood MCN, notably, a slower response to corticosteroid treatment and a higher frequency of transient hypertension and impaired renal function.

▶ The nephrotic syndrome is characterized by massive proteinuria, usually in excess of 3.5 g of protein in 24 hours, hypoalbuminemia, edema, and hyperlipidemia. Minimal-change nephropathy is the most common cause of the nephrotic syndrome in children and accounts for about 75% of all cases of the syndrome in the pediatric age group.[1] Children with MCN usually respond well to therapy with corticosteroids. Minimal-change nephropathy accounts for about 25% of the cases of nephrotic syndrome in adults. The most common cause of the nephrotic syndrome in this population is membranous nephropathy. As compared to children, adults with MCN have a delayed response to corticosteroids, and, in most instances, prolonged therapy may be required to effect complete remission. A variable proportion of adults with MCN had relapse in 3 separate studies, with follow-up periods ranging from 2.9 to 7.6 years.[2-4] In general, there are few reports regarding the long-term prognosis of adult patients with MCN.

In this report from the Department of Renal Medicine at Manchester Royal Hospital in the United Kingdom, Mak et al. reviewed the outcome of 51 patients with idiopathic adult-onset MCN seen at this medical center between 1950 and 1993. At presentation, about half of the patients had an elevated serum creatinine and hypertension. The mean follow-up for the group as a whole was 14.1 years (range 0.5 to 38.9 years). Remission of the nephrotic syndrome (partial or complete) occurred in 46%, 70%, and 92% of patients within 4, 8, and 21 weeks, respectively, of corticosteroid therapy (Figure 1). In this series, steroid resistance was on the order of 8%. Patients who experienced multiple relapses were treated with cyclophosphamide and about two-thirds of those patients were in remission after 5 years. Differences between adults and children with MCN included a lower incidence of relapses and a slower response to corticosteroids in adults, as compared with children. The results of this study indicate that adults with MCN have a good long-term outcome because progressive deterioration of renal function is relatively rare.

S. Klahr, M.D.

References

1. International Study of Kidney Diseases in Children: Early identification of frequent relapses among children with minimal change nephrotic syndrome. *J Pediatr* 101:514–518, 1982.
2. Nolasco F, Cameron JS, Heywood EF, et al: Adult-onset minimal change nephrotic syndrome: A long-term follow-up. *Kidney Int* 29:1215–1223, 1986.
3. Korbet SM, Schwartz MM, Lewis EJ: Minimal-change glomerulopathy of adulthood. *Am J Nephrol* 8:291–297, 1988.
4. Nair RM, Date A, Kimbakaran MG, et al: Minimal-change nephrotic syndrome in adults treated with alternate-day steroids. *Nephron* 47:209–210, 1987.

Immune Complex Glomerulonephritis in Patients Coinfected With Human Immunodeficiency Virus and Hepatitis C Virus
Stokes MB, Chawla H, Brody RI, et al (New York Univ; Dept of Veterans Affairs Med Ctr, New York)
Am J Kidney Dis 29:514–525, 1997   31–4

Purpose.—Patients with HIV-associated nephropathy have heavy proteinuria with rapid renal failure, "collapsing" glomerulopathy, and tubulointerstitial abnormalities. This is the most frequent diagnosis on renal biopsy of HIV-infected patients. Its etiology and pathogenesis are unknown. Previous reports described the association between hepatitis C virus (HCV) and immune complex glomerulonephritis. The clinical and pathologic findings in 12 patients with HIV and HCV coinfection and atypical features of HIV-associated nephropathy were reported.

Patients.—The patients were all IV drug users with HIV and serologic evidence of HCV coinfection. They were selected for renal biopsy because of unusual features of HIV-associated nephropathy, such as hypertension, microscopic hematuria, and cryoglobulinemia. The patients were 11 men and 1 woman (mean age, 39 years); 7 were black and 5 were Hispanic. Immune complex glomerulonephritis was present in 11 patients; the other patient had glomerulosclerosis with immune complex deposits. Although 10 of the patients had a history of past hepatitis B virus infection, none showed persistent hepatitis B surface antigenemia. None had any other known cause of immune complex glomerulonephritis.

Findings.—On renal biopsy, 5 patients had membranoproliferative glomerulonephritis, 5 had mesangial proliferative glomerulonephritis, 1 had membranous nephropathy, and 1 had "collapsing" glomerulopathy with immune complex deposits. Reverse transcription–polymerase chain reaction detected HCV RNA in renal tissue or serum, or both, in 9 of 11 patients. In addition, 4 of 8 patients who had typical clinical and pathologic features of HIV-associated nephropathy but lacked immunofluorescence evidence of immune complex deposits had HCV RNA in their renal biopsy specimens. Renal failure was present at diagnosis in 1 patient, and end-stage renal disease requiring hemodialysis developed at a mean of 6.5 months in 5 patients. The other 6 patients had stable renal function at a mean follow-up of 29 months. Results of liver function tests were abnormal in 7 patients, including 4 of the 6 with renal failure.

Conclusion.—In some patients with HIV and HCV coinfection, immune complex glomerulonephritis may be the major clinical manifestation of disease. The occurrence of immune complex glomerulonephritis in many black patients at risk for HIV-associated nephropathy may be related to the high frequency of HCV infection among black IV drug users.

▶ The clinical features of HIV-associated nephropathy include proteinuria in the nephrotic range (greater than 3.0 g/24 hr) and rapidly progressive renal insufficiency in the setting of normal-sized or enlarged kidneys on ultrasonic examination. Hypertension is rare. On renal biopsy, the combination of focal segmental glomerulosclerosis and collapse of glomerular capillaries, tubular cell degeneration, and interstitial inflammation disproportionate to the glomerular disease strongly suggests the diagnosis of HIV-associated nephropathy.

Chronic HCV infection may or may not be associated with the presence of cryoglobulins and membranoproliferative glomerulonephritis. Renal biopsy reveals a type I membranoproliferative glomerulonephritis with deposition of IgG, IgM, and C_3 in glomerular capillaries. The pathogenesis is most likely related to deposition of immune complexes in the kidney.

The report of Stokes et al. describes the clinical features of 12 patients who were IV drug users and were coinfected with HIV and HCV. In these patients, hypertension, microscopic hematuria, and cryoglobulinemia were present. Eleven patients had immune complex glomerulonephritis. Ten patients had evidence of past hepatitis B infection, but none had persistent hepatitis B surface antigenemia. The major message of this study is that, in patients with HIV who are coinfected with HCV, the picture of immune complex glomerulonephritis may predominate and change the clinical course of the nephropathy usually seen in patients with HIV infection alone.

In summary, patients with both HIV and HCV infection exhibit a range of clinical and pathologic abnormalities of the kidney, including immune complex glomerulonephritis, HIV associated nephropathy, and nonspecific changes. It is likely that not all patients with concomitant infections will have renal complications.

S. Klahr, M.D.

Thin GBM Nephropathy: Premature Glomerular Obsolescence Is Associated With Hypertension and Late Onset Renal Failure
Nieuwhof CMG, De Heer F, De Leeuw P, et al (Univ Hosp Maastricht, The Netherlands; Maasland Hosp, Sittard, The Netherlands)
Kidney Int 51:1596–1601, 1997   31–5

Background.—Thin glomerular basement membrane (GBM) nephropathy is diagnosed by the finding of a uniform thinning of the lamina densa of the glomerular basement membranes. The condition, also called familial benign hematuria, affects both sexes equally and generally has an excellent renal prognosis. A recent report of a missense mutation in collagen type IV associated with this condition raises the possibility that thin GBM nephropathy is an atypical form of Alport syndrome, a progressive renal hereditary disorder. A prospective epidemiologic study sought to discern early Alport syndrome from thin GBM nephropathy.

Patients and Methods.—Patients were participants in a study of idiopathic glomerular disease conducted between 1978 and 1984. Renal biopsy specimens were taken from patients aged 16 to 65 years who had no systemic extrarenal disease or known familial renal disorders. Included in the study were 27 patients with primary IgA nephropathy, 24 with normal renal tissue, and 19 with thin GBM nephropathy. Patients were observed for a median of 12 years for signs of disease progression: development of hypertension, increase in proteinuria, or development of uremia.

Results.—Family research conducted during follow-up revealed that 9 patients with thin GBM nephropathy had relatives with hematuria, proteinuria, and/or impaired renal function. Within 4 families, 6 elderly members had end-stage renal disease requiring dialysis. The mode of inheritance in these families appeared to be autosomal dominant. None of the 24 patients with normal renal tissue had family members with renal insufficiency. Renal biopsy specimens taken at study entry showed an increased incidence of focal global glomerulosclerosis in the GBM group, compared with normal and IgA nephropathy groups. The presence of Alport syndrome was clinically ruled out because none of the patients had hearing loss or visual abnormalities. At the end of follow-up, the incidence of hypertension in thin GBM nephropathy (7 of 18) was greater than that in healthy controls (2 of 24). Although the incidences of hypertension and increased proteinuria were comparable in the thin GBM and IgA nephropathy groups, 3 patients with IgA nephropathy had progressed to renal failure.

Conclusion.—Patients with thin GBM nephropathy are significantly more likely than those with idiopathic IgA nephropathy or normal renal tissue to have first-degree relatives with an increased incidence of focal global glomerulosclerosis and renal insufficiency. Thin GBM nephropathy, although clinically different from Alport syndrome, predisposes to premature glomerular obsolescence, hypertension, and an increased incidence of late-onset renal insufficiency. Both disorders appear to result from defects in collagen type IV–coding genes.

▶ Benign familial hematuria is characterized by the familial occurrence of persistent microscopic hematuria. In general, patients with the condition have no hearing defect and there is no progression to renal failure. To predict the benign course of the disease, additional criteria are necessary: absence of gross hematuria, the absence of proteinuria and the finding, in the kindred, of males with isolated microhematuria. Renal tissue obtained by biopsy shows thinning of the glomerular basement membrane (GBM) in approximately half of the cases and various nonspecific and minor changes in the glomerulus in the other half.

This study from the Netherlands describes 18 patients with chronic microscopic and 1 with macroscopic hematuria; all had thinning of the GBM on renal biopsy and were observed for a median of 12 years (range, 9 to 15 years). There were 4 major findings in this study: (1) the majority of patients with apparently nonfamilial hematuria actually had the familial variety; (2) thin GBM nephropathy was associated with a significantly higher incidence of renal insufficiency in the first-degree relatives and with a greater incidence of focal glomerulosclerosis than in patients with IgA nephropathy and associated hematuria, but normal findings on renal biopsy; (3) during follow-up, the incidence of hypertension was comparable to that seen in patients with idiopathic nonprogressive IgA nephropathy (and there was a decline in renal function in 3 elderly patients; and (4) none of the patients with thin GBM had hearing loss.

S. Klahr, M.D.

Myofibroblasts and Arteriolar Sclerosis in Human Diabetic Nephropathy
Pedagogos E, Hewitson T, Fraser I, et al (Royal Melbourne Hosp, Victoria, Australia)
Am J Kidney Dis 29:912–918, 1997   31–6

Background.—Myofibroblasts (MFs) may play a role in progressive interstitial fibrosis and arteriolosclerosis associated with diabetic nephropathy (DN). Biopsy specimens from 62 patients with DN (41 male and 21 female) and 17 control patients were examined to determine possible relationships.

Methods.—Myofibroblasts were detected through morphological analysis and immunostaining for α-smooth muscle actin (αSMA). Endothelial cells were stained with a modification of the avidin-biotin complex and antibodies. Arteriolar density was measured by counting interstitial arterioles. Index of arteriolosclerosis was computed as the ratio of wall surface area to total surface area. Percentage of interstitium (an index of interstitial fibrosis), percentage of collagen III, and percentage of αSMA were quantified by point counting. Rank correlation coefficients were used to relate measurements to each other and to kidney function.

Results.—In patients with DN, who had significantly greater interstitial fibrosis than control patients, αSMA staining was markedly increased ($P < 0.001$), especially in fibrotic areas (primarily periglomerular and peritubular); collagen III was similarly increased ($P < 0.001$). Index of arteriolosclerosis was greater in patients with DN ($P < 0.001$), and arteriolar density was significantly less ($P < 0.0001$), indicative of reduced blood supply. In patients with DN, αSMA correlated significantly with interstitial fibrosis ($r = 0.56$; $P < 0.001$), collagen III ($r = 0.47$; $P < 0.001$), and plasma creatinine at biopsy ($r = 0.51$; $P < 0.001$), and its percentage change at 4 years as a prognostic index ($r = 0.37$; $P = < 0.01$). Index of arteriolosclerosis showed significant correlations in patients with DN with collagen III ($r = 0.29$; $P = 0.02$), plasma creatinine ($r = 0.33$; $P = 0.01$), and glomerular filtration rate ($r = 0.39$; $P = 0.008$). Arteriolar density was strongly negatively correlated with interstitial fibrosis ($r = -0.75$; $P < 0.001$), αSMA ($r = -0.36$; $P < 0.034$), and collagen III ($r = -0.66$; $P < 0.0001$).

▶ Most glomerular diseases are accompanied by changes in the renal interstitium. Interstitial fibrosis and arteriolosclerosis occur in patients with diabetic nephropathy. Interstitial fibrosis and tubular atrophy are important histologic predictors of progressive renal disease. The study of Pedagogos et al. confirms a correlation between the severity of interstitial fibrosis and the degree of loss of glomerular filtration rate as described by others in patients with diverse renal diseases.[1-7] In this study, the authors identified myofibroblasts in the renal interstitium of patients with diabetic nephropathy, and provided information indicating that their presence correlates with the amount of interstitial fibrosis and the decrement in glomerular filtration rate.

Most studies of diabetic nephropathy have emphasized the glomeruloscle-rosis that occurs in this setting, but limited information is available regarding the relationship of vascular injury and scarring of the tubulointerstitial space. It should be noted that blood supply to the interstitium may be compromised by changes in the lumen of both capillaries and larger arteries. This study provides evidence for a significant role of myofibroblasts in the development and progression of tubulointerstitial damage in patients with diabetic neph-ropathy. Vascular abnormalities may contribute to fibroblast modulation. Additional studies will be needed to establish the role of interstitial scarring in the natural history of progression of diabetic nephropathy.

S. Klahr, M.D.

References

1. Fine LG, Norman JT: Renal growth responses to acute and chronic injury: Routes to therapeutic intervention. *J Am Soc Nephrol* 3:206S-224S, 1992.
2. Horlyck A, Gunderson HJG, Osterby R: The cortical distribution pattern of dia-betic glomerulopathy. *Diabetologia* 29:146–150, 1986.
3. Bader R, Bader H, Grund KE, et al: Structure and function of the kidney in diabetic glomerulosclerosis: Correlations between morphologic and functional parameters. *Pathol Res Pract* 167:204–216, 1980.
4. Frokjaer Thomsen O, Andersen A, Christiansen JS, et al: Renal changes in long-term type I insulin-dependent diabetic patients with and without clinical nephrop-athy: A light microscopic, morphometric study of autopsy material. *Diabetologia* 26:361–365, 1984.
5. Mauer S, Stelles M, Elles E, et al: Structural functional relationships in diabetic nephropathy. *J Clin Invest* 74:1143–1155, 1984.
6. Lane PH, Steffes MW, Fioretto P, et al: Renal interstitial expansion in insulin dependent diabetes mellitus. *Kidney Int* 43:661–669, 1993.
7. Risdon RA, Sloper JC, de Wardener HE: Relationship between renal function and histological changes found in renal biopsy specimens from patients with persistent glomerular nephritis. *Lancet* i:363–366, 1968.

Increased Renal Production of Transforming Growth Factor-β1 In Pa-tients With Type II Diabetes

Sharma K, Ziyadeh FN, Alzahabi B, et al (Thomas Jefferson Univ, Philadel-phia; Univ of Pennsylvania, Philadelphia; UMDNJ, Camden, NJ)
Diabetes 46:854–859, 1997
31–7

Purpose.—Patients with type I or type II diabetes are at risk of diabetic nephropathy. In this common complication, metabolic and vascular fac-tors may produce chronic accumulation of glomerular mesangial matrix. These processes may involve both transforming growth factor-β (TGF-β) and endothelin. Renal production of TGF-β and endothelin was assessed in patients with type II diabetes.

Methods.—The study included 14 patients with type II diabetes and 11 nondiabetic patients, all of whom were undergoing elective cardiac cath-eterization. Both groups underwent measurement of TGF-β and endothe-

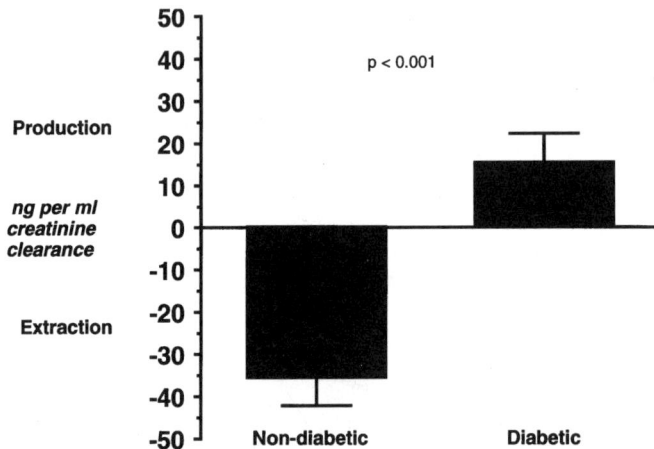

FIGURE 2.—Net renal transforming growth factor-β_1 mass values factored per creatinine clearance (mL · min^{-1} · 1.73 m^{-2}) in nondiabetic and diabetic patients. Data are means ± SE. (Courtesy of Sharma K, Ziyadeh FN, Alzahabi B, et al: Increased renal production of transforming growth factor-β_1 in patients with type II diabetes. *Diabetes* 46:854–859, 1997.)

lin levels in the aortic and renal vein blood and in urine. Net mass balance across the kidney was calculated by measurement of renal blood flow.

Results.—The results showed net production of immunoreactive TGF-β_1 by the kidneys in patients with diabetes, at a mean rate of 830 ng/min. However, patients without diabetes had net renal extraction of circulating TGF-β_1, at a mean rate of −3,479 ng/min. Mean bioassayable levels of TGF-β in urine were 2.435 ng/mg creatinine in diabetic patients and 0.569 ng/mg in nondiabetic patients. There was no significant difference between groups in renal production of immunoreactive endothelin.

Conclusions.—Patients with type II diabetes have enhanced net renal production of TGF-β_1, whereas nondiabetic controls show net renal extraction of this cytokine. Elevated production of TGF-β by the kidney may play an important role in the development of diabetic nephropathy. Longitudinal studies are needed to determine whether to renal TGF-β production is a useful marker of risk and/or progression of diabetic nephropathy.

▶ Diabetic nephropathy is the major cause of end-stage renal disease (ESRD) requiring dialysis or transplantation in the United States. About 35% of patients with newly diagnosed ESRD have diabetic nephropathy as a cause of renal insufficiency. Hyperglycemia and hypertension are important risk factors for the progression of renal disease in patients with type 1 diabetes. Diabetic nephropathy is characterized by the progressive accumulation of extracellular matrix components in the glomerular structures and the interstitial space, and ischemic changes in the vascular tree. Several reports indicate that TGF-β plays a major role in glomerular and tubulointerstitial fibrosis.[1] The TGF-β_1 stimulates matrix protein synthesis (collagens, laminin, fibronectin) and inhibits matrix degradation both by increasing the activity of metalloproteinase inhibitors and by decreasing the activity of metalloproteinases. Transforming growth factor-β, is also a chemoattractant for fibroblasts and can stimulate the proliferation of these cells. Sharma et al. demonstrate that the production of TGF-β$_1$ protein was increased in the kidneys of most of the study patients (10 of 14; 71%) with type II diabetes. By contrast, all 11 nondiabetic patients studied had net renal extraction of circulating TGF-β$_1$ (Fig 2). However, plasma levels of circulating TGF-β$_1$ were lower in diabetic patients, compared with nondiabetic patients. Additional studies are needed to define more clearly the potential role of TGF-β$_1$ in the progression of renal disease in patients with diabetic nephropathy.

S. Klahr, M.D.

Reference

1. Border WA, Noble NA: TGF-β in kidney fibrosis: A target for gene therapy. *Kidney Int* 51:1388–1896, 1997.

Increased Incidence of Glomerulonephritis Following Spleno-renal Shunt Surgery in Non-cirrhotic Portal Fibrosis
Dash SC, Bhuyan UN, Dinda AK, et al (India Inst of Medical Science, New Delhi)
Kidney Int 52:482–485, 1997   31–8

Introduction.—The spleno-renal shunt (SRS) is useful in controlling variceal hemorrhaging in patients with non-cirrhotic portal fibrosis (NCPF). Glomerulonephritis (GN) has been reported in patients with NCPF, especially after SRS surgery. The prevalence and characteristics of glomerular changes and the relationships of these renal lesions with portal hypertension were prospectively evaluated in patients with NCPF.

Methods.—Two-hundred patients with NCPF and 200 with extrahepatic portal obstruction (EHPO) underwent SRS, splenectomy, and anastomosis of the splenic vein to the left renal vein. The mean age of patients with NCPF was 28 years, and the mean age of patients with EHPO was 19 years. Patients were followed up for 5 years. Left renal biopsy specimens were obtained during surgery and throughout follow-up in patients who had significant proteinuria.

Results.—Seven percent of patients with NCPF had mild proteinuria, and their biopsy specimens showed mild mesangial proliferative GN (mes-PGN); 93% had normal biopsy results at the time of surgery. After insertion of an SRS, nephrotic syndrome developed in 28% within 5 years (Table 1). Microhematuria increased from 6% at baseline to 25% after 4 years. Renal histologic evaluations 18.5% with mesangiocapillary glomerulonephritis, 9% with mes-PGN, 3% with minimal change nephropathy, and 1.5% with chronic sclerosing GN. Granular deposition of IgA and serum complement C3 was detected by immunofluorescence. In glomerular deposits, IgA2 was the predominant form of Ig, which indicated that IgA in the immune complexes was derived from the gastrointestinal tract. Electron dense deposits in the mesangium were detected via electron

TABLE 1.—Renal Function Data in Noncirrhotic Portal Fibrosis Before and After Spleno-renal Shunting Operations in 200 Patients

	Pre-operative	1 Month	1 Year	2 Years	3 Years	Post-operative 4 Years	5 Years
Proteinuria % of patients having > 300 mg/24 hrs	7	8.5	11.5	26	27.5	29	32
Mean $U_{Pr} \times V$ g/24 hr							
M =	0.56 ± 0.09	0.6 ± 0.13	1.1 ± 0.28	2.5 ± 0.45	3.5 ± 0.46	3.8 ± 0.51	3.6 ± 0.56
N =	14	17	23	52	55	58	64
Hematuria % 200 patients	0	6	18	18	20	25	22
Average C_{Cr} (ml/month)*							
M =	79 ± 14	61 ± 5.0	60 ± 8.0	48 ± 9.0	41 ± 12	38 ± 16	32 ± 14
N =	14	17	23	52	55	58	64
Serum creatinine mg/dl	1.0 ± 0.1	1.0 ± 0.3	1.4 ± 0.4	1.5 ± 0.4	2.7 ± 1.4	2.8 ± 1.6	3.3 ± 1.7

*In patients in whom glomerulonephritis developed.

Abbreviations: C_{cr}, creatinine clearance; M, mean value; N, number of patients; U_{Pr}, incidence of proteinuria.

(Reprinted by permission of Blackwell Science, Inc., from Dash SC, Bhuyan UN, Dinda AK, et al: Increased incidence of glomerulonephritis following spleno-renal shunt surgery in non-cirrhotic portal fibrosis. *Kidney Int* 52:482–485, 1997.)

microscopy. Patients with EHPO who underwent SRS did not have renal disease at baseline, nor did they have renal disease during 5 years of follow-up. In patients with NCPF, 50% with GN progressed to renal failure in 5 years and 46.6% continued to have proteinuria. Low serum complement C3 (40%) and circulating immune complexes (14.8%) were detected in patients with GN.

Conclusion.—The rate of GN is increased after SRS in patients with NCPF, but not in those with normal livers. The IgA nephropathy type of GN is most common in patients with NCPF. Perhaps GN in patients with NCPF is the result of defective hepatic reticuloendothelial function aggravated by shunting procedures.

▶ This study from India compares 2 groups of patients admitted to the hospital for the insertion of spleno-renal shunts; there were 200 patients with biopsy-proved noncirrhotic portal fibrosis and 200 with extrahepatic portal obstruction. After the shunt, 28% of the patients with noncirrhotic portal fibrosis had nephrotic syndrome within 5 years and had a decrease in renal function (Table 1). By contrast, none of the 200 patients with extrahepatic portal obstruction had renal disease during the 5-year follow-up period. The pathogenesis of GN in patients with noncirrhotic portal fibrosis is not clear. In cirrhosis, glomerular disease has been ascribed to the presence of hepatitis B surface antigen. This was apparently not the cause of glomerular disease in these patients. In experimental animals, the injection of colloidal carbon together with oral immunization produces deposition of IgA in the mesangium. This is probably related to saturation of the reticuloendothelial system in the liver. It has been shown that the function of the hepatic reticuloendothelial system is altered in noncirrhotic portal fibrosis, but not in extrahepatic portal obstruction. The shunt procedure may enhance the post-systemic circulation and partly bypass the reticuloendothelial system in the liver. This may result in excessive levels of circulating immune complexes in the circulation, which may then lead to immune complex glomerular disease.

S. Klahr, M.D.

Involvement of Neutrophil Elastase in Crescentic Glomerulonephritis
Oda T, Hotta O, Taguma Y, et al (Natl Defense Med College, Saitama, Japan; Sendai Shakaihoken Hosp, Japan; Tohoku Univ, Sendai, Japan)
Hum Pathol 28:720–728, 1997   31–9

Introduction.—The pathogenesis of crescentic glomerulonephritis (GN) is not completely understood. Earlier observations suggest involvement of neutrophils in the renal tissue damage of this severe form of GN. Renal tissues and urine samples from 30 patients with crescentic GN were analyzed to determine the presence of neutrophil elastase (NE), a powerful tissue destructive proteinase of neutrophils.

Methods.—Surgical biopsies were examined for neutrophils and localized NE, using an immunohistochemical technique with antibodies specific

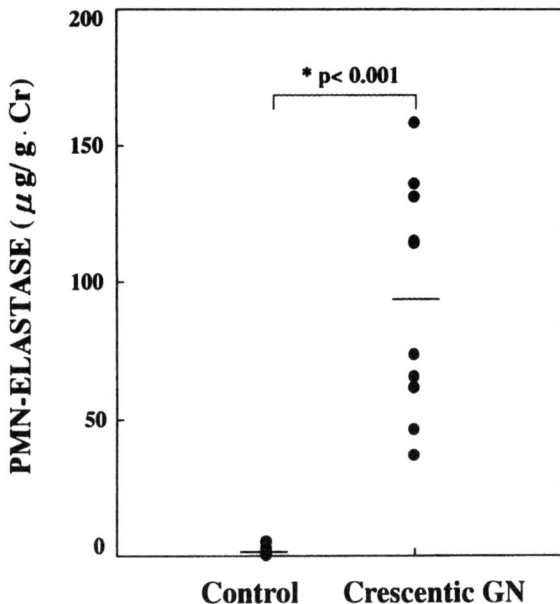

FIGURE 7.—Enzyme-linked immunosorbent assay measures of urinary NE-α1–Pl complex levels, corrected for urinary creatinine levels, from 10 crescentic GN patients and 10 healthy volunteers. The difference between mean levels is statistically significant (P < 0.001). (Courtesy of Oda T, Hotta O, Taguma Y, et al: Involvement of neutrophil elastase in crescentic glomerulonephritis. *Hum Pathol* 28:720–728, 1997.)

for neutrophils and NE. Chloroesterase staining was also used to detect neutrophils.

Results.—Neutrophil infiltration was rarely observed, and NE was localized in neutrophil cytoplasm in normal controls. In patients with crescentic GN, neutrophils were abundant and infiltrated the glomerulus and interstitium; infiltrating neutrophils were often aggregated. Neutrophil elastase was localized in the cytoplasm of neutrophils and was seen extracellularly in granular or diffuse patterns in glomerular necrotizing lesions, crescents, ruptured portions of Bowman's capsules, and periglomerular and perivascular sites of the interstitium. Urinary concentrations of NE in patients with crescentic GN were significantly greater, compared with controls (Fig 7).

Conclusion.—Neutrophil elastase is a significant factor in renal tissue damage, particularly in the formation of glomerular necrotizing and crescentic lesions and periglomerular interstitial lesions of crescentic GN.

▶ Crescentic glomerulonephritis (GN) is a severe and rapidly progressive disease that may cause end-stage renal failure in a few weeks or months. The pathogenesis of this entity has not been completely elucidated. In this study, Oda et al. have examined the potential role of neutrophil elastase, one of the most potent proteinases of neutrophils, in the pathogenesis of crescentic glomerulonephritis. Renal tissues obtained by needle biopsy for diagnostic purposes from 30 patients with crescentic GN were used in this study. Crescentic GN was characterized by a prominent infiltration and aggregation of neutrophils and extracellular granular and diffuse localization of neutrophil elastase. The affected patients also had a high concentration of neutrophil elastase in the urine (Fig 7). Thus, neutral elastase appears to have a major role in kidney damage, particularly in the formation of crescentic and necrotizing lesions in the glomeruli and lesions in periglomerular interstitium.

The new insight into the potential mechanisms of the pathogenesis of crescentic GN may result in the development of rational therapies for this disorder.

S. Klahr, M.D.

32 Other Diseases of the Kidney

Gitelman's Syndrome (Bartter's Variant) Maps to the Thiazide-Sensitive Cotransporter Gene Locus on Chromosome 16q13 in a Large Kindred[1]
Pollak MR, Delaney VB, Graham RM, et al (Brigham and Women's Hosp, Boston; New York Med College, Valhalla; Victor Chang Cardiac Research Inst, Darlinghurst, NSW, Australia)
J Am Soc Nephrol 7:2244–2248, 1996   32–1

Background.—Gitelman's syndrome (GS), a variant of Bartter's syndrome, is characterized by hypokalemia, metabolic alkalosis, hypomagnesemia, inappropriate kaliuresis and magnesiuresis, and hypocalciuria. A defect in distal renal tubular sodium chloride handling is believed to be responsible for the clinical phenotype of GS. The involvement of the renal thiazide-sensitive NaCl cotransporter gene in GS was investigated.

Methods and Findings.—Genetic linkage studies were performed in the largest kindred with GS reported to date, with 17 members in 2 generations. A human homolog of rat thiazide-sensitive cotransporter was cloned and mapped to chromosome 16q13. All the family members were genotyped at loci in this region. No recombinants were observed between the GS phenotype and inheritance of D16S408 alleles, with a lod score of 3.88 at $Q = 0$. By contrast, there were recombinants between GS and the flanking markers D16S419 and D16S400. The gene responsible for GS in this family was localized to a 15-centimorgan region on chromosome 16q.

Conclusions.—These findings suggest that the thiazide-sensitive cotransporter is defective in this kindred with GS. The classification of the different variants of Bartter's syndrome by their molecular defect will enable more rational treatment.

▶ Bartter's syndrome is characterized by metabolic alkalosis with hyperaldosteronism and severe hypokalemia. Renin levels are increased, and there is hyperplasia and hypertrophy of the juxtaglomerular apparatus. Patients with Bartter's syndrome are also refractory to the increase in blood pressure, which is seen in normal individuals given angiotensin II. Most of these patients have elevated levels of prostaglandin E_2 in the urine. Patients with

Gitelman's syndrome, a variant of Bartter's syndrome, have metabolic alkalosis and hypokalemia, as well as hypomagnesemia and hypocalciuria. By contrast, patients with Bartter's syndrome have hypercalciuria. Studies conducted in patients with Gitelman's syndrome suggest that the observed cation changes are due to a defect in the sodium-chloride cotransport in the distal convoluted tubule. A thiazide-sensitive, sodium chloride cotransporter has recently been cloned. This transporter is expressed in the convoluted portion of the distal tubule, the site at which thiazide diuretics inhibit sodium reabsorption and stimulate calcium reabsorption. This report examines the possible role of the renal thiazide-sensitive NaCl cotransporter gene in Gitelman's syndrome. A linkage analysis study in the largest known kindred with Gitelman's syndrome was performed. In this kindred the following findings were present: growth retardation, tetany, hypotension, hyperkalemia, hypomagnesemia, inability of the kidney to conserve potassium and magnesium, and hypocalciuria. The human thiazide-sensitive cotransporter gene and the gene responsible for Gitelman's syndrome in this kindred both map to chromosome 16q13. However, additional studies are needed to explore the potential substitutions or deletions present in the defective gene and to show that the function of the resulting protein is altered. Further definition of the role of the thiazide-sensitive cotransporter has important implications for potential therapy in subjects with Gitelman's syndrome.

S. Klahr, M.D.

Localization of a Single Binding Site for Immunoglobulin Light Chains on Human Tamm-Horsfall Glycoprotein
Huang Z-Q, Sanders PW (Univ of Alabama, Birmingham)
J Clin Invest 99:732–736, 1997   32–2

Introduction.—Patients with multiple myeloma commonly have a severe complication known as cast nephropathy, or "myeloma kidney." It results from binding between filtered monoclonal light chains (LC) and Tamm-Horsfall glycoprotein (THP), the coaggregation of which causes casts that obstruct flow in the distal nephron. Toward designing new treatments to reduce the incidence of cast nephropathy, a study to identify the light chain-binding site on human THP was conducted.

Methods and Results.—Human THP was deglycosylated and limited trypsin digestion was performed. The trypsin digestion studies were done in the presence and absence of a nephrotoxic LC that binds LP. This LC resulted in protection of a 29.6-kd band against trypsin digestion. The band was localized between the sixth and two hundred eighty-seventh amino acid residues of THP on NH_2-terminal amino acid sequencing and amino acid studies. Within this fragment were found 6 peptides that were tested as inhibitors of binding or aggregation of nephrotoxic LCs with THP. Binding and aggregation were completely inhibited by the peptide AHWSGHCCL, which was localized from amino acids 225–233. A cystine residue had to be present in AHWSGHCCL for optimal inhibition of binding to occur. For optimal inhibition, the entire sequence had to be present. The effects of pH on binding were accounted for by the histidine residue.

Conclusions.—A 9-amino acid sequence responsible for LC binding on THP is identified. Knowing the LC-binding site on THP opens the way to further study of the interaction between these 2 proteins, and may produce an approach to preventing cast nephropathy in patients with multiple myeloma.

▶ Multiple myeloma is characterized by the presence of malignant clones of B lymphocytes that produce intact immunoglobulins or light chains in excess. The peak incidence of multiple myeloma occurs in humans between the ages of 50 and 70 years. Renal failure occurs in about 50% of patients with multiple myeloma. Renal failure in this setting may result from deposition of casts (Bence Jones proteins - light chains) in the tubules, as well as hypercalcemia, hyperuricemia, dehydration, and infections (pyelonephritis). Cast nephropathy, or myeloma kidney, is the most common lesion resulting from deposition of light chains in the renal tubules, particularly the distal nephron. Casts develop in part because light chains bind and co-aggregate with THP, which is synthesized by cells of the thick ascending limb of the loop of Henle. Deposition of these casts in the distal renal tubule obstructs the flow of filtered fluid through the nephron and leads to renal failure. Both kappa and lambda light chains share a binding site on the THP. This study by Huang and Sanders was designed to localize the light chain-binding site on THP. They found that the binding site was localized to a linear sequence of 9 amino acids of the THP. The same authors have shown previously that modification of THP by colchicine inhibited aggregation with light chains[1] and prevented cast formation in a rat model of cast nephropathy.[2] The authors point out that identification of the light chain-binding site on THP should help the development of strategies designed to inhibit the interaction of the protein with light chains. This may lead to the development of compounds that may ameliorate or prevent "cast nephropathy," a severe renal complication of multiple myeloma.

S. Klahr, M.D.

References

1. Huang Z-Q, Sanders PW: Biochemical interaction of Tamm-Horsfall glycoprotein with Ig light chains. *Lab Invest* 73:810–817, 1995.
2. Sanders PW, Booker BB: Pathobiology of cast nephropathy from human Bence Jones protein. *J Clin Invest* 89:630–639, 1992.

End-stage Renal Disease Among Silica-exposed Gold Miners: A New Method for Assessing Incidence Among Epidemiologic Cohorts

Calvert GM, Steenland K, Palu S (Natl Inst for Occupational Safety and Health, Cincinnati, Ohio)

JAMA 277:1219–1223, 1997   32–3

Background.—The cause of end-stage renal disease (ESRD) is often not known. There are few data on the possible etiologic role of occupational or environmental exposures. Several lines of evidence suggest that silica has nephrotoxic effects. The incidence of ESRD was studied in a cohort of gold miners exposed to silica.

Methods.—The retrospective cohort study included 2,412 men who had worked in an underground gold mine for at least 1 year between 1940 and 1965. Estimated silica exposures were over the current Occupational Safety and Health Administration Permissible Exposure Limit before 1951, but within the limit after workplace interventions in the early 1950s. All subjects were alive in 1977. Miners treated for ESRD were identified through the ESRD Program Management and Medical Information System (PMMIS). The incidence of ESRD in this cohort was assessed and compared with that of the general population.

Results.—Eleven of the miners were treated for ESRD. The risk was significantly higher than that of the general population (standardized incidence ratio, [SIR] 1.37). The SIR was even higher for nonsystemic ESRD (i.e., that resulting from glomerulonephritis or interstitial nephritis). This figure rose to 7.70 for miners who had worked for 10 years or longer underground.

Conclusion.—Underground gold mine workers exposed to silica have a significantly increased incidence of ESRD. The risk is particularly high for ESRD caused by glomerulonephritis. This is the first known study to examine ESRD risk by occupational group. The ESRD PMMIS should be useful in assessing ESRD risk among workers exposed to other potentially nephrotoxic substances.

▶ The population with ESRD represents a growing fraction of the total number of Medicare beneficiaries in the United States. Between 1976 and 1991, the ESRD component of the total Medicare population increased fivefold. During the same time period, Medicare expenditures for ESRD increased from 3.2% to 5.2% of the total Medicare budget. Diabetes and hypertension are the major causes of ESRD. Scanty information is available regarding the etiologic role of potential occupational and environmental toxins in the development of renal disease. Among elements that have nephrotoxic potential, cadmium, lead, and gold are well recognized. Some drugs (analgesics and antibiotics) and other compounds also have been shown to be nephrotoxic.

This study assessed the association between silica exposure and ESRD in a cohort of 2,412 male gold miners. The authors conclude that exposure to silica is associated with an increased risk for ESRD, particularly ESRD associated with glomerulonephritis. Previous studies from Britain[1, 2] in patients exposed to silica suggested that renal tubular dysfunction appears initially and is followed by glomerular injury. Studies in experimental animals[3] suggest that silica induces interstitial nephritis by deposition of crystals in the renal parenchyma.

The odds ratio for development of ESRD in someone who has worked long term as a sandblaster is 3.8-fold, compared with matched controls. In an accelerated form of silicosis, known as silicoproteinosis, silicon dust appears to be indirectly involved in the development of rapidly progressive glomerulonephritis.[4]

The authors of this article point out the limitations of their methods in the discussion section. They do not discuss, however, the potential role of gold, per se, in the increased incidence of ESRD in this population of miners.

S. Klahr, M.D.

References

1. Lee HS, et al: A study of silica nephrotoxicity in exposed silicotic and non-silicotic workers. *Br J Ind Med* 49:35–37, 1992.
2. Lee HS, Phoon WH: Further evidence of human silica nephrotoxicity in occupationally exposed workers. *Br J Ind Med* 50:907–912, 1993.
3. Dobbie JW, Smith MJB: Silicate nephrotoxicity in the experimental animal: The missing factor in analgesic nephropathy. *Scott Med J* 27:10–16, 1982.
4. Osorio AM, Thun MJ, Novak RF, et al: Silica and glomerulonephritis. *Am J Kidney Dis* 9:224–230, 1987.

Vascular Expression of Polycystin
Griffin MD, Torres VE, Grande JP, et al (Mayo Clinic and Mayo Found, Rochester, Minn)
J Am Soc Nephrol 8:616–626, 1997   32–4

Introduction.—Patients with autosomal dominant polycystic kidney disease (ADPKD) are at increased risk for a variety of vascular abnormalities, but it has not been determined whether these vascular manifestations result directly from the genetic defect responsible for ADPKD. Tissue specimens from patients with ADPKD and controls were examined for the expression of polycystin, a large protein of unknown function encoded by the gene *PKD1* responsible for most cases of ADPKD.

Methods.—Tissue specimens obtained at autopsy included control abdominal and thoracic aorta, iliac, renal, mesenteric, and cervicocephalic arteries from 8 individuals who had died in accidents; sections of intracranial aneurysms from 10 patients with ADPKD; and sections from 13 age- and gender-matched patients without ADPKD. Additional sections were obtained from 2 patients with ADPKD who had thoracic aortic dissections and from 1 patient with dolichoectatic basilar, vertebral, and internal carotid arteries.

Results.—All control arteries showed moderate-to-weak immunostaining for polycystin; the staining pattern was greatly enhanced by partial digestion of tissue slices with the nonspecific proteases trypsin and pronase. Similar enhancement was seen with specific elastase digestion, but digestion with elastase did not enhance the staining for smooth-muscle actin. Specimens of intracranial aneurysms, aortic dissections, and dolichoectatic arteries from patients with ADPKD showed immunostaining of variable intensity for polycystin in arterial smooth-muscle cells and myofibroblasts, together with disruption of elastic laminae. Staining patterns were not significantly altered by further elastase digestion. Intracranial aneurysms from patients without ADPKD also showed a variable degree of immunostaining with polycystin antisera in the same distribution.

Conclusion.—Polycystin is expressed in the vascular smooth muscle of the elastic and large distributive arteries, and may play a role in maintaining the normal functional synergy between arterial smooth-muscle cells and adjacent elastic tissue. Findings suggest that vascular complications in ADPKD are not secondary but are directly linked to the underlying genetic defect.

▶ Approximately 500,000 people in the United States carry a mutant gene for ADPKD, making it one of the most common inherited disorders. The disorder affects several systems. With ADPKD, there is progressive cyst formation in the kidney and other organs, a tenfold to 20-fold increased risk of subarachnoid hemorrhage, compared with the general population, and an increased risk for a variety of pathologic vascular conditions. The etiology of these vascular diseases is not well understood, and some of them have been attributed to the development of hypertension and degenerative vascular involvement in these patients.

The major finding in this report is the detection, using immunohistochemical techniques, of polycystin within the smooth-muscle cells of arteries of normal adults. Polycystin is a large protein encoded by the *PKD1* gene, the mutations of which have been implicated in the development of ADPKD. The presence of polycystin in arterial walls indicates that the vascular disorders seen in these patients with ADPKD could be genetic manifestations of ADPKD rather than secondary events. Genetic malfunction, per se, may account for the development of arterial aneurysms (particularly in the circle of Willis), concentric dilation of vessels (dolichoectasias), aortic root dilation, and dissection of the thoracic aorta.

The authors of this report hypothesize that polycystin has a role in maintaining the normal interaction between arterial smooth-muscle cells and the adjacent elastic tissues, and that subtle disturbances of this interaction in patients with ADPKD lead to potentially serious pathology of the arterial wall. Obviously, additional studies are needed to understand the mechanism by which polycystin impairs the normal biology of the arterial wall.

S. Klahr, M.D.

Endothelin-1 Transgenic Mice Develop Glomerulosclerosis, Interstitial Fibrosis, and Renal Cysts but not Hypertension

Hocher B, Thöne-Reineke C, Rohmeiss P, et al (Free Univ of Berlin; Univ of Heidelberg, Germany; Schering Research Labs, Berlin; et al)
J Clin Invest 99:1380–1389, 1997   32–5

Introduction.—Endothelins have vasoconstrictive abilities and also cause a variety of biological activities in nonvascular tissues. To determine whether an endogenous activation of the paracrine endothelin system is a cause or a consequence of glomerular injury, the human endothelin-1 (*ET-1*) gene was transferred into the germline of mice.

Methods.—Human *ET-1* transgenic mice were produced by microinjection of linear human *ET-1* genomic DNA fragments into 1-cell embryos obtained from hormone-primed NMRI females mated the night before injection with NMRI males. Viable eggs were transferred to the oviducts of pseudopregnant NMRI mice. Southern blot analysis and polymerase chain reaction of DNA isolated from tail biopsy specimens were used to identify transgenic mice. Three independent transgenic lines (238, 260, and 856) were established; lines 238 and 856 were selected for further analysis.

Results.—Northern blot analysis identified transgene expression in the brain, lungs, and kidneys of both transgenic mouse lines in equal amounts. With the more sensitive reverse transcriptase–polymerase chain reaction with human-specific ET-1 primers, lower levels of transgenic expression were detected in other organs. None of the nontransgenic littermates exhibited transgene expression. Renal overexpression of ET-1 in transgenic mice was associated with an age-dependent development of renal cysts and renal fibrosis without hypertension. In both transgenic mouse lines, pronounced renal fibrosis led to a significantly decreased glomerular filtration rate, leading to fatal kidney disease.

Conclusion.—The transgenic lines produced here provide a new animal model of *ET-1*-induced renal pathology leading to renal fibrosis and fatal kidney disease. This process was not related to systemic hypertension, suggesting that an activated renal ET system is a blood-pressure–independent factor for the progression of renal fibrosis to end-stage renal disease.

► Endothelins are powerful vasoconstrictors. There are 3 different isoforms of endothelin, one of which, ET-1, has been implicated in the progression of renal disease.[1] Endothelins are produced by several renal cells, including the tubules, which can secrete abundant amounts of ET-1 and lesser quantities of endothelin-3. The endothelin system in the kidney participates in the regulation of renal blood flow, glomerular filtration rate, and tubular reabsorption of sodium and water. Endothelin-1 can stimulate proliferation of mesangial cells and appears to participate in matrix protein synthesis in the kidney. The report abstracted here describes the pathologic changes that occur in the kidney of transgenic mice expressing the human ET-1 gene.

The overexpression of human ET-1 in mouse kidney resulted in the development of renal cysts and renal fibrosis (glomerulosclerosis and interstitial fibrosis) in the absence of hypertension. The pronounced fibrosis of the kidney caused a significant, age-dependent decrease in glomerular filtration rate, leading to death of the transgenic mice resulting from uremia. Previous studies have suggested a correlation between activation of the endothelin system and renal injury. In humans and in animals with experimental renal disease, an activated renal endothelin system (ET-1) caused by hypoxia, reduction of renal mass, administration of cyclosporine, or inflammatory kidney disease, such as lupus nephritis, seems to correlate with renal damage. The development of these transgenic animal studies provides a tool for studying the underlying mechanism by which endothelin causes renal disease.

S. Klahr, M.D.

Reference

1. Kohan D: Endothelins in the kidney: Physiology and pathophysiology. *Am J Kidney Dis* 22:493–510, 1993.

Enalaprilat Inhibits Hydrogen Peroxide Production by Murine Mesangial Cells Exposed to High Glucose Concentrations
Ruiz-Muñoz LM, Vidal-Vanaclocha F, Lampreabe I (Cruces Hosp, Spain; Basque Country Univ, Lejona, Vizcaya, Spain)
Nephrol Dial Transplant 12:456–464, 1997   32–6

Introduction.—An experimental study was designed to test the hypothesis that enalaprilat, an angiotensin-converting enzyme (ACE) inhibitor, might have a modulatory effect on in vitro hydrogen peroxide production by cultured murine mesangial cells exposed to high glucose. Although ACE inhibitors are known to prevent the progression of chronic renal failure, their mechanism of action is not fully understood.

Methods.—Mesangial cells were exposed to 5.5- (basal), 30-, and 50-Mm glucose for 8 hours. Added to the 3 glucose concentration were 10, 50, and 100 ng/mL of enalaprilat. Other assays tested control groups of mesangial cells in the presence of mannitol. The scavenger activity of reactive oxygen metabolites was studied by adding catalase (100 ng/mL) to controls. A second study examined the influence of angiotensin II and saralasin on cells exposed to basal glucose concentrations, and of staurosporine in cells in the presence of elevated glucose. A microfluorimetric method not previously reported for cultured mesangial cells was used to demonstrate glucose-dependent hydrogen peroxide production.

Results.—After the first hour of the assay, the production of hydrogen peroxide by mesangial cells exposed to 50-mM glucose was significantly increased, compared with cells exposed to 5.5- and 30-mM glucose. This did not occur with 50-mM mannitol, and at no time did hydrogen peroxide production in the presence of 30-mM differ significantly from that with 5.5-mM. The addition of 100 ng/mL–enalaprilat to cells with 50-mM glucose significantly inhibited production of hydrogen peroxide over the

8-hour assay period. A similar response was obtained with 100 ng/mL–catalase. Angiotensin II and saralasin (both at 1 µM) did not alter hydrogen peroxide production by cells exposed to 5.5-mM glucose. Staurosporine (1 µM), however, a protein kinase C antagonist, caused hydrogen peroxide generation to be significantly decreased in the presence of 50-mM glucose.

Conclusion.—Recent studies suggest that glucose-induced oxidative stress plays a role in vascular complications and chronic renal damage in diabetes mellitus. The antioxidant effect of enalaprilat on cultured mesangial cells in these experiments was not linked to ACE inhibition, but may be related to inhibition of the protein kinase C system.

▶ Angiotensin-converting enzyme inhibitors are frequently used for the treatment of arterial hypertension and cardiac failure. These compounds can also improve myocardial sclerosis, attenuate postischemic myocardial dysfunction, reduce glomerulosclerosis, and decrease age-related renal interstitial fibrosis in different experimental models of renal disease. The mechanisms underlying these developoments are not well understood. They may include effects on hemodynamic events, stimulation of the synthesis of cytoprotective prostaglandins, the expression of certain cytokines and chemokines, and decreased activation of nuclear factor κ B.

Several studies, including this one, indicate that ACE inhibitors may also play a role as scavengers of free radicals. In this article, Ruiz-Muñoz et al. note that glucose-induced oxidative stress has recently been proposed as playing a role in the vascular complications and chronic renal damage that occur in patients with diabetes mellitus. This study demonstrates a glucose-dependent production of hydrogen peroxide by cultured mesangial cells.

Enalaprilat, the soluble active form of the ACE inhibitor enalapril, decreased the production of hydrogen peroxide. At basal and high glucose concentrations, this drug significantly diminished hydrogen peroxide production in a catalase-like manner, although the amount of inhibition with catalase was more extreme than that obtained with enalaprilat. Even at low concentrations, this drug had a significant modulating effect on the constitutive production of hydrogen peroxide by cells with basal glucose levels. Other studies have shown that the ACE inhibitors enalapril and captopril enhance antioxidant defenses in mouse tissues,[1] as well as changes of lipid peroxides and antioxidative factor levels in the blood of patients.[2] The enhancement of antioxidant defenses could be a mechanism by which ACE inhibitors protect against oxidative damage to cell components. This effect may contribute to the pharmacologic effects of these antihypertensive compounds.

S. Klahr, M.D.

References

1. De Cavanagh EMV, Fraga CG, Ferder L, et al: Enalapril and captopril enhance antioxidant defenses in mouse tissues. *Am J Physiol* 272:F514–F518, 1997.
2. Diordjević VB, Pavlović D, Pejović M, et al: Changes of lipid peroxides and antioxidative factor levels in blood of patients treated with ACE inhibitors. *Clin Nephrol* 47:243–247, 1997.

Prevalence and Predictors of Renal Artery Stenosis in Patients With Myocardial Infarction

Uzu T, Inoue T, Fujii T, et al (Natl Cardiovascular Ctr, Osaka, Japan)
Am J Kidney Dis 29:733–738, 1997   32–7

Background.—Renal artery stenosis (RAS), an important cause of both end-stage renal disease and secondary hypertension, may be correctable. To determine the prevalence and predictors of RAS in the population of patients with atherosclerosis, autopsy data from patients older than 40 years who had evidence of myocardial infarction related to significant coronary artery disease were retrospectively examined.

Methods.—During the 12-year period from 1981 to 1992, 297 of 1,788 autopsy cases met inclusion criteria. Demographic data, smoking history, hypertension, hypercholesterolemia, diabetes, renal function, and proteinuria were determined from medical records. At autopsy, coronary vessels were sectioned for examination of stenosis, which was characterized as to

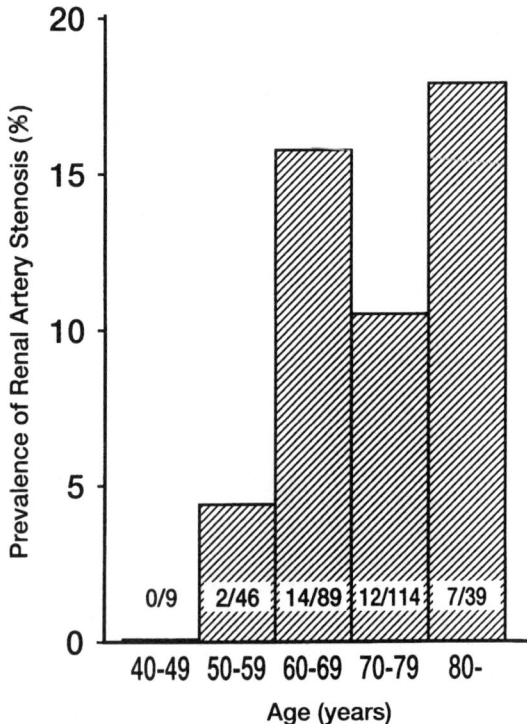

FIGURE 1.—The prevalence of renal artery stenosis and age in autopsy patients with myocardial infarction. The number of patients with renal artery stenosis and the total number of patients are the numerator and denominator, respectively, within each column. (Courtesy Uzu T, Inoue T, Fujii T, et al: Prevalence and predictors of renal artery stenosis in patients with myocardial infarction. *Am J Kidney Dis* 29:733–738, 1997.)

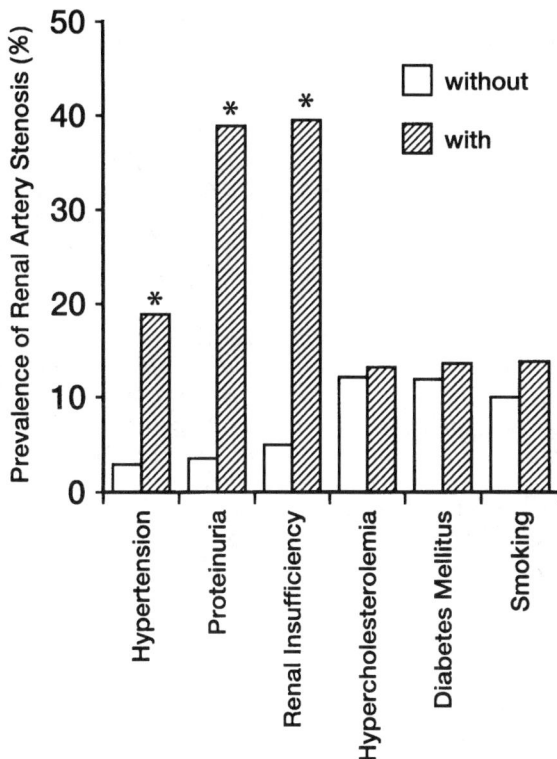

FIGURE 2.—The prevalence of renal artery stenosis in autopsy patients with myocardial infarction: Comparison between 2 groups with and without clinical characteristics such as hypertension, proteinuria, renal insufficiency, hypercholesterolemia, diabetes, and smoking. *P < 0.001. (Courtesy Uzu T, Inoue T, Fujii T, et al: Prevalence and predictors of renal artery stenosis in patients with myocardial infarction. *Am J Kidney Dis* 29:733–738, 1997.)

severity. Bilateral renal arteries were dissected to check for significant (75% or greater) stenosis.

Results.—Renal insufficiency was noted in 23% of patients for whom data were available; proteinuria was noted in 32%. Thirty-five patients (12%) showed significant (75% or greater) RAS. Infarct location did not differ between those with and without RAS. Prevalence of RAS varied with age, as shown in Fig 1; only 4% of patients younger than 60 years had significant RAS, compared with 14% of patients older than 60 years. Bilateral stenosis was found in 10 patients, all older than 60 years. Potential risk factors studied are shown in Fig 2. Renal artery stenosis was more common among patients with hypertension (19%, P < 0.001), proteinuria (39%, P < 0.001), and renal insufficiency (39%, P < 0.001). Extent of coronary artery occlusion was also related to RAS. As the number of coronary vessels with significant (75% or greater) stenosis increased, so did the likelihood of renal stenosis, and severity of occlusions in patients with 3–vessel disease showed a similar pattern. Hypertension, proteinuria, renal insufficiency, age, and number of significantly stenosed coronary arteries were found by multiple logistic regression to be independent predictors. Sex, hypercholesterolemia, diabetes, and smoking history were not.

▶ In this study from Japan, autopsies on patients older than 40 years with myocardial infarction revealed a 12% incidence of significant renal artery stenosis, defined as a narrowing of the artery equal to or exceeding 75% of the luminal area. The condition, mainly the result of atherosclerotic disease, was more prevalent with advancing age (Fig 1). Renal artery stenosis was found in 3% of patients without hypertension and in 19% of patients with hypertension.

Other studies have shown that renal artery stenosis is a common cause of end-stage renal disease, particularly in patients older than 50 years.[1, 2] It may account for 5% to 20% of patients with end-stage renal disease who are older than 50 years. In this retrospective study, regression analysis indicated that the presence of hypertension, proteinuria, or renal insufficiency significantly increased the risk of renal artery stenosis 4.8- , 11.8-, and 5.7-fold, respectively (Fig 2). The severity of narrowing of coronary vessels and the affected number of coronary vessels also correlated significantly with the presence of renal stenosis in this cohort of patients with atherosclerosis.

S. Klahr, M.D.

References

1. Scoble JE, Maher ER, Hamilton G, et al: Atherosclerotic renovascular disease causing renal failure. *Clin Nephrol* 31:119–122, 1989.
2. Corradi B, Malberti F, Farina M, et al: Chronic renal failure due to atheromatous renovascular disease in the elderly. *Contrib Nephrol* 105:167–171, 1993.

Crystalluria and Urinary Tract Abnormalities Associated With Indinavir
Kopp JB, Miller KD, Mican JM, et al (Natl Inst Diabetes and Digestive and Kidney Diseases, N IH, Bethesda, Md)
Ann Intern Med 127:119–125, 1997   32–8

Background.—The protease inhibitor indinavir has become the most widely prescribed antiretroviral agent in the United States. Indinavir therapy carries a 4% incidence of nephrolithiasis. Because distinctive urinary crystals were recently observed in patients taking indinavir, along with urinary tract symptoms, patients receiving indinavir were studied to determine the makeup of the urinary crystals, the frequency of asymptomatic crystalluria, and the incidence of urinary tract symptoms.

Methods.—The study included 240 adult patients who received indinavir in the course of clinical trials of HIV infection conducted at the National Institutes of Health. The patients had received indinavir for a mean of 30 weeks, at a maximum dose of 2,400 mg/day in 3 or 4 divided doses. Urinalysis was performed in a subgroup of 142 patients without symptoms to determine the incidence of crystalluria. The urinary crystals and stones were evaluated by high-performance liquid chromatography and mass spectrometry. Patients with urologic symptoms underwent clinical evaluation.

Results.—Twenty percent of asymptomatic patients had distinctive crystals on urinalysis, consisting of platelike rectangles and fan-shaped or starburst forms. The indinavir composition of these crystals was confirmed by mass spectrometry and high-performance liquid chromatography. None of 40 patients who were not taking indinavir had similar crystals. The incidence of urologic symptoms in the overall study group of 240 patients was 8%, including a 3% incidence of nephrolithiasis. The remaining 5% of patients had crystalluria associated with dysuria or with back or flank pain. Four patients with crystalluria and back or flank pain syndrome showed radiographic signs of intrarenal sludging.

Conclusions.—Patients taking indinavir may have characteristic crystals in the urine. Indinavir crystalluria is linked to a spectrum of urologic findings, including dysuria and urinary frequency, dysuria with flank or back pain and intrarenal sludging, or classic renal colic. When patients taking indinavir have urologic symptoms, they can generally be treated with hydration and drug withdrawal. Later, indinavir therapy may be restarted.

▶ In the last year, a substantial decrease in mortality has occurred in patients with HIV infection. This has been attributed to better clinical care of these patients and to the use of new drugs, such as protease inhibitors. Indinavir, a protease inhibitor, is the most widely prescribed drug among this class of therapeutic agents. However, indinavir has been shown to be associated with renal stones in 4% of the patients taking this drug.[1, 2] Such stones have been shown to contain indinavir crystals.[3] This study from the National Institutes of Health identified 19 patients with urinary tract disease among 240 patients receiving indinavir. Seven of these 19 symptomatic patients had renal colic. Seven others had dull back pain or flank pain, and 3 of the patients also had dysuria. Asymptomatic crystalluria was detected in 20% of patients treated with indinavir. The authors remarked that, of the 4 protease inhibitors now in use, indinavir appears to be the most often prescribed, because it is effective, well tolerated, and has pharmacologic advantages. Nevertheless, because of the findings of crystalluria and stone formation with the use of this drug, patients taking indinavir should be appropriately hydrated and may have to discontinue using it temporarily. Monthly urinalysis is advisable to detect the presence of crystalluria.

S. Klahr, M.D.

References

1. Gulick R, Mellors J, Havlir D, et al. Potent and sustained antiretroviral activity of indinavir in combination with zidovudine and lamivudine [abstract]. Third Conference on Retroviruses and Opportunistic Infections. Washington, D.C.: LB7, 1996.
2. Crixivan (indinavir sulfate)—U.S. package insert. West Point, PA: Merck & Co, 1996.
3. Daudon M, Estepa L, Viard JP, et al: Urinary stones in HIV-1 positive patients treated with indinavir. *Lancet* 349:1294–1295, 1997.

Homo- and Heterodimeric Interactions Between the Gene Products of PKD1 and PKD2

Tsiokas L, Kim E, Arnould T, et al (Harvard Med School, Boston)
Proc Natl Acad Sci U S A 94:6965–6970, 1997   32–9

Introduction.—The PKD1 and PKD2 genes are now known to be responsible for most cases of autosomal dominant polycystic kidney disease. Polycystin, a large glycoprotein that appears to play a role in cell-cell or cell-matrix interactions, is encoded by PKD1, whereas a protein homologous to a voltage-activated calcium channel and to PKD1 is encoded by PKD2. However, the way in which mutations of either protein lead to autosomal polycystic kidney disease is unknown. PKD1 and PKD2 have overlapping expression patterns, similar disease presentations, and predicted protein structures consistent with a role in signal transduction. Whether PKD1 and PKD2 are associated through a common signal transduction pathway was investigated.

Findings.—The experimental study demonstrated interaction of PKD1 and PKD2 through their C-terminal cytoplasmic tails. PKD1 was upregulated as a result of this interaction, but PKD2 was not. Homodimers were formed by the cytoplasmic tail of PKD2, but not PKD1. This occurred through a coiled-coil domain distinct from the region required for interaction with PKD1.

Conclusions.—This study demonstrates interaction between PKD1 and PKD2 through their C-terminal cytoplasmic tails. Thus, a common signaling pathway may be essential for normal tubulogenesis, and PKD2 may be required for stable expression of PKD1. Moreover, mutations in PKD2 could interfere with the function of PKD1, leading to a disease presentation similar to that expected with mutations of PKD1.

▶ Autosomal dominant polycystic kidney disease (PKD) is a genetically heterogeneous disease with loci in chromosome 16p13.3 (the PKD1 gene) and chromosome 4q21–23 (the PKD2 gene). Both genes have been cloned and are widely expressed in different tissues. Based on the overlapping expression patterns of these 2 mutated genes, the similar disease presentations, and the predicted protein structures that are compatible with a role in signal transduction, Tsiokas et al. hypothesized that PKD1 and PKD2 are closely associated in a signal transduction pathway. This study shows that the C-terminal cytoplasmic tails of PKD1 and PKD2 interact. This results in upregulation of PKD1, but not PKD2. In addition, the cytoplasmic tail of PKD2, but not PKD1, formed homodimers through a region different from the domain required for interaction with PKD1. Thse findings are consistent with a scenario in which mutations in the PKD2 could affect the action of PKD1 and, therefore, result in a disease presentation similar to that of PKD1 through distinct molecular lesions of a common signal pathway that operates in normal tubulogenesis.

S. Klahr, M.D.

Identification of the Tuberous Sclerosis Gene *TSC1* on Chromosome 9q34

van Slegtenhorst M, de Hoogt R, Hermans C, et al (Erasmus Univ, Rotterdam, The Netherlands; Univ College of London; Univ of Bath, England, et al)
Science 277:805–808, 1997   32–10

Introduction.—Tuberous sclerosis complex (TSC) is an autosomal dominant disorder characterized by widespread growth of distinctive tumors known as hamartomas. Malignancy is rare in TSC, but the manifestations of cortical tubers (brain hamartomas) may be devastating (epilepsy, mental retardation, autism, attention deficit-hyperactive disorder, or a combination of these conditions). The TSC-determining loci are located on chromosomes 9q34 (*TSC1*) and 16p13 (*TSC2*). *TSC1* and *TSC2* may function as tumor suppressor genes. The *TSC1* gene has been identified from a 900-kilobase region containing at least 30 genes. The 8.6-kilobase *TSC1* transcript is widely expressed, encoding a protein of 130 kd (hamartin) with homology to a putative yeast protein whose function is not known. A search for large deletions and rearrangements was conducted to determine further positional information.

Methods.—Several techniques were used to determine genes in the *TSC1* region: exon trapping, cDNA selection, expressed sequence tag, mapping, and whole-cosmid hybridization. The entire contig was sequenced and amplified.

Results.—Thirty-two distinctive mutations were detected in *TSC1*. Of these, 30 were truncating, and the 2105delAAAG mutation was observed in 6 apparently unrelated patients. In 1 of these 6 patients, a somatic mutation in the wild-type allele was detected in a TSC-associated renal carcinoma, which suggested that hamartin acts as a tumor suppressor.

Conclusion.—The mechanism by which loss of hamartin expression causes TSC lesions has not been identified. Being able to identify *TSC1* will allow analysis of the function of both hamartin and tuberin, and may give further insight into the molecular pathogenesis of TSC.

▶ Angiomyolipomas (hamartomas), composed of heterotopic mesenchymal tissue, were initially described in association with TSC. The hamartomas may occur in multiple organ systems, particularly in the brain, lungs, heart, and kidneys. They rarely progress to malignancy. Clinically, hamartomas may be seen as isolated entities or in association with mental retardation, epilepsy, and adenoma sebaceum in patients with TSC. The tuberous sclerosis gene was found to be linked to the ABO locus on chromosome 9 in 1987. This paper in *Science* identifies and characterizes the tuberous sclerosis gene (*TSC1* transcript, 8.6 kilobase) present on chromosome 9q34, which was located in a region containing at least 30 genes. The gene is widely expressed and encodes a protein (hamartin). Certain mutations have been observed in *TSC1*, consisting of small deletions, small insertions, and point mutations. The authors suggest that *TSC1* functions as a tumor suppressor. The mechanism by which loss of the product of this gene (hamartin) produces the lesions of TSC is unknown. However, the identification of the gene will enable analysis of the function of both hamartin and another protein, tuberin, and perhaps will provide further clues as to the pathogenesis of the derangements that occur in TSC.

S. Klahr, M.D.

Antimicrobial Prophylaxis Prior to Shock Wave Lithotripsy in Patients With Sterile Urine Before Treatment: A Meta-analysis and Cost-effectiveness Analysis
Pearle MS, Roehrborn CG (Univ of Texas, Dallas)
Urology 49:679–686, 1997   32–11

Objective.—Urosepsis is a rare but serious complication of shock wave lithotripsy (SWL) for renal and ureteral calculi. Preoperative antimicrobial agents are routinely given before SWL in high-risk patients. However, there is controversy as to whether antimicrobial prophylaxis should be given in low-risk patients with sterile preoperative urine. With the use of published data, the efficacy and cost-effectiveness of antimicrobial prophylaxis before SWL in patients with a sterile pretreatment urine culture were analyzed.

Methods.—Fourteen studies of antimicrobial prophylaxis for SWL were identified by literature search: 8 prospective, randomized, controlled trials (RCTs) comparing active treatment with placebo or no treatment (including 885 subjects) and 6 non-RCT clinical series (including 597 subjects). The RCTs were subjected to meta-analysis, with the main outcome of diagnosed urinary tract infection (UTI) after SWL. Two strategies were compared in cost analysis: a prophylactic strategy in which every patient received prophylaxis and treatment was given for UTIs developing after SWL, and a treatment-only strategy in which post-SWL UTIs were treated by various antimicrobial combinations. The meta-analysis was used to determine the median probability of post-SWL UTIs.

Results.—In the reported studies, post-SWL UTIs occurred in 0% to 28% of control patients and 0% to 8% of patients receiving prophylaxis. Bayesian analysis was performed to combine the placebo and no-drug treatment arms of 6 RCTs. This produced a median 6% probability of post-SWL UTI, compared with 2% median probability in the drug treatment arms. The relative risk of post-SWL UTIs for patients receiving prophylaxis was 0.45 (95% confidence interval 0.22–0.93). There were some cost variations, depending on the antimicrobial regimens used. However, prophylaxis added little to the overall cost of SWL and was cost-beneficial when the costs of serious UTIs requiring inpatient care were considered.

Conclusions.—Giving prophylactic antibiotics before SWL to patients with sterile pretreatment urine reduces the rate of post-SWL UTIs. Prophylaxis is a cost-effective strategy when the costs of inpatient treatment for episodes of sepsis and acute pyelonephritis are accounted for. This cost-effectiveness is based on prophylaxis in the form of an inexpensive antimicrobial, such as sulfamethoxazole/trimethoprim, vs. an expensive one, such as ciproflaxin.

▶ Urinary tract infection is a common and potentially serious complication of obstructive uropathy. Acute pyelonephritis with fever, costovertebral angle pain and tenderness, or bacteremia may be the presenting clinical picture. Obstructive uropathy is often related to urinary tract calculi. Patients with renal or ureteral calculi are now frequently treated by SWL. One of the potential complications of this procedure, although rare, is the release of bacteria from the stones as they are fragmented. The combination of transient ureteral obstruction caused by fragments of calculi, plus trauma to the tissue as a consequence of shock wave therapy, may promote UTI and lead to bacteriuria. In this report, the authors have utilized meta-analysis of 8 prospective, randomized trials that examined the efficacy and cost-effectiveness of routine antimicrobial prophylaxis prior to shock wave lithotripsy in patients whose urine was sterile prior to the procedure. The authors conclude that antibiotic prophylaxis before SWL is efficacious in reducing the rate of UTI after such a procedure. The authors also suggest that such antibiotic prophylaxis in this setting is cost-effective.

S. Klahr, M.D.

33 Acute Renal Failure

Parenteral Ketorolac: The Risk for Acute Renal Failure
Feldman HI, Kinman JL, Berlin JA, et al (Univ of Pennsylvania, Philadelphia; Univ of Medicine and Dentistry of New Jersey, New Brunswick)
Ann Intern Med 126:193–199, 1997   33–1

Background.—Parenteral administration of ketorolac tromethamine has been associated with acute renal failure. The risk of this complication, however, has not been quantified. The risk for acute renal failure associated with ketorolac was compared with that associated with opioid use.

Methods.—Thirty-five hospitals in the Philadelphia area participated in the retrospective cohort study. Data on a total of 10,219 courses of parenteral ketorolac and on 10,145 courses of parenteral opioids were analyzed. Acute renal failure was defined by a 50% or greater increase in serum creatinine concentration, and either an absolute increase of 44.2 µmol/L or more for levels less than 132.6 µmol/L at baseline or an absolute increase of 88.4 µmol/L or more for levels 132.6 µmol/L or more at baseline. A secondary definition required a physician's diagnosis.

Findings.—The overall incidence of acute renal failure after either ketorolac or opioid administration was 1.1%. Multivariate adjusted rate ratios comparing ketorolac with opioids were 1.09 overall, 1.00 for less than 5 days of treatment, and 2.08 for more than 5 days of treatment. Findings were similar when the secondary definition of acute renal failure was used.

Conclusions.—Overall, acute renal failure was not common in this cohort. The rate of renal failure after 5 days or less of ketorolac treatment was not greater than after opioid administration. However, the rate of acute renal failure associated with ketorolac may be increased among patients receiving analgesics for more than 5 days.

▶ Nonsteroidal antiinflammatory drugs (NSAIDs) are well known to cause acute renal failure (ARF).[1, 2] It has been reported that NSAID-associated ARF accounts for 37% of the ARF associated with drugs and for 7% to 10% of all cases of ARF. In addition, NSAID administration can cause interstitial nephritis, the nephrotic syndrome, hyperkalemia, and sodium and water retention. Inhibition of prostaglandins by these drugs may also cause a modest elevation in blood pressure. All NSAIDs are administered orally. Recently, ketorolac tromethamine has been approved for parenteral use as an analgesic in the United States. In this retrospective study, the risk for ARF associated with ketorolac was studied.The incidence of ARF was low in a group of patients receiving ketorolac in the hospital. Indeed, the incidence of ARF was no different from that of patients receiving opioids for analgesia. However, the authors suggested that parenteral ketorolc administration may be associated with a greater risk for ARF when therapy is prolonged (greater than 5 days). The results of this study should be interpreted with caution, since it was not a prospective, randomized clinical trial. Also, it may be prudent not to prolong the administration of ketorolac beyond 5 days.

S. Klahr, M.D.

References

1. Schlondorff D. Renal complications of nonsteroidal anti-inflammatory drugs. *Kidney Int* 44:643–653, 1993.
2. Kleinknecht D, Landais P, Goldfarb B. Analgesic and non-steroidal, anti-inflammatory, drug-associated acute renal failure: A prospective collaborative study. *Clin Nephrol* 25:275–281, 1986.

Production of Heparin Binding Epidermal Growth Factor-like Growth Factor in the Early Phase of Regeneration After Acute Renal Injury
Sakai M, Zhang M-Z, Homma T, et al (Vanderbilt Univ, Nashville, Tenn; Scios Inc., Mountain View, Calif)
J Clin Invest 99:2128–2138, 1997   33–2

Introduction.—Recent studies report that renal epithelial cells dedifferentiate and become capable of proliferating in response to acute injury. Locally produced growth factors may mediate this process, and exogenous administration of these growth factors accelerates recovery of renal function. Heparin-binding epidermal growth factor-like growth factor (HB-EGF) messenger RNA was recently found to be induced in the rat kidney after acute ischemic injury. Whether bioactive HB-EGF protein is also produced in response to renal injury, resulting from either ischemia/reperfusion or aminoglycosides, was examined.

Methods.—Unilateral ischemic renal injury was produced in male Sprague-Dawley rats, which were subsequently killed and the kidneys removed for analysis. Heparin-binding proteins were purified from homogenates of postischemic kidneys by heparin-affinity column chromatography, using elution with a 0.2–2.0 M gradient of NaCl. Three cell lines responsive to EGF were used for mitogenic assays.

Results.—Within 6 hours of ischemic injury, a single peak of proteins that eluted at 1.0–1.2 M NaCL was detected. The eluate fraction stimulated DNA synthesis in quiescent Balb/c3T3, RIE, and NRK-52E cell lines. All of these lines are responsive to the epidermal growth factor family of mitogenic proteins. Experiments also confirmed that the EGF receptor of A431 cells was tyrosine phosphorylated by this eluate peak. Immunoblotting with a polyclonal antibody against the rat HB-EGF indicated that the eluate peak contained immunoreactive proteins of 22 and 29 kD mol wt, a finding consistent with reported sizes of the secreted form and the membrane anchored form, respectively, of HB-EGF. The distal tubes of injured kidneys were the primary site of HB-EGF production.

Conclusion.—Results demonstrate that HB-EGF, a member of the EGF superfamily of growth factors that signal through EGF receptor tyrosine phosphorylation, is produced as a bioactive protein in rat kidneys of acute renal failure models. In this setting, HB-EGF appears to act as a growth factor during renal regeneration. Sublethally injured distal tubules may be the major source of this growth factor.

▶ Acute renal failure occurs in the setting of ischemia/reperfusion of the kidney or as a consequence of nephrotoxins. Regeneration of the tubular epithelium requires hyperplasia and differentiation of cells. These events are mediated by locally produced growth factors, including EGF, insulin-like growth factor 1 (IGF-1), and hepatocyte growth factor (HGF), among others.

This study demonstrates that HB-EGF is produced as a bioactive protein in rats with acute renal failure. The protein purified in this study was detected as early as 6 hours after the onset of renal ischemia, mainly in distal tubules. This endogenous protein may be an important factor in the repair, proliferation, and regeneration of tubular cells after acute renal injury.

Exogenous administration of EGF, IGF-1, or HGF has been shown to accelerate the repair of tubular epithelium in rat models of acute renal failure. These factors hasten recovery of renal function and restore normal cortical morphology in rats when administered within 24 hours of ischemic injury. The exogenous administration of HB-EGF should, presumably, result in accelerated repair of damaged epithelium caused by acute renal failure. Positive results of studies designed to explore this premise will result in HB-EGF being added to the list of growth factors that may accelerate the healing process of the tubular epithelium in acute renal failure.

S. Klahr, M.D.

Endothelin and Atrial Natriuretic Peptide Levels Following Radiocontrast Exposure in Humans
Clark BA, Kim D, Epstein FH (Beth Israel Hosp, Boston; Harvard Med School, Boston; Brockton-West Roxbury VA Hosp, Newton, Mass)
Am J Kidney Dis 30:82–86, 1997   33–3

Introduction.—Intravenous radiocontrast exposure causes vasoconstriction of the renal vascular bed. Sometimes, this can lead to acute renal failure. Factors affecting this complication include the volume of contrast administered and the underlying disease, such as renal failure and diabetes, or both conditions. The occurrence of renal failure may involve alterations in circulating vascular regulators, such as endothelin and atrial natriuretic peptide (ANP). Patients with normal renal function and patients with underlying renal failure or diabetes were studied to determine how the administered volume of radiocontrast affects endothelin and ANP levels.

Methods.—The analysis included 19 nondiabetic patients undergoing arteriography. Seven received a large volume of contrast, (i.e., 150 mL or more), while 12 received a smaller volume. Circulating endothelin and ANP levels were compared for these 2 groups. The same measurements were made in a separate study of 8 patients with underlying diabetes mellitus or renal insufficiency, or both conditions.

Results.—In the patients with normal renal function, large-volume contrast exposure was associated with a significant increase in circulating endothelin levels, from 12.3 to 19.4 pmol/L. There was no significant change after small-volume contrast exposure (from 13.9 to 12.2 pmol/L). Levels of ANP increased from 43 to 75 pg/mL in the large-volume contrast group and from 33 to 106 pg/mL in the small-volume group; both changes were significant.

The patients with renal failure or diabetes, or both conditions, received a relatively small volume of contrast, 112 mL. Their mean endothelin level started high at 25.7 pmol/L and increased to 55.4 pmol/L. Similarly, their ANP level started at 211 pg/mL and increased to 323 pg/mL. None of the patients had a significant alteration in serum creatinine after contrast exposure.

Conclusions.—Circulating endothelin and ANP levels increase in patients exposed to a large volume of IV radiocontrast. In patients with underlying renal insufficiency or diabetes, both of these values are increased to begin with and have a greater tendency to increase after radiocontrast exposure. Radiocontrast exposure may produce an increase in endothelin, contributing to renal vasoconstriction. However, this may be counterbalanced by a simultaneous increase in ANP.

▶ The IV or intra-arterial administration of radiocontrast agents for diagnostic purposes is associated with vasoconstriction of the renal vascular tree and, in some instances, with the development of acute renal failure. Nonionic contrast materials do not appear to be any less nephrotoxic than ionic agents. Certain underlying conditions (previous renal insufficiency, dehydration, or diabetes) increase the risk of development of acute renal failure after the administration of radiocontrast agents.

There are few studies of the effects of radiocontrast material administration on the levels of circulating endothelin in humans.[1] This study of Clark et al. examines the effect of the volume of radiocontrast administered on the levels of endothelin (a powerful vasoconstrictor) and ANP (a vasodilator). The authors found an increase in the levels of both after the administration of radiocontrast. Patients with underlying renal disease or diabetes had higher basal levels of both vasoactive substances and a greater tendency to have increased endothelin levels after administration of radiocontrast. The authors suggest that endothelin may contribute to renal vasoconstriction after radiocontrast administration. However, simultaneous increases in the levels of ANP may offset the effects of endothelin and protect renal function in most cases.

S. Klahr, M.D.

Reference

1. Hentschel M, Gildein P, Brandis M, et al: Endothelin is involved in the contrast media induced nephrotoxicity in children with congenital heart disease. *Clin Nephrol* 43 (Suppl 1): S12–S15, 1995.

34 Chronic Renal Failure

Homocysteinemia and Vascular Disease in End-stage Renal Disease
Dennis VW, Robinson K (Cleveland Clinic Found, Ohio)
Kidney Int 50:S-11–S-17, 1996   34–1

Background.—Homocysteine is increasingly regarded as an important factor in vascular diseases, whether or not renal failure is present. It is an intermediate amino acid, formed during metabolism of the sulfur-containing essential amino acid methionine and cleared by the kidneys. Homocysteine levels may be increased in patients with chronic renal failure or with deficiencies of folate, vitamin B_{12}, or vitamin B_6. These 3 vitamins are involved in normal methionine metabolism. Homocysteine concentrations were studied in patients with end-stage renal disease.

Findings.—The study included 176 patients with end-stage renal disease who were being managed by peritoneal dialysis or hemodialysis. Compared with a 10.1 µmol/L value in normal individuals, patients with renal failure had an average homocysteine concentration of 26.6 µmol/L. One hundred forty-nine patients had homocysteine values exceeding the 95th percentile for normal individuals, for an overall 85% prevalence of homocysteinemia. Homocysteine was negatively correlated with folate, indicating continued responsiveness despite impairment. Elevated homocysteine concentrations were linked to an increased risk of atherosclerotic and thrombotic complications. This relationship was independent of traditional risk factors and duration of dialysis. For patients with concentrations of homocysteine in the upper 2 quintiles, the odds ratio for vascular events compared to the lower 3 quintiles was 2.9, with adjustment for age, sex, hypertension, diabetes, hypercholesterolemia, smoking, and time on dialysis.

Discussion.—Homocysteinemia appears to be an independent risk factor for vascular events in patients with end-stage renal disease managed by peritoneal dialysis or hemodialysis. More research is needed to identify the mechanism by which high homocysteine concentrations lead to vascular damage in patients with renal failure. It also remains to be determined whether high homocysteine concentrations in end-stage renal disease can be corrected, and whether such correction influences the risk of atherosclerotic and other vascular events.

▶ Prospective and case-control studies indicate that an elevated level of plasma homocysteine is an important risk factor for atherosclerotic vascular disease.[1, 2] Homocysteine is a sulfur-containing amino acid formed during the metabolism of methionine, an essential amino acid. The mean value for homocysteine is about 10 μmol/L and the level for the 95th percentile is about 16 μmol/L. In this report, plasma levels of homocysteine averaged 26.6 ± 1.5 μmol/L in patients with end-stage renal failure receiving peritoneal dialysis or hemodialysis. Other reports[1, 2] indicate that elevated plasma levels of homocysteine are an independent risk factor for vascular disease in patients with end-stage renal disease. Thus, in addition to smoking, hypertension, and hypercholesterolemia, homocysteine level is a major determinant of vascular disease. Chronic renal failure and absolute or relative deficiencies of folate, vitamin B_{12}, or vitamin B_6 are the major causes of increased plasma levels of homocysteine. Fortunately, it has been shown that folic acid administration decreases homocysteine levels in the plasma of patients with chronic renal insufficiency, even when the plasma levels of folate are normal or increased.

S. Klahr, M.D.

References

1. Graham IM, Daly LE, Refsum HM, et al: Plasma homocysteine as a risk factor for vascular disease: The European concerted action project. *JAMA* 277:1775–1781, 1997.
2. Bostom AG, Lathrop L: Hyperhomocysteinemia in end-stage renal disease: Prevalence, etiology, and potential relationship to arteriosclerotic outcomes. *Kidney Int* 52:10–20, 1997.

Lipoprotein(a) Induces Glomerular Superoxide Anion Production
Greiber S, Kreusel M, Pavenstädt H, et al (Univ Hosp of Freiburg, Germany; Univ Hosp of Würzburg, Germany)
Nephrol Dial Transplant 12:1330–1335, 1997   34–2

Introduction.—Lipoprotein (a) [Lp(a)] is an independent risk factor for atherosclerotic disease and is thought to accelerate the progression of renal disease. Earlier reports of tissue culture trials indicate that the biological effects of Lp(a) are inhibitable by oxygen radical scavengers. Reactive oxygen metabolites (ROM) are significant mediators of renal disease. The effects of native and oxidized Lp(a) on the generation of ROM superoxide anion in isolated glomeruli were evaluated and compared with the effects of native LDL (nLDL) and oxidized LDL cholesterol (oxLDL).

Methods.—In isolated rat glomeruli lucigenin chemiluminescence assay was used to evaluate the effect of native and oxidized Lp(a) and LDL on ROM production.

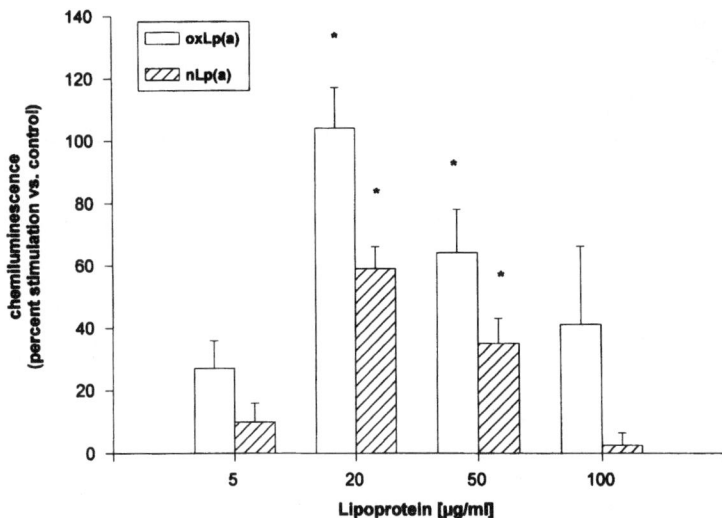

FIGURE 2.—Effects of various concentrations of nLp(a) and oxLp(a) on chemiluminescence in Glm. Increase in peak luminescence from lipoprotein-stimulated and control Glm was recorded. Data were expressed as percent increase of chemiluminescence vs control Glm. Each bar represents the mean ± SEM from 6 to 10 experiments for each concentration. A significant induction of ROM production vs control is indicated (P < 0.001, student's paired t-test). (Courtesy of Greiber S, Kreusel M, Pavenstädt H: Lipoprotein(a) induces glomerular superoxide anion production. *Nephrol Dialy Transplant* 12: 1330–1335, 1997. Reprinted by permission of Oxford University Press.)

Results.—A moderate dose-dependent stimulation of glomerular ROM production was produced by native Lp(a), with maximum ROM production induced by 20 μg/mL nLp(a) (Fig 2). The Lp(a)-induced chemiluminescence was totally inhibited by the cell permeable oxygen radical scavenger Tiron (10 Mm). Oxidized Lp(a) (20 μg/mL) created a more pronounced stimulation of ROM production. Glomerular production was significantly affected by oxLDL 50 μg/mL, but not by nLDL. The protein kinase C inhibitor bis-indolyl malemide (BIM) inhibited Lp(a)⁻ stimulated ROM production; BIM 10⁻6 M inhibited 52% and BIM 10⁻5 M inhibited 94% ROM production was also inhibited when intracellular CAMP levels were increased by forskolin.

Conclusion.—Lp(a) and oxLp(a) induce the activation of ROM in glomeruli by a pathway sensitive to inhibition of protein kinase C and increased intracellular CAMP levels.

▶ Disturbances of lipoprotein metabolism are seen frequently in patients with renal insufficiency. There also is evidence in experimental animals that hyperlipidemia may accelerate the progression of renal disease. The evidence in humans for a role of hyperlipidemia in the progression of renal disease is not uniformly convincing. However, in a retrospective analysis of nondiabetic patients with proteinuria, hypercholesterolemia, and hypertriglyceridemia, the rate of loss of renal function was nearly twofold greater than it was in the control patients. Lipoprotein(a), an independent risk factor for atherosclerosis, also may accelerate the rate of progression of renal disease. In one series, serum levels of lipoprotein(a) were increased in nephrotoxic patients, and glomerular deposits of lipoprotein(a) correlated with a faster progression of renal disease.[1] In this study, Greiber et al. report that both native and oxidized lipoprotein(a) stimulate the production of reactive oxygen metabolites (Fig 1). This stimulation appears to occur through a protein kinase C pathway. Elevation of cyclic AMP intracellularly also decreases the generation of reactive oxygen metabolites, which clearly have been shown to cause damage to renal tissue.

S. Klahr, M.D.

Reference

1. Sato H, Suzuki S, Ueno M, et al: Localization of apolipoprotein(a) and B-100 various renal diseases. *Kidney Int* 43:430–435, 1993.

Effect of Angiotensin-converting Enzyme Inhibitors on the Progression of Nondiabetic Renal Disease: A Meta-analysis of Randomized Trials
Giatras I, for the Angiotensin-Converting-Enzyme Inhibition and Progressive Renal Disease Study Group (New England Med Ctr, Boston; Tufts Univ, Boston)
Ann Intern Med 127:337–345, 1997   34–3

Introduction.—Reports vary regarding the effect of angiotensin-converting enzyme (ACE) inhibitors in delaying the decline in renal function in nondiabetic renal disease. The effect of ACE inhibitors on the development of end-stage renal disease caused by factors other than diabetes mellitus was assessed with meta-analysis.

Methods.—A MEDLINE search of english-language medical literature was conducted, and unpublished studies were analyzed to identify all randomized trials comparing ACE inhibitors with other antihypertensive agents. All reports included at least 1 year of planned follow-up investigation. No investigations of diabetic renal disease or renal transplants were evaluated. A total of 1594 patients from 10 trials were included. Data were collected regarding end-stage renal disease, death, drop out, and blood pressure.

Results.—Of 806 patients receiving ACE inhibitors, 52 (6.4%) end-stage renal disease developed in 52 (6.4%). Of these, 17 (2.1%) died. Of 788 controls subjects, end-stage renal disease developed in 72 (9.19%) and 12 (1.5%) died. Pooled relative risks were 0.70 and 1.24, respectively, for end-stage renal disease and death (Figure). The reports were not significantly heterogeneous. Declines in weighted mean systolic and diastolic blood pressure during follow-up were 4.9 and 1.2 mmHg greater, respectively, in patients taking ACE inhibitors.

Conclusion.—Compared with other antihypertensive agents, ACE inhibitors are more effective in decreasing the development of end-stage nondiabetic renal disease. Mortality is not increased with ACE inhibitor use.

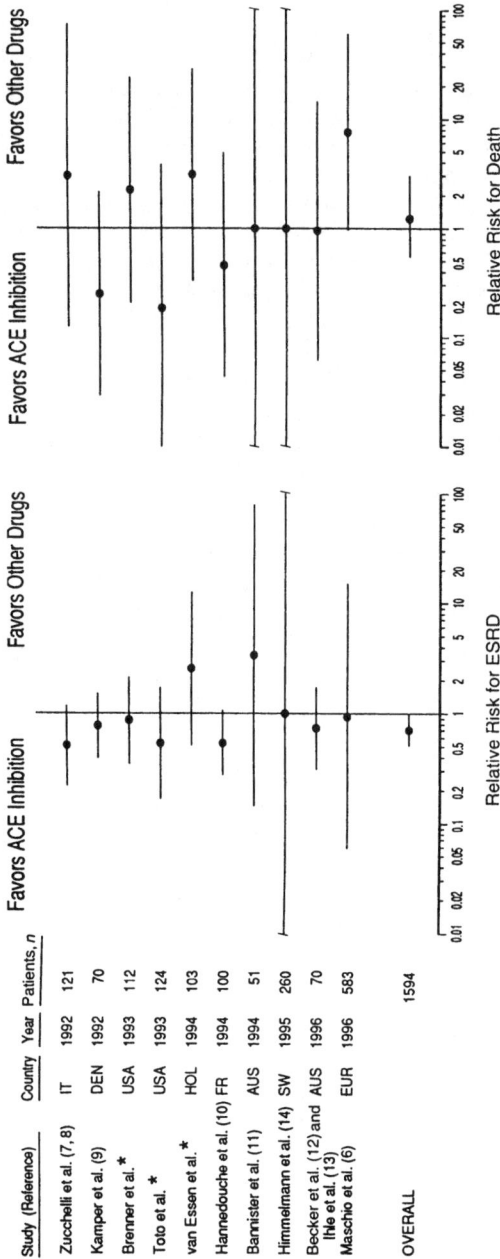

FIGURE.—Effect of angiotensin-converting enzyme (ACE) inhibition on risk for end-stage renal disease (ESRD) and death in patients with nondiabetic renal disease. Data are the relative risk with 95% CIs on a logarithmic scale. The pooled relative risk for end-stage renal disease was 0.70 (95% CI, 0.51 to 0.97), indicating a significantly lower risk in the ACE inhibitor group. The result of the test for heterogeneity among studies was not significant (p < 0.75 and > 0.2), indicating that the relative risk did not significantly differ among studies. The pooled relative risk for death was not significant (1.24 [CI, 0.55 to 2.83]), and the result of the test for heterogeneity among studies was not significant (P > 0.2). The year of publication, or approximate year of completion, of the unpublished studies is given. Interrupted lines indicate that the CIs extend to infinity because no events occurred in these studies. * = Unpublished data provided by study investigators. *Abbreviations:* AUS = Australia; DEN = Denmark; EUR = Europe; FR = France; HOL = the Netherlands; IT = Italy; SW = Sweden; USA = United States. (Courtesy of Giaturas I, for the Angiotensin-Converting-Enzyme Inhibition and Progressive Renal Disease Study. *Ann Intern Med* 127:337–345, 1997.)

It is not known if this is because of decreased blood pressure from ACE inhibition or other factors.

▶ The authors of this article used a meta-analysis of the effect of angiotensin-converting enzyme (ACE) inhibitors on the progression of renal disease. Enalapril was used in 7 of the 10 studies included in this meta-analysis; captopril, cilazapril, and benazepril were used in one study each. Patients with diabetic nephropathy were excluded from study. Patients receiving ACE inhibitors (806) were compared with those receiving other antihypertensive medications (788). The conclusion of the study was that ACE inhibitors are more effective than other antihypertensive agents in reducing the development of end-stage renal disease in nondiabetic patients.

The mechanisms that make ACE inhibitors superior to other antihypertensive medications in slowing the progression of renal disease were not addressed in this study. It is known that ACE inhibitors decrease proteinuria to a greater extent than other antihypertensive drugs in patients with comparable levels of blood pressure. In addition to decreasing blood pressure and proteinuria, ACE inhibitors inhibit the development of interstitial fibrosis by suppressing a number of cytokines and growth factors.[1] ACE inhibitors have also been shown to be effective in slowing the progression of renal disease in patients with diabetic nephropathy.[2, 3]

Mortality was comparable between the groups receiving ACE inhibitors and those receiving other antihypertensive medications: 2.1% in those receiving ACE inhibitors compared with 1.5% in those receiving other antihypertensive drugs (Fig).

S. Klahr, M.D.

References

1. Klahr S, Morrissey JJ: Comparative study of ACE inhibitors and AII receptor antagonists in interstitial scarring. *Kidney Int* 52(Suppl 63):S-111–S-114, 1997.
2. Lewis JE, Hunsicker LG, Bain RP, et al: The effect of angiotensin-converting enzyme inhibition on diabetic nephropathy. *N Engl J Med* 329:1456–1462, 1993.
3. Viberti G, Mogenson CE, Groop LC, et al: Effect of captopril on progression to clinical proteinuria in patients with insulin-dependent diabetes mellitus and microalbuminuria. European Microalbuminuria Captopril Study Group. *JAMA* 271:275–279, 1994.

Urinary and Serum Type III Collagen: Markers of Renal Fibrosis
Soylemezoglu O, Wild G, Dalley AJ, et al (Northern Gen Hosp Trust, Sheffield, England)
Nephrol Dial Transplant 12:1883–1889, 1997   34–4

Introduction.—Progressive glomerulosclerosis and tubulointerstitial fibrosis characterize the progression of chronic renal failure. Increased deposition of a wide range of extracellular matrix components within scarred kidneys cause such fibrosis. To diagnose renal fibrosis and monitor its progression, attempts have been made to measure changes in circulating collagens, fibronectin, and laminin. In patients with a variety of nephropathies who had renal biopsy, measurements of a wide range of circulating and urinary extracellular matrix components, including collagen III and IV and fibronectin, were taken to determine their value in diagnosing renal disorders.

Methods.—There were 40 patients who had a renal biopsy because of a range of subacute and chronic nephropathies. Measurements were taken of their serum and urinary levels of collagens III (amino terminal peptide of procollagen III) and IV, as well as fibronectin. Correlations were made with clinical, biochemical, and histologic parameters. To determine the predictive value of circulating and urinary extracellular matrix components for the severity of renal fibrosis, multiple regression analysis was applied.

Results.—Patients with nephropathies had increased circulating and urinary levels of collagens III and IV, but not fibronectin, when compared with healthy volunteers. Kidney biopsy samples also revealed increased immunoreactivity for these extracellular matrix components when compared with normal kidneys. There was a strong association between the severity of renal interstitial fibrosis and circulating and urinary procollagen III.

Conclusion.—Indicators for the extent of renal fibrosis are measurements of urinary collagen III and, to a lesser extent, serum collagen III. These may have diagnostic implications and may prove useful in monitoring disease progression.

▶ Chronic renal disease, once established, tends to progress to end-stage renal failure. The hallmark of progressive renal disease is a relentless decrease in glomerular filtration rate (GFR). Diverse pathogenetic mechanisms (immunologic disorders, vascular disease, and metabolic abnormalities such as diabetes) may lead to fibrosis and expansion of the tubulointerstitial compartment. In this process, diverse renal structures are replaced by collagen, fibroblasts, and mesenchymal matrix, resulting in disruption of normal renal function. The mechanisms underlying the increase in extracellular matrix components have not been completely elucidated, but they may relate to changes in the synthesis and degradation of collagens.

In this study, the authors suggest, and I concur, that measurement of collagen III in the urine may be a useful indicator of renal fibrosis. As they point out, such a measurement, once appropriately standardized, may help in making the diagnosis of chronic renal disease and may be useful in monitoring the progression of renal disease, as well as the response to potential therapy, such as administration of an ACE inhibitor.

S. Klahr, M.D.

Simplified Screening for Microalbuminuria

Pegoraro A, Singh A, Bakir AA, et al (Univ of Illinois, Chicago; West Side Veterans Administration Hosp, Chicago; Hektoen Inst, Chicago)
Ann Intern Med 127:817–819, 1997   34–5

Introduction.—Measuring levels of urinary albumin, or microalbuminuria is a means of diagnosing early renal involvement in diabetes and several other conditions. Radioimmunoassay is usually necessary for early detection, which can be expensive and is not always available. However, simpler methods have been devised to perform the screenings to save time and money. Three such methods were evaluated. The Micral-Test immunoassay (Boehringer Mannheim) is based on the color shift of a monoclonal antibody to human albumin labeled with colloidal gold. The sulfosalicylic acid test involves 5 drops of 20% sulfosalicylic acid added to 3 mL of urine in 1 test tube with turbidity indicating proteinuria. Chemstrips (Boehringer Mannheim) are chemically impregnated dipsticks.

Methods.—A total of 221 patients had screening for microalbuminuria by means of urine specimens tested with Micral-Test immunoassay strips. They were also tested for protein with sulfosalicylic acid testing and dipsticks (Chemstrips). As a standard for comparison, radioimmunoassay for albumin was used for all specimens.

Results.—Micral-Test had a negative predictive value of 99% when less than 20 mg/L was considered the upper limit of normal for albumin concentration. Sulfosalicylic acid testing had a negative predictive value of 95%, and Chemstrips had a negative predictive value of 96%. With both sulfosalicylic acid and Chemstrips, results for 74 specimens were negative. When combined, the negative predictive value of sulfosalicylic acid and Chemstrips was 99%.

Conclusion.—The combination of Chemstrips and sulfosalicylic acid testing was as good as, and less expensive than, Micral-Test to rule out microalbuminuria. Because thousands of patients with diabetes and other diseases, such as essential hypertensin and AIDS, need such testing, these findings have considerable economic implications.

▶ A number of studies in the last few years have uncovered several clinical predictors of progression of chronic renal disease. Among the strongest predictors is degree of proteinuria. In the Modification of Diet in Renal Disease (MDRD) study,[1] patients with proteinuria in excess of 3 g/24 hr had a more rapid decline in glomerular filtration rate than those with less than 1 g of protein/24 hr. In patients with diabetes and renal disease, the degree of microalbuminuria is also a predictor of progressive renal disease. This study tested the efficacy of three simple tests for the detection of microalbuminuria. Two of these methods were relatively inexpensive and reliable in out microalbuminuria. The authors suggest, and I agree, that the combination of the sulfosalicylic acid test and chemically impregnated dipsticks

(Chemstrips) are as good as, and less expensive than, an immunoassay test (Micral-Test) in ruling out the presence of microalbuminuria.

S. Klahr, M.D.

Reference

1. Peterson JC, Adler S, Burkart, JM et al: MDRD Group: Blood pressure control, proteinuria, and the progression of renal disease: The Modification of Diet in Renal Disease Study. *Ann Intern Med* 123:754–762, 1995.

35 Hypertension

Accuracy of the Diagnosis of Hypertensive Nephrosclerosis in African Americans: A Report From the African American Study of Kidney Disease (AASK) Trial
Fogo A, and the AASK Pilot Study Investigators (Vanderbilt Univ, Nashville, TN; Case Western Reserve Univ, Cleveland, OH; Morehouse School of Medicine, Atlanta, GA; et al)
Kidney Int 51:244–252, 1997   35–1

Background.—Compared with white Americans, black Americans have an excess of hypertension and end-stage renal disease presumed to be caused by hypertension. The African American Study of Kidney Disease (AASK) Trial assessed the effects of antihypertensive treatments and 2 levels of blood pressure control on the rate of decline of glomerular filtration rate (GFR) in blacks with presumed hypertensive renal disease.

Methods.—Eighty-eight eligible participants were assessed initially by renal biopsy to evaluate underlying lesions. The subjects were nondiabetic blacks, aged 18 to 70 years, with GFR between 25 and 70 ml/min/L.73 m² and with no marked proteinuria. Forty-three subjects did not undergo

TABLE 2.—Biopsy Lesions

	Mild	Moderate	Severe	Total
		Severity of vascular lesion		
Arteriolosclerosis ± arteriosclerosis	10	15	8	33
Arteriolosclerosis ± arteriosclerosis + segmental glomerulosclerosis	3	1	1	5
Additional lesions				
Global glomerulosclerosis				35
Segmental glomerulosclerosis				5
End stage kidney				1
Mesangiopathic glomerulonephritis				1
GBM thickening −				1
Cholesterol embolus				2

Abbreviation : *GBM*, glomerular basement membrane.
(Courtesy of Fogo, and the AASK Pilot Study Investigators: Accuracy of the diagnosis of hypertensive nephrosclerosis in African Americans: A report from the African American Study of Kidney Disease (AASK) Trial. *Kidney Int* 51:244–252, 1997. Reprinted by permission of Blackwell Science, Inc.)

biopsy because of contraindications or refusal. Adequate renal biopsy specimens were acquired from 39 of the remaining 46 patients.

Findings.—Thirty-eight of the 39 biopsy specimens showed arteriosclerosis and/or arteriolosclerosis (Table 2). Both had a mean severity of 1.5 on a scale of 0 to 3+. Moderate interstitial fibrosis was observed. Five biopsy specimens showed segmental glomerulosclerosis. In 1 patient, biopsy and clinical findings suggested idiopathic focal segmental glomerulosclerosis. In addition, 1 patient had mesangiopathic glomerulonephritis; 1, basement membrane thickening suggesting diabetic nephropathy; and 2, cholesterol emboli. Arteriolar and arterial sclerosis were closely associated. They also correlated with interstitial fibrosis and the reciprocal of serum creatinine. Global glomerulosclerosis involved an average of 43% of glomeruli. The extent of this lesion was not associated with the degree of arteriolar and arterial thickening but was correlated with systolic blood pressure, the reciprocal of serum creatinine, serum cholesterol, and interstitial fibrosis.

Conclusions.—The clinical diagnosis of hypertensive nephrosclerosis, based on careful clinical and laboratory assessment, is very accurate. Renal biopsy specimens obtained from nondiabetic hypertensive African Americans, with mild-to-moderate renal insufficiency in the absence of marked proteinuria, are highly likely to show renal vascular lesions consistent with the clinical diagnosis of hypertensive neophrosclerosis.

▶ High blood pressure is found in approximately 25% of the population (65 million persons) of the United States. Hypertensive nephrosclerosis is a major cause of end-stage renal disease (ESRD) in blacks. Although blacks constitute 12% of the population of the United States, they account for 28% of patients with ESRD requiring dialysis. It has been reported that the rate of developing ESRD is fourfold greater in blacks than in whites. Furthermore, blacks account for approximately 41% of new patients admitted to ESRD programs with the diagnosis of hypertensive nephrosclerosis. This diagnosis is mainly made on clinical grounds. This study used renal biopsy specimens in an effort to substantiate the accuracy of the diagnosis of hypertensive nephrosclerosis in African Americans. Of the 46 biopsy specimens obtained, 39 were adequate for histologic studies. Thirty-eight specimens demonstrated the presence of arteriolosclerosis or arteriosclerosis (Table 2). Arteriolar thickening was present and hyaline deposits were observed in arterioles or arteries. Interstitial fibrosis was moderate. From these observations, the authors suggest that the clinical diagnosis of hypertensive nephrosclerosis made on the grounds of careful clinical and laboratory evaluation is highly accurate in blacks. (The incidence of other glomerular diseases clearly defined by sound clinical criteria is exceedingly low in patients of all races and ethnic backgrounds.) The reasons for the high incidence of hypertensive nephrosclerosis in blacks are not clear; however, some studies have suggested that, at comparable levels of blood pressure, the kidneys of black patients are more susceptible to injury than those of whites.

S. Klahr, M.D.

A Short-term Antihypertensive Treatment-induced Fall in Glomerular Filtration Rate Predicts Long-term Stability of Renal Function

Apperloo AJ, de Zeeuw D, de Jong PE (Univ Hosp Groningen, The Netherlands)
Kidney Int 51:793–797, 1997   35–2

Objective.—In patients with renal impairment, initial fall in glomerular filtration rate (GFR) caused by antihypertensive treatment may lead to concern about progressive renal function loss. Because the fall in GFR may be the result of lowered intraglomerular pressure, it may indicate long-term effectiveness of treatment. Renal hemodynamic response in patients with varying degrees of renal function impairment before treatment, during treatment with either atenolol or enalapril, and after withdrawal of treatment was studied.

Methods.—Mean arterial pressure, GFR, and effective renal plasma flow were measured before, every 24 weeks during the 4-year treatment period, and 12 weeks after discontinuing therapy with either atenolol or enalapril in 40 (19 female) nondiabetic patients, average age 49.3 years. Treatment effects were analyzed statistically.

Results.—Blood pressure fell during treatment, but returned to pretreatment levels after therapy was discontinued. Whereas the initial change in GFR varied from −11 to 11 mL/min, GFR decreased slowly but significantly during the 4-year follow-up. After therapy was discontinued, GFR rose an average of 2.2 mL/min. The initial fall and subsequent rise after

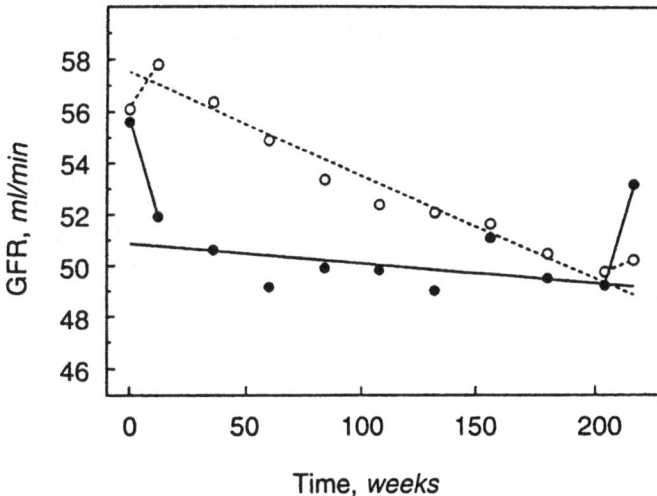

FIGURE 2.—Time course of GFR before, during, and after withdrawal of antihypertensive treatment in group A and group B. Group A (*filled circles*) are patients who initially showed a distinct fall in GFR, and group B (*open circles*) are patients in whom GFR did not fall after start of treatment. The change in GFR after start and withdrawal of treatment is indicated as well as the slope of GFR during treatment. *Abbreviation*: GFR, glomerular filtration rate. (Courtesy of Apperloo AJ, de Zeeuw D, de Jong PE: A short-term antihypertensive treatment-induced fall in glomerular filtration rate predicts long-term stability of renal function. *Kidney Int* 51:793–797, 1997. Reprinted by permission of Blackwell Science, Inc.)

withdrawal of GFR were correlated. Patients with a steeper GFR fall had a more stable course during the follow-up. Patients were divided into 2 groups: group A had a fall in GFR initially, whereas group B had a stable GFR initially (Fig 2). Group A had a fall in filtration fraction initially, whereas group B did not. Posttreatment GFR was significantly different from baseline in group B, but not in group A because of the rise in GFR in group A.

Conclusion.—Glomerular filtration rate was more stable in the long run in patients that experienced an initial fall in GFR during treatment with antihypertensive drugs.

▶ Hypertension is both a cause and a consequence of renal disease. Systemic hypertension is a major risk factor in the progression of chronic renal disease. Epidemiologic, retrospective, and prospective studies indicate that lowering blood pressure (BP) is associated with a slower loss of renal function. Results from the Modification of Diet in Renal Disease (MDRD) study found an association between the level of BP and the rate of decline in GFR in patients with chronic renal disease.[1, 2] The MDRD Study also provided evidence that, even among patients with BPs below 107 mm Hg (equivalent to a BP of 140/90), there was also a loss of renal function. This suggests that the conventional BP control goal selected to reduce the risk of cardiovascular sequela may not be low enough to protect the kidney.

In the MDRD study, patients were assigned to 1 of 2 BP goals, 107 mm Hg (usual level of control of BP) or 92 mm Hg (lower than usual level of control of BP). There was a greater decrease in GFR initially (first 4 months after starting hypertensive therapy) in the group assigned to the low BP goal. This initial decrease in GFR has been considered an unwanted effect of treatment with antihypertensive medications. The study by Apperloo et al. in The Netherlands prospectively examined the renal hemodynamic response in 40 nondiabetic patients with varying degrees of renal function impairment, before antihypertensive treatment and after withdrawal of that treatment. Patients were given atenolol or enalapril for a 4-year period. An initial fall in GFR occurring after the onset of antihypertensive treatment in patients with a mild or moderate renal function impairment was associated with a slower loss of renal function over time. This initial fall in GFR is reversible after discontinuation of antihypertensive therapy of long duration. It is likely that the decrease in GFR resulting from antihypertensive medications represents a hemodynamic event that is reversible and, as such, predicts a beneficial effect on the progression of renal disease (Fig 2).

S. Klahr, M.D.

References

1. Klahr S, Levey AS, Beck GJ, et al: The effects of dietary protein restriction and blood pressure control on the progression of chronic renal disease. *N Engl J Med* 330:877–884, 1994.

2. MDRD Group: Blood pressure control, proteinuria, and the progression of renal disease: The Modification of Diet in Renal Disease Study. Prepared by Peterson JC, Adler S, Burkart, JM, et al. *Ann Intern Med* 123:754–762, 1995.

The Vascular Effects of L-Arginine in Humans: The Role of Endogenous Insulin
Giugliano D, Marfella R, Verrazzo G, et al (Second Univ of Naples, Italy)
J Clin Invest 99:433–438, 1997   35–3

Objective.—L-arginine is the physiologic precursor of nitric oxide. Nitric oxide has demonstrated effects on vascular tone, and increasing the availability of L-arginine reduces peripheral arterial resistance while inhibiting platelet aggregation. L-arginine also stimulates insulin secretion from pancreatic beta cells. The hemodynamic and rheologic effects of L-arginine, including the possible contribution of endogenous insulin, were studied in humans.

Methods.—Three studies were performed in 10 healthy young adults. Study I examined the effects of infusion of L-arginine, 1 g/min for 30 minutes. In study II, the subjects received infusions of L-arginine plus octreotide, 25 μg as an IV bolus plus 0.5 μg/min, to block endogenous insulin and glucagon secretion. In this study, basal insulin and glucagon were replaced as well. In study III, in addition to L-arginine, octreotide, and basal glucagon, the subjects also received an insulin infusion designed to reproduce the insulin response observed in study I. The role of endogenous insulin in the hemodynamic and rheologic effects of L-arginine was investigated.

Results.—The effects of L-arginine infusion included reductions in systolic and diastolic blood pressure (mean reduction, 11 and 8 mm Hg, respectively), a 20% reduction in platelet aggregation, a 1.6 centipois reduction in blood viscosity, and a 97 mL/min increase in leg blood flow. Heart rate and plasma catecholamine level increased as well. In study II, the subjects had continued suppression of plasma insulin levels at baseline. Except for plasma catecholamines, their vascular response to L-arginine was significantly reduced. The insulin infusion given in study III re-established the plasma insulin response to L-arginine. The resulting hemodynamic and rheologic changes were similar to those observed in study I (Fig 2).

Conclusion.—In healthy adults, L-arginine infusion produces vasodilation with inhibition of platelet aggregation and blood viscosity. Endogenous insulin plays at least some role in mediating these changes. If the effect of L-arginine infusion is to stimulate nitric oxide synthesis, through the mediation of insulin or some other mechanism, it may be a useful technique for assessing endothelium-dependent vascular function under pathophysiologic conditions.

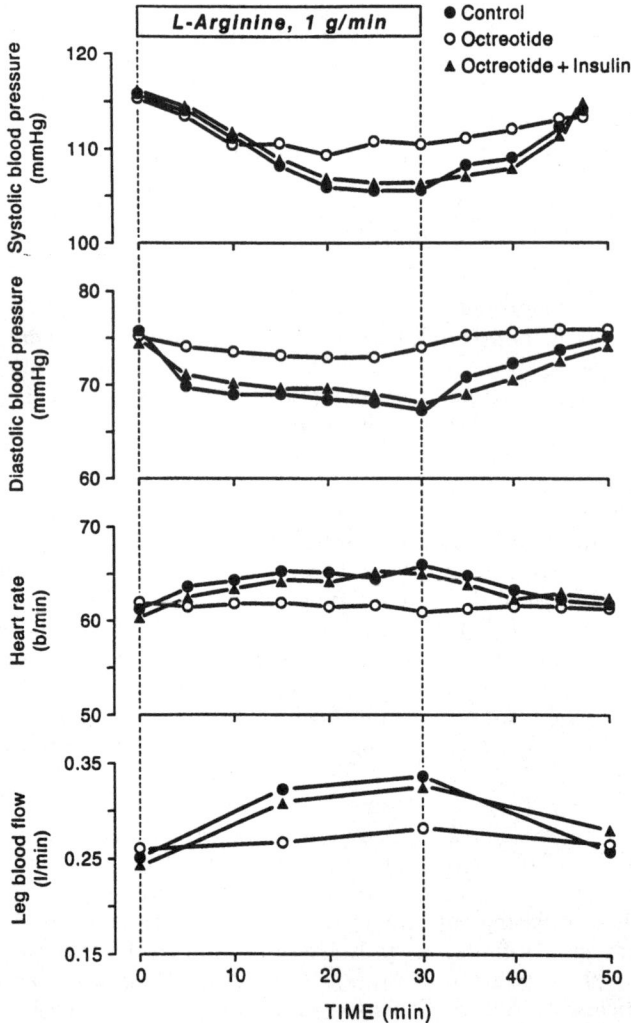

FIGURE 2.—Changes in hemodynamic parameters after L-arginine infusion in 10 healthy subjects. For clarity of presentation, the standard error of the means has been omitted. (Reproduced from *The Journal of Clinical Investigation*, courtesy of Giugliano D, Marfella R, Verazzo G, et al: The vascular effects of L-arginine in humans: The role of endogenous insulin. *J Clin Invest* 99:433–438, 1997, by copyright permission of The Rockefeller University Press.)

▶ Administration of L-arginine, the substrate for the synthesis of nitric oxide, causes peripheral vasodilation, resulting in a decrease in blood pressure and an increase in heart rate and circulating levels of catecholamines. It has been assumed that these effects of L-arginine administration were the result of increased synthesis of nitric oxide, which causes relaxation of smooth muscle by activating the formation of guanosine monophosphate.

However, this study reveals an additional mechanism by which L-arginine administration causes vasodilation.

L-arginine can stimulate directly the release of endogenous insulin from the beta cells in the pancreas. In this study, blockade of endogenous insulin secretion by octreotide markedly reduced the vascular dilation after administration of L-arginine (Fig 2). This indicates that the vascular effects of L-arginine administration are dependent, in part, on the stimulation of insulin release caused by the amino acid. Indeed, the study suggests that at least one half of the vascular response to L-arginine is mediated by endogenous insulin secretion. The other part of the response may be attributable to increased synthesis of nitric oxide. A recent report[1] indicates that insulin-induced vasodilation is mediated by nitric oxide, as this response is blunted by the administration of inhibitors of the nitric oxide synthase.

In summary, the systemic administration of L-arginine in normal individuals decreases blood pressure, inhibits platelet aggregation, and also reduces blood viscosity. A major component of the vascular effects of arginine is mediated by endogenous insulin.

S. Klahr, M.D.

Reference

1. Steinberg HO, Brechtel G, Johnson A, et al. Insulin-mediated skeletal muscle vasodilation is nitric oxide dependent: A novel action of insulin to increase nitric oxide release. *J Clin Invest* 94:1172–1179, 1994.

The Subtype 2 (AT₂) Angiotensin Receptor Mediates Renal Production of Nitric Oxide in Conscious Rats
Siragy HM, Carey RM (Univ of Virginia, Charlottesville)
J Clin Invest 100:264–269, 1997   35–4

Introduction.—It has been shown that the angiotensin AT_2 receptor modulates renal production of cyclic guanosine 3',5'-monophosphate (cGMP). The increase in cGMP may occur because angiotensin II (Ang II) acts at the AT_2 receptor to stimulate renal production of nitric oxide. Changes in renal interstitial fluid (RIF) cGMP were monitored to determine response to AT_2 receptor blockade.

Methods.—A microdialysis technique was used, and changes in RIF cGMP were observed in response to intravenous infusion of the following: the AT_2 receptor antagonist PD 123319 (PD), the AT_1 receptor antagonist Losartan, the nitric oxide synthase (NOS) inhibitor nitro-L-arginine-methyl-ester (L-NAME), the specific neural NOS inhibitor 7-nitroindazole (7-NI), and Ang II, individually or combined in conscious rats during low or normal sodium balance.

Results.—Sodium depletion caused a significant increase in RIF cGMP PD and L-NAME each reduced this increase to a similar extent. The combined administration of PD and L-NAME reduced RIF cGMP to levels seen with PD or L-NAME alone or during normal sodium intake. Angiotensin II was responsible for a twofold increase in RIF cGMP during normal sodium intake. In contrast, the RIF cGMP was not changed in the presence of PD or L-NAME, individually or combined. Compared with Ang II alone, combined administration of Ang II and either PD or L-NAME caused a significant decrease in RIP cGMP. The combined administration of Ang II, PD, and L-NAME impeded the increase in RIF cGMP caused by Ang II alone. During sodium depletion, 7-NI reduced RIF cGMP, but the decrease in cGMP in response to PD alone or PD in combination with 7-NI was greater than that with 7-NI alone. During normal sodium intake, the AngII-induced rise in RIF cGMP was blocked by 7-NI. PD alone or combined with 7-NI caused a greater inhibition of cGMP, compared with 7-NI alone. The RIF cGMP responses to L-arginine were partially inhibited by 7-NI and completely inhibited by L-NAME during sodium depletion.

Conclusion.—These findings indicate that activation of the renin–angiotensin system during sodium depletion increases renal nitric oxide production through stimulation by Ang II at the angiotensin AT_2 receptor.

▶ Most of the renal actions of angiotensin II are mediated by angiotensin 1 (AT_1) receptors, which are the most abundant type of receptors for angiotensin II in the kidney. However, the less abundant angiotensin type 2 receptors (AT_2) are also present. The actions of angiotensin II mediated by AT_2 receptors are not clearly defined. In a previous communication,[1] the authors of the present paper reported that activation of the renin–angiotensin system during sodium depletion increased cyclic guanosine 3'5'-monophosphate (cGMP) in the renal interstitial fluid. They also demonstrated that the effect was mediated by AT_2 receptors. In the current report, the authors describe the role of AT_2 receptors in the production of nitric oxide (NO) in the rat kidney. They found that activation of the renin–angiotensin system, as a consequence of sodium depletion, increases renal NO production through the effects of angiotensin II acting through the AT_2 receptors. They also report that this effect is partially the result of neural nitric oxide synthetase (NOS), as well as other NOS isoforms that participate in the production of nitric oxide through this pathway. Of course, the balance between the vasoconstrictive effects of angiotensin II and the vasodilatory effects of NO is important in regulating systemic arterial pressure and volume homeostasis.

S. Klahr, M.D.

Reference

1. Siragy HM, Carey RM. The subtype 2 (AT_2) angiotensin receptor regulates cyclic guanosine 3'5' monophosphate and AT_1 receptor-mediated prostaglandin E_2 production in conscious rats. *J Clin Invest* 97:1978–1982, 1996.

Altered Nitric Oxide Metabolism and Increased Oxygen Free Radical Activity in Lead-induced Hypertension: Effect of Lazaroid Therapy

Vaziri ND, Ding Y, Ni Z, et al (Univ of California, Irvine)
Kidney Int 52:1042–1046, 1997   35–5

Introduction.—In humans and in experimental animals, chronic exposure to low levels of lead results in arterial hypertension. There is still little understanding about the underlying mechanism of lead-induced hypertension. A previous report[1] suggested increased production of reactive oxygen species in lead-treated animals, which could have contributed to the associated hypertension by a number of different mechanisms. The possible role of reactive oxygen species and their impact on nitric oxide metabolism in lead-induced hypertension was investigated.

Methods.—During a 12-week period, male rats were treated with lead with 100 ppm in drinking water. For the next 2 weeks, they were then given either a placebo or the potent antioxidant, lazaroid (desmethyltirilazad, 5 mg/kg i.p., twice a day). They were then monitored for an additional 2 weeks and compared with 6 controls.

Results.—There was marked hypertension and a significant rise in plasma concentration of lipid peroxidation product, malondialdehyde, and a twofold reduction in urinary excretion of nitric oxide metabolites (total nitrates and nitrites) with lead administration. Blood pressure, plasma malondialdehyde and urinary nitrates and nitrites normalized

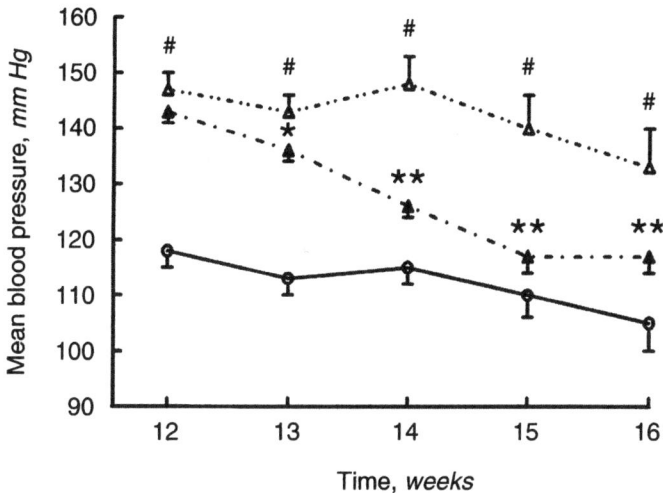

FIGURE 1.—Longitudinal measurements of mean arterial blood pressure in placebo-treated animals with lead-induced hypertension (*open triangle*), lazaroid-treated animals with lead-induced hypertension (*closed triangle*), and the normal control group (*open circle*). Lazaroid therapy was carried out for 2 weeks (weeks 13 and 14). $P = < 0.01$ vs. other groups (ANOVA) (#); $P = < 0.05$ vs. baseline value (week 12) (*); $P = < 0.01$ versus baseline value (week 12) (**). (Courtesy of Vaziri ND, Ding Y, Ni Z, et al: Altered nitric oxide metabolism and increased oxygen free radical activity in lead-induced hypertension: Effect of lazaroid therapy. *Kidney Int* 52:1042–1046, 1997. Reprinted by permission of Blackwell Science, Inc.)

promptly with lazaroid therapy (Fig 1). With the placebo therapy, blood pressure and plasma malondialdehyde remained elevated, and there was slow recovery of urinary nitrate and nitrite excretion. During the observation period, there was no significant difference found in creatinine clearance between the study groups.

Conclusion.—Marked hypertension coupled with increased reactive oxygen species production and decreased urinary nitrate and nitrite excretion resulted from chronic lead exposure. Symptoms normalized with the administration of the potent antioxidant lazaroid. In this model, the role of reactive oxygen species was supported in lead-induced hypertension.

▶ The association between lead and hypertension has been a subject of controversy. The early view that lead-induced renal injury causes hypertension has gained increased support. The administration of EDTA to mobilize lead from tissues can sometimes lower blood pressure, indicating that lead is the most probable cause of hypertension with renal failure. It has been postulated that the hypertension resulting from lead-poisoning is caused by renal damage (nephrosclerosis). This view is consistent with the observation that the clearance of creatinine decreases with increasing blood levels of lead, an effect that is independent of blood pressure. The appearance of arteriolar nephrosclerosis before hypertension develops and the relatively short duration of hypertension before renal insufficiency develops suggests that the initial renal injury from lead may be in the microvascular endothelium. Future studies are needed to establish the potential benefit of lazaroid treatment in patients with lead intoxication.

S. Klahr, M.D.

Reference

1. Gonick HC, Ding Y, Ni Z, et al: Lead-induced hypertension is related to accumulation of reactive oxygen species. *Am J Hypertens* 9:39A, 1996.

36 Transplantation

Tacrolimus Rescue Therapy for Renal Allograft Rejection: Five-Year Experience
Jordan ML, Naraghi R, Shapiro R, et al (Univ of Pittsburgh, Pa)
Transplantation 63:223–228, 1997   36–1

Introduction.—The immunosuppressant drug tacrolimus is being studied for use in renal transplant recipients. Among its other advantages, tacrolimus may be of value for salvage therapy in patients with refractory renal allograft rejection. A 74% salvage rate in refractory cases converted to tacrolimus has been reported. A larger experience with longer follow-up was evaluated.

Patients.—The 5-year experience included 169 patients who underwent tacrolimus conversion for attempted graft salvage. All patients had ongoing renal allograft rejection despite baseline cyclosporine immunosuppression. Eighty-five percent had failed therapy with high-dose corticosteroids and/or antilymphocyte agents. In each case, rejection was confirmed by biopsy. Tacrolimus conversion was carried out a median of 2 months after transplantation. Seventeen percent of patients were undergoing dialysis at the time of conversion. A "clean conversion" to tacrolimus, at a standard daily oral dose of 0.2–0.3 mg/kg/day, was used in each patient. The patients were studied for a mean of 30 months.

Outcomes.—Tacrolimus salvage was successful in 74% of the patients (Fig 1). This group had functioning grafts at follow-up, with a mean serum creatinine of 2.3 mg/dL. The salvage rate was 81% among patients previously treated with antilymphocyte agents. Forty-six percent of patients undergoing dialysis at the time of conversion had functioning grafts at follow-up, mean serum creatine, 21.5 mg/dL. In the patients with successful salvage, the mean prednisone dose was reduced from 28.0 to 8.5 mg/day, with 22% of patients currently receiving no steroids at all.

Conclusions.—Tacrolimus is an effective salvage agent for patients with refractory renal allograft rejection. It offers a new alternative to antilymphocyte preparations for patients with steroid-resistant rejection on cyclosporine-based immunosuppressant regimens.

▶ Tacrolimus (FK-506) is a macrolide antibiotic that was used initially for the prophylaxis of acute rejection after liver transplantation. It has been used more recently in kidney transplantation and in immunologically mediated

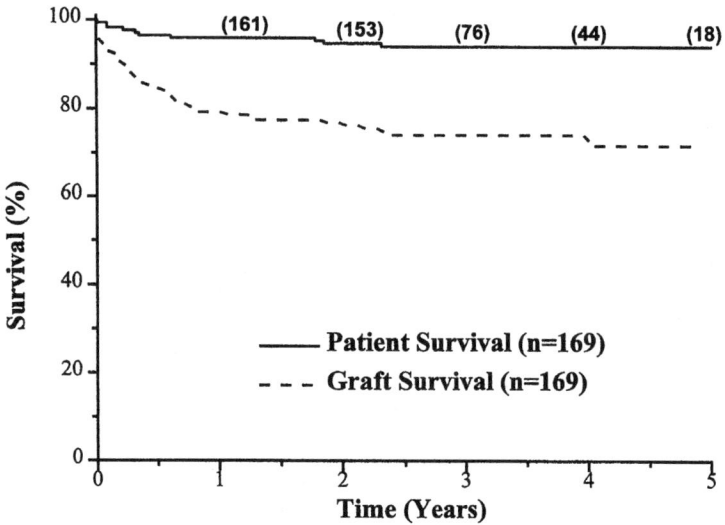

FIGURE 1.—Kaplan-Meier patient and graft survival of 169 patients converted from cyclosporine to tacrolimus therapy for refractory renal allograft rejection. Calculations are based on events from the time of conversion to tacrolimus. Numbers in parentheses indicate patients at risk at each time point. (Courtesy of Jordan ML, Naraghi R, Shapiro R, et al: Tacrolimus rescue therapy for renal allograft rejection: Five-year experience. *Transplantation* 63:223–228, 1997.)

renal diseases.[1] The drug is metabolized predominantly in the liver. Certain drugs increase the serum levels of tacrolimus by inhibiting its metabolism. These drugs include ketoconazole, erythromycin, glucocorticoids, diltiazem, and fluconazole. Other drugs (phenobarbital, rifampin) may potentially decrease tacrolimus levels by inducing the p450 pathway. Although the molecular structure of tacrolimus is dissimilar from that of cyclosporine, the 2 drugs share similar molecular targets and inhibit similar interleukin gene products.

This 5-year study from the University of Pittsburgh reports on the use of tacrolimus for rescue therapy in patients with renal allograft rejection. The criteria for successful graft salvage with this drug included one or more of the following: an improvement in the levels of serum creatinine or a return to prerejection levels; improvement on follow-up renal biopsy; and no further need for dialysis in patients who required dialysis at the time of conversion to tacrolimus. One hundred sixty-nine patients who experienced failing cyclosporine immunosuppression with ongoing rejection were switched to tacrolimus at an average of 4.3 ± 2.6 months after transplantation. At the time of the report, 159 of the 169 patients (94%) were alive and 125 of 169 patients (74%) were considered to have achieved graft rescue, according to the criteria described (Fig 1). On the basis of this experience, the authors recommend that tacrolimus be used as an alternative to the conventional compounds used for rejection episodes in patients with a kidney graft.

S. Klahr, M.D.

Reference

1. Peters DH, Fitton A, Plosker GL, et al: Tacrolimus: A review of its pharmacology and therapeutic potential in hepatic and renal transplantation. *Drugs* 46:746–794, 1993.

Risk Factors for Delayed Graft Function In Cadaveric Kidney Transplantation

Koning OHJ, Ploeg RJ, Van Bockel JH, et al (Univ Hosp Leiden, The Netherlands; Univ Hosp Groningen, The Netherlands; Univ of Leiden, The Netherlands et al)

Transplantation 63:1620–1628, 1997   36–2

Objective.—Patients receiving cadaveric kidney grafts are at risk of delayed graft function (DGF), with most studies reporting an incidence of 25% to 35%. The causes of DGF are unknown. However, several associated factors have been identified, including receiving kidneys from multiorgan donors. Donor and recipient factors affecting the occurrence of DGF were analyzed, along with the effects of DGF on long-term graft survival, in a multicenter European study.

Methods.—The study included 547 kidney allografts transplanted from multiorgan donors. The results of these transplants were compared with reported studies of kidney-only donors. Potential associated factors analyzed included many different aspects of the donor procedure, preservation quality, and posttransplant recipient-related factors.

Results.—Patients without graft failure were followed up for a median of 3.4 years. The incidence of DGF was 24%. On univariate analysis, donor factors associated with an increased risk of DGF were mean creatinine of greater than 120 µmol/L and prolonged cold ischemia time (CIT). Recipient factors were previous transplantation, no intraoperative mannitol use, poor reperfusion quality, absence of intraoperative diuresis, and pretransplant anuria or oliguria. Independent predictors after stepwise logistic regression were donor age, CIT, number of previous transplants in the recipient, and intraoperative diuresis. The posttransplant graft survival rate was 91% at 3 months, 87% at 1 year, and 72% at 4 years. Graft survival was about 10% lower for patients with DGF compared to those with immediate graft function. Compared with published data, the incidence of DGF was comparable for grafts from multiorgan and single-organ donors.

Conclusions.—Factors associated with DGF in cadaveric kidney transplants are identified. The findings suggest that giving mannitol during transplantation can reduce the risk of DGF by minimizing CIT and optimizing donor management. The evidence links DGF to a 10% increase in the risk of graft failure.

▶ Renal transplantation between close relatives, especially HLA-identical siblings, remains more successful than cadaveric renal transplantation. However, with the introduction of more effective immunosuppressive protocols, the success of kidney transplantation from cadaver donors has improved. After harvesting, kidneys can be preserved in hypothermic storage for up to 36 hours or by continuous perfusion for up to 72 hours. Delayed function of the transplanted kidney represents an important complication. Among cadaveric kidneys retrieved from multiorgan donors, stored, and shipped according to prescribed guidelines, 24% demonstratead DGF in this multicenter study, an incidence similar to that reported with transplants from kidney-only donors. In some reports of grafts from multiorgan donors, rates as great as 50% have been described.[1, 2] Delayed function of the graft immediately after transplantation and subsequently may require the use of dialysis, and it also obscures the diagnosis of graft rejection. In this multicenter study, DGF resulted in a 10% higher rate of graft failure. This report also indicates that the incidence of DGF can be reduced by the use of mannitol during transplantation. Use of mannitol apparently minimizes cold ischemia time and improves medical management of the recipient.

S. Klahr, M.D.

References

1. Rocher LL, Landis C, Dafoe DC, et al: The importance of prolonged post-transplant dialysis requirement in cyclosporin-treated renal allograft recipients. *Clin Transplant* 1:29–35, 1987.
2. Canadian Multicentre Transplant Study Group: A randomized clinical trial of cyclosporin in cadaveric renal transplantation: Analysis at 3 years. *N Engl J Med* 314:1219–1225, 1986.

37 Dialysis

The Dose of Hemodialysis and Patient Mortality
Held PJ, Port FK, Wolfe RA, et al (Univ of Michigan, Ann Arbor; Univ of Illinois, Chicago; Health Care Financing Administration, Baltimore, MD; et al)
Kidney Int 50:550–556, 1996   37–1

Background.—The association between hemodialysis dose delivered and mortality rate is not clear. Though several observational studies have shown that survival improves with higher doses, other unmeasured variables, changes in patient mix, or medical management may have affected this finding. The relationship of delivered hemodialysis dose and mortality rate was further investigated.

Methods.—Data from a U.S. national sample of 2311 patients from 347 dialysis units were analyzed. The dose beyond which more dialysis apparently does not reduce the mortality rate was also determined. Patient survival was estimated by proportional hazards regression methods, with adjustment for 21 patient comorbidity/risk factors with stratification for 9 Census regions. The measurement of treatment delivered was based on 2 alternative measures of intradialytic urea reduction, the urea reduction ratio (URR) and Kt/V, with adjustment for urea generation and ultrafiltration.

Findings.—Mortality rate has a strong, inverse association with hemodialysis dose delivered, whether measured by Kt/V or URR. The risk of death was reduced by 7%, with each 0.1 increase in delivered Kt/V. At greater than 70% URR or a 1.3 Kt/V, there were no further significant reductions in mortality rate (Fig 2).

Conclusions.—The hemodialysis dose delivered is an important predictor of mortality rate. Increasing the level of treatment is a practical, efficient means of reducing the mortality rate among patients receiving dialysis.

▶ Hemodialysis is by far the most common modality of renal replacement therapy in patients with end-stage renal disease (ESRD) in the United States. During 1993, more than 257,000 patients in the 50 states and the District of Columbia were treated for ESRD under the Medicare Program. End-stage renal disease is more common in men (54%) than in women. Over 60% of new ESRD cases are attributed to either diabetic nephropathy (35%) or

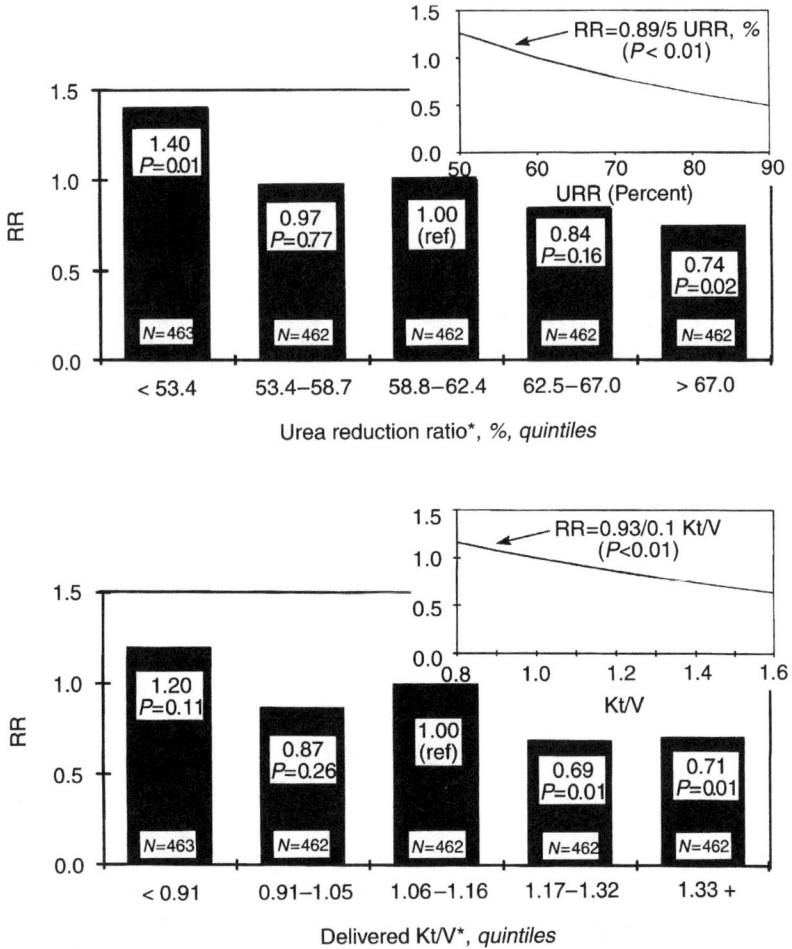

FIGURE 2.—Relative risk of mortality by delivered dose of dialysis (measured as Dugirdas corrected Kt/V) among a random sample of U.S. patients receiving dialysis for more than 1 year on Dec. 31, 1990 (N = 2311). The line represents relationship of delivered Kt/V and mortality risk, with Kt/V as a continuous variable and mean Kt/V (1.10) set as the reference (RR = 1.00). The thin portion of the line indicates segment in which correlation may be less steep. Bars represent risk of mortality for different categories of delivered Kt/V with Kt/V = 1.0 to 1.2 arbitrarily set as the reference (RR = 1.00). *From (1 − post/pre) BUN. N = 2311, thrice weekly. (Courtesy of Held PJ, Port FK, Wolfe RA, et al: The dose of hemodialysis and patient mortality. *Kidney Int* 50:550–556, 1996. Reprinted by permission of Blackwell Science, Inc.)

hypertension (28%). Patients with primary glomerular diseases constitute 11% of patients with new ESRD.

During hemodialysis, toxins, accumulated as a consequence of ESRD, and excess fluid are removed by means of the extracorporeal circulation of blood through a dialyzer (artificial kidney). Treatments are most commonly scheduled three times weekly and last 3 to 4 hours. This study examines the dose of hemodialysis and patient mortality rate. Traditionally, the removal of urea has been used as a marker of adequacy of dialysis. The amount of urea removed is related to the length of the dialysis procedure, but can be increased markedly by using a high area dialyzer and a rapid blood flow rate. With this approach, it is possible to clear the same amount of urea from plasma in 2.5 to 3 hours as was cleared in 4 to 6 hours with smaller dialyzers and lower blood flow rates. A few multicenter studies of the adequacy of dialysis therapy and subsequent mortality rates have been published. In general, in dialysis units affiliated with National Medical Care, it has been shown that the mortality rate is lower at higher doses of dialysis, measured as the urea reduction ratio. This study supports that generalization and reports on the impact of "skipped" dialysis treatments on patient survival. The authors suggest that even one "skipped" treatment per month correlates with a higher mortality rate. Although there are some limitations to this study, it appears quite clear that in a population of patients receiving dialysis, who have a relatively high mortality rate, the dose of delivered therapy affects the mortality rate substantially. Increasing the level of delivered therapy (dialysis) results in a lowering of the mortality rate (Fig 2).

S. Klahr, M.D.

Effects of Recombinant Human Growth Hormone on Muscle Protein Turnover in Malnourished Hemodialysis Patients
Garibotto G, Barreca A, Russo R, et al (Univ of Genoa, Italy; Sampierdarena and Bussana Hosps, Genoa, Italy)
J Clin Invest 99:97–105, 1997   37–2

Background.—In patients with end-stage renal disease who are receiving hemodialysis, malnutrition is an indicator of poor prognosis. One feature of chronic renal failure is resistance to anabolic hormones, which can lead to impaired growth control in uremic children and impaired protein metabolism in adults. Although recombinant human growth hormone (rhGH) therapy is widely used in growth-retarded uremic children, little is known about its effects in adults with renal diseases. The effects of rhGH treatment on muscle protein metabolism in malnourished hemodialysis patients were studied.

Methods.—The study included 6 hemodialysis patients with uremia and chronic wasting (mean, 79% of ideal body weight). In a crossover design, each patient was studied at baseline, after 6 weeks of treatment with rhGH (5 mg thrice weekly), and after a 6-week washout period. Muscle protein metabolism was assessed by evaluation of forearm [^{3}H]phenylalanine kinetics.

Results.—Treatment with rhGH was associated with a 46% reduction in forearm phenylalanine net balance (i.e., phenylalanine incorporated into muscle proteins minus phenylalanine released). There was a 25% increase in phenylalanine rate of disposal, reflecting protein synthesis, no change in phenylalanine rate of appearance, an indicator of protein degradation, and no change in forearm potassium release. Changes in insulin-like growth factor–binding protein-1 level and in the insulin-like growth factor-I/insulin-like growth factor–binding protein-3 ratio explained 15% and 47%, respectively, of the variance in forearm net phenylalanine balance. The 2 factors together explained 62% of the variance in forearm net phenylalanine balance during and after rhGH treatment.

Conclusion.—Treating malnourished hemodialysis patients with rhGH leads to an increase in muscle protein synthesis and a decrease in negative muscle protein balance during the postabsorptive state. Changes in the level of circulating free insulin-like growth factor explain the effect of rhGH in reducing net protein catabolism. However, changes in total insulin-like growth factor level have no effect.

▶ In 1993, the number of new patients treated for end-stage renal disease (ESRD) was slightly in excess of 53,000, and a total of about 220,000 patients with ESRD in the United States were being treated by renal replacement therapy (dialysis, transplantation). Malnutrition has been shown to correlate with mortality in patients undergoing hemodialysis in the United States. Decreased appetite, leading to inadequate ingestion of calories and protein, and accelerated catabolism of protein in muscle—mainly as a consequence of metabolic acidosis in patients with ESRD—are factors that contribute to the development of malnutrition. The administration of rhGH has been shown to promote positive nitrogen balance and to increase body mass in normal individuals. Treatment with rhGH has been shown to ameliorate the growth retardation of uremic children with ESRD.

The above study was designed to assess the effect of rhGH on muscle protein metabolism in 6 malnourished uremic patients undergoing hemodialysis. The findings indicate that in this small group of uremic subjects, the administration of rhGH increased muscle protein synthesis and reduced protein catabolism. Confirmation of these results in a greater number of subjects may be required before this treatment modality is recommended for uremic patients who are malnourished. Of interest is the observation that uremic subjects have elevated levels of circulating growth hormone. Despite this, pharmacologic levels of the hormone are apparently required to produce a positive nitrogen balance.

S. Klahr, M.D.

Plasma Leptin Is Partly Cleared by the Kidney and Is Elevated In Hemodialysis Patients
Sharma K, Considine RV, Michael B, et al (Thomas Jefferson Univ, Philadelphia; Cooper Univ Hosp/Univ Med Ctr, Camden, NJ)
Kidney Int 51:1980–1985, 1997   37–3

Introduction.—Leptin, a 16 kd plasma protein that is encoded by the ob gene, plays a key role in suppressing appetite in mice. It may have a similar function in humans.

There are no data available to indicate how leptin is cleared from the circulation. However, it has a short half-life, and the leptin receptor is present in the kidney, suggesting that the kidney serves as a clearance site. The kidney's role in clearing leptin from human circulation was investigated.

Methods.—A total of 14 patients, both women and men, scheduled for elective cardiac catheterization were studied. Renal function was intact in 8 patients and impaired in 6. After routine cardiac catheterization, aortic and renal vein plasma was collected for leptin measurement by radioimmunoassay. In addition, net mass balance across the kidney was calculated from renal blood flow measurements. The peripheral leptin levels of 36 patients, in a separate cohort, who had end-stage renal disease and were undergoing hemodialysis, were compared with the levels of a group of healthy controls subjects.

Results.—The net renal uptake of circulating leptin was 12% for patients with intact renal function. There was no extraction of leptin in patients with mild-to-moderate renal insufficiency. Linear regression analysis suggested that renal function, as reflected by serum creatinine, accounted for approximately 50% of the net renal extraction of leptin. Peripheral leptin levels (factored for body mass index) were 4.5 times higher in patients undergoing hemodialysis than they were in control patients. Hemodialysis with a modified cellulose membrane (Hemophane) did not clear plasma leptin.

Conclusions.—The evidence suggests that the kidney plays a role in the clearance of leptin from the human circulation. Patients undergoing hemodialysis have elevated levels of circulating free leptin, which are not reduced with cuprophane dialysis membranes. Leptin may mediate the anorexia associated with uremia. More research on leptin is needed.

▶ Leptin, a 16-kd protein secreted by fat cells, has been shown to control appetite in rodents. The role of leptin in humans, though, is not well understood. It is known that obese individuals have markedly elevated levels of leptin, and in both normal-weight and obese individuals, there is a strong correlation between serum levels of leptin and the amount of body fat.[1]

The half-life of leptin is estimated to be approximately 25 minutes. Given its short half-life and low molecular weight, it is likely that the kidney filters and metabolizes this polypeptide.

This report concludes that leptin is extracted from the circulation by the kidneys of individuals with normal renal function, and that this net extraction is decreased in patients with renal insufficiency. Leptin levels were elevated fourfold in the blood of patients with end-stage renal disease. Modified cellulose membranes used in hemodialysis did not remove leptin from the blood.

Because patients with advanced renal insufficiency develop anorexia, it would be useful to examine the potential role of different levels of leptin, along with their effects on appetite and food intake, in patients with renal insufficiency. It also would be interesting to know whether leptin levels in the circulation of such patients vary with the amount of body fat. Obviously, much needs to be learned regarding the role that leptin plays in the disease and health of humans.

S. Klahr, M.D.

Reference

1. Considine RV, Sinha MK, Heiman ML, et al: Serum immunoreactive-leptin concentration in normal-weight and obese humans. *N Engl J Med* 334:292–295, 1996.

Amino Acid Profile and Nitric Oxide Pathway in Patients on Continuous Ambulatory Peritoneal Dialysis: L-Arginine Depletion in Acute Peritonitis

Suh H, Peresleni T, Wadhwa N, et al (State Univ of New York, Stony Brook)
Am J Kidney Dis 29:712–719, 97   37–4

Objective.—Amino acids are now recognized for their important role in regulating various physiologic functions. L-arginine is an amino acid involved in the synthesis of nitric oxide (endothelium-derived relaxing factor), bacterial killing by macrophages, and polyamine production. Individuals with kidney disease have various amino acid abnormalities. Amino acid metabolism and the L-arginine–nitric oxide system were studied in patients with end-stage renal disease who were undergoing continuous peritoneal dialysis (CPD). The study was conducted during uncomplicated CPD and during episodes of acute peritonitis.

Methods.—The study included 34 patients with end-stage renal disease who were undergoing CPD. Of these, 21 were studied during uncomplicated CPD, and 13 were studied during 15 episodes of acute peritonitis. The peritoneal dialysate and serum were collected for measurement of amino acids, including L-arginine.

Results.—Patients with peritonitis had many changes in their serum amino acid profile. In patients with acute peritonitis, the mean serum L-arginine concentration was 52 µmol/L compared with 99 µmol/L in control patients. In most patients, elevated nitrite levels in dialysate during episodes of acute peritonitis suggested increased nitric oxide production. In the peritonitis group, dialysate nitrite levels were 57 µmol/L. In the control group, these levels were 36 µmol/L.

As patients recovered from peritonitis, nitric oxide generation decreased, although a few patients had low nitrite levels during acute peritonitis. In fact, the 5 patients with the lowest nitrite levels in the dialysate had a high incidence of peritonitis. Patients with peritonitis appeared to have substrate deficiency, as indicated by an increased ratio of nitrite to L-arginine in the dialysate.

Conclusions.—When peritonitis develops in a patient undergoing CPD, it leads to increased amounts of nitrite in the peritoneal fluid, along with a tendency to deplete the serum L-arginine pool. Arginine may be consumed in the process of enhanced nitric oxide production. L-arginine may be a conditionally essential amino acid in patients with acute peritonitis who are undergoing CPD.

These findings raise questions about the need for L-arginine supplementation. Although most patients are able to produce an adequate nitric oxide response to microbial invasion, a small group of patients with frequent peritonitis are not able to produce an adequate response.

▶ Although the incidence of peritonitis has decreased in patients undergoing continuous ambulatory peritoneal dialysis (CAPD), it remains a major clinical problem. The incidence of peritonitis in patients undergoing CAPD is now approximately 1 episode per patient every 12–18 months. If appropriate culture procedures are used, an organism can be isolated from the peritoneal fluid in 90% of patients who exhibit signs and symptoms of peritonitis, as well as an elevated neutrophil count. The diagnostic criteria for peritonitis include 2 of the following 3 findings:

1. Clinical evidence of peritoneal inflammation.
2. Cloudy peritoneal fluid with an elevated cell count (mainly neutrophils, > 50 µL).
3. Gram stain or culture is positive for a micro-organism in the peritoneal fluid.

Arginine is the amino acid precursor for the synthesis of nitric oxide, which can be secreted by macrophages and polymorphonuclear leukocytes. Both of these act through peroxynitrite and exhibit antimicrobial activity. Defective production of nitric oxide may lead to persistent bacterial infections. In this study, the majority of patients with acute bacterial peritonitis had increased nitric oxide production, although there was a small subset of patients who had low levels of nitrite (a marker of nitric oxide production). This, along with low levels of arginine, suggests that arginine may become critical in patients with peritonitis who are undergoing CAPD. Supplementing the diets of these patients with arginine must be considered.

S. Klahr, M.D.

Role of an Improvement in Acid-base Status and Nutrition in CAPD Patients
Stein A, Moorhouse J, Iles-Smith H, et al (Leicester Gen Hosp NHS Trust, England)
Kidney Int 52:1089–1095, 1997   37–5

Introduction.—Chronic renal failure in humans is characterized by protein malnutrition. Metabolic acidosis has been linked to renal failure and protein metabolism. Improvements have resulted with better correction of acidosis. Introduction of sodium bicarbonate helps reverse metabolic acidosis and muscle proteolysis. In the first year of treatment with continuous ambulatory peritoneal dialysis, the benefits of improved correction of acidosis were assessed.

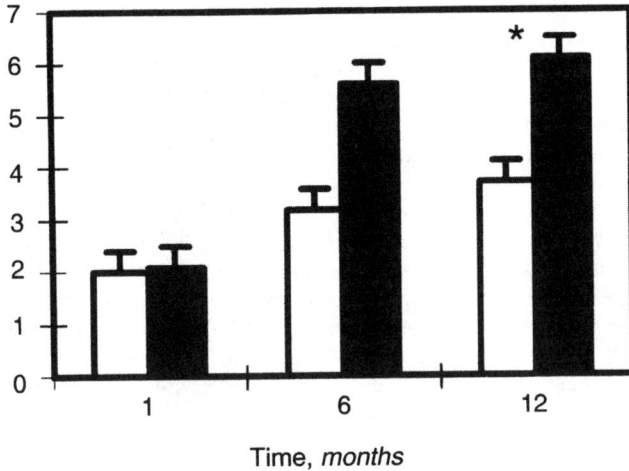

FIGURE 2.—Weight gain (kg) in high (*closed square*) and low (*open square*) alkali groups (*$P < 0.05$). (Courtesy of Stein A, Moorhouse J, Iles-Smith H, et al: Role of an improvement in acid-base status and nutrition in CAPD patients. *Kidney Int* 52:1089–1095, 1997. Reprinted by permission of Blackwell Science, Inc.)

Methods.—There were 200 continuous ambulatory peritoneal dialysis patients, and they were divided into 2 groups. One group received a high alkali dialysate (lactate 40 mmol/L) for 1 year, and the other group received a low alkali dialysate lactate (35 mmol/L) for 1 year. In the high alkali dialysate group, calcium and sodium bicarbonate were used to correct acidosis.

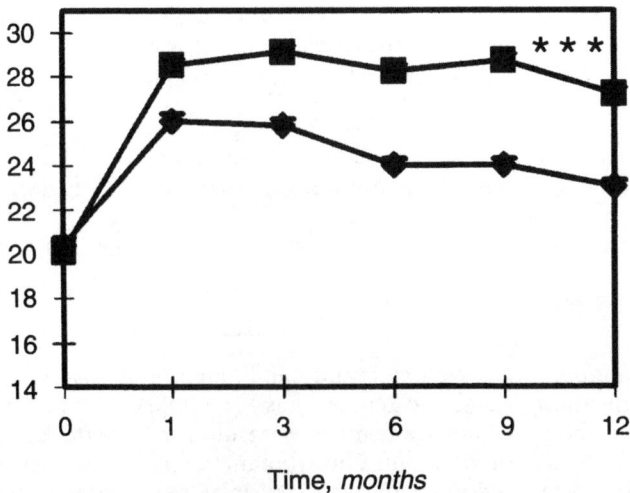

FIGURE 1.—Serum venous bicarbonate levels (mmol/L) in high (*black square*) and low (*black diamond*) alkali groups (***$P < 0.001$). (Courtesy of Stein A, Moorhouse J, Iles-Smith H, et al: Role of an improvement in acid-base status and nutrition in CAPD patients. *Kidney Int* 52:1089–1095, 1997. Reprinted by permission of Blackwell Science, Inc.)

Results.—In the high alkali dialysate group, the venous serum bicarbonate was 27.2 ± 0.3 mmol/L, and arterial pH was 7.44 ± 0.004 L. In the low alkali dialysate group, the venous serum bicarbonate was 23.0 ± 0.3 mmol/L, and the arterial pH was 7.40 ± 0.004 at 1 year. There was no significant difference in the dialysis dose at 1 year. There was a higher increase in body weight in the high alkali dialysate group (6.1 ± 0.66 kg) than there was in the low alkali dialysate group (3.71 ± 0.56 kg) (Fig 2). There was a significantly higher increase in midarm circumference in the high alkali dialysate group than there was in the low alkali dialysate group. There was no significant difference in triceps skinfold thickness. In the high alkali dialysate group, serum albumin was 37.8 ± 0.4 g/dL, and in the low alkali dialysate group, it was 38.2 ± 0.5 g/dL (Fig 1). There was no significant difference in dietary protein intake at 1 year in both groups. The high alkali dialysate group had fewer hospital admissions (1.13 ± 0.16 per patient per year) than the low alkali dialysate group (1.71 ± 0.22 per patient per year).

Conclusion.—Greater increases in body weight and midarm circumference occurred with better correction of metabolic acidosis in the first year of continuous ambulatory peritoneal dialysis. Improvement with nutritional state may be associated with the improvement in morbidity, in terms of number of hospital admissions and days in the hospital per year.

▶ In one survey of 224 patients undergoing continuous ambulatory peritoneal dialysis (CAPD) in 6 centers from Europe and North America, mild-to-moderate protein-calorie malnutrition was observed in a third of the patients, and severe malnutrition was present in an additional 8%.[1] Common manifestations of malnutrition in these patients included: anorexia, weight loss, muscle wasting, reduced body fat, and a decreased albumin level in blood.

Multiple factors may contribute to malnutrition in patients undergoing CAPD, including: loss of proteins in the dialysate, inadequate intake of proteins and calories, and increased catabolism of protein as a consequence of metabolic acidosis. The aim of this study by Stein et al. from Leicester General Hospital in the United Kingdom was to assess the potential benefits, on nutritional status and morbidity, of improved correction of metabolic acidosis in the first year of CAPD. Correction of metabolic acidosis appears to be an important therapeutic adjuvant in patients undergoing CAPD.

S. Klahr, M.D.

Reference

1. Young GA, Kopple JD, Lindholm B, et al. Nutritional assessment of continuous ambulatory peritoneal dialysis patients: An international study. *Am J Kidney Dis* 17:462–471, 1991.

38 Water, Electrolytes, and Acid-Base

Hensin, a New Collecting Duct Protein Involved in the In Vitro Plasticity
of Intercalated Cell Polarity
Takito J, Hikita C, Al-Awqati Q (Columbia Univ, New York)
J Clin Invest 98:2324–2331, 1996   38–1

Background.—There are 2 forms of intercalated cells in kidney collecting tubules: the α cell with apical endocytosis, apical H^+-ATPase, and basolateral band 3, and the β cell with reversed polarity of these proteins and no apical endocytosis. When seeded at high density, a β cell line changed into the α form. Previous research demonstrated that a partially purified 230 kd extracellular matrix protein of high-density cells can retarget band 3 from apical to basolateral domains and stimulate apical endocytosis in vitro. This protein, called *hensin*, was purified to near homogeneity.

Methods and Findings.—After purification to near homogeneity, hensin was found to belong to the macrophage scavenger receptor cysteine rich (SRCR) family. An antibody against a fusion protein produced from a partial complementary DNA recognized a 230 kd protein in rabbit kidney and in the intercalated cell line. The hensin antibody inhibited apical endocytosis expression in vitro. Hensin was secreted in a polarized fashion. It bound to the basolateral membrane and extracellular matrix. Its expression was found only in collecting tubules on immunohistochemistry of the kidney. Double immunofluorescence with hensin and peanut lectin, H^+-ATPase, or band 3 demonstrated many patterns. Most α cells had hensin staining, whereas 50% of β cells did not.

Conclusions.—Hensin, a new collecting duct protein, was described. This protein appears to be involved in the plasticity of intercalated cell polarity in vitro.

▶ The kidney has a key role in acid-base homeostasis. Transport of protons (H^+) and HCO_3^- by the renal collecting tubule is a major mechanism by which acid-base balance is regulated. The collecting tubules of the cortex and outer medulla of the kidney contain two types of cells: principal and intercalated. These latter cells are involved in acid-base transport. Intercalated cells are present in at least two forms, one that secretes H⁺ into the lumen of the tubule and another that secretes HCO_3^-. The α cell contains apical H⁺ ATPase and basolateral localization of band 3. By contrast, β cells have reversed distribution of these two proteins. A secreted factor that can reverse the polarity of intercalated cells is described. The authors have purified a protein to near homogeneity and provide evidence that it is a novel protein that may be involved in the polarity reversal of intercalated cells in vivo. The protein (named hensin) belongs to a recently described family of proteins, the scavenger receptor cysteine rich (SRCR) family. In the kidney, this protein appears to be confined to the collecting duct. Colocalization studies indicate that the protein has a heterogenous expression in intercalated cells; half of the β-intercalated cells do not express it, whereas, most of the α-intercalated cells are rich in it.

Biochemical studies have shown that although hensin is bound to membranes, it is easily removed by alkali treatment. Thus, one can hypothesize that changes in plasma pH may affect the binding of hensin to membranes and the relative secretion of H⁺ or HCO_3^- by intercalated cells of the collecting tubule of the kidney.

S. Klahr, M.D.

Upregulation of Aquaporin-2 Water Channel Expression in Chronic Heart Failure Rat
Xu D-L, Martin P-Y, Ohara M, et al (Univ of Colorado, Denver)
J Clin Invest 99:1500–1505, 1997   38–2

Introduction.—Patients with advanced congestive heart failure (CHF) usually have water retention. The recently cloned aquaporin-2 (AQP2) water channel is responsible, via vasopressin, for mediating collecting duct water permeability. This raises the possibility that the water retention of CHF could be related to upregulation of the AQP2 water channel. This hypothesis was tested in a study of rats.

Methods.—Rats underwent either ligation of the left coronary artery to induce CHF or a sham operation. About 1 month later, the animals' mean arterial pressure and cardiac output were measured. Twenty-four hours after that, the animals were killed for examination, which included measurement of mRNA and protein of AQP2. In further experiments, the effects of administering a nonpeptide V2 vasopressin receptor antagonist, OPC 31260, were studied.

Results.—Compared with sham-operated rats, the rats with experimental CHF had significantly decreased cardiac output and plasma osmolality and significantly increased plasma vasopressin. The CHF rats also had significantly increased kidney messenger RNA (mRNA) and protein AQP2. Treatment with oral OPC 31260 led to increased diuresis, decreased urinary osmolality, and increased plasma osmolality. Treated rats had significantly reduced mRNA and protein AQP2 in both the renal cortex and the inner medulla.

Conclusion.—In this rat model of CHF, upregulation of AQP2 is an early feature. Treatment with a V2 receptor antagonist inhibits AQP2 upregulation. Vasopressin may play an important role in the upregulation of AQP2 water channels and, thus, in the water retention of CHF.

▶ Hyponatremia is a common finding in patients with CHF. This is attributed to water retention as a consequence of increased water reabsorption by the kidneys. Plasma levels of arginine vasopressin (antidiuretic hormone [ADH]) are also increased in patients with CHF. It has been shown that this increase in ADH in patients with CHF was not suppressed after an acute water load.

Antidiuretic hormone increases water permeability of the principal cells of the collecting duct. Increased water permeability is achieved by the translocation of AQP2 water channels from cytosolic vesicles to the cell membrane of principal cells in the collecting duct. This usually short effect of ADH is mediated by the V2 receptor-dependent increase of cyclic adenosine monophosphate and may involve phosphorylation of the AQP2 water channel. Prolonged stimulation of water reabsorption may occur by an increase in the synthesis and insertion of AQP2 in the membrane of principal cells when elevated levels of ADH exist. Thus, in a pathophysiologic state such as CHF, characterized by elevated levels of ADH, the hormone would upregulate the synthesis of AQP2 and lead to water retention.

This experimental study from the University of Colorado, conducted in rats with induced CHF, provides evidence for a major role of antidiuretic hormone in the upregulation of AQP2 water channels and water retention in this setting. This upregulation was inhibited by the administration of a nonpeptide V2 receptor antagonist. The usefulness of V2 antagonists in the treatment of hyponatremia in patients with CHF needs to be studied.

S. Klahr, M.D.

39 Calcium, Phosphorus, and Bone

Vasectomy Is Associated With an Increased Risk for Urolithiasis
Kronmal RA, Krieger JN, Coxon V, et al (Univ of Washington, Seattle)
Am J Kidney Dis 29:207–213, 1997   39–1

Background.—In a recent multicenter study of vasectomy as a potential risk factor for coronary artery disease, an unexpected finding was an increased risk of urolithiasis. This association was further investigated in a case-control study.

Methods and Findings.—The case patients were 244 men experiencing initial episodes of urolithiasis. The age-matched control subjects were 423 men with no history of urolithiasis. Logistic regression analysis showed that among men younger than 46 years, those with vasectomies had a relative risk for urolithiasis of 1.9 compared with those without vasectomies. Among men 46 years or older, the relative risk was 0.9 for men with vasectomies. Men with vasectomies had a 2.0 relative risk of urinary calculi up to 4 years before evaluation compared with men without vasectomies. This excess risk persisted for up to 14 years after vasectomy (Table 1).

Conclusions.—In men younger than 46 years, vasectomy is associated with a 2-fold increased risk for urolithiasis, which may persist for up to 14 years after vasectomy. Given the widespread use of vasectomy for contra-

TABLE 1.—Risk of Urolithiasis Among 11,205 Men Participating in the Coronary Artery Surgery Study

Age (yr)	Person-years at Risk		No. With Urolithiasis		Relative Risk
	Vasectomy	No Vasectomy	Vasectomy	No Vasectomy	
30–34	1,190.5	53,218.5	5.5	93.5	2.63
35–39	2,090.0	49,801.0	10.5	113.5	2.20
40–44	2,548.5	44,842.0	8.5	103.5	1.45
45–49	2,289.5	37,969.5	10.0	105.0	1.57
50–54	1,537.5	28,041.5	8.0	85.0	1.72
55–64	1,184.0	24,966.0	5.0	81.0	1.30

(Courtesy of Kronmal RA, Krieger JN, Coxon V, et al: Vasectomy is associated with an increased risk for urolithiasis. *Am J Kidney Dis* 29:207–213, 1997.)

ception, this increased risk for urolithiasis may result in substantial excess morbidity.

▶ Urolithiasis is a major cause of morbidity among middle-aged men. In the United States, the annual incidence of stone disease is approximately 16/10,000 population. The male-to-female ratio is 3:1, with female patients having a proponderance of "infectious" stones. Genetic factors (enzymatic disorders) and environmental factors (diet, temperature, and humidity) influence stone formation.

Vasectomy has been considered a safe and effective method of permanent contraception. It is less expensive and is associated with much lower morbidity and mortality rates than tubal ligation. Long-term effects of vasectomy include chronic testicular pain, testicular function alterations, and epididymal obstruction. A postulated effect of vasectomy on the cardiovascular system has also been suggested. Approximately 500,000 men in the United States undergo vasectomy each year.

In 1988, Kronmal et al.[1] described a statistical relationship between vasectomy and urolithiasis (Table 1). Kronmal et al. now report the results of a case-control study specifically designed to evaluate the impact of vasectomy as a risk factor for the development of urolithiasis. The authors found that vasectomy was associated with a 2-fold increased risk for urolithiasis in men younger than 46 years of age. Although the mechanisms by which vasectomy increases the risk of urolithiasis have not been elucidated, the association between vasectomy and renal stone formation is itself an important finding. Men contemplating vasectomy for contraception should be informed of the potential risk of urolithiasis. Obviously, it will be important to delineate the mechanisms involved in the association.

S. Klahr, M.D.

Reference

1. Kronmal RA, Krieger JN, Alderman E, et al: Vasectomy and urolithiasis. *Lancet* 1:22–23, 1988.

Comparison of Dietary Calcium With Supplemental Calcium and Other Nutrients as Factors Affecting the Risk for Kidney Stones in Women
Curhan GC, Willett WC, Speizer FE, et al (Harvard Med School, Boston; Massachusetts Gen Hosp, Boston)
Ann Intern Med 126:497–504,1997   39–2

Background.—Calcium intake may affect kidney stone formation, but there is limited information about risk factors for stone formation in women. The rate of kidney stones in women is about one third the rate in men, although the reasons for this are unknown. In the past, it was assumed that a diet high in calcium increased the risk of calcium-containing kidney stones. In a large prospective study in men, a diet high in calcium was associated with a lowered risk of stone formation. The association between calcium intake and risk of stone formation in women was investigated.

Methods.—A self-administered questionnaire was completed by 91,731 women with no history of kidney stones. The subjects were participating in the Nurses' Health Study. They were between 34 and 59 years old in 1980. Follow-up was 12 years. The questionnaire was administered in 1980, 1984, 1986, and 1990.

Results.—There were 864 cases of kidney stones documented in the 903,849 person-years of follow-up. After adjustment for risk factors, there was an inverse relationship between dietary calcium and risk of kidney stones. There was a positive association between supplemental calcium and risk of kidney stones. The relative risk of stone formation was compared in women in the highest and lowest quintiles of dietary calcium intake; this risk was 0.65. The relative risk of stone formation was also compared in women who took and did not take supplemental calcium; this risk was 1.20. In 67% of the women who took supplemental calcium, the calcium was not taken with a meal, or was taken with a meal low in oxalate content. The relative risk of the other dietary factors in stone formation was compared in women in the highest and lowest quintiles of intake: the risks were 1.52 for sucrose, 1.30 for sodium, 0.61 for fluid, and 0.65 for potassium.

Discussion.—These findings suggest that a diet high in calcium may lower the risk of symptomatic kidney stone formation in women. This risk may be higher in women who take calcium supplements. Dietary calcium lowers the absorption of oxalate, and the different effects of dietary and supplemental calcium on risk of kidney stones may result from the combined amounts of calcium and oxalate consumed. Other factors in dairy products may also be involved in the lowered risk of stone formation associated with dietary calcium.

▶ Calcium is the major component of renal stones, and the pathogenesis of such stones has been linked to the excretion of calcium in the urine. Clinical wisdom dictated, therefore, that reducing urinary calcium excretion would lead to a reduction in the formation of kidney stones. In a previous study, Curhan et al.[1] found an inverse association between dietary calcium intake and risk for stone formation in men. The current report examines the role of dietary calcium intake and supplemental calcium as factors affecting the risk for kidney stones in women. The incidence of renal stones in women is one third that observed in men; the reason for this difference is currently unknown. In this study, Curhan et al. found that females ingesting a low calcium diet were at greater risk of having stones than those with higher calcium intakes. This may be attributable to reciprocal hyperoxaluria. The study also found that excess calcium ingestion (from calcium supplements) may be deleterious. Women taking calcium supplements may be at higher risk for stones, particularly if the supplements are taken between meals. In this setting, oxalate absorption may not be influenced, whereas the supplemental calcium will readily be absorbed and cause supersaturation in the urinary tract. The overall findings of this study suggest that greater ingestion of dairy products, the major source of dietary calcium, decreases the risk of kidney stones in women.

S. Klahr, M.D.

Reference

1. Curhan GC, Willett WC, Rimm EB, et al: A prospective study of dietary calcium and other nutrients and the risk of symptomatic kidney stones. *N Engl J Med* 328:833–838, 1993.

High Resolution Mapping of the Renal Sodium-Phosphate Cotransporter Gene (NPT2) Confirms Its Localization to Human Chromosome 5q35
McPherson JD, Krane MC, Wagner-McPherson CB, et al (Washington Univ, St Louis; Univ of California, Irvine; McGill Univ, Montreal)
Pediatr Res 41:632–634, 1997   39–3

Purpose.—Recent cloning studies have identified probes useful for studying the type II renal-specific Na⁺-phosphate (P_i) cotransporter (NPT2) gene, which could be involved in inherited disorders of renal P_i reabsorption. To determine whether this relationship exists, it is important to find the precise chromosomal location of the NPT2 gene. Recent studies have reported conflicting locations: chromosome 5q35 in 1 study and 5q13 in another. This study was initiated in an attempt to resolve this discrepancy.

Methods and Findings.—Three techniques were used: a human chromosome 5/rodent somatic cell hybrid deletion panel, fluorescence in situ hybridization with a PAC clone containing the NPT2 locus, and a chromosome 5–specific radiation hybrid panel. All of these techniques mapped the NPT2 gene to chromosome 5q35. The radiation hybrid panel not only confirmed the location of NPT2 but also established its position relative to other chromosome 5 loci and identified the flanking microsatellite markers D5S498 and D5S469.

Conclusion.—The NPT2 gene, which encodes the high-affinity, renal-specific brush-border membrane Na⁺-P_i cotransporter, is definitively localized to human chromosome 5q35. The conflicting results of previous studies may have occurred because hybridization was nonspecific and was not performed directly on banded chromosomes. The information provided by this study will permit linkage analysis to see whether the Na⁺-P_i cotransporter is involved in various autosomal disorders of renal phosphate wasting.

▶ About 85% of the phosphate filtered at the glomerulus is reabsorbed by the kidney under normal circumstances. This reabsorption, which plays a major role in the homeostasis of phosphate, occurs predominantly in the proximal tubule and is coupled to the reabsorption of sodium in the brush border of tubular cells. In the last few years, complementary DNAs encoding high affinity, brush-border Na^+-P_i cotransporters (NPT2) have been cloned from several mammalian species.

This paper deals with the chromosomal localization of the type II renal-specific Na^+-P_i cotransporter (NPT2) gene. The NPT2 gene has been shown to be significantly decreased in the x-linked hypophosphatemic mice, a murine homologue of human x-linked hypophosphatemia. Using 3 independent methods, the authors demonstrated that the gene encoding NPT2 maps to human chromosome 5q35. These findings will permit the use of linkage analysis to determine the causative role of this gene (NPT2) in inherited disorders of phosphate wasting by the kidney.

S. Klahr, M.D.

40 Rheumatoid Arthritis

Introduction

This year we learn that calcium and vitamin D_3 supplementation prevents bone loss in the spine secondary to low-dose corticosteroids in patients with rheumatoid arthritis (Abstract 40–1), and that proximal bursitis is a feature of active polymyalgia rheumatica (Abstract 40–2). We consider a number of treatments for rheumatoid arthritis—one that worked well in early disease with minimal toxicity (minocycline; Abstract 40–5); one that may be a useful therapeutic adjunct and appears safe (gamma-linolenic acid; Abstract 40–4); an experimental anti cytokine that is promising for established disease at least in the short run (recombinant human tumor necrosis factor receptor [p75]-Fc fusion protein; Abstract 40–6); and a draconian measure that did more harm than good (total lymphoid irradiation; Abstract 40–3).

Noted in passing: In an open-level extension study, improvement seen at 24 weeks in patients with established disease given the combination of cyclosporine and methotrexcate[1] was maintained at 48 weeks without unacceptable toxicity.[2] Also, in patients with established disease, interferon γ was no better than placebo.[3] The strongest predictors of methotrexate-induced lung injury in rheumatoid arthritis were older age, diabetes, rheumatoid pleuropulmonary involvement, previous use of disease-modifying antiinflammatory drugs, and hypoalbuminemia[4]; in addition, hydroxychloroquine retinopathy is rare.[5]

Stephen E. Malawista, M.D.

Suggested Readings

1. 1996 YEAR BOOK OF MEDICINE, p 700.
2. Stein CM, Pincus T, Yocum D, et al. Combination treatment of severe rheumatoid arthritis with cyclosporine and methotrexate for forty-eight weeks. *Arthritis Rheum* 40:1843–1851, 1997.
3. Veys EM, Menkes C-J, and Emery P: A randomized double-blind study comparing twenty-four-week treatment with recombinant interferon-γ versus placebo in the treatment of rheumatoid arthritis. *Arthritis Rheum* 40:62–68, 1997.
4. Alarcón GS, Kremer JM, Macaluso M, Weinblatt ME, *et al.* Risk factors for methotrexate-induced lung injury in patients with rheumatoid arthritis. *Ann Int Med* 127:356–364, 1997.

5. Levy GD, Munz SJ, Paschal J, Cohen HB, *et al.* Incidence of hydroxychloroquine retinopathy in 1,207 patients in a large multicenter outpatient practice. *Arthritis Rheum:* 40:1482–1486, 1997.

Calcium and Vitamin D$_3$ Supplementation Prevents Bone Loss in the Spine Secondary to Low-dose Corticosteroids in Patients With Rheumatoid Arthritis: A Randomized, Double-blind, Placebo-controlled Trial

Buckley LM, Leib ES, Cartularo KS et al (Med College of Virginia, Richmond; Univ of Vermont, Burlington)
Ann Intern Med 125:961–968, 1996   40–1

Purpose.—Patients with allergic and autoimmune diseases are commonly treated with low-dose corticosteroids. This treatment can lead to reduced bone mineral density, with a corresponding increase in the risk of fracture. Supplemental calcium and vitamin D$_3$, which improves calcium absorption, have been suggested for use in reducing bone loss. However, there are few data to support the efficacy of this intervention. Patients receiving low-dose prednisone were studied to determine whether supplemental calcium and vitamin D$_3$ can prevent bone loss.

Methods.—The randomized, controlled trial included 96 patients with rheumatoid arthritis, 65 of whom were being treated with prednisone (mean dose 5.6 mg/day, range 1 to 20 mg). The patients were randomly assigned to receive supplementation with calcium carbonate, 1,000 mg/day and vitamin D$_3$, 500 IU/day, or placebo for 2 years. At 1 and 2 years, they underwent measurement of bone mineral density in the spine and femur.

Results.—The rate of loss of bone mineral density in patients taking prednisone who were assigned to placebo was 2.0% per year in the lumbar spine and 0.9% per year in the trochanter. In contrast, patients taking prednisone who received supplemental calcium and vitamin D$_3$ had increased bone mineral density: 0.72% per year in the lumbar spine and 0.85% per year in the trochanter. This group had no increase in bone mineral density in the femoral neck or the Ward triangle, however. Patients not taking prednisone had no improvement in bone mineral density with calcium and vitamin D$_3$ supplementation.

Conclusions.—In patients receiving low-dose prednisone therapy, supplementation with calcium carbonate and vitamin D$_3$ prevents loss of bone mineral density in the spine and hip. These supplements are available over the counter and have few side effects. They may help to reduce the risk of fracture in patients who require long-term corticosteroid treatment.

▶ A task force of the American College of Rheumatology has recently made well-considered recommendations for the prevention and treatment of glucocorticoid-induced osteoporosis.[1] The recommended first-line therapies are calcium and vitamin D supplements, sex hormone replacement when appropriate, and a weight-bearing exercise program that maintains muscle mass. Thiazide diuretics and sodium restriction may be indicated to reduce hypercalciuria associated with glucocorticoid use. In patients who are not candidates for sex hormone replacement, have established osteoporosis, or are showing deterioration in bone mineral density despite these interventions, such agents as biphosphonates or calcitonin are thought to be indicated.

In a well-designed 2-year, randomized, double-blind, placebo-controlled trial of 96 patients with rheumatoid arthritis, 65 of whom were receiving treatment with corticosteroids (mean dosage, 5.6 mg/d), the current authors provide the best evidence yet for supplementation with calcium and vitamin D_3 in such patients. Unlike the more expensive active metabolite 1,25-dihydroxyvitamin D_3 (calcitriol), the parent compound at the dose employed here ([500] IU/d) is very unlikely to produce hypercalcemia and hypercalciuria. The preparation given, Os-Cal 250 + D (SmithKline Beecham), 2 tablets twice daily, also contains a total dose of 1,000 mg of elemental calcium (which the authors incorrectly refer to as calcium carbonate 1,000 mg; the latter would only contain 400 mg of elemental calcium).

As the authors point out, bone mineral density is a surrogate measure for the clinical outcomes of most interest: pain, disability, and osteoporosis-related fracture. Nevertheless, this is valuable information, and we can look forward to the extension of this work beyond 2 years, as well as to patients receiving moderate- to high-dose corticosteroid therapy.

S.E. Malawista, M.D.

Reference

1. American College of Rheumatology Task Force on Osteoporosis Guidelines: Recommendations for the prevention and treatment of glucocorticoid-induced osteoporosis. *Arthritis Rheum* 39:1791–1801, 1996.

▶ Osteoporosis is an inevitable consequence of corticosteroid excess. It affects trabecular (cancellous) bone to a greater extent than cortical bone. The major cause is a decrease in bone formation, and bone resorption does not change or increases slightly. Gastrointestinal absorption of calcium may be decreased, perhaps because of a decrease in calcitriol (1,25-dihydroxyvitamin D) formation or action. Urinary calcium excretion also may be increased, but it seems clear that the major problem is decreased bone formation.

One way to stimulate bone formation is by provision of more calcium and vitamin D, and in this study of mostly women in their 50s, modest doses of each were effective in increasing bone density in several sites. The patients' dietary calcium intake at base line was reasonable, ranging from 800 to 1,000 mg daily, but their vitamin D intake was not estimated nor was serum 25-hydroxyvitamin D measured. Perhaps the best evidence against important deficiency of either calcium or vitamin D is that the patients who had not received prednisone had no increase in bone density during the 2-year period of calcium and vitamin D treatment. These findings also lead to the conclusion that the calcium-vitamin D regimen had some rather specific "anticorticosteroid" effect.

Other regimens used to treat, or, in a few instances, to prevent, corticosteroid-induced bone loss include a combination of calcium and calcitriol, biphosphonates, and calcitonin.[1] Whether any regimen is more effective is not known, but certainly the combination of calcium and vitamin D has much to recommend it. As compared with any of the others, it is simpler, cheaper, and safer. Furthermore, it is biologically more attractive, because it should stimulate bone formation, whereas the other therapies act primarily by inhibiting bone resorption.

I think everyone treated with a corticosteroid for more than a few weeks should take 1,500 mg of elemental calcium and 800 IU of vitamin D daily. This amount of vitamin D is present in 2 tablets of most over-the-counter vitamin preparations, and combined calcium carbonate-vitamin D formulations are now available over the counter. The calcium and vitamin D should preferably be started at the same time as the corticosteroid, but later is surely better than never. Attention should of course also be paid to other measures known to increase bone density—estrogen-progestin—or slow loss of bone—smoking cessation and exercise.

R.D. Utiger, M.D.

Reference

1. Eastell R: Management of corticosteroid-induced osteoporosis. *J Intern Med* 37:439–447, 1995.

Proximal Bursitis in Active Polymyalgia Rheumatica
Salvarani C, Cantini F, Olivieri I, et al (Azienda Ospedaliera Arcispedale S Maria Nuova, Reggio Emilia, Italy; Ospedale di Prato, Italy; Azienda Ospedaliera S Orsola-Malpighi, Bologna, Italy)
Ann Intern Med 127:27–31, 1997   40–2

Introduction.—The cause of musculoskeletal symptoms in the proximal extremities of patients with polymyalgia rheumatica has not been determined. Mild synovitis characterized by infiltration of macrophages and CD4 T cells can probably explain some of the diffuse and severe musculoskeletal discomfort patients experience. Magnetic resonance imaging (MRI) of the shoulder girdle was examined in a series of consecutive patients with symptoms of active polymyalgia rheumatica.

Methods.—Thirteen patients with active symptoms of polymyalgia rheumatica, 9 patients with early symptoms of elderly onset rheumatoid arthritis, and 10 age-matched healthy controls underwent MRI of the shoulder.

Results.—Patients with polymyalgia rheumatica had a significantly higher incidence of subacromial and subdeltoid bursitis, compared to control subjects with elderly-onset rheumatoid arthritis (Figure). There was no significant difference between patients with polymyalgia rheumatica and control subjects with elderly onset rheumatoid arthritis in fre-

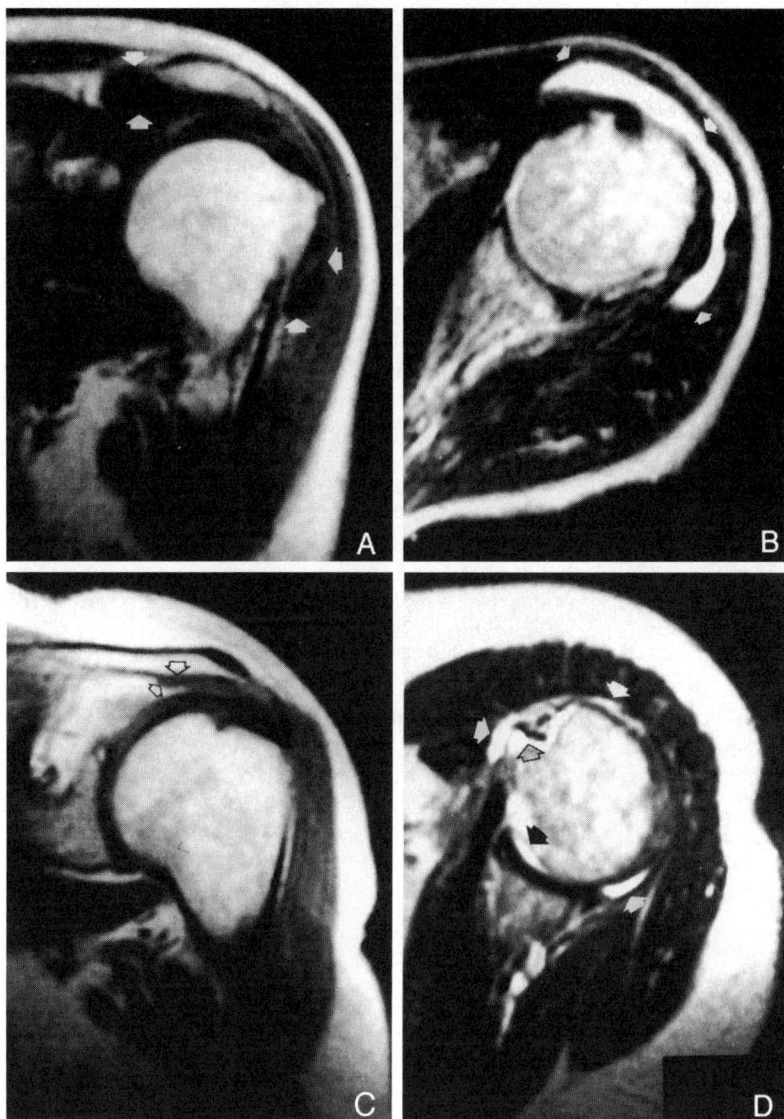

FIGURE.—Magnetic resonance images of patients with polymyalgia rheumatica. Coronal T1-weighted, **A**, and axial T2-weighted, **B**, images of the left shoulder show severe subacromial and subdeltoid bursitis (*arrows*). Coronal T1-weighted, **C**, image of the left shoulder shows mild subacromial bursitis (*arrows*). Axial T2-weighted, **D**, image of the left shoulder shows moderate subdeltoid bursitis (*solid white arrows*), mild joint effusion (*solid black arrow*), and severe tenosynovitis on the long head of the biceps (*open black arrows*). (Courtesy of Salvarini C, Cantini F, Oliveri I: Proximal bursitis in active polymyalgia rheumatica. *Ann Intern Med* 127:27–31, 1997.)

quency of synovitis of the joints and tenosynovitis of the biceps. There was no evidence of fluid accumulation in the joints, bursae, or sheaths of the long head of the biceps in healthy control subjects.

Conclusion.—Much of the diffuse and severe discomfort in the shoulder girdle of patients with polymyalgia rheumatica is probably caused by inflammation of subacromial and subdeltoid bursae in association with synovitis of the glenohumeral joints and tenosynovitis of the biceps.

▶ Polymyalgia rheumatica (PMR), generally a disease of the elderly, is characterized by aches and morning stiffness in the shoulders, neck, and pelvic girdle, and frequently by low grade fever, anorexia, weight loss, and an elevated erythrocyte sedimentation rate; the response to 10 mg of predni-sone a day is usually immediate and dramatic. Polymyalgia rheumatica often turns up in the chapter on vasculitis because of its sometime association with temporal (cranial, giant cell) arteritis, but the two are often *not* associated, and PMR is not a vasculitis *per se*. Healey and others have made a good case for PMR overlapping with a seronegative, low-dose-corticoster-oid-responsive form of rheumatoid arthritis that occurs in the elderly;[1] inapparent synovitis is well known to occur; and last year we reported on distal extremity swelling with pitting edema in this syndrome, apparently representing synovitis and tenosynovitis of regional structures.[2] With use of MRI in a case-control study including patients with early symptoms of elderly onset rheumatoid arthritis and healthy controls subjects, the authors made a good case for subacromial and subdeltoid bursitis (Figure), in association with synovitis of the glenohumeral joints and tenosynovitis of the biceps, to explain the severe proximal discomfort that afflicts patients with PMR. Thus, classical PMR appears to be only the most common presentation of a systemic, low-dose-corticosteroid-responsive, inflammatory disorder of bursae, tendons, and joints in the elderly, for which there may be multiple triggers.

S.E. Malawista, M.D.

References

1. 1993 YEAR BOOK OF MEDICINE, p 688.
2. 1996 YEAR BOOK OF MEDICINE, p 709.

Total Lymphoid Irradiation in Rheumatoid Arthritis: A Ten-Year Followup
Westhovens R, Verwilghen J, Dequeker J (Katholieke Universiteit Leuven, Belgium)
Arthritis Rheum 40:426–429, 1997   40–3

Introduction.—The earlier use of total lymphoid irradiation (TLI) in patients with rheumatoid arthritis (RA) was feared by some to increase the incidence of myeloproliferative disorders. The long-term follow-up studies

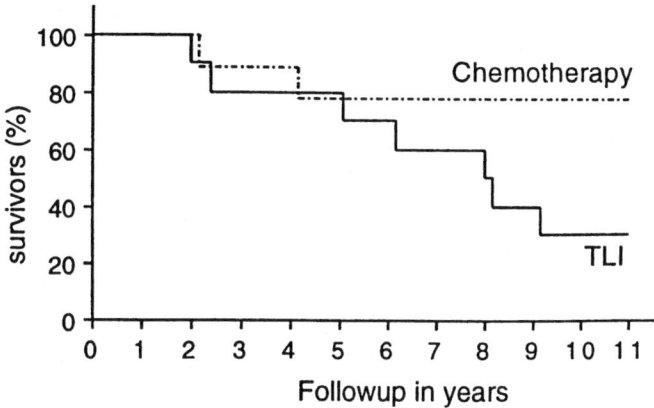

FIGURE 1.—Comparison of overall survival in rheumatoid arthritis patients treated with total lymphoid irradiation (TLI) or with combination chemotherapy. (Courtesy of Westhovens R, Verwilghen J, Dequeker J: Total lymphoid irradiation in rheumatoid arthritis: A ten-year followup. *Arthritis and Rheumatism* 40:426–429, copyright 1997, American College of Rheumatology.)

of patients with RA who underwent TLI more than 10 years previously are reported.

Methods.—From 1983 to 1984, 20 patients with severe, refractory RA unresponsive to second-line agents and corticosteroids were randomized to receive either TLI or combination chemotherapy. Patients were observed for 3 years. Short-term outcomes were good for patients in both groups. A retrospective review of 10-year follow-up studies was conducted. Medical records were available for all except 1 patient who received chemotherapy.

Results.—The most significant outcome parameter was mortality rate. Patients in the TLI group had a significant increase in late mortality, compared to patients in the chemotherapy group (70% vs. 22%) (Fig 1). At 10-year follow-up, 7 of 10 patients in the TLI group and 2 of 9 patients in the chemotherapy group had died. Sustained suppression of the CD4+ lymphocyte count was observed for up to 10 years after TLI treatment.

Conclusion.—No malignancies were seen in the first 5 years after either TLI or chemotherapy treatment. Five of 7 deaths in this series occurred in the TLI group between 5 and 10 years after treatment. Treatment with TLI was associated with increased incidence of B cell proliferation/malignancy and severe infections. Only patients in the TLI-treated group experienced sustained and pronounced depletion of peripheral blood CD4+ T cells.

▶ Total lymphoid irradiation (TLI) was a well-intentioned therapy that proved to be a disaster. We have known for some time that it did not prevent progressive erosion of joints,[1] but in the small 10-year follow-up presented here, B cell abnormalities and premature death are seen. It should be stressed that the candidates for the initial study were patients with severe, refractory rheumatoid arthritis that was unresponsive to multiple second-line agents as well as to corticosteroids; ie, the worst possible group to try to turn around clinically. Nevertheless, patients given TLI did worse than randomized control subjects who received low-dose combination chemotherapy. Seven (of 10) of the former group died, 5 of them in the second 5-year period after TLI (Fig 1). Causes of death were disease activity (at 24 months), myocardial infarction (29 months), cardiac failure (61 months), AL amyloidosis (74 months), multiple myeloma (96 months), persistent disease activity and multiple cardiac valvular insufficiency (98 months), and cardiac failure due to multiple valvular insufficiency (110 months). Both patients who died in the combination chemotherapy group had myocardial infarctions. Only 1 of the 3 surviving TLI patients was without major complications. Finally, TLI patients (and not control subjects) had a sustained and pronounced depletion of peripheral blood CD4+ T cells, and 3 of them developed B cell proliferation/malignancy (multiple myeloma, central plasmacytosis, and amyloidosis). The authors exit on the chilling note that anti-CD4+ monoclonal antibodies, currently under study in refractory rheumatoid arthritis, also induce a long-term depletion of CD4+ cells, with reversal of the CD4:CD8 ratio.

S.E. Malawista, M.D.

Reference

1. 1990 YEAR BOOK OF MEDICINE, p 630.

Gamma-Linolenic Acid Treatment of Rheumatoid Arthritis: A Randomized, Placebo-controlled Trial
Zurier RB, Rossetti RG, Jacobson EW, et al (Univ of Massachusetts, Worcester; Massachusetts Gen Hosp, Boston)
Arthritis Rheum 39:1808–1817, 1996   40–4

Objective.—Gamma-linolenic acid (GLA), a fatty acid from plant seed oil, has been shown to reduce synovitis significantly in patients with rheumatoid arthritis (RA) at a dose of 1.4 g/day. Efficacy and tolerability results of a 1-year trial of GLA treatment (2.8 g/day) in patients with RA and synovitis are presented.

Methods.—Either 2.8 g/day GLA as the free fatty acid (n = 28) or placebo (n = 28) was administered to 56 patients with RA (7 men) for 6 months in a double-blind, randomized fashion. All patients then received 2.8 g/day GLA in the following 6 months in a single-blind trial. Patients were evaluated at 3-month intervals during the study and 3 months after the end of the study.

Results.—Patients receiving GLA had moderate but significant improvement in swollen joint count and score, tender joint count and score, duration of morning stiffness, patient's global assessment and assessment of pain, and Health Assessment Questionnaire score at 6 months. Because not all measures improved with GLA vs. placebo, it is possible that the 35% oleic acid content of the sunflower seed oil placebo may have relieved some symptoms. Nonsteroidal antiinflammatory drugs (NSAIDs) and

TABLE 5.—Overall Clinical Response to Treatment of Rheumatoid Arthritis With γ-linolenic acid (GLA)

Overall response	First 6 months		Second 6 months		GLA for 12 months (n = 21)
	GLA (n = 22)	Placebo (n = 19)	GLA (n = 21)	Placebo/GLA (n = 14)	
Remission	0	0	0	0	0
Meaningful improvement	14†	4	9	5	16
No meaningful change	8	9	10	8	3
Deterioration	0	6	2	1	2

*Values are the mean absolute change on the mean (SD) percentage of change from baseline. GLA = γ-linolenic acid; MAQ = Health Assessment Questionnaire.
†P < 0.05 vs. baseline (entry), by Wilcot on sign rank test.
(Courtesy of Zurier DB, Rossetti RB, Jacobson EW, et al: Gamma-linolenic acid treatment of rheumatoid arthritis: A randomized, placebo-controlled trial. *Arthritis Rheum* 39:1808–1817, copyright 1996, American College of Rheumatology.)

prednisone doses were reduced during the trial in 7 GLA patients. GLA is converted to dihomo-GLA, which suppresses 5-lipooxygenase and 12-lipooxygenase. Although some have considered that GLA can function as an NSAID, the fact that patients with RA are better after 12 months than 6 months of treatment suggests that GLA acts more like a disease-modifying antirheumatic drug.

Conclusion.—The fatty acid GLA appears to regulate cell activation, immune responses, and inflammation in patients with RA. GLA at 2.8 g/day had a modest but significant clinical effect on RA and is well tolerated. Additional controlled studies are needed.

▶ It is bracing to read an article about a treatment for RA that has no section on adverse effects because there apparently were none. Zurier et al. have devoted themselves to analyzing the in vitro and in vivo effects of gamma-linolenic acid (GLA; 18:3 ω6), an essential fatty acid found in certain plant seed oils (borage seed oil, evening primrose oil). Its antiinflammatory properties may depend on a number of properties. These include its metabolism to the antiinflammatory/immunoregulatory eicosanoid, prostaglandin E1 (PGE_1); the inability of its metabolite, dihomo-γ-linolenic acid to be converted to inflammatory leukotrienes by 5-lipoxygenase (but rather to produce an inhibitor of both 5- and 12-lipoxygenase activity); alterations in cell membrane structure that can determine the behavior of membrane-bound enzymes and receptors (fat, not protein, is what "you are what you eat" refers to); and direct suppression of interleukin-2 production by mononuclear cells and of the proliferation of interleukin-2–dependent peripheral blood and synovial T lymphocytes.

In the current 1-year, randomized, placebo-controlled trial, the authors provide the disclaimer that GLA is not approved in the United States for the treatment of any condition and should not be viewed as therapy for any disease. However, the treated patients, who continued to take stable doses of their previous (second-line and other) agents during the study, experienced sufficient meaningful (≥25%) improvement (Table 5) that we certainly want to see more work on the adjunctive clinical effects of this apparently benign plant extract.

S.E. Malawista, M.D.

Treatment of Early Rheumatoid Arthritis With Minocycline or Placebo: Results of a Randomized, Double-blind, Placebo-controlled Trial

O'Dell JR, Haire CE, Palmer W, et al (Univ of Nebraska, Omaha; Omaha VA Hosp, Neb)
Arthritis Rheum 40:842–848, 1997   40–5

Background.—Rheumatologists currently emphasize the importance of early control of rheumatoid arthritis (RA). Evidence suggests that tetracyclines may have antiarthritic action. Thus, the efficacy of minocycline in the treatment of seropositive RA within the first year of diagnosis was investigated.

Methods.—Forty-six patients with RA were enrolled in the 6-month study. The patients received 100 mg of minocycline twice a day or placebo.

Findings.—Eighteen patients met 50% improvement criteria at 3 months and maintained at least a 50% improvement for 6 months. No significant toxicity was documented. Responders included 65% of the

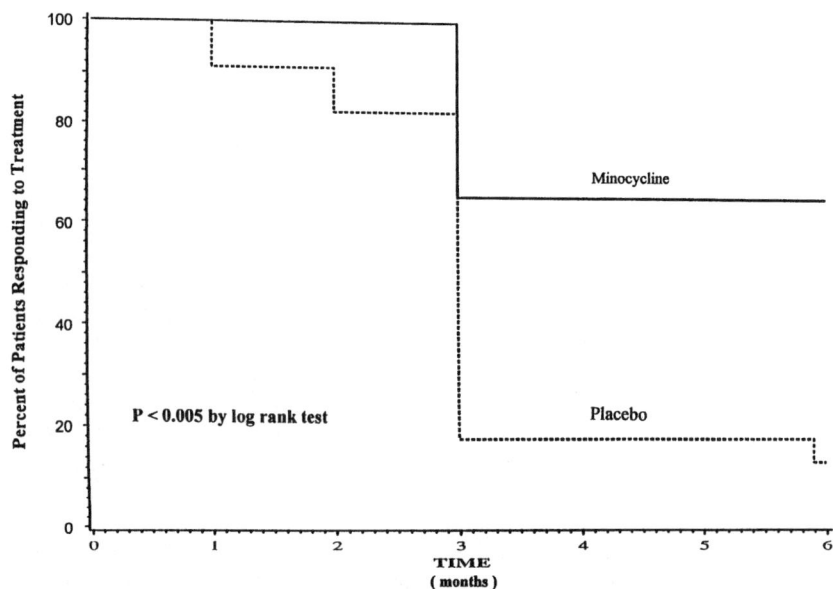

FIGURE 1.—Kaplan-Meier plot of the proportion of patients responding to treatment with either minocycline or placebo. (Courtesy of O'Dell JR, Maire CE, Palmer W, et al: Treatment of early rheumatoid arthritis with minocycline or placebo: Results of a randomized, double-blind, placebo-controlled trial. *Arthritis Rheum* 40:842–848, 1997, copyright American College of Rheumatology.)

TABLE 3.—Therapy at 1 Year: Minocycline Versus Placebo

	Patients originally in minocycline group (n = 23)	Patients originally in placebo group (n = 20)	P
No. in remission	5	1	0.13
No. improved by 50%	20	9	0.004
No. receiving DMARDs*	7	17	<0.001
No. receiving minocycline	11	3	0.023
No. receiving no therapy	5	1	0.13

*DMARDs = disease-modifying antirheumatic drugs.
(Courtesy of O'Dell JR, Haire CE, Palmer W, et al: Treatment of early rheumatoid arthritis with minocycline or placebo: Results of a randomized, double-blind, placebo-controlled trial. *Arthritis Rheum* 40:842–848, 1997.)

patients receiving minocycline and only 13% of the patients receiving placebo.

Conclusions.—Minocycline is effective in the treatment of patients with seropositive RA in the first year of disease. Further research is needed to establish optimal treatment duration and to investigate the mechanism(s) of action.

▶ In this 24-week, randomized, double-blind, placebo-controlled trial, minocycline was generally successful in patients with early (<1 year) seropositive RA, despite the authors having stacked the cards against success. First, they required 50% improvement in order for a patient to be classified as improved, instead of the 20% or 25% rate that is often used. Second, not wanting to continue placebo therapy for more than 3 months in patients with active RA, they required the 50% improvement to occur within that period as a criterion for continuation in the study. Thus, they are likely to have lost patients from the study before their response to minocycline was maximal. Nevertheless, in those remaining, the results with minocycline were maintained, and were dramatically better than those with placebo (Fig 1). Its mechanism of action is unknown.

None of these patients had previously received any long-acting agents, and only stable doses of nonsteroidal antiinflammatory (NSAIDs) were allowed during the first 6 months. During a second and open 6 months in which any medication including minocycline was allowed, the original minocycline group continued to do better than the placebo group (Table 3), although the authors note that relapses tended to occur when the drug was stopped.

In 2 earlier double-blind, placebo-controlled studies,[1] minocycline was only moderately effective, but the populations were different: the earlier groups had RA for averages of 13 and 8 years; in the former group, 95% of patients had joint erosions. Studies such as the current one, in a drug with less toxicity than most current long-acting agents, will favor the early use of minocycline in RA.

S.E. Malawista, M.D.

Reference

1. 1996 YEAR BOOK OF MEDICINE, p 702.

Treatment of Rheumatoid Arthritis With a Recombinant Human Tumor Necrosis Factor Receptor (p75)-Fc Fusion Protein
Moreland LW, Baumgartner SW, Schiff MH, et al (Univ of Alabama, Birmingham; Physician's Clinic of Spokane, Wash; Denver Arthritis Clinic, Colo; et al)
N Engl J Med 337:141–147, 1997   40–6

Introduction.—Both laboratory and clinical evidence suggest an important role for proinflammatory cytokines, particularly tumor necrosis factor (TNF), in the pathogenesis of rheumatoid arthritis, and the administration of TNF antagonists has reduced symptoms of the disease. A small number of patients with refractory rheumatoid arthritis showed some decrease in disease activity after treatment with a recombinant human TNFR p75-Fc fusion protein (TNFR:Fc). The safety and efficacy of TNFR:Fc was examined in a double-blind trial of 180 patients.

Methods.—The multicenter trial randomized patients to 1 of 4 treatment groups: placebo, 0.25 mg of TNFR:Fc per square meter of body-surface area, 2 mg of TNFR:Fc per square meter, or 16 mg of TNFR:Fc per square meter. Injections were administered subcutaneously, twice weekly for 3 months. All patients had failed to respond to 1 or more disease-modifying antirheumatic drugs. During the trial they were allowed to continue stable doses of nonsteroidal anti-inflammatory drugs and corticosteroids. Clinical response was measured by changes in composite symptoms of arthritis as defined by the American College of Rheumatology.

Results.—Patients had a mean age of 53; 77% had disease of >5 years' duration. The 4 groups were similar in baseline disease activity. Overall, 76% of patients given TNFR:Fc completed the trial, vs. 52% of those assigned to placebo. Most who withdrew did so because of inadequate control of symptoms. The completion rate was highest (93%) in the 16-mg group. Active treatment led to significant reductions in disease activity, and the effects of TNFR:Fc were dose-related. In the 16-mg group, 75% of patients had improvement of $\geq 20\%$ in symptoms, and the mean percent reduction in number of swollen or tender joints was 61%. Mild injection-site reactions and mild upper respiratory tract symptoms were the most common adverse events. No antibodies to TNFR:Fc were detected in serum samples, and there were no major abnormalities in hematologic findings or serum chemical profiles during or after the trial.

Conclusion.—Patients with refractory rheumatoid arthritis showed improvement in inflammatory symptoms after 3 months of treatment with TNFR:Fc. The benefits were significant and rapid, but disease activity increased after cessation of therapy.

▶ In this multicenter, 3-month, double-blind trial of a parenterally administered fusion protein linking the soluble TNF receptor (p 75) to the Fc portion of human IgG1 (TNFR:Fc), there was a dose-related therapeutic effect 2 by the two most important measures of inflammatory activity, the counts of swollen and tender joints. These patients had established disease, most of them for over 5 years. None of them developed antibodies or serious reactions to the treatment. Note that activity returned toward baseline when the agent was stopped.

Although the study was well done and the initial results were good, an accompanying editorial raises all the proper questions.[1] This is one of a number of approaches to anticytokine therapy in rheumatoid arthritis currently being considered. Unless this is an adjunctive therapy, to be used, for example, while slow-acting drugs are getting going, the duration of efficacy and the long-term effects of blocking the activity of TNF will have to be carefully examined. We also need to know whether this therapy is strictly antiinflammatory or whether it can prevent further destruction of joints; a study aimed at early, nonerosive disease would be most likely to answer that question. That being said, this was an excellent beginning.

S.E. Malawista, M.D.

References

1. Firestein GS, Zvaifler NJ: Anticytokine therapy in rheumatoid arthritis. *N Engl J Med* 337:195–197, 1997.

41 Systemic Lupus Erythematosus

Introduction

This chapter deals with the long-term treatment of systemic lupus erythematosus (SLE) with cyclosporin A (Abstract 41–1); a possible thrombogenic mechanism for pregnancy loss in the antiphospholipid-antibody syndrome (Abstract 41–2); ribosomal P autoantibodies in neuropsychiatric SLE (Abstract 41–3); the prevalence of antineutrophil cytoplasmic antibodies (ANCAs) in patients with connective tissue disease (Abstract 41–4); and the range of antinuclear antibodies in "healthy" individuals (Abstract 41–5).

Noted in passing: a review of the clinical associations of antiphospholipid antibodies[1] and the use of testosterone to prevent cyclophosphamide-induced azoospermia.[2]

S.E. Malawista, M.D.

References

1. Lockshin MD: Antiphospholipid antibody. *JAMA* 277:1549–1551, 1997.
2. Masala A, Faedda R, Alagna S, Satta A, et al: Use of testosterone to prevent cyclophosphamide-induced azoospermia *Ann Intern Med* 126:292–295, 1997.

Long-term Treatment of Systemic Lupus Erythematosus With Cyclosporin A
Caccavo D, Laganà B, Mitterhofer AP, et al (Univ La Sapienza, Rome)
Arthritis Rheum 40:27–35, 97   41–1

Introduction.—Cyclosporin A (CSA) has been used for many years to treat patients with connective tissue autoimmune diseases because of its selective immunosuppressive features. The efficacy of long-term treatment with CSA was evaluated in 30 patients with systemic lupus erythematosus (SLE).

Methods.—All patients had SLE that was poorly responsive or unresponsive to treatment with steroids and/or cytotoxic drugs. Disease activ-

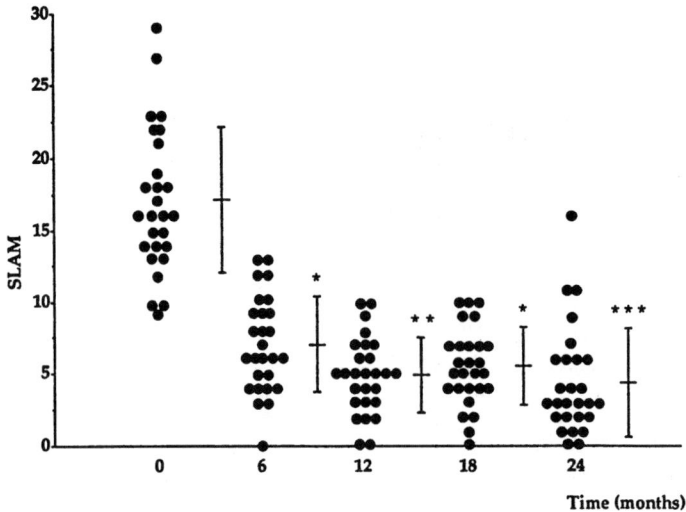

FIGURE 1.—Change in the systemic lupus activity measure (SLAM) scores in 27 patients with systemic lupus erythematosus after treatment with cyclosporin A. Closed circles represent the SLAM scores for individual patients. Bars show the ± SD. * = $P < 0.01$ vs. time 0; ** = $P < 0.01$ vs. time 0; $P < 0.05$ vs. 6 months (time 1); *** = $P < 0.01$ versus time 0; $P < 0.01$ versus time 1. (Courtesy of Caccavo D, Laganà B, Mitterhofer AP: Long-term treatment of systemic erythematosus with cyclosporin A. *Arthritis Rheumatism* 40:27–35, 1997.)

ity was prospectively assessed before initiation of CSA and at 6, 12, 18, and 24 months during follow-up using the systemic lupus activity measure (SLAM).

Results.—Twenty-seven of 30 patients were able to complete at least 24 months of CSA treatment. There was a significant reduction in mean SLAM score after 6 months of treatment that was sustained throughout treatment (Fig 1). Most clinical manifestations of SLE were notably improved within 4 to 8 weeks of initiation of CSA. Anemia, leukopenia, and

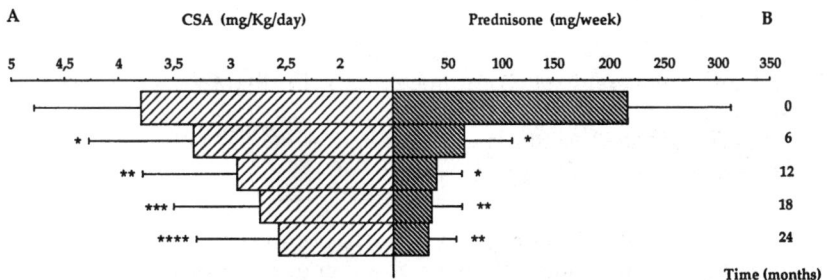

FIGURE 7.—Reduction of dosage of cyclosporin A (CSA) (A) and of steroids (B) during the follow-up of 27 patients with systemic lupus erythematosus. Columns represent the mean dosage at each time point, while bars show the SD. **A,** * = $P < 0.05$ vs. time 0; ** = $P < 0.01$ vs. time 0; *** = $P < 0.01$ vs. time 0, $P < 0.05$ vs. 6 months (time 1); **** = $P < 0.01$ vs. time 0, $P < 0.01$ versus time 1. **B,** * = $P < 0.01$ vs. time 0, ** = $P < 0.01$ vs. time 0, $P < 0.05$ vs. time 1. (Courtesy of Caccavo D, Laganà B, Mitterhofer AP: Long-term treatment of systemic erythematosus with cyclosporin A. *Arthritis Rheumatism* 40:27–35, 1997.)

thrombocytopenia were especially sensitive to CSA treatment in patients whose condition was either poorly controlled or unresponsive to steroids and/or other cytotoxic medications. Steroid dosage was decreased significantly during CSA administration (Fig 7). Serum creatinine levels did not change significantly during treatment. Side effects included 63% hypertrichosis, 23% paresthesias, 20% gastrointestinal symptoms, 17% gingival hyperplasia, 10% hypertension, 7% tremors, and 13% nephrotoxicity.

Conclusion.—Cyclosporin A may be considered effective in treating patients with SLE whose condition is poorly responsive to conventional treatment. A steroid-sparing effect and progressive disappearance of hypercortisolism were observed in patients treated with CSA. Most clinical benefits were observed within 6 months of treatment. Thus, the focus of prolonged treatment should be toward consolidating clinical results rather than achieving further improvements.

▶ The treatment of corticosteroid-resistant systemic lupus erythematosus (SLE) is not for the inexperienced or faint hearted. The current authors report considerable success over 2 years with the careful use of cyclosporin A (CSA), starting with 30 such patients, half of whom had never received cyclophosphamide or azathioprine. The 27 patients who completed the course had overall improvement in their indexes of SLE activity, mostly within the first 6 months of treatment (Fig 1; the 'SLAM' score covers symptoms occurring in the month before a given assessment, and includes 24 clinical manifestations and 8 laboratory parameters). Mean hemoglobin levels approached normal in the 20 patients in whom it was initially low; all of 6 white blood cell counts below 3,500/mm³ became normal; 6 of 7 platelet counts below 150,000/mm³ became normal, and all 4 urinary proteins of >3 g/24 hours decreased markedly within a month and continued to improve thereafter. The means of successive serum creatinine levels, a measurement of major concern with CSA therapy, were stable; however, initial hypertension or elevated serum creatinine levels were exclusions from the study. Quite impressive was the corticosteroid-sparing effect, maintained as the dose of CSA was tapered (Fig 7). Cyclosporin A was stopped in 3 patients: early, in 2 patients, because of raised serum creatinine levels or severe epigastric pain that were resistant to a decrease in dosage; in one patient, after 5 months because of tremors.

Two years is long for a clinical trial but very short in a lifetime. The authors do note preliminarily that patients appear to need continuation of CSA, even as little as 2 mg/kg/day, to avoid relapses. We look forward to the results of longer follow-up studies.

S.E. Malawista, M.D.

Pregnancy Loss in the Antiphospholipid-Antibody Syndrome—A Possible Thrombogenic Mechanism

Rand JH, Wu X-X, Andree HAM, et al (Mount Sinai School of Medicine, New York; New York Univ)
N Engl J Med 337:154–160, 1997   41–2

Background.—Patients with the antiphospholipid-antibody syndrome are at risk of arterial and venous thrombosis and recurrent pregnancy loss. However, little is known about the pathogenesis of this disorder. Annexin V is a phospholipid-binding protein that is a powerful anticoagulant. Placental villi from patients with the antiphospholipid-antibody syndrome show very low levels of annexin V, suggesting that hypercoagulability could result from reduction of surface-bound annexin V by antiphospholipid antibodies. The effects of antiphospholpid antibodies on annexin V levels on cultured trophoblasts were studied, including the effects on cell procoagulant activity.

Methods.—The investigators obtained IgG antibodies from the plasma of 3 patients with antiphospholipid-antibody syndrome and 3 normal controls. The isolated antibodies were then incubated with cultured BeWo placental trophoblast cells, primary cultured trophoblast, and human um-

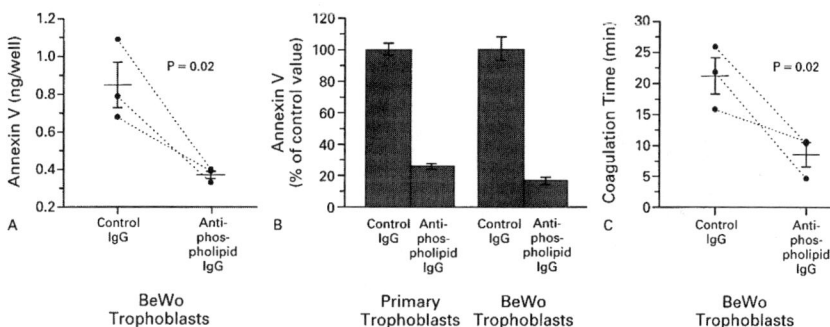

FIGURE 1.—Effects of antiphospholipid-antibody IgG on annexin V and plasma coagulation on trophoblasts. Cultured trophoblasts (from the BeWo cell line) grown to confluence were exposed to IgG preparations (2 mg per milliliter) from 3 patients and their controls for 2 hours at 4°C to inhibit the recycling of membranes and vesicles. Annexin V was then dissociated with buffer containing EGTA and measured by immunoassay. (All tests were performed in quadruplicate.) A shows that the mean (±SE) level of annexin V, indicated by the horizontal line and error bar, was significantly lower after exposure to antiphospholipid IgG than after exposure to control IgG (0.37 ± 0.02 vs. 0.85 ± 0.12 ng per well, $P = 0.02$). B shows how antiphospholipid IgG affects annexin V levels on primary culture trophoblasts and BeWo trophoblasts. (The data on the former were normalized for the DNA concentration, and both sets of data were normalized as percentages of the control values so that the 2 cell types could be shown together.) Annexin V levels on the surface of both types of trophoblasts were significantly reduced ($P < 0.001$ for both). C shows the coagulation time of plasma added to BeWo trophoblasts exposed to preparations of IgG from the 3 patients for 2 hours at 4° C, as compared with controls. In these experiments, annexin V was not dissociated from the cells. The mean (±SE) coagulation time was significantly shorter in the antiphospholipid-IgG–exposed trophoblasts than in the controls (8.7 ± 2.0 vs. 21.3 ± 2.9 minutes, $P = 0.02$). (Reprinted by permission of The New England Journal of Medicine from Rand JH, Wu X-X, Andree HAM, et al: Pregnancy loss in the antiphospholipid-antibody syndrome—a possible thrombogenic mechanism. *N Engl J Med* 337:154–160. Copyright 1997 Massachusetts Medical Society.)

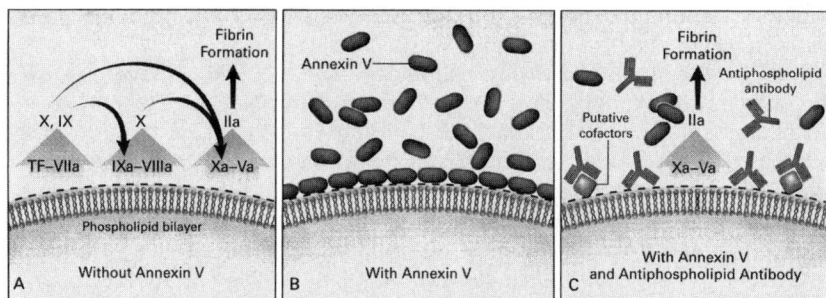

FIGURE 4.—Mechanisms of the reduction of annexin V levels and the acceleration of coagulation associated with antiphospholipid antibodies. In **A**, anionic phospholipids (minus signs) on the surface of the cell-membrane bilayer serve as potent cofactors for the assembly of 3 coagulation complexes: the tissue-factor–VIIa complex, the IXa-VIIIa complex, and the Xa-Va complex. The presence of such phospholipids thus accelerated blood coagulation. The tissue-factor–VIIa complex yields either factor IXa or factor Xa; the IXa-VIIIa complex yields factor Xa; and Xa formed from both these reactions becomes the active enzyme in the prothombinase complex (Xa-Va), which yields factor IIa (thrombin) and in turn cleaves fibrinogen to form fibrin. In **B**, when antiphospholipid antibodies are absent, annexin V forms clusters that bind with high affinity to the surface of anionic phospholipids and block the assembly of the phospholipid-dependent coagulation complexes, thereby inhibiting coagulation. In **C**, directly or through an interaction with protein-phospholipid cofactors, antiphospholipid antibodies disrupt the ability of annexin V to cluster on the phospholipid surface. This action reduces the binding affinity of annexin V and permits more anionic phospholipid to be available to form complexes with coagulation proteins. As a result, coagulation is accelerated and the development of thrombosis is promoted *TF*, tissue factor. (Reprinted by permission of The New England Journal of Medicine from Rand JH, Wu X-X, Andree Ham, et al: Pregnancy loss in the antiphospholipid-antibody syndrome—a possible thrombogenic mechanism. *N Engl J Med* 337:154–160. Copyright 1997 Massachusetts Medical Society.)

bilical vein endothelial cells. An enzyme-linked immunosorbent assay was used to measure cell surface annexin V expression. In coagulation studies, coagulation times were measured in plasma overlaid on the culture cells.

Results.—Levels of annexin V were reduced in cells exposed to antiphospholipid-antibody IgG, compared with controls: 0.37 versus 0.85 ng/well for trophoblasts and 1.6 versus 2.1 ng/well for endothelial cells (Fig 1). Mean plasma coagulation time with trophoblasts exposed to IgG from patients with antiphospholipid-antibody syndrome ws 8.7 minutes, compared with 21.3 minutes with control trophoblasts. Coagulation times were also shorter with exposed endothelial cells, 9.8 versus 14.2 minutes.

Conclusions.—Annexin V expression and plasma coagulation are decreased on cultured trophoblasts and endothelial cells exposed to antiphospholipid antibodies. Annexin V may have antithrombotic activity at the apical surface of trophoblasts and endothelial cells. The arterial and venous thrombosis occurring in antiphospholipid-antibody syndrome may result from the reduced annexin V levels at these sites (Fig 4).

▶ The authors provide evidence for a potentially important prothrombotic effect of antiphospholipid antibodies—a reduction in the quantity of the potent anticoagulant protein annexin V on the surface of placental trophoblasts (Fig 1) and vascular endothelial cells. The mechanism is diagrammed in Fig 4. Anti-annexin V antibodies, seen in some patients with SLE who have arterial or venous thrombosis, intrauterine fetal loss, or prolonged activated partial thromboplastin times,[1] may work in a similar fashion.

In an excellent accompanying editorial,[2] Cowchock would have us resist the impulse to overgeneralize these findings. She points out that what we call antiphospholipid antibodies are broadly defined as a family of antibodies binding primarily anionic phospholipids that have formed complexes with proteins; these antibodies are detectable by immunoassays or clotting tests. Their clinical importance requires evidence of pathophysiologic effects, such as thrombocytopenia, a history of thrombosis, or the presence of a lupus anticoagulant. Moreover, since clinical conditions such as thrombocytopenia and thrombosis have multiple causes, identifying these antibodies as the cause of a prolonged clotting time in a phospholipid-dependent clotting test requires confirmatory testing—at a minimum, mixing the sample with fresh plasma to rule out deficiencies of common clotting factors. The current authors did indeed obtain their IgG autoantibodies from women who had additional clinical and laboratory findings indicating abnormal coagulation. They provide valuable insight into at least 1 way in which certain antiphospholipid antibodies can cause disease.

S.E. Malawista, M.D.

References

1. Kaburaki J, Kuwana M, Yamamoto M, Kawai S and Ikeda Y: Clinical significance of anti-annexin V antibodies in patients with systemic lupus erythematosus. *Amer J Hematology* 54:209–213, 1997.
2. Cowchock S: Autoantibodies and pregnancy loss. *New Engl J Med* 337:197–198, 1997 (editorial).

Ribosomal P Autoantibodies in Systemic Lupus Erythematosus: Frequencies in Different Ethnic Groups and Clinical and Immunogenetic Associations

Arnett FC, Reveille JD, Moutsopoulos HM, et al (Univ of Texas, Houston; Natl Univ of Athens, Greece; Cornell Univ, New York)
Arthritis Rheum 39:1833–1839, 1996   41–3

Background.—Some patients with systemic lupus erythematosus (SLE) have autoantibodies to ribosomal P protein (anti-P), which have been associated in some studies with lupus psychosis and depression. To determine the prevalence of anti-P antibodies in a large, multiethnic cohort of patients with SLE, to evaluate the association between these anti-P antibodies and lupus psychosis, and to identify major histocompatability (MHC) class II alleles associated with anti-P antibodies, serum samples from a large group of patients with SLE were evaluated.

Study Design.—The study group consisted of 120 white, 127 black, 75 Hispanic, and 14 Chinese Americans who received a diagnosis of SLE at the University of Texas-Houston Health Science Center. Sera from these patients with SLE were examined, along with sera previously obtained

TABLE 2.—Frequencies of Lupus Psychosis and/or Depression in Patients With and Without Antiribosomal P Antibodies

Clinical feature	No. (%) of anti-P positive patients (n = 63)	No. (%) of anti-P negative patients (n = 283)	P	Odds ratio
Psychosis	8 (13)	9 (3)	0.005	4.43
Depression	10 (16)	5 (2)	3×10^{-5}	10.5
Either or both	17 (27)	13 (5)	$<1 \times 10^{-7}$	7.68

Note: Greek and Bulgarian patients are excluded.
(Courtesy of Arnett FC, Reveille JD, Moutsopoulos, HM, et al: Ribosomal P autoantibodies in systemic lupus erythematosus: Frequencies in different ethnic groups and clinical and immunogenetic associations. *Arthritis Rheum* 39:1833–1839, copyright 1996, American College of Rheumatology.)

from 32 Greek and 16 Bulgarian patients with SLE. Enzyme-linked immunosorbent assay (ELISA) was used to determine anti-P antibody levels in sera. Deoxyribonucleic acid oligotyping of sera was utilized to determine HLA-DR and DQ alleles.

Findings.—Anti-P antibodies were detected in 13% to 20% of patients, but were more common in Chinese patients and less common in Bulgarian patients. Lupus psychosis or depression was significantly associated with the presence of anti-P antibodies in patient sera (Table 2). The MHC class II alleles HLA-DR2, DQ6 haplotypes DRB1*1501 or 81503, DQA1*0102, and DQB1*0602 were detected at increased levels in anti-P positive white, black and Mexican-American patients with SLE. The strongest association was between HLA-DQB1*0602 and anti-P. The HLA-DQ8 specificity (DQB1*0302) was increased in both white and Mexican-American patients with SLE with anti-P who were negative for HLA-DQB1*0602 but was not increased in black Americans with SLE, in whom HLA-DQB1*0301 was increased. A shared amino acid sequence in HLA-DQB1 was strongly associated with anti-P across ethnic groups in this study group.

Conclusions.—Sera from a large, multiethnic group of patients with SLE were analyzed for antiribosomal P protein antibodies. The association of anti-P antibodies with lupus psychosis and with MHC class II alleles was also examined. The presence of anti-P in the sera of these patients with SLE was correlated with neuropsychiatric lupus. The anti-P response in patients with SLE appeared to be influenced by MHC class II alleles.

▶ Ten years ago in these pages,[1] I first reported on the possible association of anti-ribosomal P antibodies (anti-P antibodies) with lupus psychosis. There have been several papers both pro and con such an association since then. Currently, the "pros" seem to have the high ground.[2] The current work may involve the largest cohort of patients with SLE (349) studied for this association to date, and includes the widest diversity of ethnic groups. The authors found anti-P antibodies in only 13% to 20% of the various groups, but the associations with neuropsychiatric lupus (psychosis and/or depression) were significant (Table 2). No linkage was found between anti-P and anti-Ro/SS-A, anti-La/SS-B, anti-Sm, anti-Ul RNP, or anticardiolipin antibodies.

A connection between anti-P and the pathogenesis of neuropsychiatric lupus is not yet clear. However, this antibody is also associated with the development of lupus hepatitis and lupus nephritis, and, in a recent study,[3] affinity-purified anti-P was found to penetrate into living hepatoma cells in culture and cause dysfunction marked by inhibition of apolipoprotein secretion and an accumulation of intracellular fat. We can anticipate similar studies on brain cells.

S.E. Malawista, M.D.

References

1. 1988 YEAR BOOK OF MEDICINE, p 715.
2. Isshi K, Hirohata S: Association of anti-ribosomal P protein antibodies with neuropsychiatric systemic lupus erythematosus. *Arthritis Rheum* 39:1483–1490, 1996.
3. Koscec M, Koren E, Wolfson-Reichlin M, et al: Autoantibodies to ribosomal P proteins penetrate into live hepatocytes and cause cellular dysfunction in culture. *J Immunol* 159:2033–2041, 1997.

Prevalence of Antineutrophil Cytoplasmic Antibodies in a Large Inception Cohort of Patients With Connective Tissue Disease
Merkel PA, Polisson RP, Chang YC, et al (Massachusetts Gen Hosp, Boston; Harvard Med School, Boston)
Ann Intern Med 126:866–873, 1997   41–4

Introduction.—Antineutrophil cytoplasmic antibodies (ANCA)—antiproteinase 3 antibodies (anti-PR3), and antimyeloperoxide antibodies (anti-MPO)—are helpful in the diagnosis of types of vasculitis such as Wegener's granulomatosis and microscopic polyangitis. It is not unusual for connective tissue diseases to appear in the differential diagnosis of this spectrum of vasculitis. The prevalence of ANCA was analyzed for as long as 5 years in a blinded, controlled trial of a unique group of patients with various connective tissue diseases.

Methods.—Of 386 patients evaluated: 70 had systemic lupus erythematosus (SLE), 70 had rheumatoid arthritis, 45 had scleroderma, 36 had inflammatory myositis, 44 had Sjögren syndrome, and 165 had early undifferentiated connective tissue disease. Serum samples were collected from these patients and 2 control groups: a group of 200 random blood donors and 52 patients with known vasculitis and positive anti-PR3 or anti-MPO results. The presence of anti-PR3 and anti-MPO was detected by combining the results of indirect immunofluorescence tests for cytoplasmic (C-ANCA) and perinuclear (P-ANCA) patterns with results of enzyme-linked immunosorbent assays (ELISAs) directed to measure antigen.

Results.—Cytoplasmic ANCA was not detected in any patients from any group. Perinuclear ANCA was associated with the presence of antinuclear antibodies and was frequently detected in patients with SLE (31%); it was not common in other patients groups. Atypical ANCA immunofluorescence patterns were observed in 11% to 39% of groups. In 9 and 2 study patients, ELISA detected anti-PR3 and anti-MPO, respectively. During follow-up, no patients with positive ELISA results had any indication of renal vasculitis. Test specificity for vasculitis was 99.5% in patients with connective tissue disease when using a scoring system combining immunofluorescence and ELISA.

Conclusion.—Patients with connective tissue disease are known to have multiple autoantibodies. A rigorous ANCA testing system that combines immunofluorescence results with those of ELISA is highly specific for Wegener granulomatosis and related vasculitides, even in the presence of connective tissue disease.

▶ Vasculitides associated with certain ANCAs include Wegener's granulomatosis, microscopic polyangiitis, Churg-Strauss syndrome, idiopathic necrotizing and crescentic glomerulonephritis, and some related or overlapping conditions (but not, for example, Takayasu's arteritis, Henoch-Schönlein purpura, or cryoglobulinemia). The 2 diagnostically useful ANCAs are antiproteinase 3 antibodies (anti-PR3), which produce a cytoplasmic staining pattern on indirect immunofluorescence (C-ANCA; especially useful in Wegener's granulomatosis), and antimyeloperoxidase antibodies (anti-MPO), which produce a perinuclear or nuclear pattern (P-ANCA). The latter is an ethanol fixation artifact, as MPO is found in cytoplasmic (azuropil) granules, but the result is a staining pattern resembling that of antinuclear antibodies (ANA). Because ANCA-positive vasculitides and connective tissue diseases share a number of clinical features—glomerulonephritis, alveolar hemorrhage, tracheobronchitis, sinusitis, palpable purpura, arthritis, ocular inflammation, neuropathy—it would be well to be able to separate their marker antibodies. The current authors have done this, in the first comprehensive, blinded, controlled study to determine the presence of ANCA among patients in whom connective tissue disease was diagnosed according to strict criteria and to use a full set of laboratory tests for ANCA; the test specificity for vasculitis was 99.5% among patients with connective tissue disease.

Two points are worth making. First, ANCAs were applied here to a specific population and for a specific purpose. As I pointed out in last year's YEAR BOOK, both the predictive value and the false-positive rate of such tests vary with the prevalence of disease in a given population;[1] thus, if the tests were done on everyone who walked into a general practitioner's office, almost every positive result would be a false positive result. Neither ANCAs nor ANAs alone should be used for general screening, and certainly not for decisions about therapy. Second, these workers were blessed with a highly experienced ANCA testing laboratory that has honed its skills on over 20,000 samples since 1989. The reader should be sure that his laboratory can do both immunofluorescence and antigen-specific ELISA tests for anti-PR3 and anti-MPO. (In those with the facilities, another way to separate P-ANCA from

ANAs would be to fix their cells with a cross-linking agent such as paraformaldehyde rather than with ethanol; the former will result in a frank cytoplasmic pattern for 'P'-ANCA.)

S.E. Malawista, M.D.

References

1. 1997 YEAR BOOK OF MEDICINE, p 707.

Range of Antinuclear Antibodies in "Healthy" Individuals

Tan EM, Feltkamp TEW, Smolen JS, et al (Scripps Research Inst, La Jolla, Calif; The Netherlands Red Cross Blood Transfusion Service, Amsterdam; Univ of Vienna; et al)
Arthritis Rheum 40:1601–1611, 1997   41–5

Background.—Immunofluorescence microscopy (IFM) is the standard method for detecting antinuclear antibodies (ANA) in sera. To determine the range of ANA in healthy controls vs. that of patients with systemic lupus erythematosus (SLE), systemic sclerosis (SSc), Sjögren's syndrome (SS), rheumatoid arthritis (RA), or soft-tissue rheumatism (STR), the ANA Subcommittee of the International Union of Immunological Societies (IUIS) Standardization Committee conducted an international multicenter study.

Study Design.—Fifteen international laboratories with experience in conducting IFM assays for ANA in sera participated in the study. Each laboratory contributed 2–4 serum samples from healthy volunteers in each age category: 21–30 years, 31–40 years, 41–50 years, and 51–60 years. Each laboratory also contributed 2–4 serum samples from patients in each disease category: SLE, SSc, SS, RA, and STR. All IFM assays for ANA were performed on HEp-2 substrates at 1:40, 1:80, 1:160, and 1:320 dilutions of serum. Each laboratory used its own protocols for the assays.

Findings.—In the healthy population, serum samples from 31.7% of individuals from all age categories were ANA positive at 1:40, 13.3% at 1:80, 5.0% at 1:160, and 3.3% at 1:320 dilution. When compared with serum samples from patients, a low cutoff at 1:40 serum dilution would have high sensitivity and would classify most patients as positive, but would have low specificity. A high positive cutoff at 1:160 serum dilution would have high specificity, as it would exclude 95% of healthy individuals but would have low sensitivity (Table 1).

Conclusions.—The levels of antinuclear antibodies in serum from healthy volunteers and patients with a variety of autoimmune diseases were compared using IFM assays in 15 experienced international laboratories. The results show that although IFM assay for ANA is useful to recognize disease, its limitations must be appreciated. It is recommended that laboratories performing IFM ANA assays report results at both 1:40 and 1:160 dilutions and also report the percentage of healthy individuals

TABLE 1.—Operating Characteristics of Antinuclear Antibody Immunofluorescence Assays

Disease	Cutoff dilution	Sensitivity, %	Specificity, %
SLE	1:40	97.4	68.3
	1:80	97.4	87.6
	1:160	94.7	95.0
	1:320	86.8	96.7
SSc	1:40	100	68.3
	1:80	94.6	86.7
	1:160	86.5	95.0
	1:320	83.8	96.7
SS	1:40	84.2	68.3
	1:80	76.3	86.7
	1:160	73.7	95.0
	1:320	71.1	96.7
RA	1:40	48.6	68.3
	1:80	37.8	86.7
	1:160	13.5	95.0
	1:320	2.7	96.7
STR	1:40	38.5	68.3
	1:80	23.1	86.7
	1:160	7.7	95.0
	1:320	3.8	96.7

Note: Sensitivity is the percentage of patients with the disease for whom the assay result was positive at the indicated cutoff value. Specificity is the percentage of normal individuals for whom the assay result was negative at the indicated cutoff value.

Abbreviations: SLE, systemic lupus erythematosus; *SSc,* systemic sclerosis (scleroderma); *SS,* Sjögren's syndrome; *RA,* rheumatoid arthritis; *STR,* soft-tissue rheumatism.

(Courtesy of Tan EM, Feltkamp TEW, Smolen JS, et al: Range of antinuclear antibodies in "healthy" individuals. *Arthritis Rheum* 39:1833–1839, 1996.)

who are positive at these dilutions, to permit appropriate assay interpretation.

▶ In this study, almost a third (31.7%) of "healthy" individuals were ANA positive by IFM at a serum dilution of 1:40. Table 1 shows how specificity rises with positivity at higher dilutions. This, then, is another example of how the screening of inappropriate populations is likely to lead to many false positive results.

What, in fact, is the clinical and biological significance of low-titer antinuclear antibodies by IFM in individuals who appear normal, or at least without classic disease manifestations? The authors offer at least 4 possible reasons for this phenomenon: (1) low avidity cross-reaction with a tissue component that is not the true antigen; (2) a transient phenomenon such as might occur after an acute infection, now on the wane; (3) reaction with an autoantigen present in low concentration, leading to a weak fluorescent signal; and (4) antibody participating in a true autoimmune reaction, but present in low concentration. Thus, low-titer antibody on IFN is not necessarily without clinical or biological significance but can only be interpreted properly in conjunction with the clinical condition of the blood donor followed over time.

S.E. Malawista, M.D.

42 Spondyloarthropathy and Reactive Arthritis

Introduction

In this chapter, we examine the diagnosis of spondyloarthropathy vs. fibromyalgia in women (Abstract 42–1), the pathology of toe dactylitis in spondyloarthropathy (Abstract 4–2), and the symptoms of diffuse idiopathic skeletal hyperostosis (Abstract 42–3).

S.E. Malawista, M.D.

The Overdiagnosis of Fibromyalgia Syndrome
Fitzcharles M-A, Esdaile JM (McGill Univ, Montreal; Univ of British Columbia, Vancouver, Canada)
Am J Med 130:44–50, 1997   42–1

Introduction.—Fibromyalgia syndrome (FM) is characterized by musculoskeletal pain, affects mostly middle-aged women, and has no known cause or consistently successful treatment. Because the diagnosis is based upon clinical findings, there is concern that overdiagnosis may occur and other conditions may not be considered. The cases reported here suggest that other diagnoses should be ruled out in the setting of ill-defined musculoskeletal pain.

Methods.—During 1995, 321 patients were newly referred to a rheumatologist for evaluation. Final working clinical diagnoses included soft-tissue rheumatic complaints (30%), degenerative arthritis (25%), inflammatory arthropathy (19%), and other miscellaneous conditions (26%). Thirty-five of 96 patients thought to have soft tissue rheumatism were diagnosed with FM, but 11 were found to have previously unrecognized spondyloarthropathy.

Results.—The 11 patients with spondyloarthropathy, all women, had a mean age of 42 and a mean duration of symptoms of 15 years. Nine had current prominent spinal pain together with either enthesopathy, or psoriasis or ulcerative colitis. All patients had limited mobility in at least the spinal region, and most experienced prolonged morning stiffness. Despite previous evaluations by at least 1 specialist in musculoskeletal syndrome, all had received a definite or probable diagnosis of FM. Radiographic sacroiliitis was observed in 7 patients. Previous treatment, consisting of analgesics and low-dose antidepressants, brought little response. Once spondyloarthropathy had been diagnosed, however, most patients had some pain relief from therapeutic dosages of nonsteroidal anti-inflammatory drugs or sulphasalazine.

Discussion.—Although patients with FM have widespread musculo-skeletal pain, laboratory tests and bone and joint radiographs are normal. Symptoms of spondyloarthropathy may overlap considerably with those of FM, and spondyloarthropathy has been thought to be less common in women than it actually is (male to female ratio 2 to 3:1). Thus spondyloarthropathy should be considered in women with an ill-defined pain syndrome, prominent spinal pain and associated enthesopathy, or a history or family history of seronegative-associated disease.

▶ This article could equally well be called, "The Underdiagnosis of Spondyloarthropathy in Women." Most internists do not realize that radiologic sacroiliitis is no longer an absolute requirement for diagnosis, that spondyloarthropathy in women can be subtle—despite pain and subsequent functional impairment, they are more likely to have cervical spine symptoms, and less severe radiographic abnormalities—and that the estimated ratio of males to females has fallen from 10:1 to 2 or 3:1. The current diagnostic criteria of the European Spondyloarthropathy Study Group include *inflammatory spinal pain*—age of onset under 40 years, insidious onset, duration at least 3 months, association with morning stiffness, improvement with exercise—*or synovitis*—asymmetrical, predominantly in the lower limbs—*and one or more of the following*: positive family history; psoriasis; inflammatory bowel disease; urethritis, cervicitis, or acute diarrhea within 1 month before arthritis; alternate buttock pain; enthesopathy (spontaneous pain or tenderness at the site of tendon insertion, or at the Achilles tendon or plantar fascia); or sacroiliitis.

Criteria for fibromyalgia require the presence of widespread musculo-skeletal pain for at least 3 months and tenderness at at least 11 of 18 specific soft tissue points on manual palpation. As pointed out by the authors, both conditions frequently occur with a long history of ongoing, ill-defined pain, sleep disturbance, and prominent symptoms on awakening. However, in fibromyalgia the pain tends to be diffuse and muscular; in spondyloarthropathy, it tends to be spinal, intense, and localized to fairly specific sites in the neck, mid-thoracic, anterior chest wall, or lumbar regions. Similarly, the symptoms that awaken patients with spondyloarthropathy from sleep are likely to be more spinal and specific than is the case in fibromyalgia. Distinguishing between the 2 conditions is important therapeutically. In spondyloarthritis, spinal mobilization exercises and nonsteroidal antiinflammatory agents (NSAIDs) are effective; they are not generally useful in fibromyalgia.

S.E. Malawista, M.D.

Toe Dactylitis in Patients With Spondyloarthropathy: Assessment by Magnetic Resonance Imaging

Olivieri I, Barozzi L, Pierro A, et al (S Orsola-Malpighi Hosp, Bologna, Italy)
J Rheumatol 24:926–930, 1997   42–2

Introduction.—It has recently been shown with ultrasonography and magnetic resonance imaging (MRI) that finger dactylitis is caused by flexor tenosynovitis and that enlargement of the joint capsule is not necessary for producing the typical sausage-like digit. Toes were examined with MRI to determine if the same conclusions are valid for toe dactylitis.

Methods.—Twelve sausage-like toes (Fig 1) and corresponding contralateral toes of 7 consecutive patients meeting Amor criteria for seronegative spondyloarthropathy underwent MRI evaluation (Fig 2) of the metatarsophalangeal (MTP), proximal interphalangeal (PIP), and distal interphalangeal (DIP) joints. Pathologic and corresponding contralateral normal toes were examined by a rheumatologist.

Results.—Fluid collection was detected with MRI in the flexor synovial sheaths of all dactylitic toes. Compared to normal contralateral toes, the plantar bone-to-skin distance was significantly increased in dactylitic toes because of sheath distension. In normal toes, the peritendinous soft tissues were significantly thicker compared to toes with dactylitis. The extensor synovial sheaths were involved in 4 of 12 dactylitic toes. Only 2 of 36 MTP joints showed capsule distension. The MRI showed 100% sensitivity and specificity for flexor sheath involvement, but lacked sensitivity for extensor synovial sheaths. Specificity was low for joint capsule distension.

Conclusion.—Toe dactylitis may be similar to finger dactylitis in that it is caused by flexor tenosynovitis. It is possible that synovitis of MTP, PIP, and DIP joints may not be necessary for the sausage-like appearance. Physical examination is adequate for the diagnosis of toe dactylitis.

▶ Show a rheumatologist a "sausage-like" finger or toe (dactylitis; Fig 1), and he/she will immediately begin looking for other evidence of a seroneg-

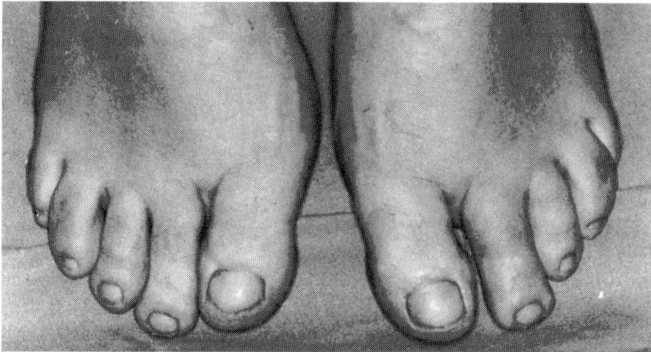

FIGURE 1.—Dactylitis of the 2nd toe of the left foot. (Courtesy of Olivieri I, Barozzi L, Pierro A: Toe dactylitis in patients with spondyloarthropathy: Assessment by magnetic resonance imaging. *J Rheumatol* 24:926–930, 1997.)

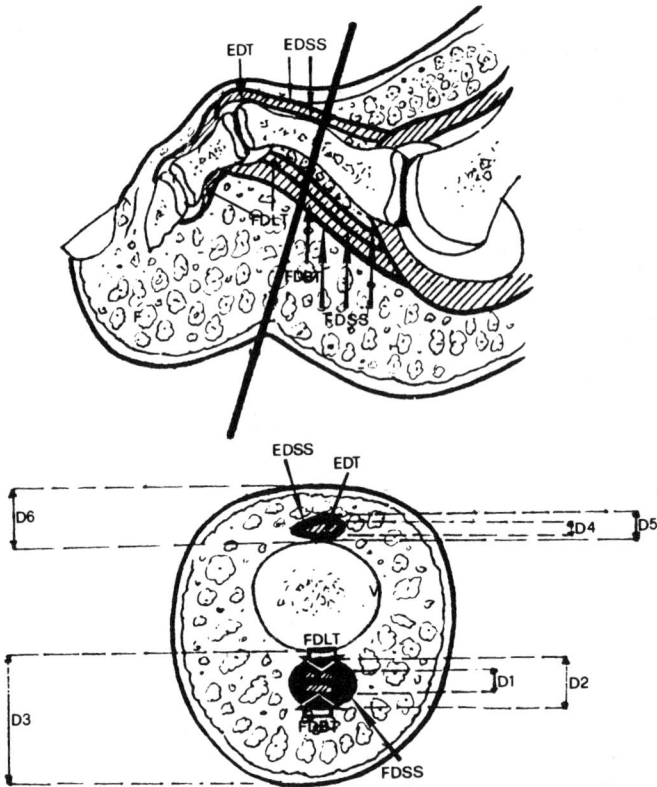

FIGURE 2.—Diagram of measurements of the flexor and extensor tendons, flexor and extensor synovial sheaths, and peritendinous soft tissues. D1 = flexor tendon diameter; D2 = flexor digitorum synovial sheath diameter; D3 = plantar bone to skin distance; D4 = extensor tendon diameter; D5 = extensor digitorum synovial sheath diameter; D6 = dorsal bone to skin distance; EDT = extensor digitorum tendon; EDSS = extensor digitorum synovial sheaths; FDBT = flexor digitorum brevis tendon; FDLT = flexor digitorum longus tendon; FDSS = flexor digitorum synovial sheaths. (Courtesy of Olivieri I, Barozzi L, Pierro A: Toe dactylitis in patients with spondyloarthropathy: Assessment by magnetic resonance imaging. *J Rheumatol* 24:926–930, 1997.)

ative spondyloarthropathy, and especially for psoriatic arthritis. Using magnetic resonance imaging (MRI) of toes, and previously of fingers,[1] the authors have shown that dactylitis is primarily a flexor tenosynovitis, as indicated by distension of tendon sheaths (Fig 2). Swelling of joint capsules, previously thought to accompany flexor tenosynovitis, is only a sometime thing; extensor tenosynovitis may also be present in the toes. This information will not change our approach to the affected digits—with MRI as the gold standard, flexor tenosynovitis can be identified on physical examination with 100% sensitivity and specificity—it is simply a matter of knowing more precisely the pathologic anatomy of what we are looking at.

S.E. Malawista, M.D.

Reference

1. Olivieri I, Barozzi L, Favaro L, et al: Dactylitis in patients with seronegative spondyloarthropathy: Assessment by ultrasonography and magnetic resonance imaging. *Arthritis Rheum* 39:1524–1528, 1996.

A Controlled Study of Diffuse Idiopathic Skeletal Hyperostosis: Clinical Features and Functional Status
Mata S, Fortin PR, Fitzcharles M-A, et al (Montreal Gen Hosp; Queen Elizabeth Hosp, Vancouver, Canada; McGill Univ, Montreal; et al)
Medicine 76:104–117, 1997   42–3

Introduction.—Diffuse idiopathic skeletal hyperostosis (DISH) is characterized by spinal and peripheral enthesopathy, a disorder at the site of insertion of a tendon, ligament, or articular capsule into the bone (enthesis; enthesitis when inflamed). The clinical and laboratory manifestations of DISH were compared with those of healthy control subjects and patients with lumbar spondylosis.

Methods.—All research subjects underwent standardized clinical evaluation, musculoskeletal examination, the Arthritis Impact Measurement Scales, Health Assessment Questionnaire, physical disability scale, an overall back disease rating scale, and laboratory testing of blood samples.

Results.—There were 56 patients with DISH, 43 patients with spondylosis, and 31 healthy research subjects. Patients with DISH were more likely to give a history of upper extremity pain, medial epicondylitis of the elbow, enthesitis of the patella or heel, or dysphagia, compared to patients with spondylosis. Compared to healthy control subjects, patients with DISH had more extremity and spinal stiffness and pain. They also weighed more while young, had a greater body mass index, and greater reduction in neck rotation and thoracic movements, compared to research subjects in both control groups. Patients with DISH and control subjects with spondylosis had similar levels of spinal disability and physical disability. There were no significant between-group differences in laboratory testing.

Conclusion.—Diffuse idiopathic skeletal hyperostosis may be considered a distinct disorder with signs and symptoms that separate it from other spinal problems. Patients with DISH may experience major disability.

▶ I have pointed out that DISH (diffuse idiopathic skeletal hyperostosis; ankylosing hyperostosis; Forestier/Rotes-Querol disease) is not uncommon in the elderly, and may be picked up on a routine 2-way chest radiograph.[1] The radiologic picture is one of flowing calcification and ossification along the anterolateral aspect of at least 4 contiguous vertebral bodies, with relative preservation of disc height. When the subject is asymptomatic, no further action is required.

Patients in the current study were not discovered randomly; they came from a major hospital outpatient department and from two private rheumatology practices. In an exhaustive analysis of 56 patients with DISH, the authors concluded that this is a distinct disorder with clinical findings that may result in important disability. It is not extraordinary that symptoms occur; this is after all a noninflammatory condition characterized by the ossification of paravertebral ligaments and peripheral entheses (entheses are the sites of insertion of tendon, ligament, or articular capsule into bone). And indeed, as noted in the abstract, these patients had a constellation of symptoms that differed from those both of individuals with spondylosis of the lumbar spine and of healthy control subjects.

S.E. Malawista, M.D.

Reference

1. 1995 YEAR BOOK OF MEDICINE, p 797.

43 Sclerosing Syndromes

Introduction

Here we consider the significance of palpable tendon friction rubs in systemic sclerosis (Abstract 43–1).

S.E. Malawista, M.D.

The Palpable Tendon Friction Rub: An Important Physical Examination Finding in Patients With Systemic Sclerosis
Steen VD, Medsger TA Jr (Georgetown Univ, Washington, DC; Univ of Pittsburgh, Pa)
Arthritis Rheum 40:1146–1151, 1997   43–1

Objective.—Systemic sclerosis (SSc: scleroderma) includes limited cutaneous SSc (lcSSc) and diffuse cutaneous SSc (dcSSc). Distinguishing these 2 variants early is important because of the increased morbidity of dcSSc. The frequency and significance of palpable tendon friction rubs have been used to differentiate between the 2 variants in clinical examinations.

Methods.—Between January 1, 1972, and December 31, 1991, 1,305 patients with SSc were evaluated at the University of Pittsburgh and classified as having lcSSC or dcSSc according to standard methods. As part of the examination, the examiner places his or her fingers across the tendon area and has the patient move the underlying joint (Fig 1). If friction rub is present, a squeaking sensation will be noted. Visceral involvement and serologic results were noted at each visit. All data were entered into a database and used to determine the prognostic significance of tendon friction rubs. Patients were studied for an average of 6.3 years.

Results.—Tendon friction rubs were found in 368 (28%) patients on the first visit and in an additional 105 (8%) patients in subsequent visits. Whether categorized as SSC or by individual variant, patients with tendon friction rubs had a significantly shorter disease duration, and a significantly shorter 5-year cumulative survival from the first symptom. Patients with SSc as a class with tendon friction rubs had a significantly higher percentage of diffuse scleroderma. Patients with SSc and dcSSc with tendon friction rubs had significantly more cardiac and renal involvement. Patients with SSc and lcSSc had a significantly higher percentage of antitopoisomerase I antibody. Multiple regression analysis was used to deter-

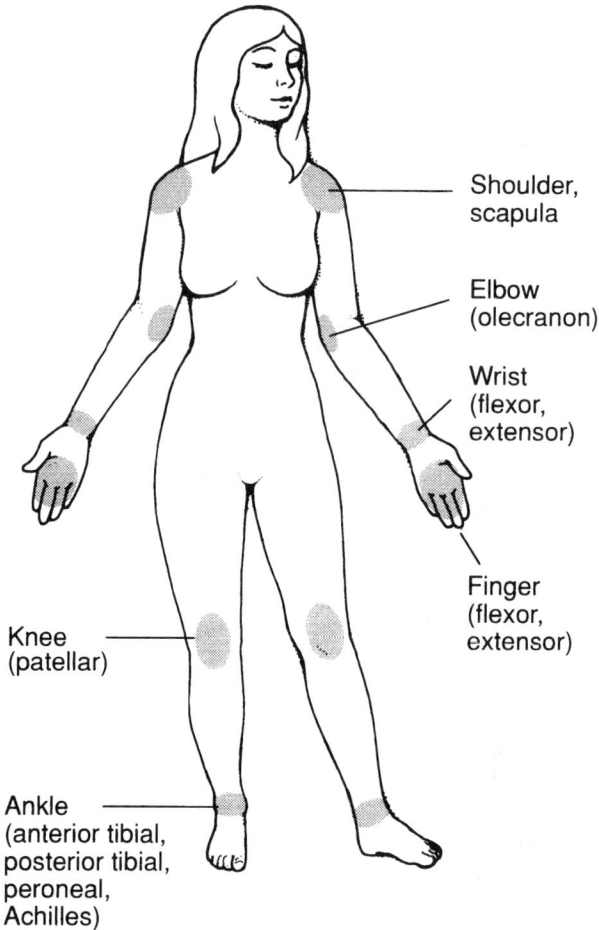

FIGURE 1.—Sites where tendon friction rubs can most commonly be palpated. (Courtesy of Stenn VD, Medsger TA Jr: The palpable tendon friction rub: An important physical examination finding in patients with systemic sclerosis. *Arthritis Rheum* 40:1146–1151, copyright 1997, American College of Rheumatology).

mine the best predictors of progression to dcSSc with truncal skin thickening. Multiple regression analysis was also used to determine factors predictive of death in dcSSc.

Conclusion.—The tendon friction rub distinguished dcSSc from lcSSc. It is simple, easily performed, inexpensive, and identifies patients at risk of severe disease. The test should be routinely included in rheumatologic examinations.

▶ Palpable tendon friction rubs in SSc were first described by Westphal in 1876. Although noted since then and frequently mentioned in textbooks, their frequency and diagnostic and prognostic significance in SSc has not previously been reported.

In the current study of 1,305 new patients with SSc with diffuse or limited scleroderma seen between 1972 and 1991, 368 (28%) had tendon friction rubs on the initial visit, and an additional 105 (8%) on a subsequent visit. The most common sites for palpable tendon friction rubs are shown in Figure 1, especially the flexor and extensor tendons of fingers and wrists and the anterior tibial and peroneal tendons. The rubs are known to be associated with thickening and fibrinous deposits on the surface of the affected tendon sheaths, with relatively little inflammatory reaction. Patients were often aware of these rubs on joint motion; they were sometimes painful. Rubs are best elicited during active maximal range of motion of the underlying joint by the patient, with the palmer aspect of the examiner's fingers over the tendon area of interest; the rub consists of a leathery, rubbing, "squeaking" sensation. The mean maximum number of tendon friction rubs at any single examination was 5; only 14% of the patients had a maximum of just 1 rub. These were early findings—60% of the patients with rubs had symptoms for less than 2 years, and of 175 patients re-examined more than 5 years later, only 20% still had them.

Tendon rubs had a positive predictive value for the diagnosis of diffuse scleroderma of 93% and a negative predictive value of 97%. As expected in diffuse SSc, these early findings were strongly correlated with other symptoms and signs of diffuse disease—more severe skin thickening, more frequent heart and kidney involvement, and decreased survival. Thus, palpable tendon friction rubs are simple and important signs.

S.E. Malawista, M.D.

44 Crystal-associated Arthritis

Introduction

In this chapter, we consider intradermal urate tophi (Abstract 44–1) and the use of intramuscular triamcinolone acetonide in pseudogout (Abstract 44–2).

Noted in passing: As uncovered in three patients with anorexia nervosa, the rare finding of premenopausal tophaceous gout (especially in the absence of obesity, renal insufficiency, and hypertension) should raise the question of longtime covert diuretic abuse.[1]

S.E. Malawista, M.D.

Reference

1. Hayem G, Delahousse M, Meyer O, Palazzo E, Chazerain P, Kahn M-F: Female premenopausal tophaceous gout induced by long-term diuretic abuse. *J. Rheumatol* 23:2166–2167, 1996.

Intradermal Urate Tophi
Fam AG, Assaad D (Univ of Toronto)
J Rheumatol 24:1126–1131, 1997
44–1

Introduction.—Intradermal urate tophi are rare cutaneous manifestations of chronic gout. Six cases were reviewed to examine the clinical features of intradermal urate tophi and identify risk factors associated with its development.

Methods.—The 6 patients, 5 men and 1 woman with a mean age of 59.8, were studied over a 10-year period (1987 to 1996). Data obtained include the duration and pattern of gouty attacks, the presence of risk factors for gout and intradermal tophi, treatment with antigout drugs, and concomitant medications. Tophi were sought in the olecranon, prepatellar or bunion bursae, Achilles tendon, ear pinnae, toes, and fingers. Aspirates were examined by compensated polarized light microscopy for the presence of monosodium urate (MSU) crystals, a sign of gouty tophi. Laboratory studies were also performed, and 1 patient with hyperpigmentation underwent purine enzyme studies and had biopsies examined by ordinary and polarizing light microscopies.

Results.—The mean duration of gout in the patients was 10 years. Attacks were frequent in 2 cases (up to 12 per year) and less frequent in 4 (up to 3 per year). Intradermal urate crystal deposits appeared as small, superficial, pustule-like lesions located on the thighs and legs of 1 patient,

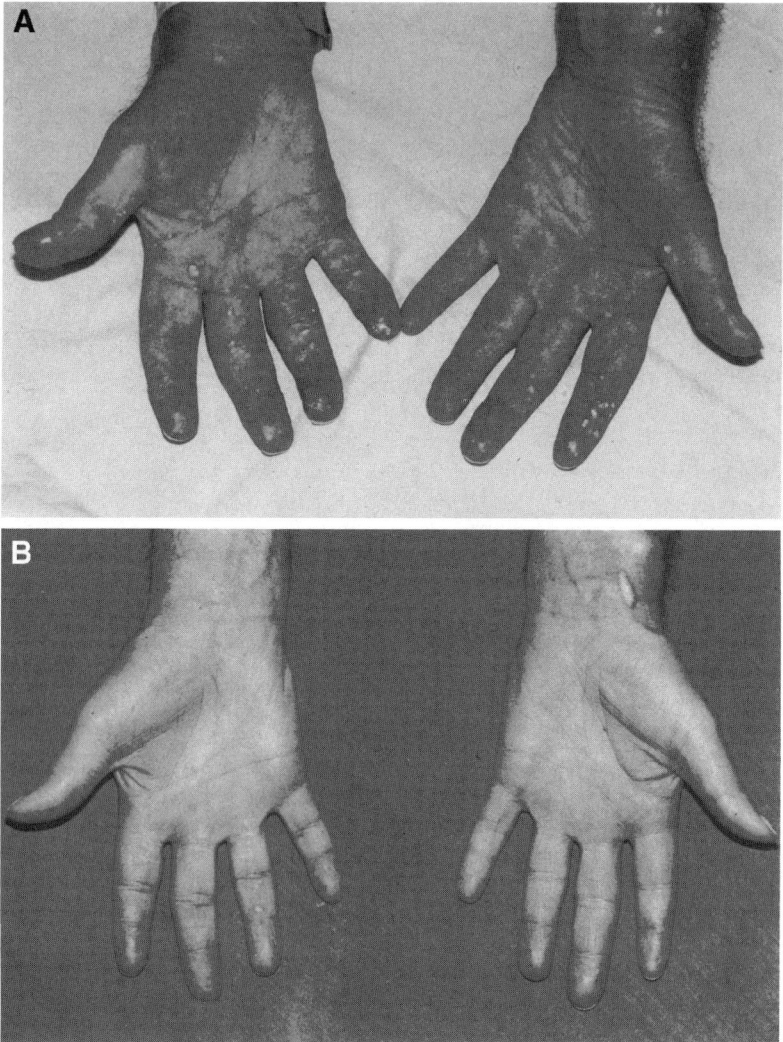

FIGURE 3.—A. Right hand in 1990, showing multiple, superficial, small, white intradermal, tophaceous lesions on the fingers (Patient 2). B. Follow-up photograph (1994) showing resolution of intradermal tophi (Patient 2). (Courtesy of Fam AG, Assaad D: Intradermal urate tophi. *J Rheumatol* 24:1126–1131, 1997.)

the fingertips and thumbtips of 4 (Fig 3), and on the second left toetip of 1. Lesions in 1 patient were associated with an unusual skin hyperpigmentation. Superimposed inflammatory episodes occurred in all patients and were accompanied by increasing pain, swelling, and erythema of the intradermal tophi. All intradermal tophi exhibited negatively birefringent, needle-shaped, MSU crystals. The mean pretreatment serum urate was 570.6 μmol/L. Among the risk factors for gout and intradermal tophi present in patients were renal failure (all 6) and hypertension and chronic diuretic therapy (4 of 6). Other risk factors identified were alcohol abuse, myeloma, a positive family history, and chronic low-dose acetylsalicylic acid.

Conclusion.—Intradermal urate tophi are far less common than subcutaneous tophi in patients with gout. The intradermal tophi may ulcerate and become inflamed, and patchy skin pigmentation is also possible. Risk factors were renal insufficiency, hypertension, and chronic diuretic use.

▶ Intradermal tophi that may drain urate sludge or become intermittently inflamed are rare but dramatic. As one would expect, they tend to be associated with situations in which the serum urate concentrations are chronically elevated—renal insufficiency, hypertension, and chronic diuretic use. These lesions are treatable with appropriate measures to counter hyperuricemia (Fig 3). The patient whose hands are depicted was a 34-year-old renal transplant recipient undergoing long-term hemodialysis, who had had gout for 3 years when first seen. He responded to 150 mg daily of allopurinol after first having had to be desensitized to it.[1]

S.E. Malawista, M.D.

Reference

1. 1993 YEAR BOOK OF MEDICINE, p 714.

Prospective Use of Intramuscular Triamcinolone Acetonide in Pseudogout
Roane DW, Harris MD, Carpenter MT, et al (David Grant Med Ctr, Travis Air Force Base, Calif; Wilford Hall Med Ctr, Lackland Air Force Base, Tex)
J Rheumatol 24:1168–1170, 1997   44–2

Introduction.—Although nonsteroidal antiinflammatory drugs (NSAIDs) are standard therapy for pseudogout, many patients with the disease are elderly and have contraindications to NSAIDs. A group of older patients with pseudogout was treated with intramuscular (IM) triamcinolone acetonide in order to assess the safety and efficacy of this agent as an alternative to NSAIDs.

Methods.—Eligible patients had documented pseudogout and were seen at the rheumatology service within 5 days of symptom onset. Fourteen patients were enrolled, 10 women and 4 men with a mean age of 73 years. They were treated with 60 mg triamcinolone acetonide suspension IM and evaluated at day 1–2 postinjection, day 3–4, day 10–14, and day 30. Those whose initial response was inadequate were eligible for a second injection on day 1–2. Response was evaluated by patient and physician global assessment through use of a visual analog scale and by assessment of joints for warmth, erythema, nonpainful range of motion, and circumference.

Results.—Twelve of the 14 patients had contraindications to NSAIDs. The most commonly affected joints were the knee, ankle, and wrist. Ten patients had a monoarticular attack and 4 had from 2 to 6 involved joints. All patients responded well to triamcinolone, with >50% improvement in the global assessment. Six patients received a second injection on day 1–2. There were no instances of medication toxicity, and no patient experienced a rebound attack during the follow-up period.

Conclusion.—Agents currently used to treat pseudogout include NSAIDs, especially indomethacin, intra-articular glucocorticoids, and oral colchicine, but these agents may have side effects or are impractical to administer for polyarticular attacks. These elderly patients responded well to IM triamcinolone acetate, which may prove to be a safe and effective alternative to NSAIDs and intra-articular corticosteroids.

▶ When nonsteroidal antiinflammatory drugs (NSAIDs) are contraindicated, as they often are in the elderly population at risk for pseudogout, the most favored treatments are intraarticular corticosteroids and intravenous colchicine. However, the former may be impractical when attacks are polyarticular, and the latter is limited by unfamiliarity with its usage to many physicians. In this open prospective study, the current authors offer 1 or 2 intramuscular doses of 60 mg of a suspension of triamcinolone acetonide as an effective and reasonable safe alternative. They do note that single intramuscular injections of this drug can impair the hypothalamic-pituitary-adrenal (HPA) axis for at least 3 to 4 weeks. An effective and gentler treatment, especially for elderly patients with multiple medical problems, is ACTH.[1]

S.E. Malawista, M.D.

Reference

1. 1995 Year Book of Medicine, p 809.

45 Vasculitis

Introduction

Here we review color duplex ultrasonography in the diagnosis of temporal arteritis (Abstract 45–1), the use of azathioprine in Behçet's syndrome (Abstract 45–2), and aspects of relapsing polychondritis (Abstract 45–3). Noted in passing: A review of small-vessel vasculitis.[1]

Stephen E. Malawista, M.D.

Reference

1. Jennette JC, Falk RJ: Small-vessel vasculitis. *N Engl J Med* 337:1512–1523, 1997.

Color Duplex Ultrasonography in the Diagnosis of Temporal Arteritis
Schmidt WA, Kraft HE, Vorpahl K, et al (Clinic of Rheumatology, Berlin; Klinikum Buch, Berlin)
N Engl J Med 337:1336–1342, 1997   45–1

Introduction.—A temporal-artery biopsy is usually recommended to confirm the clinical diagnosis of temporal arteritis, but the procedure may lead to complications, and false-negative findings can occur if the biopsy is taken from an area without lesions. A prospective study of patients with clinically suspected active temporal arteritis or polymyalgia rheumatica assessed the value of color duplex ultrasonography (US) in diagnosing temporal arteritis.

Methods.—Thirty patients met at least 3 of the 5 criteria for temporal arteritis. Biopsy was performed in 27 patients and yielded positive findings in 21, negative findings in 4, and insufficient material for analysis in 2. Symptoms of both temporal arteritis and polymyalgia rheumatica were present in 16; 2 had symptoms of temporal arteritis alone and 2 of polymyalgia rheumatica alone. Thirty-seven patients met 3 or more criteria for polymyalgia rheumatica, and 15 patients with negative histologic findings received a diagnosis other than temporal arteritis or polymyalgia rheumatica. Controls were 30 patients with rheumatoid arthritis but no signs of temporal arteritis. Two color duplex US studies performed in each case were read before the biopsies.

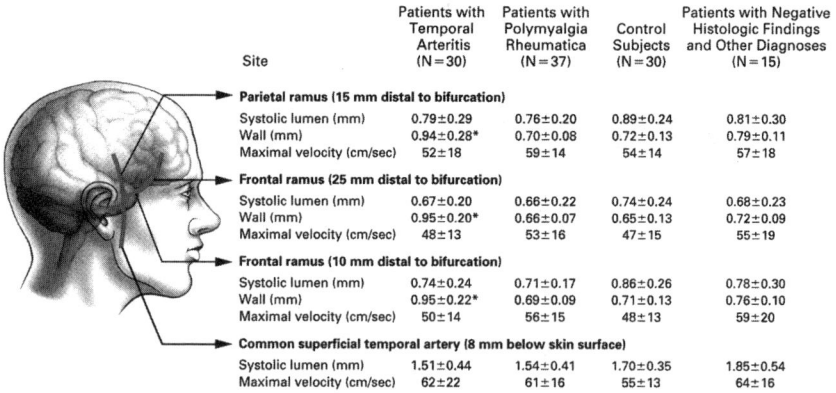

Site	Patients with Temporal Arteritis (N = 30)	Patients with Polymyalgia Rheumatica (N = 37)	Control Subjects (N = 30)	Patients with Negative Histologic Findings and Other Diagnoses (N = 15)
Parietal ramus (15 mm distal to bifurcation)				
Systolic lumen (mm)	0.79±0.29	0.76±0.20	0.89±0.24	0.81±0.30
Wall (mm)	0.94±0.28*	0.70±0.08	0.72±0.13	0.79±0.11
Maximal velocity (cm/sec)	52±18	59±14	54±14	57±18
Frontal ramus (25 mm distal to bifurcation)				
Systolic lumen (mm)	0.67±0.20	0.66±0.22	0.74±0.24	0.68±0.23
Wall (mm)	0.95±0.20*	0.66±0.07	0.65±0.13	0.72±0.09
Maximal velocity (cm/sec)	48±13	53±16	47±15	55±19
Frontal ramus (10 mm distal to bifurcation)				
Systolic lumen (mm)	0.74±0.24	0.71±0.17	0.86±0.26	0.78±0.30
Wall (mm)	0.95±0.22*	0.69±0.09	0.71±0.13	0.76±0.10
Maximal velocity (cm/sec)	50±14	56±15	48±13	59±20
Common superficial temporal artery (8 mm below skin surface)				
Systolic lumen (mm)	1.51±0.40	1.54±0.41	1.70±0.35	1.85±0.54
Maximal velocity (cm/sec)	62±22	61±16	55±13	64±16

FIGURE 1.—Measurement of the superficial temporal arteries. Plus-minus values are means ±SD of the right and left sides. The arterial wall was defined to include the intima, media, adventitia, and temporal fascia. Asterisks indicate a significant difference ($p < 0.01$ by the Mann-Whitney U test) between the patients with temporal arteritis and the other three groups. (Reprinted by permission of The New England Journal of Medicine from Schmidt WA, Kraft HE, Vorpahl K, et al: Color duplex ultrasonography in the diagnosis of temporal arteritis. *N Engl J Med* 337:1336–1342, copyright 1997, Massachusetts Medical Society.)

Results.—In patients with temporal arteritis the diameter of the artery wall was significantly larger than in the other groups (Fig 1). The US studies of 22 (73%) patients with temporal arteritis showed a dark halo around the lumen of the temporal arteries, and the halos disappeared after corticosteroid treatment (mean 16 days). Stenoses or occlusions of temporal-artery segments were present in 80% of patients; 93% had stenoses, occlusions, or a halo. None of the US studies of patients without temporal arteritis showed a halo, but stenoses or occlusions were observed in 7%. The interrater agreement was ≥95% for each of the 3 types of abnormalities identified at US.

TABLE 2.—Sensitivity and Specificity of Duplex Ultrasonography of the Temporal Arteries for the Diagnosis of Temporal Arteritis and to Confirm Histologic Findings

FINDING	DIAGNOSIS*		CONFIRMATION OF HISTOLOGIC FINDINGS†	
	SENSITIVITY positive tests/total (%)	SPECIFICITY negative tests/total (%)	SENSITIVITY positive tests/total (%)	SPECIFICITY negative tests/total (%)
Halo	22/30 (73)	82/82 (100)	16/21 (76)	24/26 (92)
Stenosis or occlusion	24/30 (80)	76/82 (93)	18/21 (86)	23/26 (88)
Halo, stenosis, or occlusion	28/30 (93)	76/82 (93)	20/21 (95)	22/26 (85)

*Thirty patients had temporal arteritis, and 82 patients had been given other diagnoses.
†Twenty-one patients had positive histologic findings, and 26 patients had negative histologic findings (4 in the temporal-arteritis group, 7 in the group with polymyalgia rheumatica, and 15 with other diagnoses).
(Reprinted by permission of The New England Journal of Medicine from Schmidt WA, Kraft HE, Vorpahl K, et al: Color duplex ultrasonography in the diagnosis of temporal arteritis. *N Engl J Med* 337:1336–1342, Copyright 1997, Massachusetts Medical Society.)

Conclusion.—Color duplex US visualizes characteristic signs of temporal arteritis with a sensitivity and specificity (Table 2) that may provide a diagnosis without the need for temporal-artery biopsy. A dark halo is the most specific sign; patients with strong clinical evidence of temporal arteritis but no clear halo should still undergo biopsy.

▶ Color duplex ultrasonography combines the imaging capabilities of B-mode US with the flow-velocity determinations of Doppler US, permitting assessment of both the arterial anatomy and the flow characteristics of a vessel at specific sites. Examples of measurements of the superficial temporal arteries are seen in Fig 1. In patients with temporal arteritis, the authors find helpful the presence of a hyperechoic halo on US (Table 2), which they believe represents edema because such halos appear intimal, while major cellular infiltrates, seen on histologic analysis, are generally deeper.

As for when US might replace temporal artery biopsy, the authors are appropriately modest in their recommendations: they would require typical clinical signs of temporal arteritis and a clearly demonstrable halo, unless there is reason to suspect another form of vasculitis. However, because new procedures tend to drive out optimal clinical assessment, the textured view of an accompanying editorial[1] is especially welcome. The editorialists wonder how much better US is than a careful physical examination—i.e., that it needs to be formally compared with an evaluation for redness, tenderness, and thickening. They point out that US may not be helpful in the patients who present the most difficult diagnostic challenge—those with systemic illness but no definite signs on physical examination, whose arteries may not yet have detectable physical alterations. And because the results of temporal artery biopsy alone predict the likelihood of giant cell arteritis in over 90% of cases, any new test has a high standard to meet. Finally, while recognizing the diagnostic potential of temporal artery color duplex US, they believe the ultimate goal to be the development of a sensitive indicator that will identify inflammation anywhere in the vascular tree, and suggest that serum or cellular markers that indicate inflammation within blood vessels are more likely to fulfill this requirement.

S.E. Malawista, M.D.

Reference

1. Hunder GG, Weyand CM: Sonography in temporal arteritis. *N Engl J Med* 337:1385–1386, 1997 (editorial).

Azathioprine in Behçet's Syndrome: Effects on Long-term Prognosis
Hamuryudan V, Özyazgan Y, Hizli N, et al (Univ of Istanbul, Turkey)
Arthritis Rheum 40:769–774, 1997   45–2

Background.—Behçet's syndrome is a multisystem vasculitis with associated ocular involvement, arterial lesions, and neurologic disease. Most serious in male and young affected persons, it can result in disability and

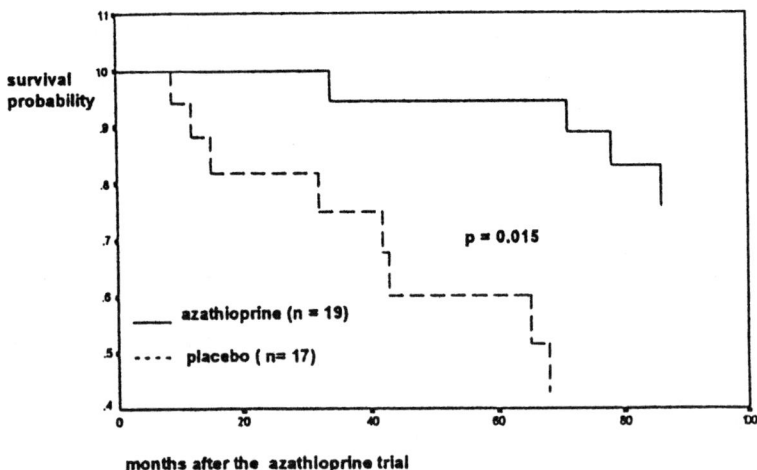

FIGURE 1.—Probability of emergence of a 2-line drop in visual acuity of the right eye, regardless of the duration of eye involvement before entry into the azathioprine trial. (Courtesy of Hamuryudan V, Özyazgan Y, Hizli N, et al: Azathioprine in Behçet's syndrome: Effects on long-term prognosis. *Arthritis Rheum* 40:769–774, copyright 1997, American College of Rheumatology.)

death. The effectiveness of immunosuppressive drugs in Behçet's syndrome has been demonstrated in controlled trials. Before the use of these drugs, blindness occurred after onset of uveitis in 3 to 4 years. Azathioprine at 2.5 mg/kg/day has been shown to be superior to placebo in maintaining visual acuity and preventing new eye disease in Behçet's syndrome. There are few data on the effect of azathioprine on the long-term prognosis of Behçet's syndrome.

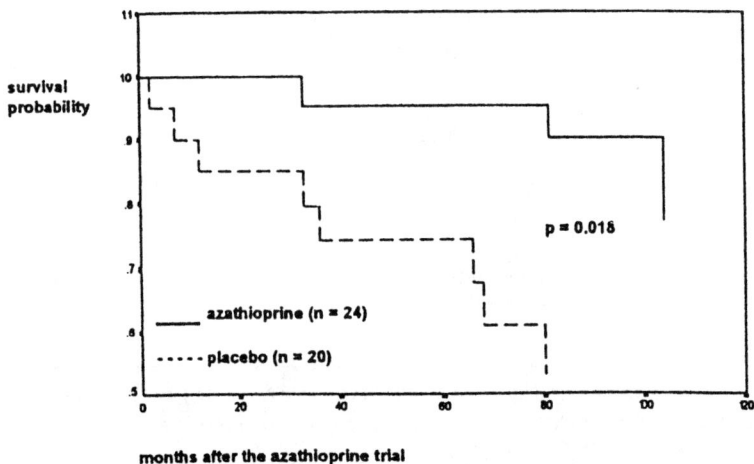

FIGURE 5.—Probability of emergence of blindness, regardless of the duration of eye involvement before entry into the azathioprine trial. (Courtesy of Hamuryudan V, Özyazgan Y, Hizli N, et al: Azathioprine in Behçet's syndrome: Effects on long-term prognosis. *Arthritis Rheum* 40:769–774, copyright 1997, American College of Rheumatology.)

TABLE 2.—Distribution of Severe Extraocular Involvement During the
Follow-up Period

Group	Complication (n)
Group 1 placebo	Pulmonary artery aneurysm (1), vena cava superior syndrome (1)
Group 1 AZA	None
Group 2 placebo	Pulmonary arterial aneurysm (1), carotid artery aneurysm and secondary amyloidosis (1), neurologic involvement (5)
Group 2 AZA	Neurologic involvement (2)

Note: Group 1 patients had no eye involvement at entry into the original trial; group 2 patients had eye involvement at entry into the original trial.
Abbreviation: AZA, Azathioprine.
(Courtesy of Hamuryudan V, Özyazgan Y, Hizli N, et al: Azathioprine in Behçet's syndrome: Effects on long-term prognosis. *Arthritis Rheum* 40:769–774, copyright 1997, American College of Rheumatology.)

Methods.—The effect of azathioprine on the long-term prognosis of Behçet's syndrome was studied in 73 male patients from a previous randomized, double-blind, placebo-controlled trial of azathioprine a mean of 94 months before.

Results.—The emergence of blindness and a 2-line drop in visual acuity of the right eye occurred significantly more often in patients originally given placebo than in patients originally given azathioprine, despite treatment given when needed in both groups during follow-up (Fig 1) (Fig 5). There were more extraocular complications in patients given placebo (Table 2). The benefits of azathioprine were especially noted in patients with eye involvement of short duration before the study.

Discussion.—Patients with Behçet's syndrome given early treatment with azathioprine had a more positive long-term prognosis than did patients given placebo. Better outcomes were associated with earlier treatment during the course of eye involvement.

▶ The original syndrome described in 1937 by Hulusi Behçet, a Turkish dermatologist, included oral and genital aphthous ulcerations and hypopyon iritis. It is now recognized as a multisystem vasculitis that can include recurrent synovitis, erythema nodosum-like lesions, and neurologic disease. Many drugs have been used empirically for this disorder.[1-3] The current study is a long-term (mean, almost 8 years) follow-up of patients from a 2-year randomized, double-blind, placebo-controlled trial of azathioprine at 2.5 mg/kg/day, with or without corticosteroids, in which the drug was effective in controlling disease progression, especially that of eye disease.

In the current study, the treated patients did better from the standpoints of both visual acuity (Fig 1) and blindness (Fig 5). Moreover, patients treated before eye involvement was evident tended to have less subsequent extraocular involvement than those treated after (Table 2), making the authors wonder whether preemptive immunosuppressive therapy may be indicated in individuals at high risk for severe disease (male and young). A difficult question.

S.E. Malawista, M.D.

References

1. 1985 YEAR BOOK OF MEDICINE, p 782.
2. 1986 YEAR BOOK OF MEDICINE, p 708.
3. 1991 YEAR BOOK OF MEDICINE, p 708.

Relapsing Polychondritis: Clinical and Immunogenetic Analysis of 62 Patients

Zeuner M, Straub RH, Rauh G, et al (Univ of Regensburg, Germany; Ludwig-Maximilian Univ, Munich)
J Rheumatol 24:96–101, 1997
45–3

Background.—Relapsing polychondritis is an extremely rare inflammatory disorder, believed to be of autoimmune origin, that affects cartilaginous structures throughout the body. Relapsing polychondritis generally occurs between the ages of 40 and 60 in men and women. In about 30% of cases, relapsing polychondritis is associated with other rheumatic or autoimmune diseases. Clinical manifestations have been described in about 300 patients. Most earlier studies summarize case reports, but these studies should be interpreted carefully, because many case reports describe only severe or extraordinary cases. This is the first analysis of patients currently under clinical observation. Diagnosis of relapsing polychondritis is based on clinical findings, with patients often having elevated sedimentation rate and mild anemia. There may be an association with HLA-DR4.

Methods.—Participants were recruited from 15 rheumatic disease units in university hospitals and other tertiary referral centers in Germany, Switzerland, and The Netherlands. Data from 26 female and 36 male patients were analyzed. The median patient age at diagnosis was 46.6 years. HLA-DR specificities were identified in 60 patients, and these frequencies were compared to those in healthy control subjects.

Results.—Of all patients, 58 had auricular chondritis, 31 had ocular symptoms, and 35 had nasal involvement (Table 1). Patients also had involvement of joints, respiratory system, skin, cardiovascular system, CNS, and kidneys. There were 22 patients with associated diseases, such as systemic lupus erythematosus or rheumatoid arthritis. There was a significant association between susceptibility to relapsing polychondritis and HLA-DR4. No difference in frequency or distribution of DRB1*04 subtype alleles was seen between patients and control subjects. There was a negative association between extent of organ involvement and HLA-DR6.

Discussion.—In these patients, the immunogenetic findings and overlapping clinical symptoms with other autoimmune or rheumatic diseases indicate that immunologic mechanisms may be involved in the pathogenesis of relapsing polychondritis. Auricular chondritis was seen more often than in previous studies, but saddle-nose deformity, arthritis, and microhematuria were seen less often.

TABLE 1.—Clinical Manifestations in 62 Patients With Relapsing Polychondritis

Clinical Manifestations	Manifestations at Presentation, n (%)	Cumulative Manifestations, n (%)
Auricular chondritis	34 (54.8)	58 (93.5)
Hearing loss	7 (11.3)	12 (19.4)
Vertigo	6 (9.7)	14 (22.6)
Nasal chondritis	18 (29.0)	35 (56.5)
Laryngotracheal involvement	8 (12.9)	19 (30.6)
Ocular symptoms	20 (32.3)	31 (50.0)
Arthritis	12 (19.4)	33 (53.2)
Skin manifestations	6 (9.7)	15 (24.2)
Cardiovascular involvement	1 (1.6)	14 (22.6)
Renal involvement	1 (1.6)	4 (6.5)
Central nervous system involvement	0	6 (9.7)

(Courtesy of Zeuner M, Straub RH, Rauh G, et al: Relapsing polychondritis: Clinical and immunogenetic analysis of 62 patients. *J Rheumatol* 24:96–101, 1997.)

▶ Relapsing polychrondritis is a rare systemic inflammatory disease affecting cartilage. I include it here as a reminder, because the diagnosis is clinical and the disorder may be superimposed on other rheumatic diseases, such as systemic lupus erythematosus or rheumatoid arthritis, as it was in 36% of the cases reported here. Entry into this study required proven inflammatory episodes involving at least 2 or 3 sites (auricular, nasal, laryngotracheal cartilage) or 1 of these sites together with 2 other manifestations, such as ocular inflammation, hearing loss, vestibular dysfunction, or seronegative inflammatory arthritis.

These were unselected patients recruited during 5 years from 15 rheumatic disease units in university hospitals and other tertiary referral centers in Germany, Switzerland, and The Netherlands; their clinical manifestations are shown in Table 1. Note the frequency of auricular chondritis, typically seen as red and tender but sparing the (noncartilaginous) ear lobes. In contrast, saddle-nose deformity, arthritis, and microhematuria, which bear poor prognoses, were much less common, as were life-threatening cardiovascular or respiratory problems. Perhaps this is because these patients are being studied currently, rather than retrospectively, when they might have had more time to express the grimmer textbook manifestations of this illness.

S.E. Malawista, M.D.

46 Infectious Arthritis

Introduction

This chapter addresses the diagnosis and monitoring of Whipple's disease by means of polymerase chain reaction (Abstract 46–1); the persistence of parvovirus B19 DNA in synovial membranes of young patients with or without chronic arthropathy (Abstract 46–2); the duration of tick attachment as a predictor of the risk of Lyme disease in endemic areas (Abstract 46–3); ceftriaxone versus doxycycline in the treatment of acute disseminated Lyme disease (Abstract 46–4); and simultaneous human granulocytic ehrlichiosis and Lyme borreliosis (Abstract 46–5).

Noted in passing: Two position papers of the American College of Physicians addressing laboratory evaluation in the diagnosis of Lyme disease,[1, 2] and the demonstration of culture-confirmed infection and reinfection with *Borrelia burgdorferi*.[3]

Stephen E. Malawista, M.D.

References

1. American College of Physicians: Guidelines for laboratory evaluation in the diagnosis of Lyme disease. *Ann Intern Med* 127:1106–1108, 1997.
2. Tugwell P, Dennis DT, Weinstein A, et al: Laboratory evaluation in the diagnosis of Lyme disease. *Ann Int Med* 127:1109–1123, 1997.
3. Nowakowski J, Schwartz I, Nadelman RB, et al: Culture-confirmed infection and reinfection with *Borrelia burgdorferi*. *Ann Intern Med* 127:130–132, 1997.

Diagnosis and Monitoring of Whipple Disease by Polymerase Chain Reaction

Ramzan NN, Loftus E Jr, Burgart LJ, et al (Mayo Clinic and Mayo Graduate School of Medicine, Rochester, Minn; State Univ of New York, Syracuse; Standard Univ, Calif; et al)
Ann Intern Med 126:520–527, 1997
46–1

Background.—Whipple's disease is a systemic bacterial infection with associated diarrhea, abdominal pain, fever, lymphadenopathy, chronic arthralgia, weight loss, and occasional central nervous system involvement that can include dementia, lethargy, and motor and sensory deficits. Diagnosis can be made by recognition of bacillary organisms in a small-bowel biopsy specimen that are positive on periodic-acid-Schiff testing and negative on acid-fast testing. Whipple's disease can go undiagnosed in patients who never develop gastrointestinal symptoms, or it can be misdiagnosed as rheumatoid arthritis or sarcoidosis. Although antibiotic treatment has been used, about a third of patients have recurrent disease. There is no current test for cure.

Methods.—A retrospective laboratory-based evaluation was made of stored tissue specimens from 30 patients with Whipple's disease that was clinically diagnosed and histologically confirmed, and from 8 patients with suspected Whipple's disease, but without definitive histological evidence of disease. Pretreatment and posttreatment small bowel and lymph node biopsy specimens were tested by polymerase chain reaction for *Tropheryma whippelii* DNA.

Results.—In 29 of the 30 patients with histologically confirmed disease, and in 7 of the 8 patients with suspected disease, results of polymerase chain reaction were positive. Posttreatment small-bowel biopsy specimens were obtained from 17 patients; the results of polymerase chain reaction were positive in 12 cases. When the results of these 12 patients were correlated with therapeutic outcome, it was noted that 7 of the 12 patients had relapse during follow-up or did not respond to treatment. None of the 5 patients with negative polymerase chain reaction results of posttreatment biopsy specimens had relapse. There was no correlation between posttreatment histology and clinical outcome.

Discussion.—Polymerase chain reaction is highly sensitive and specific in the diagnosis of Whipple's disease, identification of inconclusive cases, and monitoring of treatment response. Negative results of polymerase chain reaction may indicate a low risk of relapse. Positive results of polymerase chain reaction that remain positive during treatment may predict a poor outcome. Histopathologic evaluation of posttreatment specimens does not predict relapse or cure.

▶ Although most patients with Whipple's disease have weight loss, diarrhea, and abdominal pain, gastrointestinal symptoms may be preceded by a host of other complaints including pleuritis, lymphadenopathy, cardiac valvular lesions, fever, wasting, central nervous system or eye problems, and, of special interest to the rheumatologist, longstanding arthritis. Classical diagnosis depends on the recognition in a small-bowel biopsy specimen of periodic-acid-Schiff positive, acid-fast negative, bacillary organisms. In the current study, the authors found polymerase chain reaction (PCR) amplification of specific DNA sequences of *Tropheryma whippelii* in 29 of 30 stored tissue specimens from patients with histologically confirmed disease and in 7 of 8 from those with suspected disease (and from no blinded controls—very important when PCR is being used). The tissues were formalin-fixed and paraffin-embedded, and yet contained enough of the targeted DNA sequences for successful amplification.

Like Lyme disease, Whipple's disease is a disorder in which there are no clear points to indicate when all the organisms are dead, making the evaluation of antibiotic therapy difficult. Therefore, it was of special interest that in 17 posttreatment small-bowel biopsies (mean duration of follow-up, almost 10 years), PCR on specimens from 12 patients were positive, and that 7 of those 12 subsequently had relapses (or never responded to treatment), versus no relapses among 5 patients whose follow-up specimens were PCR negative. The critical question for a given tissue and agent is how long it takes DNA to be degraded once an organism is dead. In a mouse model of Lyme disease, both PCR and culture became negative in bladder and skin immediately after a 5-day course of antibiotics.[1] Rapid degradation in human tissues and diseases would make PCR a useful way to evaluate therapeutic efficacy. While such work is being pursued, the clinical question is, should one worry more about a patient whose PCR does not become negative after treatment? Stated that way, the answer is clearly "yes."

S.E. Malawista, M.D.

Reference

1. Malawista SE, Barthold SW, Persing DH: Fate of *Borrelia burgdorferi* DNA in tissues of infected mice after antibiotic treatment. *J Infect Dis.* 170:1312–1316, 1994.

Persistence of Parvovirus B19 DNA in Synovial Membranes of Young Patients With and Without Chronic Arthropathy
Söderlund M, von Essen R, Haapasaari J, et al (Univ of Helsinki; Rheumatism Found Hosp, Heinola, Finland; Central Military Hosp, Helsinki)
Lancet 349:1063–1065, 1997   46–2

Background.—Human parvovirus B19 is associated with many diseases, such as erythema infectiosum, fetal hydrops and other complications of pregnancy, acute aplastic or hypoplastic crises in individuals who are hematologically predisposed, and chronic anemia in individuals who are immunocompromised. Parvovirus arthropathy is generally transient, but can be chronic and meet the diagnostic criteria of rheumatoid arthritis or juvenile chronic arthritis. Parvovirus B19 DNA has been found in the bone marrow and joint fluids and synovial membranes of patients with transient or chronic arthropathies.

Methods.—Tissue samples were examined for parvovirus B19 DNA by polymerase chain reaction. There were 37 children between ages 2 and 16 years with chronic unexplained arthritis, and 27 young adults between ages 19 and 24 years with joint trauma who served as control subjects. The timing of parvovirus infection was analyzed serologically.

Results.—Polymerase chain reaction showed that all specimens of synovial fluid, bone marrow, and blood were negative for B19 DNA. B19 DNA analysis was done in samples of synovial membrane in 29 of the pediatric patients, 8 of whom had B19 DNA in the synovial membrane. Results were positive for B19 DNA in synovial membrane in 13 of the 27

TABLE.—Results of Paired Samples of Synovial Membrane B19 DNA and
IgG Antibodies to B19

B19 DNA	B19-IgG antibodies		
	+	−	Total
+	18	0	18
−	2	26	28
Total	20	26	46

(Courtesy of Söderlund M, von Essen R, Haapasaari J: Persistence of parvovirus B19 DNA in synovial membranes of young patients with and without chronic arthropathy. *Lancet* 349:1063–1065, copyright 1997, The Lancet Ltd.)

control subjects. Serum IgG antibodies to B19 were found in all individuals with B19 DNA in synovial membrane (Table).

Discussion.—These findings show that B19 DNA can be found in synovial membrane of patients with chronic arthropathy and of healthy individuals. These results also indicate that the diagnostic criteria for parvovirus arthropathy should be re-evaluated.

▶ There is a *déjà vu* quality here. Like parvovirus, rubella is also associated with transient, early-rheumatoid-arthritis-like polyarthralgias or polyarthritis. Over a decade ago, it was rubella virus that had also begun to be recovered from joints and lymphoreticular tissues of patients with chronic arthritis.[1–4] However, the sheer variety of the syndromes—Still's disease, erosive polyarthritis, pauciarticular and polyarticular juvenile rheumatoid arthritis, typical ankylosing spondylitis[1, 4]—militated against a primary etiologic role of the virus in any of them. I said then, "I favor the view that inflammatory joints are places where rubella virus can persist comfortably. "Hot" joints are generally well below core body temperature. We know that the virus can persist in primary human synovial cultures maintained at 32° C, an appropriate temperature for peripheral joints, without killing cells and without cellular production of interferon.[3] At 37° C, virus in such cultures disappears in about a month. Thus, inflamed joints have temperatures and tissues that support the persistence of rubella *in vitro.* "

There are some differences in the case of parvovirus B19: Evidence for virus came from polymerase-chain-reaction (PCR) amplification of specific genomic DNA primers, not from recovery of virus; synovial tissue was positive but not synovial fluid; and attempts to grow parvovirus in synoviocyte cultures have so far been unsuccessful. The current authors found PCR positivity in 28% (8 of 29) of children with chronic arthritis, but also in 48% (13 of 27) of healthy young adults who underwent arthroscopy or arthrotomy for joint trauma. They paid careful attention to avoiding false positives, and the presence of B19-IgG antibodies correlated well with PCR positivity (Table). The implication is of course that once again the virus in question is likely to be a fellow traveler rather than an etiologic agent.[5]

S.E. Malawista, M.D.

References

1. 1983 YEAR BOOK OF MEDICINE, p 657.
2. 1985 YEAR BOOK OF MEDICINE, p 792.
3. 1986 YEAR BOOK OF MEDICINE, p 720.
4. 1987 YEAR BOOK OF MEDICINE, p 792.
5. Kingsley G: Microbial DNA in the Synovium: A Role in Aetiology or a Mere Bystander? *Lancet* 349:1038–1039, 1997 (editorial).

Duration of Tick Attachment as a Predictor of the Risk of Lyme Disease in an Area in Which Lyme Disease Is Endemic

Sood SK, Salzman MB, Johnson BJB, et al (Albert Einstein College of Medicine, New Hyde Park, NY; Natl Ctr for Infectious Diseases, Fort Collins, Colo; State Univ of New York, Stony Brook)
J Infect Dis 175:996–999, 1997   46–3

Introduction.—There is controversy over the practice of administering antibiotic prophylaxis after a tick bite in areas in which Lyme disease is endemic. Although organ involvement can result in serious illness, the incidence of infection after an individual tick bite is low and treatment of symptomatic disease is effective. A prospective study of persons with tick bites sought to determine whether prolonged attachment correlates with a high risk of infection.

Methods.—Eligible patients had been bitten by a deer tick in the 72 hours preceding study entry, submitted the tick, and underwent serologic testing. Those receiving an antibiotic were excluded, and antibiotics were administered only when erythema migrans developed. Sera were obtained on the day of tick submission and 4 to 6 weeks later. An incident case of *Borrelia burgdorferi* infection was defined as either the occurrence of erythema migrans between the time of the tick bite and the second visit, or seroconversion by electroimmunoassay (EIA) and immunoblot, or both. Ticks submitted were analyzed for *B. burgdorferi* DNA. Duration of tick attachment was determined from the scutal index of engorgement.

Results.—The 312 individuals who reported a tick bite submitted 316 specimens; 303 were ticks and 229 were the deer tick (*Ixodes scapularis*). Polymerase chain reaction assay performed on 227 *I. scapularis* ticks identified 32 as positive for *B. burgdorferi*. Paired sera and an intact tick were available for 105 study participants (109 bites). There were 4 cases of *B. burgdorferi* infection (3.7% of bites), 3 of which occurred when duration of attachment was ≥72 hours. Risk of infection (Fig 1) was significantly higher from nymphal *I. scapularis* attached ≥72 hours (18%) when compared with all other *I. scapularis* bites (2%).

Conclusion.—The odds of infection with *B. burgdorferi* increase considerably with longer duration of attachment. Identification of the tick and its sex and stage could also help to characterize an individual's risk of

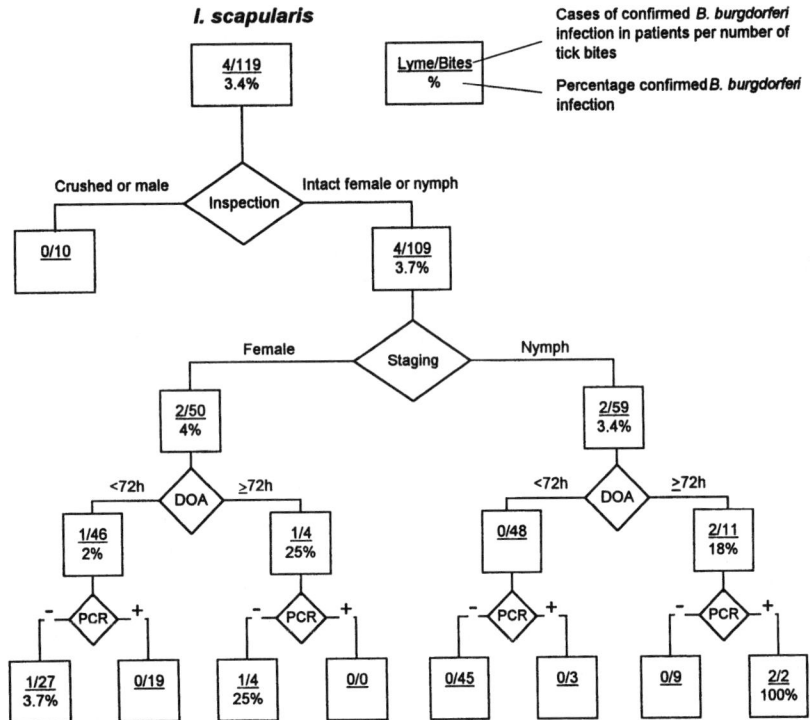

FIGURE 1.—Prevalence of *Borrelia burgdorferi* infection by type of *Ixodes scapularis* bite. Shown only are subjects who completed paired serologic testing. Excludes larvae. *Abbreviations: DOA*, duration of attachment; *PCR*, polymerase chain reaction. (Courtesy of Sood SK, Salzman MB, Johnson BJB, et al: Duration of tick attachment as a predictor of the risk of Lyme disease in an area in which Lyme disease in endemic. *J Infect Dis* 175:996–999, 1997. Copyright © 1997 by The University of Chicago.)

infection. Thus, antibiotic prophylaxis might be advised for those with nymphal or female *I. scapularis* and duration of attachment ≥72 hours.

▶ *B. burgdorferi*, the spirochete that causes Lyme disease, resides in the midgut of *Ixodes scapularis (dammini)*, the deer tick. When the tick engorges, the spirochetes are activated and eventually make their way to the tick's salivary glands, whence they travel to the host. The journey from the midgut takes time; in animal studies, there is an exponential increase in the risk of *B burgdorferi* infection only after 48–72 hours of tick attachment.

How does one decide whether a tick bite should be treated? Most people do not know how long a tick has been feeding on them, but this can be estimated by the "scutal index," computed as the ratio of body length to the maximum width of the scutum. The accuracy of this index is based on an exponential increase in the body length during the blood meal, and an inflexible scutum.

In the current study, using this estimate of feeding time, the authors found that engorgement for ≥72 hours increased the risk of infection from about 2% to 4% overall, to 18% for a nymphal bite and 25% for a female bite (Fig

1). Here, then, is their approach to a tick bite: (1) examine the specimen to rule out non-deer ticks, which constituted 27.5% of ticks in the current study, (2) assign stage and sex of the ticks, (3) estimate length of attachment of I. scapularis nymphs or adult females (the primary vectors of Lyme disease), and (4) consider treating those feeding for ≥72 hours. If all such subjects in the study had been given antibiotic prophylaxis, there would have been treatment of only 13% (25/193) of deer tick bites in which duration of attachment could be determined, or 8% (25/316) of all specimens submitted as possible deer ticks. In contrast, polymerase chain reaction did not predict who would become infected.

There are caveats. For safety's sake, keep an eye on the site of the tick bite for a month (some workers would do only this, because the cure rate of early *erythema chronicum migrans* is very high). Also, note that these strategies depend both on seeing the tick that is engorging (most people do not) and on not missing another tick engorging at another site.

S.E. Malawista, M.D.

Ceftriaxone Compared With Doxycycline for the Treatment of Acute Disseminated Lyme Disease

Dattwyler RJ, Luft BJ, Kunkel MJ, et al (State Univ of New York, Stony Brook; Danbury Hosp, Conn; Middelfort Clinic, Eau Claire, Wis; et al)
N Engl J Med 337:289–294, 1997   46–4

Introduction.—Previous studies of patients with erythema migrans, the earliest and most easily recognized sign of Lyme disease, grouped patients with localized disease together with patients who had acute disseminated *Borrelia burgdorferi* infection. A prospective study was designed to determine whether patients with acute disseminated infection should be treated differently from those with localized infection.

Methods.—The randomized, open-label study compared parenteral ceftriaxone (2 g once daily for 14 days) with the usual treatment for localized Lyme disease, oral doxycycline (100 mg twice daily for 21 days), in patients with erythema migrans lesions and acute disseminated disease but without meningitis. A diagnosis of disseminated disease was based on the finding of multiple erythema migrans lesions or objective evidence of organ involvement. Patients were evaluated clinically and underwent serologic testing at baseline and follow-up visits.

Results.—Sixty-eight patients were randomized to parenteral ceftriaxone and 72 to oral doxycycline; 58 in the ceftriaxone group and 62 in the doxycycline group completed the 9 months of evaluation. The 2 groups were generally well matched for age, sex, and severity of symptoms at baseline. Ninety-nine patients (71%) were positive for *B. burgdorferi* on ELISA at study entry. Clinical cure rates were virtually equivalent: 85% in the ceftriaxone group and 88% in the doxycycline group. Only 1 patient in each group had objective evidence of treatment failure at the final evaluation, but residual, usually mild symptoms were present in both

TABLE 3.—The Most Common Persistent Symptoms at the Last Follow-up Visit, According to Treatment Group*

SYMPTOM	CEFTRIAXONE (N = 18)			DOXYCYCLINE (N = 10)		
	MILD	MODERATE	SEVERE	MILD	MODERATE	SEVERE
			no. of patients			
Arthralgia	11	2	1	4	1	1
Backache	2	0	0	1	0	0
Fatigue	5	1	0	4	1	0
Headache	1	1	0	0	0	0
Irritability	3	1	0	0	0	0
Malaise	5	0	0	1	0	0
Myalgia	3	0	1	1	1	1
Stiff neck	2	0	0	0	0	0

*Some patients had more than 1 symptom.
(Reprinted by permission of The New England Journal of Medicine from Dattwyler RJ, Luft BJ, Kunkel MJ, et al: Ceftriaxone compared with doxycycline for the treatment of acute disseminated Lyme disease. N Engl J Med 337:289–294, copyright 1997, Massachusetts Medical Society.)

groups (Table 3). There were more drug-related adverse events in the ceftriaxone group (57%) than in the doxycycline group (43%), and the incidence of diarrhea was significantly higher with ceftriaxone treatment (37% versus 6%). Only 4 patients in each group withdrew from the study because of adverse side effects.

Discussion.—Oral doxycycline and parenterally administered ceftriaxone were equally effective treatment for acute disseminated Lyme disease. Both agents were well tolerated, produced an excellent clinical response, and prevented late manifestations of the disease. Persistent symptoms were common, however, particularly in the ceftriaxone group.

▶ These authors specifically address acute disseminated infection with B. burgdorferi—i.e., the horse was clearly out of the barn—unlike previous studies that lumped together patients with early disseminated disease with those whose infection was apparently confined to the site of the tick bite. Thus, of 140 patients, 94% had multiple EM lesions; others, definite organ involvement (but meningitis was an exclusion). With parenteral ceftriaxone, 2 g daily for 14 days or oral doxycycline, 100 mg bid for 21 days, only 1 patient in each group was considered a treatment failure. Over several months, the 2 regimens were equally effective in preventing the late manifestations of disease. It was curious that at last follow-up (usually 9 months after treatment), more patients in the ceftriaxone group reported persistent symptoms, which were usually mild and did not interfere with daily activities (Table 3).

With regard to cost-effectiveness of oral vs. intravenous therapy, the authors of an article in the same issue[1] concluded that for most patients with early Lyme disease or with Lyme arthritis,[2] intravenous therapy appears to be no more effective than oral therapy, is more likely to result in serious complications, and is substantially more expensive. However, intravenous therapy is preferable for patients who also have objective neurologic findings—meningitis or radiculopathy in association with early Lyme disease (possibly excepting those with facial palsy alone), or encephalopathy or polyneuropathy in association with Lyme arthritis.

S.E. Malawista, M.D.

References

1. Eckman MH, Steere AC, Kalish RA, et al: Cost effectiveness of oral as compared with intravenous antibiotic therapy for patients with early Lyme disease or Lyme arthritis. N Engl J Med 337:357–363, 1997.
2. 1995 YEAR BOOK OF MEDICINE, p 820.

Stimultaneous Human Granulocytic Ehrlichiosis and Lyme Borreliosis
Nadelman RB, Horowitz HW, Hsieh T-C, et al (New York Med College, Valhalla)
N Engl J Med 337:27–30, 1997   46–5

Introduction.—The deer tick, *Ixodes scapularis*, has been found in several locales to be infected with both *Borrelia burgdorferi* and with the agent of human granulocytic ehrlichiosis (HGE). Dual infection in humans may change the natural history of each disease and affect the choice of antimicrobial therapy. Cultivation of the agent of HGE is now possible, thus allowing proof of coinfection to be established. The case reported here demonstrates that simultaneous infection with *B. burgdorferi* and the agent of HGE occurs in humans.

> *Case Report.*—A man, 47, was seen with symptoms of fever, headache, myalgia, arthralgia, and generalized weakness. He had been in good health until these symptoms appeared several weeks earlier, 1 month after he had removed a small tick from his right thigh. A faint, pink circular rash suggestive of erythema migrans was present on the patient's right flank, and his white-cell and platelet counts were lower than normal; liver function assays yielded several mildly abnormal results. Treatment with doxycycline (100 mg twice daily for 14 days) resolved the patient's symptoms, and he recovered completely. Blood specimens obtained before treatment were cultured to determine the presence of HGE. Skin biopsy tissue was examined for *B. burgdorferi* infection.

Results.—The organism in the cell culture was confirmed, both by polymerase chain reaction (PCR) and immunofluorescence microscopy, to be the agent of HGE. Direct PCR amplification of the skin-biopsy specimen and the visualization of motile spirochetes by fluorescence microscopy confirmed the presence of *B. burgdorferi*.

Discussion.—Findings in this case provide convincing evidence that coinfection with *B. burgdorferi* and the agent of HGE does occur in humans. The patient exhibited clinical and laboratory features characteristic of both infections. Coinfection may occur through the bite of a single tick harboring both infections, or through bites from different ticks each with a separate infection.

▶ Last year[1] I reported that in patients with atypical or particularly severe Lyme disease, one should look for coinfection with *B. microti,* the causative agent of the malaria-like illness, babesiosis. I pointed out that a third tick-borne infection to consider in patients with a summer musculoskeletal flu-like syndrome, again delivered by the same tick, is HGE.[1, 2] This illness, reminiscent of Rocky Mountain spotted fever without the spots, is caused by an obligate intracellular coccobacillus resembling rickettsia that infects granulocytic blood cells. I present the current study to emphasize that HGE is among us—here in a co-infection with the Lyme spirochete—and to indicate how its presence is currently established.

Erythema migrans is diagnostic for Lyme disease. Common to both illnesses are fever, headache, myalgia, arthralgia, and weakness, as well as abnormalities of liver function. Cough is much more suggestive of HGE, and leukopenia and thrombocytopenia are characteristic. Inclusions in neutrophils in HGE (morulae) may be hard to find; only 3 cells in 1,000 had them in the current study. Since both Lyme disease and HGE respond to doxycycline but only Lyme disease responds to amoxicillin, in adults the former antibiotic will probably drive out the latter as the treatment of choice for Lyme disease.

Although HGE is often referred to as an emerging disease, it may be more properly thought of as already emerged but largely unrecognized until now. For example, in a PCR study of *I. scapularis* ticks collected in 1995,[2] about half of 100 adult ticks contained DNA characteristic of one or the other agent (about a quarter of them, DNA from both agents; 20-odd percent of 73 nymphs also contained DNA from each agent). Moreover, the percentages were not much lower from 100 adult ticks preserved in alcohol since 1984 (*B. Burgdorferi,* 45%; HGE, 32%; both, 19%).

S.E. Malawista, M.D.

References

1. 1997 YEAR BOOK OF MEDICINE, p 719.
2. Schwartz I, Fish D, Daniels TJ: Prevalence of the rickettsial agent of human granulocytic ehrlichiosis in ticks from a hyperendemic focus of Lyme disease. *N Engl J Med* 337:49–50, 1997.

47 Other Topics

Introduction

Subjects of rheumatologic interest lying outside the seven categorical chapters include the use of intermittent etidronate to prevent corticosteroid-induced osteoporosis (Abstract 27–9); the effect of calcium and vitamin D supplementation on bone density in men and women aged at least 65 years (Abstract 27–7); the relation of quadriceps weakness to osteoarthritis of the knee (Abstract 47–1); the treatment of primary amyloidosis with colchicine alone, melphalan and prednisone, or all three (Abstract 12–10); and acute rheumatic fever in adults (Abstract 47–2).

Noted in passing: Reviews of sarcoidosis,[1] corticosteroid therapy in severe illness,[2] and the management of multiple sclerosis[3]; and a controlled trial of an educational program to prevent low back injuries which enhanced understanding without reducing the likelihood of a disabling injury[4] (the accompanying editorial is eloquent[5]).

Stephen E. Malawista, M.D.

References

1. Newman LS, Rose CS, Maier LA: Sarcoidosis. *N Engl J Med* 336:1223–1234, 1997.
2. Lamberts AJJ, Bruining HA, DeJong FH: Corticosteroid therapy in severe illness. *N Engl J Med* 337:1285–1292, 1997.
3. Rudick RA, Cohen JA, Weinstock-Guttman B, et al: Management of multiple sclerosis. *N Engl J Med* 337:1604–1611, 1997.
4. Daltroy LH, Iversen MD, Larson MG, et al: A controlled trial of an educational program to prevent low back injuries. *N Engl J Med* 337:332–338, 1997.
5. Hadler NM: Workers with disabling back pain. *N Engl J Med* 337:341–343, 1997.

Quadriceps Weakness and Osteoarthritis of the Knee
Slemenda C, Brandt KD, Heilman DK, et al (Indiana Univ, Indianapolis)
Ann Intern Med 127:97–104, 1997   47–1

Objective.—The role of quadriceps weakness in the pathology of disease has not been well studied, particularly in asymptomatic patients with radiographic evidence of osteoarthritis of the knee. The relation among lower extremity muscle strength, lower extremity lean tissue mass, and osteoarthritis of the knee in patients aged 65 years or older was studied to determine if quadriceps weakness occurs before or after joint pain or is mediated by tissue atrophy or by physiologic mechanisms that may inhibit muscle contraction.

Methods.—A cross-sectional prevalence study was conducted with 462 community-dwelling volunteers (226 men) aged 65 years or older. Standing anteroposterior and lateral radiographs of both knees were obtained, and knee pain and function were assessed using the Western Ontario and McMaster Universities Arthritis Index. The strength of each leg was evaluated using an isokinetic dynamometer, and lower extremity lean tissue mass was determined using total-body dual-energy x-ray absorptiometry.

Results.—Men were significantly heavier and taller, and had greater lower extremity strength and lean tissue mass in the lower extremities than women did. Men and women with osteoarthritis were heavier and had significantly more functional impairment than their counterparts with normal radiographs and no knee pain. Participants with osteoarthritis had significantly more lower extremity weakness, 20% lower extensor strength, but similar or more lean tissue mass of the involved lower extremity, compared with participants with normal radiographs. The prevalence of osteoarthritis increases and strength decreases with age. Each 10-lb increase in knee-extension strength lowered the risk of radiographic osteoarthritis by 20% and lowered the risk of symptomatic arthritis by 29%. An increase in strength of 19% for men and 27% for women lowered with risk of osteoarthritis by 20% and 30%, respectively.

Conclusion.—Quadriceps weakness in asymptomatic individuals with osteoarthritis may be the result of muscle dysfunction and may predispose

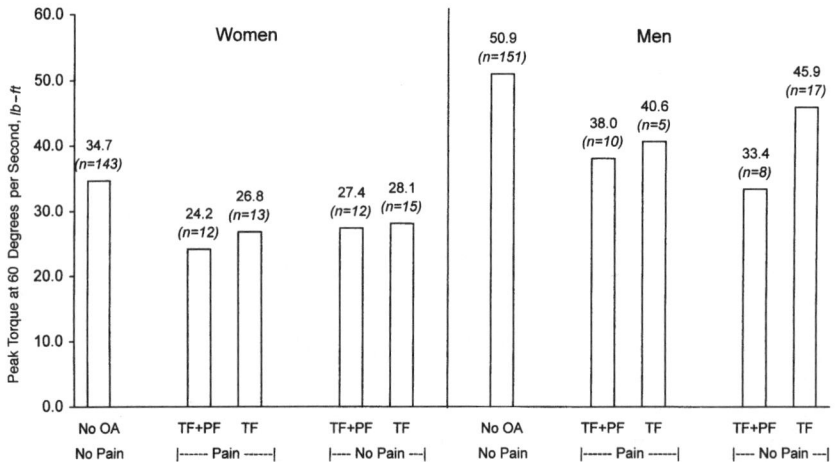

FIGURE.—Left leg strength, measured as peak extensor torque at 60 degrees per second, related to sex, topographic localization of radiographic changes of osteoarthritis, and the presence of recent knee pain. The numbers at the top of each bar represent the mean peak torque, and the numbers in parentheses represent numbers of participants. Strength was generally greater in the right than in the left leg, but the magnitude of the differences in right leg strength among participants was similar to the magnitude of the differences in left leg strength. *OA* = osteoarthritis, *PF* = patellofemoral, *TF* = tibiofemoral.

them to damage to knee cartilage and other tissue. Whether quadriceps strengthening exercises can delay or prevent osteoarthritic damage should be evaluated in a randomized, placebo-controlled trial.

Clinical Significance.—Quadriceps weakness in patients with asymptomatic osteoarthritis of the knee may increase their risk of knee pain, disability, and progressive joint damage.

▶ The key finding in this community-based study is that quadriceps weakness may be present in patients who have radiographic evidence of osteoarthritis without knee pain or muscle atrophy (Figure). The implication is that weakness of knee extensors may be a risk factor for the initiation as well as the progression of damage to articular cartilage and other tissues in the knee with osteoarthritis. A more general discussion of the role of muscle in osteoarthritis is found in an accompanying editorial.[1]

An alternative explanation is that there is subclinical cross-talk between damaged joint and quadriceps muscle in asymptomatic individuals with osteoarthritis. Although the between-leg differences in strength in participants with unilateral osteoarthritis were similar to those with bilateral disease, the sample in the former group were small; a larger series might answer this which-came-first question. In any case, exercise aimed at increasing leg strength has been shown to improve knee pain and function in osteoarthritis in the short term. Studies of the longer-term effects on such parameters as the development or progression of pathologic changes and on the risk of pain or disability are in order.

S.E. Malawista, M.D.

Reference

1. Brandt KD: Putting some muscle into osteoarthritis. *Ann Intern Med* 127:154–156, 1997.

Acute Rheumatic Fever in Adults: A Resurgence in the Hasidic Jewish Community
Feuer J, Spiera H (Mount Sinai Med Ctr, New York)
J Rheumatol 24:337–340, 1997   47–2

Background.—Acute rheumatic fever in children has recently reemerged in the United States. It was traditionally believed that acute rheumatic fever in adults was rare and that carditis was uncommon and mild. Carditis of acute rheumatic fever is defined as a new organic heart murmur, enlarging heart, congestive heart failure, or pericarditis. It is important to know if carditis is present when one is administering antibiotic prophylaxis.

Methods.—The medical records of 12 adult patients with acute rheumatic fever were reviewed. There were 5 men, and most patients were between ages 21 and 38 years; one patient was 50 years old. Nine patients were Hasidic Jews.

Results.—Three patients had a childhood history of rheumatic fever. At disease onset, 10 patients had fever. All patients had antecedent sore throat, and 3 patients had throat cultures positive for B-hemolytic streptococcus. Four patients had carditis, one of whom had carditis in childhood and at age 30. The chief complaint of these patients was arthritis. The knees, ankles, wrists, and the small joints of the hands and feet were the most commonly affected joints. Three of 4 patients had murmurs or gallops. One patient with pericarditis developed florid congestive heart failure. All patients with carditis responded to treatment with nonsteroidal antiinflammatory drugs or acetylsalicylic acid. Steroid treatment was needed in 3 patients to control severe arthritis.

Discussion.—These findings indicate that acute rheumatic fever in adults is no longer uncommon and is frequently seen in Hasidic Jews. Acute rheumatic fever in adults may often be associated with carditis. It is important to adhere to the guidelines for penicillin prophylaxis because of the high incidence of carditis and the disabling nature of the arthritis.

▶ Since the importance of penicillin prophylaxis for acute rheumatic fever was recognized, this disorder has declined in incidence in the Western world, to the point where reminders are necessary of its continued sporadic appearance and of the damage it can do, principally to the heart. Tocsins are occasionally sounded—for example, an article and editorial in the *New Engl J Med* a decade ago regarding an epidemic around Salt Lake City[1]—after which relative silence ensues, easily leading to inattention. The current authors collected a dozen adult patients over 5 years who fit the Jones criteria for rheumatic fever, largely from a private Manhattan rheumatology practice; 4 patients had carditis. Nine were Hasidic Jews, whose households contained 2 to 8 children under age 18, with a mean of 4 per household, vs. a mean of < 2 in the United States overall (the average family size in the Utah outbreak was 6.5, and 65% of patients shared their bedrooms with others). Human leukocyte antigen typing among the patients, and recovery and serotyping of the triggering Group A streptococci, were not reported. At a time when so many acute joint complaints are thoughtlessly treated for Lyme disease (in which symmetrical, small-joint involvement is very unusual), it is well to keep in mind that acute rheumatic fever is still among us, and that it can occur in adults.

S.E. Malawista, M.D.

Reference

1. 1998 YEAR BOOK OF MEDICINE, p 757.

PART SEVEN

THE CHEST

JAMES R. JETT, M.D.

Introduction

I selected the 41 articles in this section from a list of 250 articles selected by the various editors of the YEAR BOOK OF PULMONARY DISEASE. Each of these editors has chosen articles on topics within their particular area of expertise; all editors are heavily involved in clinical medicine at their respective institutions. These articles have been selected for their clinical usefulness or their implication for the future, and I have tried to balance the topics. In brief, the articles selected address issues related to nicotine addiction, lung cancer, malignant pleural effusion, chronic obstructive pulmonary disease, cystic fibrosis, lung volume reduction surgery, asthma, interstitial lung disease pulmonary thromboembolism/pulmonary hypertension, tuberculosis, HIV, bacterial infections, intensive care medicine and sleep. If you have a particular interest in one of these areas and would like to find more articles on the topic, then I suggest that you review the YEAR BOOK OF PULMONARY DISEASE or other relevant year books including the YEAR BOOK OF CRITICAL CARE MEDICINE and the YEAR BOOK OF INFECTIOUS DISEASE. If you choose to read these abstracts and their accompanying comments, I am certain that you will take away a number of "clinical pearls" that will be useful to you in your practice and aid you in teaching. I encourage you to pull some of the articles that are of particular interest to you and review them critically. You may very well find that you disagree with the major points made by the abstracter or the commentator. If so, feel free to write to the commentator with your point of view. This book is meant to be an educational experience, both for the reader and the editors. We would value your input.

James R. Jett, M.D.

48 Nicotine

Cost-effectiveness of Treating Nicotine Dependence: The Mayo Clinic Experience
Croghan IT, Offord KP, Evans RW, et al (Mayo Clinic, Rochester, Minn)
Mayo Clin Proc 72:917–924, 1997   48–1

Background.—Cigarette smoking is involved in more than 19% of all deaths in the United States. Each year, approximately 17 million Americans attempt to stop smoking but less than 10% are successful. The cost per net year of life gained for patients treated for nicotine dependence at the Mayo Nicotine Dependence Center (NDC) from 1988 through 1992 was estimated in a cost-effective study.

Methods.—Nonphysician counselor services provided to NDC patients included a 1-hour consultation, the development of an individual treatment plan, and a relapse-prevention follow-up program. The study group consisted of 5,544 NDC adult patients with the following information available: demographics, smoking history, interventions, and 6-month smoking status. The years of life gained were computed with respect to age, sex, initial smoking rate, and 6-month status using mortality rates from the American Cancer Society's 25-State Cancer Prevention Study (ACS-CPS II). The average cost of the intervention per patient was $396.

Results.—The smoking cessation rate was 22.2% in this study group. The estimated net years of life gained for all NDC patients, with a 5% rate of discount for benefits, was 0.058. There was a cost of $6,828 for each net year of life gained.

Conclusions.—This study demonstrates that a smoking cessation program can be successfully provided to patients in a cost-effective manner. The use of nonphysician healthcare professionals is important in controlling the costs of the program.

► It is estimated that smoking accounts for more than 400,000 deaths per year in the United States alone. Annually, 17 million U.S. smokers attempt to stop smoking on their own—7.6% are successful.[1] This low success rate clearly reflects the tremendous addictiveness of nicotine. As physicians, it is our responsibility to advise patients of the hazards of smoking; however, all too often we stop there and fail to go into a discussion of "how to do it." This article should give us encouragement and renew our spirit to fight our old nemesis, tobacco. The success rate of smoking cessation at 1 year was

517

22.2% after consultation by a member of the NDC, and a standard follow-up program. Some, but not all, patients received nicotine replacement therapy with a patch or gum. The cost-effectiveness of this intervention was $6,828 per year of life gained, and this estimate did not include the savings to the patient in terms of future cigarette purchases or the savings to society in terms of the decrease in future illnesses secondary to smoking. The next time you see smokers in your office, advise them to quit smoking and give them information about how to enroll in a smoking cessation program in your community. If you can get them to enroll, approximately 1 in 5 will be cured of their addiction. That is far better than we do with the pulmonary diseases induced by this agent.

J.R. Jett, M.D.

Reference

1. Hatziandreu EJ, Pierce JP, Lefkopoulo M et al: Quitting smoking in the United States in 1986. *J Natl Cancer Inst* 82:1402–1406, 1990.

A Comparison of Sustained-Release Bupropion and Placebo for Smoking Cessation

Hurt RD, Sachs DPL, Glover ED, et al (Mayo Clinic and Mayo Foundation, Rochester, Minn; Palo Alto Ctr, Calif; West Virginia Univ, Morgantown; et al)
N Engl J Med 337:1195–1202, 1997   48–2

Introduction.—Because nicotine appears to act as an antidepressant in some smokers, antidepressant medications may be of value as nicotine-replacement therapy for smoking cessation. Results of clinical trials, however, have been mixed. A double-blind, placebo-controlled trial was designed to evaluate the efficacy and safety of a sustained-release form of bupropion as an aid to smoking cessation.

Methods.—Volunteers for the trial were recruited from 3 centers. Of the 742 evaluated individuals, 615 met study criteria. Those eligible for the study had smoked an average of 15 or more cigarettes a day for the past year, wanted to stop smoking, and were in generally good health. Smokers with a history of major depression were included, but not those with current depression. Randomization was to placebo or bupropion at a dose of 100, 150, or 300 mg/day for 7 weeks. The target quit date was 1 week after the start of treatment. Participants received brief counseling weekly during treatment and several times during follow-up. Self-reports of smoking cessation were confirmed by a carbon monoxide level in expired air of 10 ppm or less.

Results.—After 7 weeks of treatment, rates of smoking cessation were 19.0% in the placebo group, 28.8% in the 100-mg group, 38.6% in the 150-mg group, and 44.2% in the 300-mg group (Table 2). Rates of cessation had fallen to 12.4%, 19.6%, 22.9%, and 23.1%, respectively, at 1 year. Only the 300-mg and 150-mg groups had significantly better cessation rates than the placebo group. For the 103 participants who were

TABLE 2.—Point-Prevalence Smoking-Cessation Rates Confirmed by Carbon Monoxide Measurement

Time after Target Quitting Date	Percentage of Subjects Not Smoking				P Value*			
	Placebo (N = 153)	100 mg of Bupropion (N = 153)	150 mg of Bupropion (N = 153)	300 mg of Bupropion (N = 156)	Overall	Placebo vs. 100-mg dose	Placebo vs. 150-mg dose	Placebo vs. 300-mg dose
6wk†	19.0	28.8	38.6	44.2	<0.001	0.04	<0.001	<0.001
3 mo	14.4	24.2	26.1	29.5	0.01	0.03	0.01	<0.001
6 mo	15.7	24.2	27.5	26.9	0.06	0.06	0.01	0.02
12 mo	12.4	19.6	22.9	23.1	0.06	0.09	0.02	0.01

Note: Point prevalence was estimated weekly.

*The P values given are from analyses that did not include site as a covariate; therefore, they can be obtained directly from the given cessation rates. In logistic-regression analyses that included site as a covariate, the same differences were found to be statistically significant. The overall P value is for the simultaneous comparison of all 4 groups treated categorically. When dose was treated as a continuous variable, a significant dose effect was detected at all times (P less than 0.001 at week 6, $P = 0.003$ at 3 months, $P = 0.02$ at 12 months). The pairwise dose comparisons presented were identified a priori, and the corresponding P values are unadjusted.

†Week 6 was the final week of study medication.

(Reprinted by permission of *The New England Journal of Medicine*, courtesy of Hurt RD, Sachs DPL, Glover ED, et al: A comparison of sustained-release bupropion and placebo for smoking cessation. *N Engl J Med* 337:1195–1202, copyright 1997, Massachusetts Medical Society.)

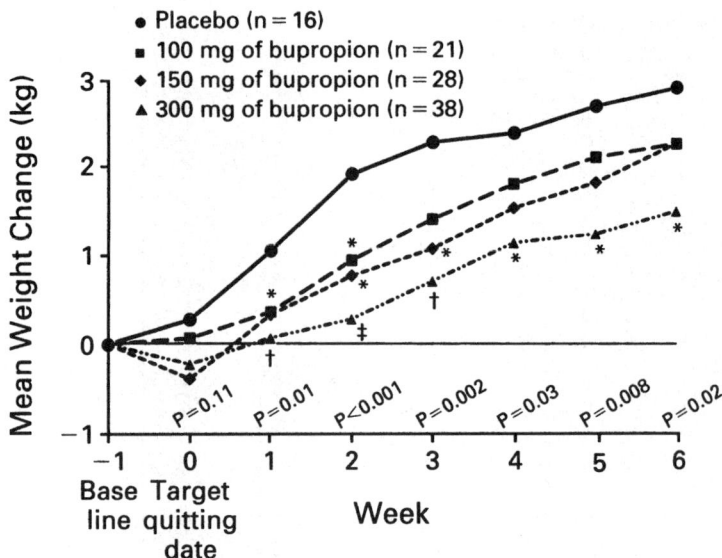

FIGURE 2.—Mean change in weight from base line through the end of treatment among 103 subjects who were continuously abstinent. Weight was analyzed at the end of each week. The mean weight change was significantly greater than zero (P less than 0.05 by the 1-sample t-test) at weeks 1 through 6 in the placebo group, at weeks 2 through 6 in the 100-mg and 150-mg groups, and at weeks 3 through 6 in the 300-mg group. The P values shown are for the effect of dose assessed with a linear regression model in which absolute change in weight was the dependent variable and dose was the independent variable. Asterisks (0.01 less than P less than or equal to 0.05), daggers (0.001 less than P less than or equal to 0.01), and the double dagger (P less than or equal to 0.001) indicate a significant difference (by the 2-sample t-test) from placebo. The number of subjects with data available is the same for all periods except week 5, for which data were missing for 1 subject in the 150-mg group. Treatment was started at base line. (Reprinted by permission of *The New England Journal of Medicine*, courtesy of Hurt RD, Sachs DPL, Glover ED, et al: A comparison of sustained-release bupropion and placebo for smoking cessation. *N Engl J Med* 337:1195–1202, copyright 1997, Massachusetts Medical Society.)

continuously abstinent during the treatment phase, mean weight gain after 7 weeks (Fig 2) was negatively associated with dose (2.9 kg in the placebo group, 2.3 kg in the 100-mg and 150-mg groups, and 1.5 kg in the 300-mg group). Mean weight gain at 6 months (5.5 kg, 6.6 kg, 4.4 kg, and 4.5 kg, respectively) in the 59 individuals who were continuously abstinent during this period was not significantly associated with dose. Treatment had no effect on depression, as measured by Beck Depression Inventory scores. Adverse events occurred at similar rates in the 4 groups and caused 37 participants to stop treatment prematurely.

Conclusion.—Although many study participants were smoking at 1-year follow-up, bupropion proved to be an effective treatment for smoking cessation. The 300-mg dose (150 mg twice a day) is recommended as the most effective dose and the one associated with lower weight gain during the treatment phase.

▶ In recent years, there has been a proliferation of smoking cessation aides and forms of nicotine replacement (gum, patch, spray). The overall success rate with these methods is approximately 20% at 1 year. There have been attempts at treatment with other nonnicotine-containing agents, but without much success. Bupropion may very well revolutionize the treatment of nicotine addiction. After only 7 weeks of treatment, the smoking cessation rate was 23% at 1 year for the 150-mg and 300-mg bupropion (Table 2). Bupropion, originally marketed as an antidepressant, is a weak inhibitor of neuronal uptake of norepinephrine and dopamine, but it has an effect on serotonin. This could be responsible for its efficacy in smoking cessation. An additional attractive feature of the drug in this study was that with the highest dose tested and the one recommended for future treatment, there was the least weight gain at the end of 7 weeks (Fig 2). However, in the 59 subjects who were continuously abstinent from the target quitting date to the 6-month follow-up visit, the mean weight gain varied from 5.5 kg in the placebo group to a low of 4.4 kg in the 150-mg group and 4.5 kg in the 300-mg group (P = NS). Weight gain continues to be problematic and at least 1 reason voiced by smokers for not quitting.

This study opens up many exciting new possibilities. As the authors point out, the optimal duration of treatment with bupropion is not known but will certainly be tested. Additionally, trials are already underway to combine bupropion and nicotine replacement. Preliminary results with this combination are very encouraging, but we must wait for the completed reports. Finally, for the most refractory and hard core nicotine addicts, we have used a 1-week inpatient treatment program at the nicotine dependence center with encouraging results.[1] The recent 1-year cessation rate with this program is 43%.

J.R. Jett, M.D.

Reference

1. Hurt RD, Dale LC, Offord KP et al: Inpatient treatment of severe nicotine dependence. *Mayo Clin Proc* 67:823–828, 1992.

49 Lung Cancer

The Changing Radiographic Presentation of Bronchogenic Carcinoma With Reference to Cell Types
Quinn D, Gianlupi A, Broste S (Marshfield Clinic, Marshfield, Wis)
Chest 110:1474–1479, 1996   49–1

Background.—Chest radiography and radiographic patterns as indicators of cell type continue to be the basic methods of diagnosing lung cancer. However, much of the reference data come from a Mayo Clinic review published in 1969, representing lung cancer in an earlier era. Since that time, a marked increase in lung cancer incidence in women has occurred, as well as a shift in the relative frequency of cell types. Therefore, a contemporary series of patients was reviewed and compared with the earlier Mayo Clinic series.

Methods.—Three hundred forty-five patients found to have lung cancer between 1990 and 1992 were included in the series. Two radiologists unaware of cell type interpreted the radiographs.

Results.—In the current series, 49% of the patients had adenocarcinoma as a peripheral tumor, compared with 72% in the earlier series. Squamous cell carcinoma as a peripheral tumor was seen in 43% of those in the current series and in 31% of the control series. No significant differences were found between adenocarcinoma and squamous cell disease presenting as peripheral or central in origin in the 2 series.

Conclusions.—Adenocarcinoma has increased in relative frequency among patients with lung cancer. The percentage of patients with peripheral primary tumors has declined, whereas that of patients with central tumors has increased. There has been a relative increase in squamous carcinoma as peripheral mass presentation. No significant difference exists between these cell types in the proportions presenting as peripheral masses or central tumors on chest radiographs.

▶ It is estimated that in 1997 women will account for 45% of the 178,000 new cases of lung cancer in the United States.[1] In recent years, adenocarcinoma has replaced squamous cell carcinoma as the most frequent histologic type. The age-adjusted rates of lung cancer increased by 30% from 1973–1977 to 1983–1987.[2] The largest percentage increases were observed for small cell carcinoma and adenocarcinoma. In addition to the changing demographics, this article confirms the change in roentgenographic presentation based on cell type. We can no longer accurately guess the cell type on the basis of the chest radiograph's appearance. However, this will not change our clinical practice because almost all patients with lung cancer need histologic proof of diagnosis if any treatment is going to be instituted.

J.R. Jett, M.D.

References

1. Parker SL, Tong T, Bolden S, et al: Cancer statistics, 1997. *CA: A Journal for Clinicians* 47:5–27, 1997.
2. Travis WD, Travis LB, Devesa SS: *Lung Cancer* 75:191–202, 1995.

Peripheral Lung Cancer: Screening and Detection With Low-dose Spinal CT Versus Radiography
Kaneko M, Eguchi K, Ohmatsu H, et al (Natl Cancer Ctr Hosp, Tokyo; Natl Cancer Ctr East Hosp, Chiba, Japan)
Radiology 201:798–802, 1996   49–2

Background.—In Japan, mass screening for lung cancer is performed annually in more than 500,000 people in about 80% of local communities. Lung cancer recently became the leading cause of cancer death among Japanese men, surpassing death from gastric cancer. More than half of lung cancers in Japan are adenocarcinoma. Although early detection of peripheral cancer is indicated to reduce mortality rates, many studies have reported the pitfalls of radiographic screening. The current study compared low-dose spiral computed tomography (CT) with radiography of the chest in the screening and detection of small peripheral lung cancers in a high-risk population.

Methods.—A total of 3,457 examinations were performed in 1,369 persons at high risk for lung cancer. The studies included posteroanterior and lateral radiographs and low-dose spiral CT scans, obtained twice a year between September 1993 and April 1995.

Findings.—Overall peripheral lung cancer was detected on 0.3% of the examinations. Chest radiographic results were negative in 11 of these 15 patients. Tumors were detected only by low-dose spiral CT. Low-dose spiral CT and chest radiography had detection rates of 0.43% and 0.12%, respectively. Ninety-three percent of the tumors identified were stage I.

Conclusions.—In this high-risk population, low-dose spiral CT was a more effective screening tool for peripheral lung cancer than was chest radiography. Additional large-scale studies are needed to further define the efficacy and cost-effectiveness of low-dose spiral CT in a randomized, controlled population.

▶ Routine screening for lung cancer is not recommended by the American Cancer Society or the U.S. Preventive Service Task Force. This recommendation is based on the 3 screening trials at Memorial Sloan Kettering, Johns Hopkins, and Mayo Clinic conducted in the 1970s and early 1980s. Those trials compared screening with sputum cytology and chest roentgenogram vs. yearly chest roentgenogram alone (2 centers) or the 1-time recommendation of chest radiograph and sputum cytology yearly (recommended but patient not reminded to undergo tests). None of the 3 studies showed a reduction in lung cancer mortality rate in the group with combined modality screening compared with the control arm.

It is clear that patients with symptomatic lung cancer have a worse survival rate than those in whom the cancer is detected in an asymptomatic phase. All of us have a few patients who are cured from their lung cancer (5-year survivors), and in most of these individuals the lung cancer was detected by chance before symptoms occurred. Since the prior screening studies were performed, we have learned that chronic obstructive pulmonary disease is an independent risk factor for lung cancer (independent of smoking history).[1] Two recent papers on lung volume reduction surgery identified incidental lung cancers in 2%–3% of all patients undergoing lung volume reduction surgery. These cancers were detected on the routine CT scans performed in the preoperative evaluation.[2]

This article is one of the first studies to address the issue of screening for lung cancer with spiral CT scanning, and it looks very promising. Issues that must be dealt with include the cost of the test and the radiation dose involved (equivalent to about 10 chest roentgenograms).

The issue of screening for lung cancer is ripe for reevaluation using newly determined risk factors such as chronic obstructive pulmonary disease, family history and sex, and new tools such as spiral CT scanning, autoflourescence bronchoscopy[3], and molecular markers detected in the sputum. I predict that screening for lung cancer will be recommended in 10 years, if not sooner.

J.R. Jett, M.D.

References

1. Kennedy TC, Proudfoot SP, Franklin WA, et al: Cytopathological analysis of sputum in patients with airflow obstruction and significant smoking histories. *Cancer Res* 56:4673–4678, 1996.
2. Pigula FA, Keenan RJ, Ferson PF, et al: Unsuspected lung cancer found in workup for lung reduction surgery. *Ann Thorac Surg* 61:174–176, 1996.
3. Lam S, MacAulay C, Hung J, et al: Detection of dysplasia and carcinoma in situ with a lung imaging fluorescence endoscopic devise. *J Thorac Cardiovasc Surg* 105:1035–1040, 1993.

Lung Nodule Enhancement at CT: Prospective Findings
Swenson SJ, Brown LR, Colby TV, et al (Mayo Clinic and Mayo Found, Rochester, Minn)
Radiology 201:447–455, 1996   49–3

Introduction.—The noninvasive identification of benign lung nodules could reduce the number of resections by thoracotomy or thoracoscopy and lead to considerable cost savings. To determine the value of CT in

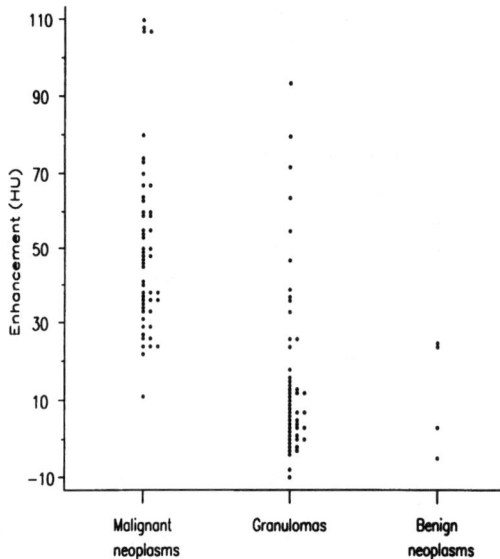

FIGURE 4.—Distribution of enhancement in Hounsfield units for each of the 3 types of lesions. On the basis of the Wilcoxon rank sum test, the median enhancement for the malignant neoplasms was statistically significantly higher than that for the granulomas and benign neoplasms ($P < 0.001$). (Courtesy of Swenson SJ, Brown LR, Colby TV, et al: Lung nodule enhancement at CT: Prospective findings. *Radiology* 201:447–455, 1996. Radiological Society of North America.)

distinguishing benign from malignant nodules, solitary indeterminate pulmonary nodules in 141 patients were imaged with spiral CT.

Methods.—The nodules measured 7 to 30 mm in diameter and were relatively spherical. Excluded were nodules with benign patterns of calcification or fat on thin-section CT images. Preenhancement analysis consisted of 3-mm-collimation spiral scans through the entire nodule. After contrast material (iopamidol) was administered, serial, 5-second, 3-mm-collimation spiral acquisitions were performed at four 1-minute intervals. Patients in whom a clinical or pathologic diagnosis of the nodule could not be obtained and those whose studies were not technically adequate were excluded, leaving 107 patients for analysis. A nodule with an enhancement of 25 Hounsfield units (HU) or more was considered to have substantial enhancement. Twenty-four histologic specimens were graded after immunoperoxidase vascular staining with antibody to factor VIII-associated antigen.

Results.—There were 51 malignant neoplasms, 51 granulomas, and 4 benign neoplasms. The malignant group included 12 adenocarcinomas, 11 bronchial carcinoids, and 8 squamous cell carcinomas. Histologic proof of diagnosis was obtained in only 7 granulomas, and 44 were considered granulomas because there was no radiologic evidence of growth during a follow-up of at least 2 years. Both the median enhancement (Fig 4) and the median diameter of malignant neoplasms were significantly higher than those of granulomas and benign neoplasms. With 20 HU as the threshold

Parameter	Estimate (%)	95% CI
Sensitivty	98	90, 100
Specificity	73	59, 84
Positive predictive value	77	65, 87
Negative predictive value	98	87, 100
Accuracy	85	77, 91
Prevalence of malignancy	49	39, 59

Abbreviation: CI, confidence interval.
(Courtesy of Swenson SJ, Brown LR, Colby TV, et al: Lung nodule enhancement at CT: Prospective findings. *Radiology* 201:447–455, 1996. Radiological Society of North America.)

for a positive test result, the sensitivity of CT enhancement was 98%, the specificity was 73%, and the accuracy was 85% (Table 5). There was a statistically significant relationship between degree of enhancement and the amount of central vascular staining.

Conclusion.—The protocol used here allows satisfactory enhancement of pulmonary nodules with a diameter of 7 to 30 mm. With iodinated contrast material, malignant neoplasms enhance significantly more than granulomas and benign neoplasms. Enhancement also indicates vascularity.

► In an ideal world, all solitary malignant pulmonary nodules would be resected, all benign lesions would be left alone, and patients would not have to undergo unnecessary surgery. In reality, it is estimated that 25% to 35% of solitary pulmonary nodules that are resected are benign.[1,2] Recent reports using positron emission tomography have suggested that it has 80% to 90% sensitivity and specificity for diagnosing malignant solitary pulmonary nodules.

In this large series, the authors reported a sensitivity of 98% and specificity of 73%. Thus, a nodule that does not enhance by 20 HU is extremely unlikely to be malignant (false negative) and can be carefully observed. My major caution is that all clinicians must be satisfied that the use of this technique in their institution might not be as sensitive or specific as that reported by the authors of this Mayo Clinic study. Currently, a multicenter trial is underway to determine the variability of these results in other institutions.

J.R. Jett, M.D.

References

1. Midthun DE, Swensen SJ, Jett JR: An approach to the solitary pulmonary nodule. *Mayo Clin Proc* 68:378–385, 1993.
2. Lung Cancer Study Group: Randomized trial of lobectomy versus limited resection for T1N0 non–small cell lung cancer. *Ann Thorac Surg* 60:615–623, 1995.

50 Malignant Effusion

Thoracoscopic Talc Poudrage Pleurodesis for Malignant Effusions
Viallat J-R, Rey F, Astoul P, et al (Paoli Calmettes Inst, Marseilles, France; La Conception Hosp, Marseilles, France)
Chest 110:1387–1393, 1996   50–1

Background.—A renewed interest in talc pleurodesis has recently been expressed in North America. The efficacy and safety of thoracoscopic talc poudrage for pleurodesis in patients with malignant effusions were reported.

Methods.—Thoracoscopy was performed for diagnosis and subsequent talc pleurodesis in 215 patients and for pleurodesis only in 145 patients. Two hundred seventy-two patients had pleural metastases, and 88 had mesothelioma. Mean follow-up was 12 months.

Findings.—Thirty-three critically ill patients died in the first month and were not included in the final analysis. These patients had illnesses that should have contraindicated the procedure. Of the remaining patients, 90.2% had a successful pleurodesis at 1 month and 82.1% had a lifelong pleural symphysis. Adverse effects were fever in 9.8%, empyema in 2.5%, pulmonary infection in 0.8%, and malignant invasion of the scar in 1 patient. In addition, 1 patient died with end-stage disease 3 days after the procedure (Table 2).

Conclusions.—Thoracoscopic talc poudrage is effective and safe for lifelong pleurodesis. It should be done early in the course of malignant effusions to avoid the risk of respiratory failure. The use of no more than

TABLE 2.—Results of Talc Pleurodesis at 1 Month*

	Mesotheliomas† (n=85)‡	Pleural Metastases† (n=242)‡	Overall (n=372)‡
Complete response, %	78.8	88.5	85.9
Partial response, %	5.9	3.7	4.3
Failure, %	15.3	7.8	9.8
Total, %	100	100	100

Complete response, normal or subnormal radiograph; *partial response*, residual pleural fluid (<500 mL), not requiring further tapping; *failure*, all other causes.
†$P = 0.085$. Comparison of mesotheliomas and pleural metastases did not show any significant difference.
‡No. of evaluable patients.
(Courtesy of Viallat J-R, Rey F, Astoul P, et al: Thoracoscopic talc poudrage pleurodesis for malignant effusions. *Chest* 110:1387–1393, 1996.)

5 gm of talc for malignant effusions and 1 to 2 gm for pneumothoraces is recommended.

▶ The debate on the best modality for treatment of malignant pleural effusion continues. This article is the largest series that I am aware of that analyzes the results of thoracoscopy and talc poudrage. The long-term results with lifetime pleural symphysis of 82% is excellent. In this group of patients with a terminal malignancy, ongoing problems with management of the malignant pleural effusion greatly detracts from their quality of life. Thus, it is best to control the effusion as quickly and efficiently as possible. My own experience with talc poudrage has been similar to that reported here. I would agree that these patients should be treated earlier rather than later. My practice is to proceed with pleurodesis if the patient has to be tapped on a second occasion for symptomatic relief.

To date, it has not been proven that talc pleurodesis by thorascopy and poudrage is superior to talc slurry by chest tube at the bedside. Currently, there is an ongoing multicenter trial in North America to evaluate this question. The results of that trial should be available sometime in 1998. Another important result of this ongoing trial will be clarification of the issue of hypoxic respiratory failure or acute respiratory distress syndrome as a sequelae of talc pleurodesis. Until now we have seen only sporadic reports of this complication, and it appears to be more common when higher doses of talc (10 gm) are used. Most centers performing talc pleurodesis currently use a total talc dose of 3–5 gm.

J.R. Jett, M.D.

51 Chronic Obstructive Pulmonary Disease

Outcomes Following Acute Exacerbation of Severe Chronic Obstructive Lung Disease
Connors AF Jr; Dawson NV, Thomas C, et al (Case Western Reserve Univ, Cleveland, Ohio; Duke Univ, Durham, NC; Marshfield Med Research Found/ Marshfield Clinic, Wis; et al)
Am J Respir Crit Care Med 154:959–967, 1996   51–1

Objective.—Most previous studies of the outcomes of chronic obstructive pulmonary disease (COPD) have been in small numbers of patients from a single hospital, focusing on hospital mortality. Little is known about how an acute exacerbation of COPD affects functional status or quality of life after recovery, or about the resources used in caring for such exacerbations. The long-term outcomes of acute exacerbations of COP, including the clinical factors associated with survival, were prospectively studied.

Methods.—The study cohort consisted of 1,016 adult patients from 5 hospitals admitted with an exacerbation of COPD. All had breathlessness, respiratory failure, or change in mental status caused by COPD as their man reason for admission, as well as a $PaCO_2$ of 50 mm Hg or greater. Patient outcomes evaluated were survival, hospital and ICU length of stay, intensity of care, functional status, health status, health utility, and quality of life.

Findings.—The patients as a group were elderly and ill; 78% had at least 2 co-existing illnesses. The index exacerbation was associated with infection in 51% of cases, usually a respiratory infection, and with congestive heart failure in 26% of cases. Estimated probability of death within 2 months was 20%. Most patients had increased heart and respiratory rates and severe hypoxemia and hypercarbia, with a median $PaCO_2$ of 56 mm Hg. Eighty-nine percent of patients survived to hospital discharge. However, survival decreased to 80% at 2 months and 67% at 6 months. Kaplan-Meier survival was 57.5% at 1 year and 51% at 2 years (Fig 1). Factors associated with reduced survival were mechanical ventilation and an ICU stay. Eighty-one percent of patients who survived to hospital discharge were discharged home.

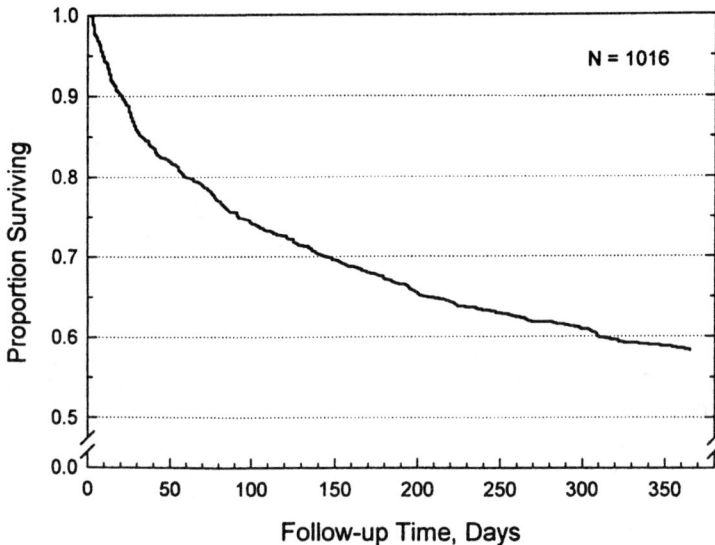

FIGURE 1.—One-year survival for 1,016 patients with severe acute exacerbation of COPD, The Kaplan-Meier survival estimates over the 365 d after study entry are shown. Although moderate hospital mortality (11%) was seen, there was considerable mortality in the months after the index admission. (Courtesy of Connors A Jr, for the Support Investigators: Outcomes following acute exacerbation of severe chronic obstructive lung disease. *Am J Respir Crit Care Med* 154:959–967, official journal of the American Thoracic Society, copyright 1996, American Lung Association.)

Fifty percent of patients discharged from the hospital were readmitted within 6 months, and 22% were readmitted more than once. Mortality was increased significantly for patients requiring readmission. In their initial hospitalization, 53% of patients spent time in the ICU (median stay 2 days) and 35% were mechanically ventilated. Thirty-eight percent of total hospital days were spent in the ICU. The total cost for the patients during their index hospitalizations was $16.4 million, with a median cost of $7,400. By 6 months, 54% of patients required assistance with activities of daily living. Just 21% considered themselves to be in good to excellent health. In a multivariate model, survival was independently related to severity of illness, body mass index, age, prior functional status, PaO_2/FiO_2, congestive heart failure, serum albumin, and cor pulmonale.

Conclusions.—Though hospital survival is relatively good for patients hospitalized for an exacerbation of COPD, the risk of death rises in the subsequent months. Patients who survive are at risk of readmission to the hospital or nursing home admission. They are likely to be dependent in activities of daily living, and their quality of life is poor. The multivariate model developed in this study can predict a patient's probability of survival using readily available clinical information.

▶ This is a valuable study for several reasons. It is a very large study, including more than 1,000 patients, and it is prospective. The population is selected: only hypercapnic COPD patients with acute exacerbations requiring hospitalization, many of whom had other medical problems, were studied. Nevertheless some important results emerge. While hospital mortality is only 11 per cent, nearly half the patients are dead within 2 years after the hospitalization. Costs of care were high with high rates of ICU admission and half of patients surviving to discharge requiring readmission. In addition, quality of life during this time is rated as fair or poor by a majority of patients. The value of a study such as this is 2-fold. It allows caretakers on the one hand and patients on the other to use the individual patient data to make a realistic assessment of the patient's prognosis. This may assist in the discussions of advanced directives or other end-of-life decisions.

J.R. Maurer, M.D.

Reducing Length of Stay for Patients Hospitalized With Exacerbation of COPD by Using a Practice Guideline
Kong GK, Belman MJ, Weingarten S (Univ of California, Los Angeles)
Chest 111:89–94, 1997   51–2

Background.—Recent research suggests that patients with chronic obstructive pulmonary disease may stay in the hospital longer than necessary. In a retrospective study, a practice guideline for patients hospitalized for exacerbation of COPD appeared to have the potential to save hospital days without compromising quality of care through early discharge of low-risk patients. A prospective assessment of this practice guideline for low-risk COPD patients was performed.

Retrospective Study.—The retrospective study included 250 consecutive patients hospitalized for exacerbation of COPD. The practice guideline stated that patients with none of a list of complications after 72 hours in the hospital could be considered low-risk and considered for early discharge. Those with major complications during the first 72 hours were excluded. According to the guideline, 95% of patients were considered low-risk.

Prospective Study.—The guideline was prospectively studied over a 12-month period, with alternating months between guideline and control periods. This study included 124 patients. In contrast to the retrospective study, only 19% were identified as low risk. For those patients so identified, the length of stay was not significantly reduced. In both the control and intervention groups, the length of stay for COPD exacerbation declined over time.

Conclusions.—The practice guideline evaluated in this study seemed to have potential to reduce hospital stay in patients with COPD. However, on prospective examination, the guideline did not reduce length of stay and may even have increased costs. Clinical practice guidelines should be tested prospectively before widespread implementation.

▶ One of the offshoots of the near universal move to managed care is the development of clinical practice guidelines which are generally felt to represent an acceptable standard of practice in dealing with whatever the condition the guidelines addresses. These are derived as much as possible from existing literature (evidence-based) and from expert opinion. They are usually not, however, validated by prospective studies before they are published in professional journals. This study illustrates the potential pitfalls of the endorsement of clinically unvalidated guidelines. Perhaps prospective "validation" of proposed guidelines should be required before endorsement of these guidelines especially when they are likely to affect large numbers of patients and be widely followed by managed care organizations.

J.R. Maurer, M.D.

Attitudes Regarding Advance Directives Among Patients in Pulmonary Rehabilitation
Heffner JE, Fahy B, Hilling L, et al (St. Joseph's Hospital, Phoenix, Ariz; Univ of Ariz, Tucson; Mt. Diablo Med Ctr, Concord, Calif)
Am J Respir Crit Care Med 154:1735–1740, 1996   51–3

Introduction.—Advance directives (ADs) enable patients to communicate their wishes at the end of life and designate surrogates for substituted judgment. Despite efforts to promote ADs, patients usually do not ask about them and physicians often fail to bring up the subject. A survey of patients with chronic lung conditions was designed to assess their knowledge, opinions, and attitudes about end-of-life issues.

Methods.—Patients surveyed were enrolled in pulmonary rehabilitation programs, one in Arizona and another in California. All outpatient adults attending the programs were eligible for the study. A total of 105 patients received a 41-item, self-directed questionnaire to complete at home. In addition to demographic and health-status information, the survey gathered responses about attitudes, beliefs, understanding, health concerns, and preferences regarding life-support interventions and ADs.

Results.—All 105 eligible patients completed the questionnaire. Although drawn from only 2 sites, few patients were under the care of the same physician. The mean patient age was 67.6; 61.9% were married and 68.5% had some college education. Chronic obstructive pulmonary disease was present in 86.7%, and 61.9% had previously been hospitalized for complications of their lung condition. Most worried about their health (94.3%) and had formulated opinions (93.8%) about undergoing intubation. Overall, 41.9% had completed a living-will document. Older age made it more likely that a patient had a living will or a durable power of attorney document. Although 98.9% expressed a desire for patient-physician AD discussions, only 19.0% had such discussions and only 14.3% thought that their physicians understood their end-of-life wishes. Most patients said that baseline health status or likely clinical outcome would govern the decision for life-support interventions. About half (49.5%) wanted the decision to be based on their explicit AD documents; 38.1% would leave the decision to their appointed surrogate.

Conclusion.—Most of these patients with chronic lung conditions had definite opinions about end-of-life issues, including ADs and life-support intervention preferences. Patients want to discuss these topics with their physician, but few physicians initiate the discussion.

▶ Physicians still feel uncomfortable discussing end-of-life plans with their patients! In this article, more than 98% of patients answering a questionnaire wanted information about end-of-life issues; however, less than 20% actually had these discussions and most preferred to have these discussions with their physicians. Ideally, either the patient or physician could initiate such discussions (which virtually always reduce the anxiety and distress at the time of dying), but patients expect the physician to take this role. And the physician often does not. The authors suggest that education regarding advance directives could be disseminated as part of pulmonary rehabilitation programs. This is a good idea, as we need to be more sensitive to meeting all of the patient's needs. It would also be a good idea to offer ongoing education and techniques for physicians who, because of their own discomfort, avoid these end-of-life topics.

J.R. Maurer, M.D.

Adverse Effects of Corticosteroid Therapy: A Critical Review
McEvoy CE, Niewoehner DE (Univ of Minnesota, Minneapolis)
Chest 111:732–743, 1997   51–4

Introduction.—For the treatment of chronic obstructive pulmonary disease (COPD), inhaled and systemic corticosteroids are commonly prescribed. Regarding efficacy of steroid therapy in COPD, there is insufficient evidence, despite their frequent use. Long-term, large studies assessing the clinical outcomes of corticoid treatment for stable or acute COPD are yet to be conducted. The purported adverse systemic effects associated with the use of corticosteroids in the treatment of COPD are reviewed.

Systemic corticosteroids.—Some of the adverse events of corticosteroid therapy include osteoporosis, adrenal insufficiency, cataract formation, dermal thinning, diabetes, hypertension, psychosis, infection, and hyperadrenocorticism. Skeletal decalcification as a characteristic feature of adrenal hyperplasia is seen, and osteoporosis is the most feared complication. Long-term administration of corticosteroids clearly affects hypothalamic-pituitary-adrenal function, but the magnitude of the effects is uncertain. Peptic ulcer disease does not seem to be associated with systemic corticosteroid use, but patients with an associated history of tobacco use should be further investigated. A previous study showed a dose-dependent relationship with acute psychiatric reactions, particularly acute psychosis or inappropriate euphoria. A modest increase in lethal and nonlethal infections has been associated with systemic corticosteroids. A significant increase in the number of newly diagnosed cases of diabetes mellitus has been linked with systemic corticosteroid therapy.

Inhaled corticosteroids.—Inhaled corticosteroids may have less potential for serious adverse effects than systemic corticosteroids. Local reactions caused by their deposition in the oropharynx are the most common adverse effects of inhaled corticosteroids, such as dysphonia, oropharyngeal candidiasis, wheezing, and cough. In adult asthmatics taking inhaled corticosteroids, positive throat cultures for Candida species are commonly found. Simple measures such as spacer devices, mouth rinsing, and reduction in dosage can usually help to manage these topical phenomena. A few case reports have linked inhaled corticosteroids with insomnia, depression, mania, euphoria, nightmares, and somnolence.

Conclusion.—The clinician must evaluate whether the benefits of such therapy outweigh the potential for adverse events while awaiting the results of more definitive prospective trials. A grater risk for adverse events is seen in the population of patients with COPD who generally are older, less active, and have significant tobacco histories. Assessments of risk should be made on a disease-specific basis as different diseases may place patients at greater or lesser risk of corticosteroid complications.

▶ The controversy of whether either oral or inhaled corticosteroids, particularly given chronically, are of proven benefit in patients with COPD rages on. These authors begin with the premise that very little proof exists regarding the benefits of these drugs and then go on to examine the evidence documenting the myriad toxicities, especially of the oral steroids. Unfortunately, very little of the side-effect literature is disease-specific, making it difficult to comment directly on the impact in COPD patients. Nevertheless, it does give one pause while considering the potential for precipitating significant morbidity in this elderly group of patients in whom steroid side effects may create significant changes in quality of life. Quite appropriately, the authors make a plea for disease-specific studies to better delineate the impact of steroid toxicity in the chronic lung disease population.

J.R. Maurer, M.D.

Cystic Fibrosis

A Prognostic Model for the Prediction of Survival in Cystic Fibrosis
Hayllar KM, Williams SGJ, Wise AE, et al (King's College Hosp, London; Charing Cross Hosp, London; Brompton Natl Heart and Lung Hosp, London)
Thorax 52:313–317, 1997   51–5

Introduction.—The cornerstone of treatment for endstage cystic fibrosis (CF) is double-lung, heart-lung, or heart-lung-liver transplantation. An accurate prediction of survival is needed to optimize the timing and results of transplantation. Predictors of short- and medium-term survival in patients with CF were examined to create a prognostic model which allows accurate prediction of survival.

Methods.—Data was gathered prospectively in a cohort of 403 patients (cohort A) with CF who were recruited between 1967–1987. A prognostic model was generated after determining variables that accurately predict survival. The model was validated with cohort A, then subsequently validated in a further cohort of 100 patients with CF recruited between 1988–1993.

Results.—During the study period, 188 (50.4%) patients in cohort A died. Factors significantly correlated with survival were: percentage predicted forced expiratory volume in one second, percentage predicted forced vital capacity, short stature, high white cell count, and chronic liver disease (presence of hepatomegaly). These variables accurately predicted 1 year survival in cohort A and cohort B.

Conclusion.—This prognostic model may be useful in predicting prognosis in other patient cohorts with CF. This should add valuable information to criteria used to judge short- and medium-term management of patients with CF.

▶ Since the publication of the article by Kerem et al[1]. delineating prognostic factors in cystic fibrosis patients, the selection of these patients for lung transplantation has become much more sophisticated, as has the ability to counsel patients on their expected survivals. Subsequent articles have sought to better define and refine the factors identified by Kerem et al. Hayllar et al.[2] report on a cohort of United Kingdom cystic fibrosis patients. This study identified 2 factors not previously associated with poor survivals: high white blood cell counts documented in stable patients and and hepatomegaly (presumably a marker of chronic liver disease). The large epidemiologic study of Rosenfeld et al.[3] in which approximately 85 percent of all U.S. cystic fibrosis patients seen between 1988 and 1992 were included. The most important impact of this study was to confirm the earlier finding of Kerem et al, of excess mortality in females aged less than 20 years, a point which has been challenged by some.

J.R. Maurer, M.D.

References

1. Kerem E, Reisman J, Corey M, et al: Prediction of mortality in patients with cystic fibrosis. *N Engl J Med* 326:1187–1191, 1992.
2. Hayllar KM, Williams, Wise AE, et al: A prognostic model for the prediction of survival in cystic fibrosis, *Thorax* 52:313–337, 1997.
3. Rosenfeld M, Davis R, FitzSimmons S, et al: Gender gap in cystic fibrosis mortality. *Am J Epidemiol* 145:791–803, 1997.

52 Lung Volume Reduction Surgery

Results of 150 Consecutive Bilateral Lung Volume Reduction Procedures in Patients With Severe Emphysema
Cooper JD, Patterson GA, Sundaresan RS, et al (Washington Univ, St Louis, Mo)
J Thorac Cardiovasc Surg 112:1319–1330, 1996   52–1

Background.—Chronic obstructive pulmonary disease causes significant morbidity and mortality in patients with emphysema. The intermediate-term outcomes of bilateral lung volume reduction in highly selected patients with emphysema were reported.

Methods.—One hundred fifty bilateral lung volume reduction procedures were performed between January 1993 and February 1996. Criteria for patient selection were severe dyspnea; increased lung capacity; and a pattern of emphysema consisting of regions of severe destruction, hyperinflation, and poor perfusion. Patient age ranged from 36 to 77. Mean 1-second forced expiratory volume was 25% of the predicted; total lung capacity, 142% of predicted; and residual volume, 283% of predicted. Using a linear stapler and bovine pericardial strips attached to buttress the staple line, the surgeon excised 20% to 30% of the volume of each lung. Supplemental oxygen was needed in 93% of the patients, continuously or with exertion.

Findings.—The mortality rate at 90 days was 4%. Extubation at the end of the procedure was possible in all but 1 patient. With experience, length of hospital stay declined. The last 50 patients had a median stay of 7 days. The major complication was prolonged air leakage. At 6 months, the 1-second forced expiratory volume was increased by 51% and the residual volume decreased by 28%. The partial pressure of arterial oxygen rose by a mean 8 mm Hg. Seventy percent of the patients who had needed continuous supplemental oxygen before surgery no longer needed it. The improvements in measured pulmonary function were accompanied by a significant decline in dyspnea and improved quality of life. These benefits were well maintained at 1 and 2 years.

Conclusion.—In highly selected patients with severe emphysema, lung volume reduction provides benefits that can only be achieved otherwise by lung transplantation. Preoperative rehabilitation is essential.

Bilateral Lung Volume Reduction Surgery for Advanced Emphysema: A Comparison of Median Sternotomy and Thoracoscopic Approaches
Kotloff RM, Tino G, Bavaria JE, et al (Univ of Pennsylvania, Philadelphia)
Chest 110:1399–1406, 1996   52–2

Background.—At the authors' center, lung volume reduction surgery in patients with advanced emphysema has been performed by median sternotomy (MS) and by video-assisted thoracoscopic surgery (VATS), according to individual surgeons' preferences. The short-term outcomes of the procedures done by MS and VATS were compared.

Methods.—Eighty patients underwent surgery by MS and 40 by VATS. In all patients, preoperative assessment included pulmonary function testing, arterial blood gas determination, and a 6-minute walk test. Pulmonary function testing and the walk test were repeated 3 to 6 months after surgery.

Findings.—At the end of surgery, all patients were extubated, but 17.5% of those in the MS group and 2.5% in the VATS group later needed reintubation. Mortality rates at 30 days were 4.2% and 2.5% in the MS and VATS groups, respectively. Although this difference was nonsignificant, the total in-hospital mortality rate was 13.8% for the MS group and

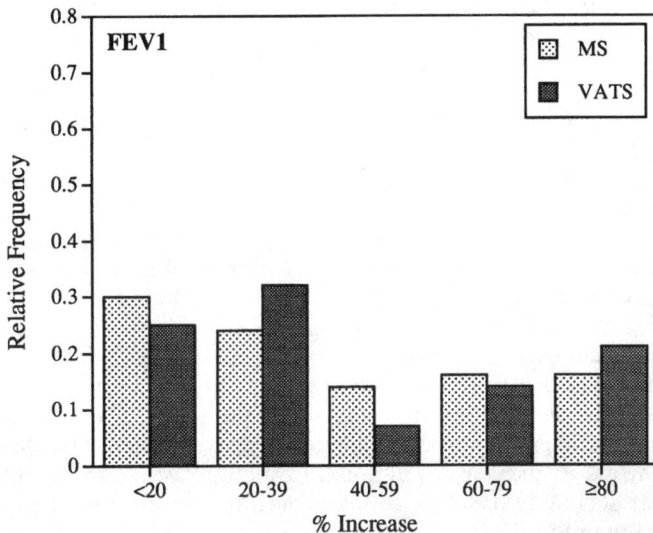

FIGURE 1.—Distribution of postoperative changes in forced expiratory volume in 1 second (FEV_1). *Abbreviations: MS*, median sternotomy; *VATS*, video-assisted thoracoscopic surgery. (Courtesy of Kotloff RM, Tino G, Bavaria JE, et al: Bilateral lung volume reduction surgery for advanced emphysema. *Chest* 110:1399–1406, 1996.)

remained unchanged in the VATS group. Deaths occurred mainly among elderly patients. The 2 groups did not differ significantly in the duration of air leaks or length of hospital stay. The functional outcomes associated with the 2 methods were similar (Fig 1).

Conclusion.—Bilateral lung volume reduction surgery by MS and VATS results in comparable improvement in pulmonary function and exercise tolerance. Video-assisted thoracoscopic surgery is associated with a significantly reduced incidence of respiratory failure and a trend toward lower in-hospital mortality. Thus, this may be the preferred technique, especially in high-risk patients.

▶ Selection is only 1 of the many questions regarding volume reduction surgery that remain to be answered. Of most importance to many is: "If it works, how long does the improvement last?" A second major question is: "What is the best surgical approach?" These 2 articles address some aspects of both issues. The group from Washington University was 1 of the first to report large numbers using the MS approach and, in this report, includes follow-ups of up to 2 years. They provide data on hospital stay, suggesting that experience with the procedure may be important in outcomes and reduced hospital stays.

The second article compares VATS and MS. Early outcomes are comparable in this study, but the follow-up is very short. Note that prolonged air leak is the most common complication listed in both articles and seems to be a problem with either type of procedure. Again, more patients and longer follow-up are needed to adequately compare surgical techniques and outcome durability.

J.R. Maurer, M.D.

53 Asthma

Changes in Peak Flow, Symptom Score, and the Use of Medications During Acute Exacerbations of Asthma
Chan-Yeung M, Chang JH, Manfreda J, et al (Univ of British Columbia, Vancouver, Canada; Univ of Manitoba, Winnipeg, Canada)
Am J Respir Crit Care Med 154:889–893, 1996   53–1

Background.—Few studies have investigated the value of serial peak expiratory flow rate (PEF) measures for early detection of an acute exacerbation and monitoring compared with symptom diaries. A panel study of the effects of environmental exposures on patients with asthma included the keeping of symptom and medication-requirement diaries as well as twice-daily measures of PEF for 1 year.

Methods.—Forty-one patients and matched controls participated in the panel study. Changes in symptoms, PEF, and the use of medications during acute exacerbations of asthma were analyzed. Data from 9 to 7 days before the onset of an acute exacerbation comprised the baseline data, with which data from the subsequent 14 days were compared. A PEF decrease of 30% from the patient's best reading was 1 criterion for acute exacerbation. Others included any unscheduled visit to a physician or emergency department or hospitalization for treatment of asthma, asthma symptom increases during the day and night for more than 48 hours not responding to usual medications, and the initiation or doubling of the dose of orally given or inhaled steroids for any of the foregoing reasons.

Findings.—Significant symptomatic increases occurred before a significant decrease in PEF. No patient had a decline of more than 30% in PEF before the onset of symptoms. Daily PEF variation was not significantly greater than baseline (Table 2).

Conclusions.—Peak expiratory flow rate monitoring is not as sensitive as a symptom diary for revealing acute exacerbations of asthma. A 30% reduction in PEF is too stringent a criterion for defining an acute exacerbation.

▶ Considerable emphasis has been recently placed on the utility of measuring peak flows in patients with asthma to improve treatment and alert patients and physicians to impending exacerbations at an earlier stage. Numerous patient education plans spend a considerable amount of time and effort to encourage patients to routinely perform peak flows. However,

TABLE 2.—Comparison of Proportion of Individuals With Varying
Maximal Decrease in Mean Peak Expiratory Flow and Morning Peak
Expiratory Flow on Days 6 to 14 of Acute Exacerbation

Maximal	% Subjects	
Decrease in PEF	Mean PEF	Morning PEF
< 10%	21.6	27.0
10–20%	27.0	29.7
20–30%	24.3	16.2
> 30%	27.0	27.0

(Courtesy of Chan-Yeung M, Chang JH, Manfreda J, et al: Changes in peak flow, symptom score, and the use of medications during acute exacerbations of asthma. *Am J Respir Crit Care Med* 154:889–893, official journal of the American Thoracic Society, copyright 1996, American Lung Association.)

several recent studies have called into question the utility of peak flows in following the status of patients with asthma chronically.

This study further supports these earlier ones by determining that neither the daily peak flow nor the change in peak flow throughout the day is an accurate predictor of exacerbations of asthma. This observation continued to hold true even when the threshold for exacerbations was dropped to 20% decrease in peak flow, with only 51% of exacerbations meeting that criterion. In fact, patient symptoms, as recorded in a diary, more accurately predict the development of an exacerbation. Although this study had a much more controlled set of symptom scores than patients would have reported otherwise, it certainly raises the question of whether time and money might more wisely be spent on the development and implementation of patient symptom diaries, rather than routine monitoring of peak flow.

S.E. Wenzel, M.D.

A Controlled Trial of Immunotherapy for Asthma in Allergic Children
Adkinson NF Jr, Eggleston PA, Eney D, et al (Johns Hopkins Univ, Baltimore, Md; Johns Hopkins School of Hygiene and Public Health, Baltimore, Md)
N Engl J Med 336:324–331, 1997   53–2

Background.—Few clinical trials of multiple-allergen treatment for perennial allergic asthma have been performed. The additive benefit of broad-spectrum immunotherapy was investigated in the current randomized, placebo-controlled study.

Methods.—One hundred twenty-one children with moderate-to-severe, perennial asthma and allergies were included. All were receiving daily medication for asthma. Subcutaneous injections of a mix of up to 7 aeroallergen extracts or placebo were given, as well as maintenance injections for 18 months or more. Medications were adjusted every 2–3 weeks based on peak flow rates and symptoms.

Findings.—Median medication scores decreased from 5.4 to 4.9 in the immunotherapy group and from 5.2 to 5 in the placebo group (a nonsignificant between-group difference). The number of days of oral corticosteroid use was comparable in the 2 groups. Thirty-one percent of the immunotherapy group and 28% of the placebo group had partial or complete remission of asthma. The groups did not differ in their use of medical care, symptoms, or peak flow rates.

Conclusions.—In these children with perennial asthma and allergies receiving appropriate medical treatment, immunotherapy with injections of allergens for more than 2 years was not beneficial. These findings are not consistent with common clinical opinion and previous research.

▶ Immunotherapy (IT) with allergen extracts has been used for the prophylactic management of allergic diseases in children and adults for more than 80 years. Although a previously published meta-analysis had suggested that IT was moderately effective in improving objective parameters of asthma,[1] the number of large, placebo-controlled studies of sufficient duration evaluating the efficacy of IT in perennial (year-round) asthma is scarce. The current study evaluated 121 children with allergies and asthma to determine whether there was any added benefit of IT to conventional pharmacotherapy for asthma. This was a carefully done study that stabilized patients on an optimal medical regimen for more than 1 year. Patients were evaluated with skin-prick reactivity and radioallergoabsorbant (RAST) testing and were randomized to a placebo or IT arm (based on their responses) for the next year. The responses for all outcome parameters (including medication use and methacholine reactivity) in the 2 groups were nearly identical, which suggested that IT had no impact on perennial, moderate asthma when given concurrently with standard medical care.

However, 2 important caveats must be mentioned. The first is that no children in this study were treated with cockroach extracts—allergens that, increasingly, have been thought to be at least as important as the house dust mite in perennial allergies. Therefore, a large portion of the causative allergens "may" have been missed. Secondly, when subgroup analysis was performed, there were "suggestions" that treating younger children with milder asthma may have a favorable impact on the disease. Whether IT could prove to be preventive for the development of more severe chronic disease will require further study. Therefore, although this study once again suggests that IT is not effective in moderate-to-severe perennial asthma, further studies are still necessary, including those to determine whether certain subgroups with mild, short-duration asthma may benefit from early intervention. Until that time, IT cannot be recommended as a treatment for perennial asthma.

S.E. Wenzel, M.D.

Reference

1. Abramson MJ, Puy RM, Weiner JM. Is allergen immunotherapy effective in asthma? *Am J Respir Crit Care Med* 151; 969–974, 1995.

Incidence and Outcomes of Asthma in the Elderly: A Population-based Study in Rochester, Minnesota

Bauer BA, Reed CE, Yunginger JW, et al (Mayo Clinic, Rochester, Minn)
Chest 111:303–310, 1997   53–3

Objective.—Asthma sufferers older than 65 may be underdiagnosed and undertreated. Results of a community-based retrospective cohort study of 102 Rochester, Minnesota, residents diagnosed between 1964 and 1983 with asthma or asthmatic symptoms after age 65, describes their clinical characteristics, use of health services, and long-term survival.

Methods.—Medical records of 102 elderly patients diagnosed with asthma or asthmatic symptoms were reviewed, and 4 patients were excluded because of evidence of chronic obstructive pulmonary disease (COPD). Incidence rates were determined for four 5-year time periods for age groups 65 to 74, 75 to 84, and 85 years and older. Results were analyzed statistically.

Results.—Of the 98 patients (46 men) accepted into the study, 61 were aged 65 to 74 years, 30 were aged 75 to 84 years, and 7 were aged 85 or older. More than half of the patients had a smoking history. The most frequently reported symptoms were wheezing, dyspnea, and cough. The overall age- and sex-adjusted incidence of asthma was 95/100,000. The age-adjusted incidence for males was 126/100,000 and for females was 74/100,000. The age-adjusted incidence was 103/100,000 for ages 65 to 74, 81/100,000 for ages 75 to 84, and 58/100,000 for those aged 85 or older. Men were significantly more likely to have asthma than women. Elderly asthmatic patients had a higher than average utilization of healthcare services. Less than half of the patients had pulmonary function tests, 25% had peak flow measurements, few had allergy skin tests and serum IgE determinations, 15% had an allergy consultation, and 20% had a pulmonary consultation. Less than one-third had pulmonary function test results. About 80% of elderly asthmatic patients had 1 or more ambulatory visits for asthma, 40% had unscheduled ambulatory visits. 22% had emergency department visits, and 42% were hospitalized for asthma. Survival at 1, 5, and 10 years was 95%, 72%, and 57%, respectively. Observed survival was similar to expected survival.

Conclusion.—Although asthma is common in the elderly, pulmonary function tests are performed infrequently. Diagnostic evaluation should be pursued more aggressively, particularly in light of the increased utilization of health services by these elderly patients. Observed survival of these patients was similar to expected survival.

▶ Newly diagnosed asthma in the elderly is poorly understood, with very few data to help understand epidemiology or pathogenesis. The authors performed a retrospective chart analysis of medical records in the Rochester, Minnesota, area, looking for cases of definite and "probable" asthma in the population over 65 years of age. Although the study has flaws based on the retrospective study design and the criteria for classifying chronic obstructive pulmonary disease vs. asthma in patients with a smoking history (of which 54% of the identified individuals had at least some history), the study is an initial attempt to further define the population of elderly patients who wheeze. Interestingly, the evaluation of many of these patients appeared to be very limited, with only a few undergoing pulmonary function or allergy testing. Most complained of symptoms arising after an upper respiratory infection. In the patients who did undergo spirometry, little evidence for reversible obstruction existed, implying that either a large percent of COPD patients with fixed airflow limitation were included or that asthma in patients of 65 years of age may tend to present with a more irreversible process. This population also appeared to have a high health care utilization, with 42% of the population requiring a hospitalization in the year of follow-up, but without an effect on mortality rates. The combination of high health care utilization and underutilization of evaluation (and potentially appropriate treatment) may imply that asthma (and, perhaps, COPD) in the elderly is underdiagnosed, underappreciated, and undertreated.

S.E. Wenzel, M.D.

Effect of Long Term Treatment With Salmeterol on Asthma Control: A Double-blind, Randomised Crossover Study
Wilding P, Clark M, Thompson Coon J, et al (City Hosp, Nottingham, England; Univ Hosp, Nottingham, England)
BMJ 314:1441–1446, 1997   53–4

Objective.—Some studies indicate that administration of β_2 agonist treatment for asthma as required according to symptoms and peak expiratory flow measurements is more effective than regular administration of the drug. The long term efficacy and safety of salmeterol was studied in patients with mild to moderate asthma who took salmeterol and placebo for 6 weeks each.

Methods.—Morning and evening peak expiratory flow was measured in 101 asthmatic patients (50 females), aged 19 to 60 years, taking at least 200 γ beclomethasone dipropionate or budesonide twice daily. Patients received either 50 γ twice daily or placebo for 6 months and then crossed over to the opposite treatment arm after a 1-month washout period. Patients adjusted their inhaled steroid use according to predetermined criteria based on symptoms and peak expiratory flow.

Results.—There were 87 patients who completed the study. Inhaled steroid use was a significant 17% lower in salmeterol users than in placebo users. Salmeterol patients initially using ≤600 γ inhaled steroid reduced their steroid use by 19% compared with placebo patients (329 vs. 404 γ). Salmeterol patients initially using >600 γ inhaled steroid reduced their steroid use by 14% compared with placebo patients. There was no significant difference between groups with respect to exacerbations or oral steroid treatments. Morning and evening peak expiratory flow, forced expiratory volume, and forced vital capacity were significantly higher in

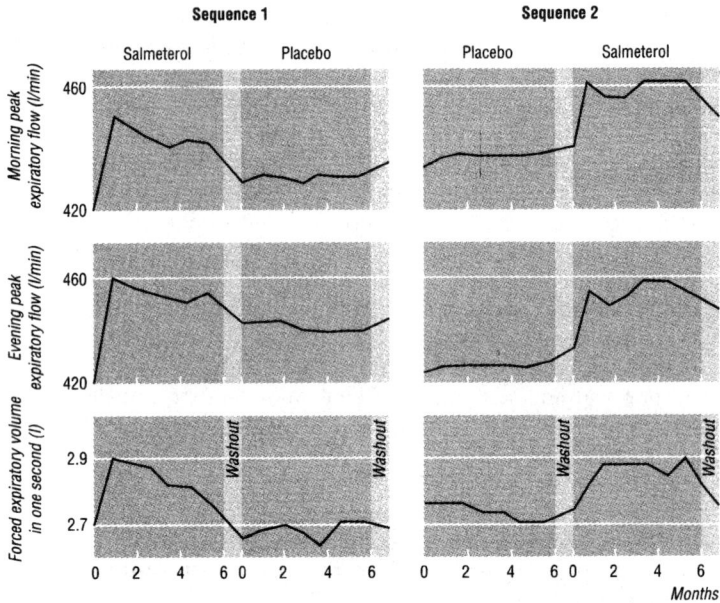

FIGURE 2.—Mean morning and evening peak flow and forced expiratory volume in 1 second during treatment with salmeterol and placebo, according to whether salmeterol was given first (sequence 1) or second (sequence 2). (Courtesy of Wilding P, Clark M, Thompson Coon J, et al: Effect of long term treatment with salmeterol on asthma control: A double-blind, randomised crossover study. *BMJ* 314:1441–1446, 1997, by permission of the BMJ Publishing Group.)

the salmeterol group than in the placebo group (Fig 2). Salmeterol users had more symptom-free days and nights, less bronchodilator use, and a higher response to methacholine. Serum potassium levels, heart rate, and frequency of ectopic beats of salmeterol and placebo users were similar. Two salmeterol patients and 1 placebo patient were withdrawn because of adverse events. Salmeterol patients had more palpitations.

Conclusion.—Lung function improved and asthma symptoms decreased in salmeterol patients who reduced their inhaled steroid use according to predetermined criteria.

▶ The appropriate combination of medications for the treatment of mild-moderate persistent asthma remains controversial. Several short-term studies suggest that the combination of a long-acting beta agonist, such as salmeterol (Serevent®) with a low dose of inhaled steroid is more effective in improving pulmonary function and symptoms than increasing the dose of inhaled steroids further. As salmeterol is not known to have any obvious anti inflammatory properties, concern has continued that this combination, with its potent effect on symptoms, decreases the patient's reliance on inhaled steroids, consequently decreasing the anti inflammatory effects. However, as the use of inflammation itself to monitor asthma control remains in doubt, long-term studies following clinical outcomes such as deterioration in pulmonary function testing and exacerbation rates with various treatment regimens are needed.

The Wilding, et al.'s study begins to address some of these issues. Patients "well-controlled" on moderate doses of inhaled steroids were randomized to treatment with the addition of placebo or salmeterol in a cross over design, with 6 months per treatment arm. In this "long-term" study, subjects on salmeterol were able to reduce their inhaled steroid dose by 17%, while improving forced expiratory volume in 1 second, peak flows and symptom scores as compared to placebo (Fig 2). More importantly, although not statistically different, there were fewer exacerbations on salmeterol + steroids than on placebo + steroids, despite the higher dose used. Interestingly, even with these drugs, fully 34% required oral steroids at some time during the 6 months of the study, despite entering under what was felt to be "good control." "Markers" of inflammation were not evaluated in this study.

The results of this study are interesting. Clearly, they raise concern over the idea that treatment of inflammation is the "only" approach to the treatment of asthma, suggesting that "other factors" are also important. Lastly, the surprising need for oral steroids in 34% of the patients during the 6 months of the study, suggests that even "state-of-the-art" treatment of asthma does not lead to an obliteration of exacerbations. Better pharmacologic treatment of asthma is still needed.

S.E. Wenzel, M.D.

Leukotriene Antagonist Prevents Exacerbation of Asthma During Reduction of High-dose Inhaled Corticosteroid
Tamaoki J, for the Tokyo Joshi-Idai Asthma Research Group (Tokyo Women's Med College, Japan; et al)
Am J Respir Crit Care Med 155:1235–1240, 1997   53–5

Introduction.—Although high-dose inhaled corticosteroids are increasingly prescribed for the maintenance treatment of all degrees of asthma, the safety of their long-term use is a matter of concern. A randomized trial was conducted to determine whether the leukotriene antagonist ONO-1078 (pranlukast) prevents asthma exacerbations during reduction of high-dose inhaled beclomethasone dipropionate (BDI).

Methods.—The study was conducted at 5 centers in Japan. Eligible patients had symptoms of asthma well controlled by inhaled BDI at a daily dose of 1,500 µg or more for at least 6 weeks before the study. A 2-week run-in period was followed by a 6-week double-blind treatment period during which daily doses of BDI were halved in all patients. Forty-two patients received ONO-1078 (450 mg twice daily) and 37 were given placebo. All visited the outpatient clinic each week during the run-in and treatment periods and recorded medications and symptoms daily.

Results.—The placebo and active treatment groups were similar in baseline characteristics. By the end of the treatment period, FEV$_1$ de-

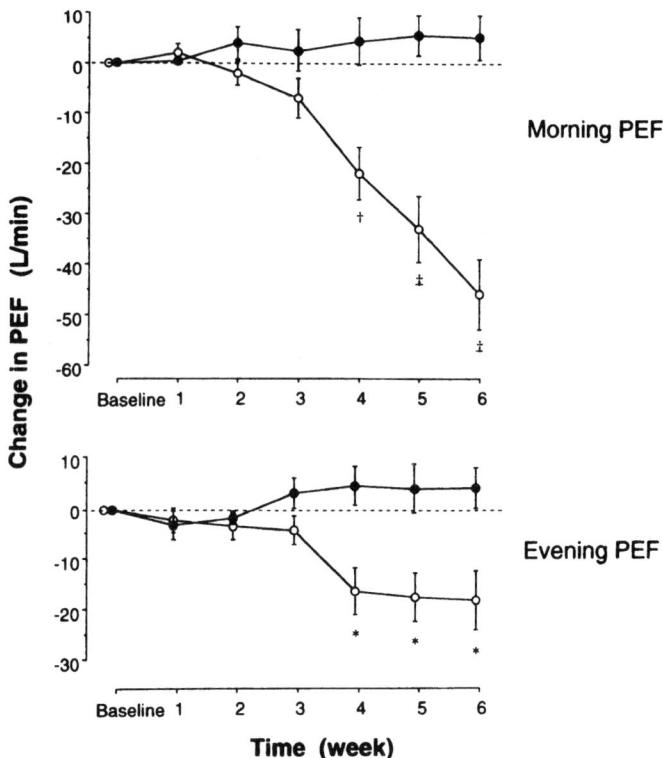

FIGURE 1.—Changes in mean morning and evening PEF during 6 wk of treatment with ONO-1078 (*closed circles*) or placebo (*open circles*). After baseline period, the dose of inhaled beclomethasone dipropionate was reduced to half in each patient. Values represent mean (± SEM) changes in weekly PEF. *p <0.05, †p <0.01, ‡p <0.001, significantly different from baseline values. *Abbreviation: PEF,* peak expiratory flow. (Courtesy of Tamaoki J, for the Tokyo Joshi-Idai Asthma Research Group: Leukotriene antagonist prevents exacerbation of asthma during reduction of high-dose inhaled corticosteroid. *Am J Respir Crit Care Med* 155:1235–1240, official journal of the American Thoracic Society, copyright 1997, American Lung Association.)

creased by a mean of 0.33 L (10.2% from baseline) in the placebo group and was unchanged in the ONO-1078 group. Mean morning peak expiratory flow (PEF) fell from baseline in the placebo group (Fig 1), to a maximal decrease of 46 L/min at week 6. In contrast, mean morning PEF was sustained above baseline throughout the treatment period in the ONO-1078 group. Mean evening PEF showed similar differences in the 2 groups. Differences in daytime and night-time asthma symptoms were less marked, but the increase in the number of daytime asthma symptoms was significantly greater at week 6 in the placebo group (Fig 2). During weeks 5 and 6, asthma symptoms woke patients in the placebo group 61% of nights, vs 46% of nights in the ONO-1078 group. The need for relief medication increased at weeks 5 and 6 in the placebo group, but not in the ONO-1078 group. Concentrations of serum eosinophil cationic protein and exhaled nitric oxide increased only in the placebo group.

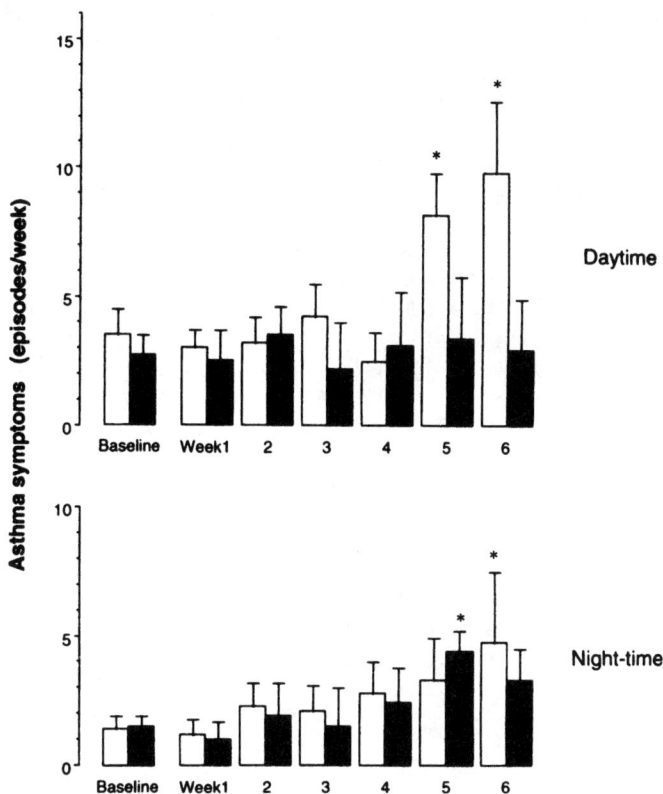

FIGURE 2.—Changes in the number of daytime and night time asthma symptoms during 6 wk of treatment with ONO-1078 (*closed columns*) or placebo (*open columns*). After baseline period, the dose of inhaled beclomethasone dipropionate was reduced to half in each patient. Values represent mean (± SEM) changes in the number of symptoms per week. *p <0.05, significantly different from baseline values. (Courtesy of Tamaoki J, for the Tokyo Joshi-Idai Asthma Research Group: Leukotriene antagonist prevents exacerbation of asthma during reduction of high-dose inhaled corticosteroid. *Am J Respir Crit Care Med* 155:1235–1240, official journal of the American Thoracic Society, copyright 1997, American Lung Association.)

Conclusion.—Recent studies indicate that the leukotriene antagonist is effective in treating allergen- and exercise-induced bronchoconstriction in patients with asthma. The findings of this study show that the cysteinyl leukotriene receptor antagonist ONO-1078 allows patients taking high doses of inhaled corticosteroid for control of asthma symptoms to reduce their steroid dose.

▶ Antiinflammatory treatment of asthma has focused on inhaled cortico-steroids, often at ever-escalating doses to improve symptoms. However, doses of inhaled corticosteroids of >1,500 g/day are not without short- and long-term side effects. Therefore, strategies have been developed to limit the steroid doses, including salmeterol, nedocromil and theophylline. However, the true "antiinflammatory" effects of any of these medications remain in question.

In the last year, drugs which modulate the inflammatory leukotriene pathway have become available in the United States. However, only minimal studies have existed regarding their abilities as "steroid-sparing" agents. The study by Tamaoki, et al., demonstrates that when inhaled corticosteroids are halved in patients taking high doses of these drugs (>1,500 g/day), a leukotriene receptor antagonist (LTRA) (ONO-1079, or pranlukast, as it is being developed in the U.S.) is capable of maintaining pulmonary function, symptom scores, and beta-agonists use as compared to placebo (Figs 1 & 2). In addition, the LTRA appeared to have a favorable effect on markers of inflammation, including seurm eosinophilic cationic protein and exhaled nitric oxide when compared to placebo. Interestingly, the effect on objective measures (peak flows, FEV_1) appeared to be greater than the effect on symptoms, especially nocturnal symptoms, where no protective effect of the LTRA was seen (Fig 2). The reasons for this dichotomy in response are unknown, but similar findings have been seen in other studies, suggesting that traditional objective measures may not accurately represent many of the pathophysiologic changes which lead to the clinical symptoms of asthma. Finally, the study was of short duration (6 weeks) and longer studies are certainly needed to evaluate effects on long-term exacerbations and urgent medical visits. However, this study preliminarily supports the beneficial effects of the combination of inhaled steroids and leukotriene modulating drugs in the treatment of asthma.

S.E. Wenzel, M.D.

Stabilization of Asthma Mortality

Sly RM, O'Donnell R (George Washington Univ, Washington, DC)
Ann Allergy Asthma Immunol 78:347–354, 1997   53–6

Background.—Asthma death rates in the United States have increased since 1978. Recent trends in asthma mortality were investigated.

Methods.—Data on asthma deaths in the 50 states and the District of Columbia were analyzed by race, age, sex, and race after age adjustment. These data were obtained from the National Center for Health Statistics and the Bureau of the Census.

Findings.—Asthma death rates increased from 0.8 per 100,000 general population in 1977 and 1978 to 2 in 1989 in the United States. In 1994, there was an increase to 2.1 per 100,000. These death rates have been much greater among white females than white males, with an increasing disparity. Asthma death rates among 5- through 34-year-olds have been much higher in blacks than whites, with no significant change between 1980 and 1994. The age-adjusted death rates for blacks of all ages rose from 1.5 in 1977 and 1978 to 3.5 in 1988 and 3.7 in 1994. The corresponding rates for whites rose from 0.5 in 1977 to 1.2 in 1989, remaining at that level through 1994. The increase in rates among blacks was significantly greater than among whites. There were significantly greater age-adjusted rates of increase for each race separately for 1979 through 1987 compared with 1988 through 1994.

Conclusions.—In most age groups, asthma death rates in the United States appear to have stabilized since 1988 at more than 50% higher than those in 1979. However, there is only a suggestion of such stabilization among persons aged 5 through 34 years, when certification of death from asthma is most accurate. Asthma death rates have been higher among blacks than whites and among white females than white males.

▶ Much has been made of the increases in asthma prevalence and mortality in the last 20 years, with asthma deaths in 1994 rising to their highest levels since 1954. However, the explanation for this phenomenon remains poorly understood. The most recent statistics may suggest that asthma mortality rates, at least, are stabilizing in certain groups in the United States, with a total asthma death rate of 1.9 to 2.1/100,000 for the years from 1988 to 1994, where the latest statistics are available. However, there remain subgroups in the total where that stabilizing trend is not yet visible, most specifically, blacks (males and females), and white females (Figs 3 & 4). These current statistics do not provide any further answers regarding cause but continue to suggest that these groups, in particular, demand special attention. It remains to be seen whether socioeconomic and environmental factors, prescribing practices, health care delivery options, or other factors are the reasons for the continued increased mortality in these groups.

S.E. Wenzel, M.D.

54 Interstitial Lung Disease

Cigarette Smoking: A Risk Factor for Idiopathic Pulmonary Fibrosis
Baumgartner KB, Samet JM, Stidley CA, et al (Univ of New Mexico, Albuquerque; Johns Hopkins Univ, Baltimore, Md; Mayo Clinic Scottsdale, Ariz; et al)
Am J Respir Crit Care Med 155:242–248, 1997   54–1

Background.—Hypotheses about the etiology of idiopathic pulmonary fibrosis (IPF) have been investigated only in descriptive reports of case series and small epidemiologic studies. The current multicenter, epidemiologic, case-control study further explored possible etiologic factors for IPF.

Methods.—Two hundred forty-eight case patients and 491 control subjects matched for sex, age, and geographic region were included. Data on potential IPF risk factors, including household, occupational, and environmental exposures to smoking, were obtained by telephone interview.

Findings.—Seventy-two percent of the patients and 63% of control subjects had a history of ever smoking. Persons who had ever smoked had a 1.6 odds ratio of IPF. The risk was increased significantly for former smokers and for current smokers with a 21- to 40-pack-year history of smoking.

Conclusions.—A history of smoking appears to increase the risk for IPF. Though no clear exposure-response patterns could be found with cumulative cigarette consumption, a trend for time since smoking cessation was noted, with the greatest risk occurring in those who had quit most recently.

▶ Idiopathic pulmonary fibrosis (IPF) is one of the most common forms of interstitial lung disease. Patients with IPF present with progressive dyspnea on exertion and/or chronic cough and have diffuse interstitial lung infiltrates on the chest radiograph. Typical inspiratory crackles (velcro crackles) are heard in most patients over the lung bases. IPF is usually progressive and is associated with a median survival of 3 to 5 years. It is characterized by inflammation in the lung parenchyma that gradually leads to diffuse fibrosis. The fibrotic process is accentuated in the bases and the peripheral zones of the lungs as seen on a high-resolution computed tomography (HRCT). The cause of this disorder is unknown, although there are speculations regarding possible environmental triggers and some familial cases exist.

This article by Baumgartner and associates is an important epidemiologic study looking for possible risk factors for idiopathic pulmonary fibrosis. This study finds cigarette smoking to be associated with the development of IPF. Aside from adding to a list of detrimental effects associated with cigarette smoking, the results of this study have some relevance in evaluating smokers. The presence of IPF may be masked on pulmonary function testing and chest radiograph when there is coexisting chronic obstructive pulmonary disease or emphysema.[1] Since restrictive and obstructive changes will tend to compensate each other, one may suspect the coexistence of IPF and chronic obstructive pulmonary disease when the patient presents with severe dyspnea that is out of proportion to the degree of spirometric abnormalities (may at times be normal) and the diffusing capacity is severely reduced.[1] Typical bibasilar inspiratory crackles will be heard even in the absence of obvious radiographic lung infiltrates.

J.H. Ryu, M.D.

Reference

1. Schwartz DA, Merchant RK, Helmers RA, et al: The influence of cigarette smoking on lung function and patients with idiopathic pulmonary fibrosis. *Am Rev Respir Dis* 144:504–506, 1991.

Lung Function Tests in Patients With Idiopathic Pulmonary Fibrosis: Are They Helpful for Predicting Outcome?
Erbes R, Schaberg T, Loddenkemper R (Chest Hosp Heckeshorn, Berlin)
Chest 111:51–57, 1997   54–2

Background.—The course of idiopathic pulmonary fibrosis (IPF) varies greatly. Predictive parameters on presentation to the hospital were investigated in 1 group of patients with IPF, with a focus on extensive lung function tests.

Methods.—Ninety patients were studied. Forty-seven were women. Assessment included standard tests of lung volumes, arterial oxygen tension, and gas exchange at rest and during bicycle exercise.

Findings.—At the initial assessment, most patients were found to have a decreased total lung capacity (TLC) of 79.2%, an arterial oxygen tension considered pathologic in 63% (when related to age), significantly reduced arterial oxygen tension with 11.8 mm Hg, and increased alveolar-arterial oxygen pressure difference with 46.4 mm Hg during bicycle exercise. Reduced survival was associated with age older than 50 years, a decreased value to more than 2 standard deviations less than the predicted values of both, and TLC alone or combined with a decreased vital capacity. Sex, parameters of gas exchange at rest, and arterial oxygen tension at rest and during bicycle exercise did not affect survival.

Conclusions.—Standard lung function testing is useful for determining the prognosis of patients with IPF. Extensive tests such as gas exchange measurements at rest and during bicycle exercise do not provide additional useful prognostic information.

▶ This study by Erbes and colleagues looks at the usefulness of pulmonary function results in assessing prognosis for patients with idiopathic pulmonary fibrosis (IPF). Although this group of patients is said to have biopsy-proven IPF, it is likely that the group reported here is a heterogeneous population. At the present time, we lack a uniform definition for IPF. Most agree that it is a condition that affects middle-aged or older individuals causing a slowly progressive fibrotic process in the lungs. Lung biopsy most commonly shows usual interstitial pneumonia, but other types of interstitial pneumonias may be seen. Clinical manifestations include progressive dyspnea on exertion, chronic cough, typical fine bibasilar crackles on lung auscultation, digital clubbing, diffuse interstitial lung infiltrates on the chest radiograph, and a restrictive defect on pulmonary function testing. Pulmonary function tests are used to objectively gauge the severity of physiologic impairment in patients with suspected lung disease. They are also used to monitor disease course and to assess response to treatment. This study suggests that total lung capacity and vital capacity measurement at presentation can provide prognostic information for patients with IPF. Although these results are at variance with some other previous studies, it seems to make sense that patients with more severe impairment will likely have a worse prognosis. In my own practice, I generally measure total lung capacity, vital capacity, diffusing capacity, oximetry at rest and exercise, and arterial blood gas study at rest on room air at baseline for patients with IPF. For follow-up visits, I mainly rely on repeated vital capacity and diffusing capacity measurements with total lung capacity and arterial blood gas study performed as needed.

J.H. Ryu, M.D.

Diffuse Lung Disease: Diagnostic Accuracy of CT in Patients Undergoing Surgical Biopsy of the Lung
Swensen SJ, Aughenbaugh GL, Myers JL (Mayo Clinic, Rochester, Minn)
Radiology 205:229–234, 1997   54–3

Introduction.—Patients with compatible clinical and radiologic findings characteristic of specific diffuse lung diseases are commonly treated without lung biopsy. A retrospective review of thin-section CT was conducted to determine whether there is a subset of patients with diffuse lung disease in whom accurate diagnosis could be made with CT only.

Methods.—Two radiologists retrospectively reviewed CT scans of 85 patients who underwent open lung biopsy or video-assisted thoracoscopic surgery. Fifty-eight of 85 patients (68%) underwent thin-section CT (1-mm collimation at 10-mm intervals with use of a high–spatial-frequency reconstruction algorithm). The 3 most likely diagnoses were listed (by consensus) in the order of probability. The radiologists rated their level of confidence in their first choice.

Results.—Of 16 possible diseases, 5 diseases accounted for 74% of all diseases in 85 patients. They were usual interstitial pneumonia, infection, lymphoproliferative disorder, bronchiolitis obliterans with organizing pneumonia, and hypersensitivity pneumonitis. The correct diagnosis was listed as 1 of the 3 choices in 79 patients (93%). The correct diagnosis was the radiologists' first choice in 54% of patients. Radiologists rated a high level of confidence in the case of 20 patients (24%), all of whom had chronic lung disease. The first choice was correct in 18 of 20 patients (90%). Usual interstitial pneumonia was predicted most frequently with the highest level of confidence.

Conclusion.—Patients with clinical and radiologic findings characteristic of a specific diffuse lung disease do not need to undergo biopsy. Diagnoses by CT and clinical findings can be made with a high level of confidence.

▶ Over the last 10 years, thin-section CT of the chest has substantially altered the diagnostic evaluation of patients with diffuse lung diseases. We have come to recognize that some of these diseases—such as usual interstitial pneumonia (idiopathic pulmonary fibrosis), sarcoidosis, and pulmonary Langerhans' cell histiocytosis are shown to have distinctive features on thin-section CT of the chest.[1] Thus, with wider use of thin-section CT in the evaluation of these patients, a decreasing number of lung biopsies have been performed in recent years.

In this article by Swensen et al., the correct diagnosis was made by the radiologist in 90% of cases when the first choice diagnosis was made with a high level of confidence after review of the thin-section CT of the chest. The disorders included were usual interstitial pneumonia, lymphoproliferative disorder, hypersensitivity pneumonitis, nonspecific interstitial pneumonia with fibrosis, eosinophilic granuloma (Langerhans' cell histiocytosis), lymphangitic carcinomatosis, and sarcoidosis. Hence, when characteristic features are seen on thin-section CT of the chest and there are clinical features consistent with the diagnosis, a lung biopsy may not be needed. In our clinical experience, usual interstitial pneumonia has been the most common clinical entity among diffuse lung diseases that we have diagnosed with thin-section CT of the chest and without biopsy confirmation.

J.H. Ryu, M.D.

Reference

1. Mathieson JR, Mayo JR, Staples CA, et al: Chronic diffuse infiltrative lung disease: Comparison of diagnostic accuracy of CT and chest radiography. *Radiology* 171:111–116, 1989.

Outcome in Sarcoidosis: The Relationship of Relapse to Corticosteroid Therapy
Gottlieb JE, Israel HL, Steiner RM, et al (Jefferson Med College, Philadelphia)
Chest 111:623–631, 1997 54–4

Introduction.—Relapse after the withdrawal of steroids is a recognized clinical pattern of sarcoidosis, but few studies have been conducted to support this clinical impression. An observational study of 337 patients with sarcoidosis compared the characteristics of those who relapsed after a period of stability with the characteristics of untreated patients.

Methods.—Patients were enrolled over a 4-year period. Those whose symptoms resolved without treatment (118) were considered to have spontaneous remission. The remaining 219 patients were given corticosteroid therapy, starting with a dose equivalent to 20 mg of prednisone daily and usually continued for at least 1 year. Symptoms resolved and did not recur after discontinuation of treatment in 103 patients (induced remission group); the 116 patients in the recalcitrant group required continued therapy because of severity of symptoms or lack of compliance. Treated and untreated patients were compared for demographic, clinical, and radiographic characteristics.

Results.—The relapse rate was 74% in the induced remission group, but only 8% in the spontaneous remission group. White patients had a lower treatment rate than African-American patients (43% vs. 76%), but relapse rates did not differ significantly in the 2 groups (20% and 28%, respectively). The rate of sustained remission in whites (58%) was twice that of African-American (29%). Although nearly half of chest radiographs (40%) showed no change in type during relapse, interstitial profusion increased significantly within types 2 and 3 (the types associated with parenchymal abnormalities). Patients with musculoskeletal complaints and those with symptoms from hepatic involvement were at highest risk for relapse. Characteristics associated with a favorable prognosis included asymptomatic chest radiographic abnormalities at entry, erythema nodosum, and peripheral adenopathy. Relapse was most common (50% of cases) between 2 and 6 months after steroids were discontinued, but 20% of patients relapsed after more than 12 months.

Conclusion.—Relapse of sarcoidosis was common among patients who received steroid therapy but rare among those who were not treated. An explanation for this marked difference is that patients whose disease was likely to be severe were identified early and the decision was made to treat. Another possibility is that corticosteroids help prolong the disease by delaying resolution.

▶ Corticosteroid therapy in sarcoidosis remains a controversial issue because of the lack of well-controlled clinical trials. Although corticosteroid therapy appears to have short-term benefits, a long-term efficacy is not clear.[1] This study shows a high relapse rate in those patients who had an induced remission with corticosteroid therapy. It is unclear whether corticosteroids prolong the course of sarcoidosis or whether those patients treated with corticosteroids had more severe and protracted disease than patients who experience spontaneous remissions. In the absence of compelling indications for treatment such as severe ocular, neurologic, or cardiac involvement, a period of observation (6 months) is reasonable for observing the course of pulmonary disease. If a spontaneous remission occurs or the disease remains stable, corticosteroid therapy may be avoided.

J.H. Ryu, M.D.

Reference

1. Newman LS, Rose CS, Maier LA: Sarcoidosis. *N Engl J Med* 336:1224–1235, 1997.

Silicosis in the 1990s
Rosenman KD, Reilly MJ, Kalinowski DJ, et al (Michigan State Univ, East Lansing)
Chest 111:779–786, 1997   54–5

Background.—Silicosis has been of concern in Michigan for over 6 decades. This study evaluated the state-based surveillance data for this disease based on reports from 1987 through 1995.

Methods.—All instances of silicosis or pneumoconiosis not otherwise specified were required to be reported to the Michigan Department of Public Health. Patients with the disease were interviewed by telephone with a standard questionnaire that asked, among other things, about work history, respirator symptoms, and smoking history. These data, plus pulmonary function testing results and a recent chest radiograph, were reviewed to see if they met the criteria for silicosis established by the National Institute of Occupational Safety and Health.

Findings.—Of the 577 patients with silicosis, 567 (98.3%) were men and 257 (44.9%) were black. Patients had worked on average 27.8 years in a job that exposed them to silica. Of the people with silicosis, simple silicosis was present in 377 (65.3%) and progressive fibrosis was present in 164 (28.4%). Nineteen (3.3%) had normal radiographs but biopsy evidence of silicosis. About 60% of the patients with silicosis had restricted or obstructed breathing, regardless of smoking status. Working in an iron foundry was the most frequent cause of silicosis, present in 79.8% of cases (Table 4). Less than 10% of the facilities that had medical surveillance provided medical screening for silicosis; about 30% performed preemployment testing only, about 30% provided no medical surveillance at all, and about 20% administered pulmonary function tests without chest radiographs. Finally, the majority of these patients (43.5%) had not applied for workers' compensation.

Conclusions.—Between 50 and 80 new cases of silicosis are reported each year in Michigan, yet this number likely underrepresents the true incidence. Thus workplace reviews, adequate controls, and reminders are

TABLE 4.—Primary Industry Where Silica Exposure Occurred for Individuals Confirmed With Silicosis for the Years 1985 to 1995

Industry (SIC Code)	No. (%) of Cases*
Manufacturing	
Primary metal industries (33)	458 (79.8)
Includes iron, steel, gray, and ductile iron foundries	
Stone, clay, glass, and concrete products (32)	28 (4.9)
Transportation equipment (37)	22 (3.8)
Includes auto bodies and boat building	
Fabricated metal products (34)	9 (1.6)
Miscellaneous (25, 26, 28, 30, 35, 38)	14 (2.4)
Includes chemicals and allied products, rubber parts, metalworking machinery, and dental equipment	
Mining	
Metal mining (10)	12 (2.1)
Nonmetallic mineral mining, except fuels (14)	2 (0.3)
Construction (15, 16, 17)	21 (3.7)
Transportation, communication, etc. services (40, 41, 47, 49, 73, 76)	6 (1.0)
Includes transportation, sanitary, and repair services	
Pipeline operations (46)	1 (0.2)
Dental laboratory (80)	1 (0.2)
Total	574 (100.0)

*For 3 workers, the industrial classification was not known.
Abbreviation: SIC, standard industrial classification.
(Courtesy of Rosenman KD, Reilly MJ, Kalinowski DJ, et al. Occupational and environmental lung disease: Silicosis in the 1990s. *Chest* 111:779–786, 1997.)

needed wherever silica is being used, particularly where sandblasting occurs. Although people with the disease had been exposed to silica for an average of 27.8 years, there were nevertheless people who began working with silica in the 1970s and 1980s who have developed silicosis. Thus silicosis remains a problem that, due to its chronic nature, will not disappear in the near future.

▶ Silicosis is a disease caused by inhalation of crystalline silica. Although the incidence has generally been decreasing in the United States, this study by Rosenman et al. shows that this disorder is not disappearing in the 1990s. In addition, there probably is a substantial number of cases that remain undiagnosed since a surveillance system of this type tends to identify individuals with advanced disease. Many workplaces do not provide adequate medical screening for workers at risk, and air quality controls are suboptimal. In addition, there are problems with compliance on the part of the workers in using safety equipment. Therefore, silicosis will likely remain a problem for years to come.

J.H. Ryu, M.D.

55 Pleural Emboli/ Pulmonary Hypertension

The Duration of Oral Anticoagulant Therapy After a Second Episode of Venous Thromboembolism
Schulman S, and the Duration of Anticoagulation Trial Study Group (Karolinska Hosp, Stockholm; et al)
N Engl J Med 336:393–398, 1997   55–1

Introduction.—Two recent multicenter trials have shown that extending the duration of oral anticoagulant therapy after a first episode of venous thromboembolism can reduce the rate of recurrence. Because the optimal duration of prophylactic oral anticoagulation after a second episode has not been determined, a multicenter trial was designed to compare the benefits of treatment for 6 months with indefinite treatment.

Methods.—During the 3-year enrollment period, 227 patients were randomly assigned to the 2 treatment groups. Eligible patients were at least 15 years old and had a second episode of acute pulmonary embolism or deep-vein thrombosis in the leg, the iliac veins, or both. Initial treatment consisted of heparin for at least 5 days; oral anticoagulation with warfarin sodium or dicumarol was usually started at the same time as heparin therapy. The target chosen for the international normalized ratio was 2.0–2.85. Patients in the 6-month group discontinued oral anticoagulant without tapering at their 6-month evaluation. Principle end points of the study were major hemorrhage, recurrent venous thromboembolism, and death.

Results.—There were 26 recurrences of venous thromboembolism during the 48 months of follow-up (Table 2). Only 3 recurrences (2.6%) were in the indefinite therapy group, compared to 23 in the 6-month group (20.7%). No recurrence took place during anticoagulation therapy (the 3 patients in the indefinite therapy group had prematurely discontinued therapy). When compared with therapy of indefinite duration, the relative risk of recurrence in the group assigned to 6 months of oral anticoagulation therapy was 8.0. Thirteen major hemorrhages occurred, 3 in the

TABLE 2.—Frequency of Principal End Points After 4 Years, According to the Duration of Assigned Treatment

END POINT	6 Mo (N = 111)	INDEFINITE (N = 116)	RELATIVE RISK (95% CI)*	P VALUE
Major hemorrhage	3 (2.7)†	10 (8.6)	0.3 (0.1–1.1)	0.084
Recurrence	23 (20.7)	3 (2.6)‡	8.0 (2.5–25.9)	<0.001
In hospitals with logbooks§	21 (22.1)	3 (3.1)	7.1 (2.2–22.9)	<0.001
Death	16 (14.4)	10 (8.6)	1.7 (0.8–3.5)	0.21

*Relative risks are expressed as the ratio of the number of patients with the specified end point to the total number of patients in the 6-month group, divided by the corresponding ratio in the indefinite treatment group.
†Two of the hemorrhages occurred after the discontinuation of oral anticoagulation.
‡All recurrences in this group occurred after the premature discontinuation of anticoagulation.
§There were 95 patients in the 6-month group and 96 in the indefinite treatment group at these 12 hospitals.
Abbreviation: CI, confidence interval.
(Reprinted by permission of The New England Journal of Medicine, from Schulman S, and the Duration of Anticoagulation Trial Study Group: The duration of oral anticoagulant therapy after a second episode of venous thromboembolism. *N Engl J Med* 336:393–398, copyright 1997, Massachusetts Medical Society.)

6-month group (2.7%) and 10 in the indefinite treatment group (8.6%). The relative risk of major hemorrhage in the 6-month group was 0.3.

Discussion.—The risk of major hemorrhagic complications has been a deterrent to the long-term use of oral anticoagulant therapy after a second episode of venous thromboembolism. There was a trend toward an increased risk of major hemorrhage with indefinite duration of therapy, but this was offset by a much lower rate of recurrent thromboembolism.

▶ The currently recommended duration of anticoagulant therapy for patients with the first episode of venous thromboembolism (VTE) is 3 to 6 months.[1] However, the duration of treatment may be shortened for patients with temporary risk factors for thromboembolic disease, e.g., recent surgery. Conversely, the duration of therapy may need to be lengthened in those patients with persistent risk factors, e.g., hereditary hypercoagulable state. The optimal duration of therapy for those patients with recurrent VTE (pulmonary thromboembolism or deep venous thrombosis) has not been entirely clear. This study by Schulman and colleagues shows prophylactic oral anticoagulation continued indefinitely to be associated with a substantially lower rate of recurrent venous thromboembolism compared to anticoagulant treatment for 6 months in those patients who have suffered a second episode of venous thromboembolism. This benefit came at the price of increased incidence of major hemorrhage. Although the relative risks will need to be assessed for individual patients, an indefinite period of anticoagulation is recommended for most patients after a second episode of venous thromboembolism.

J.H. Ryu, M.D.

Reference

1. Hyers TM, Hull RD, Wegg JG: Antithrombotic therapy for venous thromboembolic disease. *Chest* 108:335S–350S, 1995.

Pulmonary Embolism: Validation of Spiral CT Angiography in 149 Patients

van Rossum AB, Pattynama PMT, Ton ERTA, et al (Leyenburg Hosp, The Hague, The Netherlands; Leiden Univ, The Netherlands)
Radiology 201:467–470, 1996   55–2

Background.—Spiral CT angiography is a promising alternative technique for detecting and excluding pulmonary embolism (PE). To date, clinical experience with spiral CT angiography has been limited. The accuracy of spiral CT angiography for detecting PE in a large group of consecutive patients was studied.

Methods.—Spiral CT angiography and ventilation-perfusion scintigraphy were done in 149 patients with clinically suspected PE. When the findings of ventilation-perfusion scans were indeterminate, pulmonary angiography was done.

Findings.—The diagnostic quality of spiral CT angiograms was satisfactory in all patients. For observer 1, the sensitivity and specificity of spiral CT angiography for detecting PE were 94% and 96%, respectively. For observer 2, the sensitivity and specificity were 82% and 93%, respectively. Interobserver agreement was good. The technique proved effective in detecting PE in pulmonary arteries up to the segmental level but not in the smaller subsegmental branches. For both observers, 3 spiral CT angiographic findings were negative.

Conclusions.—Spiral CT angiography is an accurate technique for detecting and excluding PE. The sensitivity ranges from 82% to 94%, and the specificity from 93% to 96%.

▶ Ventilation-perfusion lung scans have played a major role in the evaluation of suspected PE. Unfortunately, in most patients who undergo ventilation-perfusion lung scanning, the result is nondiagnostic, requiring additional studies such as pulmonary angiography. Over the past 5 years, several studies have reported on the use of spiral or electron-beam CT with IV contrast in the diagnosis of PE. The reported sensitivity of this diagnostic mode has ranged from 63% to 91% and specificity of 78% to 97%.[1–3]

This study by van Rossum and associates represents one of the larger studies in this regard, with 149 patients. Taken together, the currently available data on CT angiography show this method to be useful and accurate in evaluating cases of suspected PE. One exception to this statement is a subset of patients who have thromboemboli only in subsegmental vessels, where CT angiography performs poorly compared with standard pulmonary angiography.

At present, CT angiography appears to be a reasonable alternative to ventilation-perfusion lung scanning, particularly in patients who have pre-existing lung disease and are likely to have an indeterminate ventilation-perfusion lung scan result. However, a negative CT angiogram does not entirely exclude the possibility of PE, particularly in a patient at high risk (high clinical suspicion).

J.H. Ryu, M.D.

References

1. Goodman LR, Curtin JJ, Mewissen MW, et al: Detection of pulmonary embolism in patients with unresolved clinical and scintigraphic diagnosis: Helical CT versus angiography. *AJR* 164:1369–1374, 1995.
2. Teigen CL, Maus TP, Sheedy PF II, et al: Pulmonary embolism: Diagnosis with contrast-enhanced electron-beam CT in comparison with pulmonary angiography. *Radiology* 194:313–319, 1995.
3. Remy-Jardin M, Remy J, Deschildre F, et al: Diagnosis of pulmonary embolism with spiral CT: Comparison with pulmonary angiography and scintigraphy. *Radiology* 200:699–706, 1996.

Association Between Thrombolytic Treatment and the Prognosis of Hemodynamically Stable Patients With Major Pulmonary Embolism: Results of a Multicenter Registry

Konstantinides S, Geibel A, Olschewski M, et al (Universitaetsklinik Freiburg, Germany; Krankenhaus Bruchsal, Germany; Universitaetklinik Giessen,Germany; et al)
Circulation 96:882–888, 1997

55–3

Background.—Thrombolytic therapy is associated with the resolution of major pulmonary embolism, but may also be associated with a risk of severe hemorrhagic complications. A large multicenter registry of patients with major pulmonary embolism was utilized to examine the efficacy and safety of thrombolytic therapy compared to conventional heparin anticoagulation in patients who were hemodynamically stable when seen.

Study Design.—The study group consisted of patients from the Management Strategy and Prognosis of Pulmonary Embolism Registry conducted between 1993 and 1994. During this period, 204 German centers registered 1,001 consecutive patients with a diagnosis of major pulmonary embolism. The present study included 719 patients from the registry with pulmonary hypertension and/or ventricular afterload stress on echocardiography or catheterization of the right side of the heart, but no arterial hypotension or cardiogenic shock at presentation. One group of these patients was treated with primary thrombolytic therapy and the other group with primary heparin therapy. The primary clinical end point was overall 30-day mortality.

Findings.—After diagnosis of pulmonary embolism, 169 patients received thrombolytic therapy within 24 hours. The remaining 550 patients received conventional heparin anticoagulation. In 125 of the heparin-treated patients, thrombolytic therapy was received after the initial 24 hours. The mean age of those patients who received primary thrombolytic therapy was younger than the mean age of the heparin group. The patients with thrombolytic therapy were more likely to have a history of deep vein thrombosis and less likely to have congestive heart failure and chronic pulmonary disease. The average hospital stay was about 25 days. The overall 30-day mortality was 9.6%. Overall mortality was significantly lower in the primary thrombolytic therapy group than in the heparin therapy group. Univariate analysis indicated that syncope, arterial hypotension, history of congestive heart failure, and chronic pulmonary disease were significantly associated with a higher death rate. Mortality was higher in those with dilation of the right ventricle and in those with proximal vein thrombosis. Multiple logistic regression analysis indicated that primary thrombolysis was the only clinical variable that was an independent predictor of patient outcome. Younger patients, those with arterial hypotension, those without a history of recent major surgery, and those with echocardiographically detected right ventricular enlargement particularly benefited from thombolytic therapy. Patients with postoperative pulmonary embolism had increased mortality after treatment with thrombolytic therapy. Major bleeding episodes occurred in 80 patients. The rate of major bleeding was significantly higher in the thrombolysis group. Cerebral hemorrhage was rare. One patient in each group died of a bleeding complication.

Conclusions.—This multicenter study evaluated the safety and efficacy of thrombolytic therapy in 719 hemodynamically stable patients with major pulmonary embolism. Primary thrombolytic therapy was associated with a significant reduction in overall mortality in this group. These results suggest that early thrombolytic therapy may favorably affect the clinical outcome of hemodynamically stable inpatients with major pulmonary embolism.

▶ Although this study by S. Konstantinides et al. reports a better survival rate in hemodynamically stable patients with major pulmonary embolism when treated with thrombolytic agents, the reader should note several limitations of the study. This study was based on a multicenter registry, and the assignment of patients to thrombolysis vs. heparin was nonrandomized. Indeed, there were several clinical variables that were significantly different between the 2 treatment arms when analyzed retrospectively. Patients who received thrombolytic therapy tended to be younger and were less likely to have a history of pre-existing cardiac or pulmonary disease. Although the authors state that these factors were taken into account using a multivariate regression model, one still wonders whether this type of selection bias may partly explain the better outcome for patients treated with thrombolytic therapy. In addition, the choice of the thrombolytic agent and presumably the dose and duration as well were not standardized. Furthermore, confirmation of the pulmonary embolism diagnosis was obtained in only 73% of patients by a high probability lung scan or pulmonary angiography. In the remaining patients, diagnosis was apparently based on clinical examination, arterial blood gas analysis, and echocardiography. Lastly, it is unclear why patients with severe hemodynamic compromise (cardiogenic shock or circulatory collapse) were excluded from analysis, because one would think that thrombolytic therapy may be most useful in those patients with massive pulmonary embolism. Data presented in this study do not alter the conclusion that the optimum application of thrombolytic therapy in the treatment of venous thromboembolism remains relatively undefined and that its use needs to be individualized.[1]

J.H. Ryu, M.D.

Reference

1. Hyers TM, Hull RD, Weg JG: Antithrombotic therapy for venous thromboembolic disease. *Chest* 108:335S–351S, 1995.

Brain Serotonin Neurotoxicity and Primary Pulmonary Hypertension From Fenfluramine and Dexfenfluramine: A Systematic Review of the Evidence

McCann UD, Seiden LS, Rubin LJ, et al (Natl Inst of Mental Heath, Bethesda, Md; Univ of Chicago; Univ of Maryland, Baltimore, Md)
JAMA 278:666–672, 1997   55–4

Introduction.—For the treatment of obesity for up to 12 months, the Food and Drug Administration recently approved the use of dexfenfluramine hydrochloride (N-ethyl-α-methyl-m-[trifluoromethyl]phenethylamine [Redux, Wyeth-Ayerst Laboratories, Philadelphia, Pa, and Interneuron Pharmaceuticals Inc, Lexington, Mass], the dextro or)S[+]) stereoisomer of fenfluramine. In North America, fenfluramine has become widely used. In promoting and maintaining weight loss, the use of fenfluramines when given in conjunction with Phentermine is effective. The drug was approved by a 6–5 margin after a second hearing by the Food and Drug Administration advisory committee that evaluated dexfenfluramine for issues of efficacy and safety. The safety concerns centered around the drug causing brain serotonin neuron damage in animals, including nonhuman primates, and the use of fenfluramine being linked to the development of primary pulmonary hypertension. The data on brain serotonin neurotoxicity in animals treated with fenfluramines and the evidence linking fenfluramines to primary pulmonary hypertension was systemically reviewed.

Methods.—A computerized search of MEDLINE reviewing articles from 1966 to 1997 was conducted. The types of articles reviewed concerned the long-term effects of fenfluramines on brain serotonin neurons, pulmonary function in animals and humans, and body weight.

Results.—In all the animal species tests and with all the routes of drug administration used, fenfluramines caused dose-related, long-lasting reductions in serotonin axonal markers. When one takes into account known relations between body mass and drug clearance, doses of fenfluramines that produce signs of brain serotonin neurotoxicity in animals are on the same order as those used to treat humans for weight loss. The pathological and clinical potential for neurotoxicity in humans is unknown, as no human studies have yet been conducted. The risk of developing primary pulmonary hypertension is increased with an odds ratio of 6.3, particularly when used for more than 3 months, by the use of appetite suppressants, most commonly fenfluramines.

Conclusion.—An increased risk of primary pulmonary hypertension is associated with use of fenfluramines. They also cause brain serotonin toxicity in animals, and serotonin systems play a role in mood regulation, cognition and memory, impulsivity, anxiety, sleep, aggression, and neuroendocrine function. The long-term consequences of prolonged use of fenfluramines should be addressed in future studies. The risks of fenfluramines outweigh their perceived benefits in cases in which weight loss is desired purely for personal appearance.

Valvular Heart Disease Associated With Fenfluramine-Phentermine
Connolly HM, Crary JL, McGoon MD, et al (Mayo Clinic and Mayo Found, Rochester, Minn)
N Engl J Med 337:581–588, 1997   55–5

Background.—Fenfluramine and phentermine are prescription medications that have been individually approved by the Food and Drug Administration (FDA) as appetite suppressants for the treatment of obesity. Though not approved by the FDA for use in combination, these drugs are frequently prescribed together to reduce the dosages of each agent required and thereby lower side effects. In 1996, the total number of prescriptions for these agents exceeded 18 million in the United States alone. This article describes 24 cases of unusual valvular disease in patients taking fenfluramine-phentermine.

Study Design.—All patients were identified during the course of routine evaluation. As more patients with similar clinical features were identified and an association was suspected, other physicians were consulted about cases in their own practices.

Findings.—A group of 24 women were identified with unusual valvular morphology and regurgitation by echocardiography, approximately 1 year after the initiation of fenfluramine-phentermine therapy. Pulmonary hypertension was detected in 8 of these women. Cardiac surgical intervention was required in 5 patients. At operation, the heart valves were observed to have a glistening white appearance. Histopathological findings included plaque-like encasement of the leaflets and chordal structures with intact valve architecture. These features were similar to those seen in carcinoid or ergotamine-induced valve disease.

Conclusions.—These cases suggest that the combination of fenfluramine-phentermine commonly prescribed in the United States as an appetite suppressant may be associated with valvular heart disease. Prospective studies will be required to validate this observation. The mechanism of injury and the frequency of the association have not been determined.

Nevertheless, patients considering drug treatment for obesity should be informed of the potential serious adverse effects of this drug combination.

▶ Severe cardiopulmonary complications have been reported to be associated with fenfluramine (Podamin) and dexfenfluramine (Redux). This has led to the voluntary withdrawal of the medications from the market on September 15, 1997. Pulmonologists should be familiar with the review by McCann et al. (Abstract 55–4) and the case series by Connolly et al. (Abstract 55–5). Fenfluramines have been shown to cause brain serotonin neurotoxicity in animals, and are associated with the development of pulmonary hypertension and valvular heart disease. The risk of pulmonary hypertension has been reported to be greater than 20-fold for patients using these anorexigens for greater than 3 months.[1] Most of the patients in this report (90%) were taking fenfluramines. In the case series by Connolly et al., the histopathological changes were identical to changes seen in patients with carcinoid or ergotamine-induced valvular heart disease. The circumstantial evidence suggests that the valvular lesions were induced by elevated circulating levels of serotonin. These complications occurred in patients < 50 years of age. Patients presenting with complaints of dyspnea or those patients in whom a new heart murmur is detected should be questioned carefully about the prior use of fenfluramines and an echocardiogram should be performed. In asymptomatic patients who have previously taken these drugs alone or in combination with other drugs such as phentermine, an echocardiogram should be strongly considered before having any invasive procedure.[2]

P. Strollo, M.D.

References

1. Abenhaim L, Moride Y, Brenot F, et al., for the International Primary Pulmonary Hypertension Study Group. Appetite-suppressant drugs and the risk of primary pulmonary hypertension. N Engl J Med 1996; 335:609–616.
2. FDA Press Release November 13 1997.

56 Tuberculosis

Patient's Self-interpretation of Tuberculin Skin Tests
Colp C, Goldfarb A, Wei I, et al (Beth Israel Med Ctr, New York)
Chest 110:1275–1277, 1996   56–1

Objective.—Because tuberculin (purified protein derivative [PPD]) skin tests must be interpreted within 48–72 hours, results are sometimes reported by the patient or a relative. The reliability of these reports is unknown. A prospective evaluation of patients' self-interpretation of PPD was performed in an inner-city general hospital outpatient clinic.

Methods.—Patients in the Adult Primary Care Clinic at Beth Israel Medical Center in New York City received 0.1 mL of stabilized tuberculin PPD by intradermal injection along with an anergy test consisting of a 0.1-mL injection of mumps skin test antigen when indicated. Patients were instructed in interpretation of a positive test result and told to return within 48–72 hours. Patients who returned were interviewed and given a questionnaire to assess their understanding about tuberculosis and interpretation of the skin test. Interviewers were to record patients' awareness and understanding of test results.

Results.—Of the 68 patients (25 male), average age 51 years, 45 were foreign born, 22 were Caribbean Hispanics, and 2 were Russian. Eighteen of the 59 who returned had a positive test result ranging from 10 to 20 mm induration. One patient recognized a positive test reaction, 4 noticed swelling, and 7 could not make a judgment. Twenty of 45 patients had proven anergy. Because it became apparent that patients were not aware of their positive skin test results, the last 24 patients were counseled intensively. Three patients in this group were unable to recognize their positive test reactions. Similar studies identified 37% awareness in their positive reactors. Other studies with better results excluded patients who did not return for a test interpretation or who were unable to interpret their results. Studies in college students showed excellent self-reading results. The high failure rates in this general primary care clinic are attributed in part to the foreign and less well-educated patient clientele, and, because of the frequent correct identification of positive control skin test results, to denial.

Conclusion.—Patients receiving PPD tests cannot be relied upon to interpret results correctly. Tests must be interpreted by professionals.

▶ This article once again brings home the message that if we cut corners, we are going to "get burned." Because of the hassle and inconvenience to the patients, many physicians will place a tuberculin skin test and ask the patient to telephone in the results based on a self-reading. This article clearly points out the fallacy of this approach. If we place a PPD, we should make sure that the patient comes back at 48 hours for an interpretation by a designated health professional with experience in interpreting skin tests.

J.R. Jett, M.D.

Rifampin Preventive Therapy for Tuberculosis in Boston's Homeless
Polesky A, Farber HW, Gottlieb DJ, et al (Boston Univ)
Am J Respir Crit Care Med 154:1473–1477, 1996   56–2

Background.—The Centers for Disease Control and Prevention and the American Thoracic Society have recommended prophylaxis for patients with known exposure to isoniazid (INH)-resistant tuberculosis. However, current non-INH regimens are empiric or are based mainly on data in animal models. The use of rifampin during an outbreak of INH-resistant tuberculosis was investigated.

Methods.—Two hundred four patients with documented tuberculin skin test conversions but without active tuberculosis at the time of clinical assessment for their positive skin test were eligible for prophylaxis. Seventy-one patients received no treatment, 38 were given INH, 49 received rifampin, and 37 were given rifampin plus INH.

Findings.—Active tuberculosis subsequently developed in 8.6% of persons receiving no treatment, in 7.9% given INH, and in none given rifampin or rifampin plus INH. Tuberculosis was significantly less likely to develop in the rifampin recipients than in those given no treatment (Table 2).

TABLE 2.—Incidence of Tuberculosis in Skin Test Converters by Type of Preventive Therapy

Variable	No Therapy	INH	Rifampin	Rifampin + INH	Rifampin-containing Regimen
Total no. in group	71	38	49	37	86
Total Tb, no. (%)	6 (8.4)	3 (7.9)	0	0	0
p Value†		0.62	0.04	0.08	< 0.01

*None of the 9 individuals who received a combination of antituberculosis medications developed active tuberculosis.
†p Value for comparison of each treatment group to the no-therapy group by Fisher's exact test.
(Courtesy of Polesky A, Farber HW, Gottlieb DJ, et al: Rifampin preventive therapy for tuberculosis in Boston's homeless. *Am J Respir Crit Care Med* 154:1473–1477, official journal of the American Thoracic Society, copyright 1996, American Lung Association.)

Conclusions.—Despite the limitations of the current study, the findings suggest that rifampin should be used as initial prophylaxis in persons likely to be infected by INH-resistant tuberculosis. Treatment with any rifampin-containing preventive therapy effectively prevented the development of active disease.

▶ This article addresses an issue that arises periodically. It is not a problem that is limited strictly to urban centers. A nationwide survey of drug-resistant tuberculosis in the United States in 1991 identified resistance to 1 or more drugs in 14% of cases. Resistance to INH was present in 8% of new cases of tuberculosis and 21% of recurrent cases. Streptomycin resistance was present in 6% and 8% of new and recurrent cases, respectively. Resistance to rifampin was identified in 3.5% of new and 9% of recurrent cases.[1]

Even though the study is a nonradomized trial, it provides some of the best data available to support the American Thoracic Society and Centers for Disease Control and Prevention recommendation that recent skin test convertors who were exposed to a case of INH-resistant tuberculosis should be treated with rifampin at standard therapeutic doses. The American Thoracic Society and Centers for Disease Control and Prevention recommended prophylaxis for 12 months, but this article suggests that 6 months may be adequate.

J.R. Jett, M.D.

Reference

1. Bloch AB, Cauthen GM, Onorato IM, et al: Nationwide survey of drug resistant tuberculosis in the United States. *JAMA* 271:665–671, 1994.

57 Tuberculosis and the Human Immunodeficiency Virus

Six-month Supervised Intermittent Tuberculosis Therapy in Haitian Patients With and Without HIV Infection
Chaisson RE, Clermont HC, Holt EA, et al (Johns Hopkins Univ, Baltimore, Md; Centres pour le Developpement et la Santé, Cité Soleil, Haiti)
Am J Respir Crit Care Med 154:1034–1038, 1996   57–1

Background.—Although patients infected with HIV and tuberculosis (TB) respond well to standard anti-TB treatment, the best therapy for TB in HIV disease is unknown. The outcomes of standard short-course, intermittent treatment for TB in patients with HIV infection were compared with the outcomes in patients with HIV-seronegative status with TB in a developing country.

Methods.—Four hundred twenty-seven patients in Haiti were enrolled in the prospective trial. One hundred seventy-seven patients had HIV infection. Supervised treatment consisted of isoniazid, rifampin, pyrazinamide, and ethambutol 3 times a week for 8 weeks, followed by isoniazid and rifampin 3 times a week for 18 weeks.

Findings.—Nine percent of patients with HIV-seropositive status with pulmonary or intrathoracic TB and 1% of patients with HIV-seronegative status with these forms of TB died. Eighty-one percent of patients with HIV-seropositive status and 87% of patients with HIV-seronegative status were cured. Three percent of patients with HIV-seronegative status and 5.4% of patients with HIV-seropositive status completing treatment had relapses. A life-table plot of survival at 18 months after enrollment showed that patients with seropositive status had a probability of 91% of remaining alive at 6 months, 77% at 12 months, and 66% at 18 months. Patients with seronegative status had a 97% probability of remaining alive at 18 months.

Conclusions.—These data confirm the efficacy of 6-month rifampin-containing regimens in patients with HIV-related TB. More than 90% of the current patients complied with this thrice-weekly, supervised treatment.

▶ Directly observed therapy for TB has been the major factor in the decline of TB in New York City[1] and elsewhere.[2, 3] These 2 articles have demonstrated acceptable cure rates and relapse rates in 2 impoverished settings in different parts of the world. The Spanish study treated the homeless, individuals with alcoholism, and/or IV drug-abusing patients with twice weekly therapy for the entire 6-month period. In the Haitian trial, 427 patients were treated with thrice weekly therapy for the full 6 months. Of note is that 42% were patients infected with HIV. This study demonstrated that directly observed therapy for 6 months was effective for patients with HIV-positive status and for patients with HIV-negative status. If we are going to continue our progress against this difficult disease with increasing frequency of drug resistance, then we must substantially expand directly observed therapy. The outcomes with twice or thrice weekly treatment, for some or all of the 6 months of treatment, are similar to those with daily therapy.

J.R. Jett, M.D.

References

1. Frieden TR, Fujiwara PI, Wasko RM, et al: Tuberculosis in New York City: Turning the tide. *N Engl J Med* 333:229–233, 1995.
2. Weis SE, Slocum PC, Blais FX et al: The Effect of Directly Observed Therapy on the Rates of Drug Resistance and Relapse in Tuberculosis *NEJM* 330:1179–1184, 1994.
3. Chaulk CP, Moore-Rice K, Rizzo R et al: Eleven Years of Community-Based Directly Observed Therapy for Tuberculosis *JAMA* 274:945–951, 1995.

58 Human Immunodeficiency Virus

Respiratory Disease Trends in the Pulmonary Complications of HIV Infection Study Cohort
Wallace JM, and the Pulmonary Complications of HIV Infection Study Group
(Olive View-UCLA Med Ctr, Sylmar, Calif; Research Triangle Inst, Research
Triangle Park, NC; Northwestern Univ, Chicago; et al)
Am J Respir Crit Care Med 155:72–80, 1997   58–1

Background.—Many complications of human immunodeficiency (HIV) infection occur in the respiratory tract. Understanding the patterns of respiratory complications over time would be useful for anticipating the resources needed to care for persons with HIV infection. Trends in the incidence of specific respiratory illnesses were studied in a multicenter cohort of patients with progressive HIV disease during a 5-year period.

Respiratory Disease Trends in HIV Infection Study Cohort.—Upper respiratory tract infections were the most common respiratory disorders. However, the incidence of lower respiratory tract infections rose as CD4 counts decreased. The main lower respiratory infection in patients with study entry CD4 counts of ≥ 200 cells/mm^3 was acute bronchitis. Acute bronchitis, bacterial pneumonia, and *Pneumocystis carinii* pneumonia occurred at high rates, with no apparent time trends in patients with entry CD4 counts of <200 cells/mm^3, despite chemoprophylaxis in >80% of the patients after the first year. The rate of other pulmonary opportunistic infections increased with time in these patients (Table 2).

Conclusions.—Trends in respiratory disorders associated with HIV infection are determined by the disease stage and influenced by transmission category. Acute bronchitis is prevalent in all stages of HIV infection, whereas the incidence rates of bacterial pneumonia and *P. carinii* increase continuously during disease progression to an advanced stage. Patients with advanced disease have a high incidence of acute bronchitis, bacterial

TABLE 2.—Disease Resolution According to Cox Regression Model

	Year 1	Year 2	Rate* No. Episodes Year 3	Year 4	Year 5
Any respiratory illness	69 (765)	61 (625)	68 (611)	71 (556)	87 (431)
Upper respiratory tract infections*	47 (518)	35 (360)	40 (358)	40 (318)	52 (256)
Lower respiratory tract infections	21 (233)	25 (251)	26 (237)	28 (219)	34 (167)
Bronchitis	13 (146)	14 (144)	13 (116)	14 (110)	14 (70)
Bacterial pneumonia	3.9 (43)	4.7 (48)	6.1 (55)	6.4 (50)	7.3 (36)
P. carinii pneumonia	2.8 (31)	4.3 (44)	5.8 (52)	5.8 (46)	9.5 (47)
Tuberculosis	0.5 (6)	0.6 (6)	0.5 (4)	0.5 (4)	1.0 (5)
Other opportunistic	0.6 (7)	0.9 (9)	1.1 (10)	1.1 (9)	1.8 (9)
Pulmonary vascular disorders	0.1 (1)	0.4 (4)	1.0 (9)	1.5 (12)	0.8 (4)
Pulmonary neoplasms	0.3 (3)	0.5 (5)	0.6 (5)	0.5 (4)	0.6 (3)
Infiltrative disorders	0.9 (10)	0.5 (5)	0.2 (2)	0.4 (3)	0.2 (1)

Note: Prognostic variables included in the model were sex, race, age, number and duration of lesions before enrollment, surface area of lesions, and severity of pain at baseline.
*$P < 0.05$.
(Courtesy of Whitley RJ, and the National Institute of Allergy and Infectious Diseases Collaborative Antiviral Study Group: Acyclovir with and without prednisone for the treatment of herpes zoster. *Ann Intern Med* 125:376–383, official journal of the American Thoracic Society, copyright 1996, American Lung Association.)

pneumonia, and *P. carinii* pneumonia despite the widespread use of chemoprophylaxis.

▶ Pulmonary complications are common in patients with HIV. Although most of these complications are infectious in nature, a variety of noninfectious processes can also occur. Therefore, evaluation of a respiratory illness occurring in a patient with HIV infection can sometimes be challenging. Most opportunistic infections occur when a patient's CD4 count drops to >200 cells/mm.[3] This study by Wallace and associates is a longitudinal study involving a large number of patients. It provides important data regarding the incidence rates of various respiratory disorders, infectious and noninfectious, over a 5-year observation period. These observations should be useful in preventive care of patients with HIV as well as in evaluating respiratory illnesses in these patients.

J.H. Ryu, M.D.

Predictors of *Pneumocystis carinii* Pneumonia in HIV-infected Persons
Stansell JD, for the Pulmonary Complications of HIV Infection Study Group
(Univ of California, San Francisco; Research Triangle Inst, Research Triangle Park, North Carolina; Hahnemann Univ, Philadelphia; et al)
Am J Respir Crit Care Med 155:60–66, 1997   58–2

Background.—*Pneumocystis carinii* pneumonia (PCP) has become the most common serious opportunistic infection complicating the course of HIV infection. Early in the AIDS epidemic, PCP accounted for almost two thirds of index AIDS diagnoses, a proportion that has since declined to about 40%. The main reason for this decrease is the recognition of certain risk factors associated with *P. carinii* infection and the use of prophylactic regimens. Predictors of PCP were investigated in a prospective, multicenter, observational cohort study.

Methods and Findings.—The status of 1,182 HIV-infected patients was followed for approximately 52 months, and 145 episodes of PCP occurred. A low CD4 count was associated with the risk of PCP. Subtle changes in diffusing capacity for carbon monoxide also were found to be associated with PCP. A univariate analysis revealed that patients with CD4 counts exceeding 200 µL were at risk for recurrent, undiagnosed fevers; night sweats; oropharyngeal thrush; and unintentional weight loss. Patients with CD4 counts of less than 200 µL who were not receiving preventive treatment were 9 times more likely to have PCP within 6 months than patients receiving prophylactic therapy. The risk for PCP was one third as great in black patients as it was in white patients. In a multivariate analysis, low CD4 lymphocyte count, use of prophylaxis, racial differences, and declining diffusing capacity for carbon monoxide were found to affect risk.

Conclusions.—These findings strongly support the current recommendations for anti-*Pneumocystis* prophylaxis in persons with CD4 lymphocyte counts of less than 200 µL. Furthermore, the criteria for such treatment may need to be expanded to include persons with specific symptoms and findings associated with HIV infection whose CD4 lymphocyte levels exceed 100 µL.

▶ Patients with HIV infection are at risk for a variety of infectious and noninfectious pulmonary complications. Most opportunistic infections occur when CD4 cell counts fall below 200 µL. Prophylaxis for PCP in HIV-infected patients at risk has decreased the proportion of new AIDS cases with an index diagnosis of PCP. Nonetheless, it remains the most common cause of acute lung disease in patients with AIDS.[1, 2] This prospective multicenter study clarifies the risk factors for PCP in HIV-infected subjects. It is important to note that 5.2% of subjects developing PCP never had a CD4 cell count below 200 µL. The authors report that this subgroup of patients can be identified by the presence of oral thrush or recurrent fevers, night sweats, and unintentional weight loss. Therefore, patients with these symptoms or signs should be given PCP prophylaxis, even if their CD4 cell count is above 200 µL. Although declining diffusing capacity was associated with the development of PCP, I agree with the authors' conclusion that routine determinations of diffusing capacity in this setting are unlikely to be cost-effective.

J.H. Ryu, M.D.

References

1. Logan PM, Primack SL, Staples C, et al: Acute lung disease in the immunocompromised host. Diagnostic accuracy of the chest radiograph. *Chest* 108:1283–1287, 1995.
2. Kuhlman JE: Pulmonary manifestations of acquired immunodeficiency syndrome. *Semin Roentgenol* 29:242–274, 1994.

59 Bacterial Infections

The Continued Emergence of Drug-resistant *Streptococcus pneumo-niae* in the United States: An Update From the Centers for Disease Control and Prevention's Pneumococcal Sentinel Surveillance System
Butler JC, Hofmann J, Cetron MS, et al (Ctrs for Disease Control and Prevention, Atlanta, Ga)
J Infect Dis 174:986–993, 1996   59–1

Introduction.—The most common cause of purulent meningitis, community-acquired pneumonia, bacteremia, and acute otitis media is *Streptococcus pneumoniae*. Although penicillin had been prescribed for treatment of life-threatening pneumococcal infections for more than 40 years, in the 1990s drug-resistant strains emerged, including those with reduced susceptibility to multiple antibiotics. There was a more than 60-fold increase in isolates resistant to penicillin in 1992 compared to 1979–1987. The continuing emergence of penicillin-nonsusceptible strains of *S. pneumoniae* in the United States was documented, along with the appearance of resistance in a greater number of pneumococcal serotypes.

Methods.—At 12 hospitals in 11 states, serotyping and antimicrobial susceptibility testing were done on all pneumococcal isolates. The broth microdilution method was used to do the antimicrobial susceptibility testing. The isolates were classified as resistant, intermediate, or susceptible to each drug tested. Six major classes of drugs were tested, including β-lactams and carbapenems, trimethoprim-sulfamethoxazole, macrolides, ofloxacin, tetracycline, or chloramphenicol. Relative risks and confidence intervals were calculated.

Results.—There was 14.1% penicillin-nonsusceptible *S. pneumoniae* and 3.2% penicillin-resistant among 740 isolates. In this group, 25.5% were nonsusceptible to more than 1 antimicrobial agent. Among children younger than 6 years, the penicillin-resistant *S. pneumoniae* were more prevalent (18.4%) than among the patients that were 18 years or older (11.7%). There was also a higher prevalence among white persons (16.2%) than among black persons (12.1%). Up to 89% of penicillin-resistant *S. pneumoniae* were serotypes in the 23-valent pneumococcal vaccine, and penicillin-resistant *S. pneumoniae* represented 15 serotypes. There has been a substantial increase in the prevalence of strains that were nonsusceptible or resistant to penicillin, erythromycin, and trimethoprim-sulfamethoxazole, whereas those nonsusceptible or resistant to tetracycline have remained constant.

Conclusion.—In the United States, the proportion of isolates with reduced susceptibility and the number of serotypes of nonsusceptible strains are increasing. To treat and prevent disease caused by these strains, improved local surveillance for penicillin-resistant *S. pneumoniae* infections, judicious use of antibiotics, and development and use of effective pneumococcal vaccines will be required.

▶ Possibly more ominous than the identification of new organisms as causes of community acquired are the increasing reports of multiple drug resistance of organisms that once were exquisitely sensitive to common antibiotics. Butler et al. report on surveys of 12 hospitals in 11 states; more than 17 percent of 740 isolates were either penicillin nonsusceptible or penicillin resistant. Pneumococcal strains which develop penicillin resistance often develop multidrug resistance and become very difficult to treat. Clavo-Sanchez et al[1] state that nearly one half of clinically significant infections caused by *S. pneumoniae* were caused by resistant organisms. In this prospective, five hospital study of patients infected with *S. pneumoniae* the authors were able to identify risk factors for drug-resistant organisms. Despite the increasing awareness of growing antibiotic resistance by this and other organisms, the ongoing often indiscriminate use of antibiotics in the setting of minimal indications is particularly distressing.

J.R. Maurer, M.D.

Reference

1. Clavo-Sánchez AJ, Girón-Quintero J, López-Prieto D, et al: Multivariate analysis of risk factors for infection due to penicillin-resistant and multidrug-resistant Streptococcus pneumoniae: a multicentre study. *Clin Infect Dis* 24:1052–1059, 1997.

A Prediction Rule to Identify Low-risk Patients With Community-acquired Pneumonia
Fine MJ, Auble TE, Yealy DM, et al (Univ of Pittsburgh, Pa; Massachusetts Gen Hosp, Boston; Harvard Med School, Boston; et al)
N Engl J Med 336:243–250, 1997   59–2

Background.—About 4 million new cases of adult community-acquired pneumonia are seen in the United States each year. Hospital admission rates vary from region to region, which indicates that admission criteria may be inconsistent. Physicians tend to overestimate the risk of death, and patients at low risk are often hospitalized. Accurate, objective models for identifying low-risk patients with pneumonia may improve decisions about hospitalization.

Methods.—A prediction rule for patients with community-acquired pneumonia was derived from analyzing data from almost 14,200 adult inpatients. Patients were categorized into 5 classes by risk of 30-day hospital mortality. The prediction rule was validated with data from more than 38,000 inpatients and almost 2,300 additional inpatients and outpatients. In step 1 of the prediction rule, patients at low risk of death are identified from history and findings from physical examination. In step 2, the other patients are classified by findings from step 1 plus laboratory and radiographic data.

Results.—Mortality rates were similar in the 5 risk classes in the 3 patient cohorts. Mortality was 0.1% to 0.4% in class I, 0.6% to 0.7% in class II, and 0.9% to 2.8% in class III. There were only 7 deaths among 1,575 patients in the 3 lowest risk classes from the group of almost 2,300 inpatients and outpatients; only 4 of these 7 deaths were pneumonia related. Risk class was significantly associated with risk of hospitalization among outpatients and with use of intensive care and number of days admitted among inpatients.

Discussion.—This prognostic model accurately identified patients with community-acquired pneumonia with a low risk of death. This rule may help physicians make better decisions about hospitalizing patients with pneumonia. The predictor variables are well defined and may be evaluated at the initial examination, and patients can be assigned to the lowest risk class by information from the history and initial examination.

▶ As health care costs become more and more important, a host of approaches—from the development of clinical practice guidelines to the identification of outcome predictors have been proposed to assist in identifying appropriate cost efficient management strategies.

This article proposes a version of an outcome predictor which the authors call a prediction rule. Physicians can follow a decision tree at each step plugging in patient/disease characteristics which should be readily accessible. Physical signs and comorbidities have certain point values. Total point values place a patient in 1 of 5 risk classes; if the patient fits into a low-risk class presumably he can be treated as an outpatient thus saving considerable cost. This type of system might be very useful especially when validated by a huge cohort as in this instance.

J.R. Maurer, M.D.

Intrapleural Streptokinase Versus Urokinase in the Treatment of Complicated Parapneumonic Effusions: A Prospective, Double-blind Study
Bouros D, Schiza S, Patsourakis G, et al (Univ of Crete, Greece)
Am J Respir Crit Care Med 155:291–295, 1997   59–3

Introduction.—An estimated 1 million people a year in the United States have parapneumonic pleural effusions (PPE) in association with bacterial pneumonias. Two forms, complicated PPE (CPE) and pleural empyema, can lead to sepsis and death. Treatment of CPE and pleural empyema with fibrinolytics is reported to be safe and effective, but few studies have compared the various available agents. This prospective study examined outcome in patients given streptokinase (SK) or urokinase (UK).

Methods.—Fifty consecutive patients with CPE or pleural empyema were randomized to either SK (25 patients) or UK (25 patients). The 2 groups were similar in median age, gender distribution, proportions with CPE and pleural empyema, and clinical findings. All had inadequate drainage through chest tube (<70 mL/24 hr). The 2 drugs were diluted in 100 mL normal saline and infused intrapleurally through the test tube at daily doses of 250,000 IU of SK and 100,000 IU of UK. Patients were followed for a mean period of 12 months with clinical examinations, chest radiographs, and/or US or CT of the thorax.

Results.—The number of SK or UK instillations ranged from 3 to 12. Both groups showed a significant increase in the mean volume drained in the first 24 hours after instillation (380 mL for the SK group and 420.8 mL for the UK group). The total mean volume of fluid drained was 1,596 for the SK group and 1,510 for the UK group. Two patients administered SK experienced high fever as an adverse reaction, and 2 in each group failed to show clinical and radiologic improvement and required surgical intervention. All patients who responded to the therapy were doing well at follow-up. The mean total cost of the drug higher in the UK group ($320) than in the SK group ($180). Duration of hospitalization after the start of fibrinolytic therapy was slightly longer with SK (mean 11.28 days versus 10.48 days with UK).

Conclusion.—Both UK and SK enhanced the drainage of plural fluid in patients with CPE or pleural empyema. Fibrinolytic agents can reduce the need for surgery in such cases without jeopardizing subsequent surgical intervention when the therapy fails. Because of the potential for dangerous allergic reactions to SK, UK is recommended as the fibrinolytic agent of choice.

▶ Fibrinolytic agents have been sporadically used for many years in complicated parapneumonic effusions and empyemas to lyse adhesions and potentially reduce the need for open drainage procedures. However, it has only been in the 1990s that the use of these agents has been widely advocated and clinically applied. As a result, to date anecdotal studies have outnumbered well-designed studies not only to assess outcomes using these agents, but also to compare the relative benefits and negative aspects of the different agents. In this prospective study comparing the 2 most commonly used agents, streptokinase and urokinase, the authors found similar success rates in both groups. While the drug cost of urokinase was about twice that of streptokinase, the hospital stay of patients receiving urokinase was slightly lower making the cost differential very small. Since the incidence of adverse reactions is higher with streptokinase (nearly 10% in this series), urokinase seems to be a reasonable choice in most situations.

J.R. Maurer, M.D.

60 Intensive Care Medicine

Effects of a Medical Intensivist on Patient Care in a Community Teaching Hospital
Manthous CA, Amoateng-Adjepong Y, Al-Kharrat T, et al (Yale Univ, Bridgeport, Conn; Univ of Chicago)
Mayo Clin Proc 72:391–399, 1997   60–1

Introduction.—Questions remain about the medical intensivist's role in critical care administration. In particular, there are few data on the value of having a full-time, hospital-based intensivist in the community hospital setting. The impact of adding a trained intensivist on patient care and educational outcomes in a community teaching hospital was evaluated.

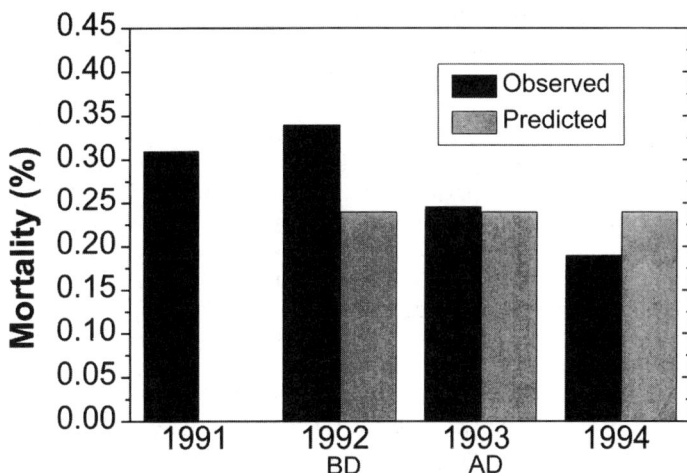

FIGURE 2.—Observed mean in-hospital mortality (*dark bars*) for patients admitted to the medical intensive-care unit during the periods before (1991 through 1992) (*BD*) and after (1993 through 1994) (*AD*) integration of a full-time intensivist director. Projected mortalities based on acuity of illness (acute physiology and chronic health evaluation or APACHE II scores) for 1992 through 1994 are demonstrated by the *light bars*. (Courtesy of Manthous CA, Amoateng-Adjepong Y, Al-Kharrat T, et al: Effects of a medical intensivist on patient care in a community teaching hospital. *Mayo Clinic Proc* 72:391–399, 1997.)

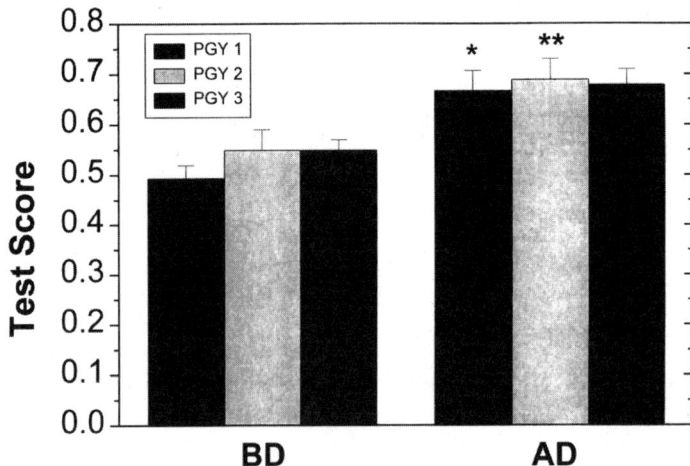

FIGURE 3.—Mean critical-care in-service examination scores for the year after integration of a full-time intensivist director and institution of a formal critical-care curriculum. * = End of first year after-director (*AD*) values tended to be higher than beginning of second year before-director (*BD*) values (*P* = 0.14). ** = End of second year AD values were significantly higher than beginning of third year BD values (*P* < 0.05). *PGY* = postgraduate year.

Methods.—The retrospective study analyzed data on patients admitted to the medical ICU of a community teaching hospital before and after the hiring of a medical intensivist as full-time director of critical care. There were 459 patients in the year before the director was hired (BD) and 471 patients in the year after the director was hired (AD). The 2 groups were compared for mortality and lengths of stay. The scores of residents on a standardized critical care examination were compared for the same 2 periods.

Results.—The BD and AD groups were similar in terms of case mix and illness severity scores. Mortality in the ICU was 21% in the BD period versus 15% in the AD period. At the same time, in-hospital mortality dropped from 34% to 25%. For most disease categories, disease-specific mortality was reduced in the AD period. More detailed analysis was performed in the subgroup of patients with pneumonia. Again, there were no differences in patient characteristics or severity of illness. Pneumonia-specific mortality decreased from 46% to 31%, across illness severity categories.

Mean length of hospital stay decreased from 23 days in the BD period to 18 days in the AD period. Mean ICU stay decreased from 5 to 4 days. The residents' critical care in-service test scores improved from 54% to 68%. For residents at a comparable level of treatment, scores were significantly higher in the AD period than in the BD period.

Conclusions.—Adding a medical intensivist to the staff of a community hospital is linked to improvements in patient and educational outcomes. Though no cause-and-effect conclusions can be drawn, the findings suggest that the costs of providing full-time intensivist coverage may be justified at many hospitals. Reduced mortality most likely results from improved staff education and proficiency in the ICU, or improved ICU organization and coordination between disciplines.

▶ According to Manthous et al., all that training in critical care may be useful after all. This retrospective review supports the notion that a full-time medical intensive care unit (MICU) director favorably affects patient mortality (Fig 2) and housestaff education (Fig 3). Until a prospective investigation is funded and published, this appears to be the "best evidence" for having a full time MICU director on the faculty in a teaching hospital. The obvious additional question is: "Is there value added by having in-house supervision by critical care specialists twenty four hours per day?" Further investigations as well, are required to examine this equally important question.

P. Strollo, M.D.

Effect on the Duration of Mechanical Ventilation of Identifying Patients Capable of Breathing Spontaneously
Ely EW, Baker AM, Dunagan DP, et al (Wake Forest Univ, Winston Salem, NC; Lynchburg Pulmonary Associates, Va; Mayo Clinic, Jacksonville, Fla)
N Engl J Med 335:1864–1869, 1996   60–2

Introduction.—Clinical judgment alone does not accurately predict timing of successful discontinuation of mechanical ventilation. It is possible that if patients could be screened daily with a trial of spontaneous breathing, physician behavior could be altered to discontinue mechanical ventilation earlier in appropriate patients.

Methods.—Three hundred adult patients receiving mechanical ventilation in medical and coronary intensive care units were randomized to either an intervention or control group (149 and 151, respectively). Patients in the intervention group were screened daily by physicians, respiratory therapists, and nurses to identify those capable of breathing spon-

---

TABLE 2.—Comparison of Outcomes Between Study Groups

END POINT	INTERVENTION GROUP (N = 149) median no. of days (interquartile range)		CONTROL GROUP (N = 151)		P VALUE
Weaning time*	1	(0–2)	3	(2–7)	<0.001
Mechanical ventilation	4.5	(2–9)	6	(3–11)	0.003
Intensive care	8	(4–18)	9	(5–16)	0.17
Hospital care	14	(9–26)	15.5	(6–30)	0.93

*Weaning time was defined as the number of days from the time the patient had a successful screening test to the discontinuation of mechanical ventilation.
(Reprinted by permission of The New England Journal of Medicine, courtesy of Ely EW, Baker AM, Dunagan DP, et al: Effect on the duration of mechanical ventilation of identifying patients capable of breathing spontaneously. *N Engl J Med* 335:1864–1869, copyright 1996, Massachusetts Medical Society.)

taneously. Physicians were notified by a preprinted message on the medical record when the patient had successfully completed a 2-hour trial of spontaneous breathing. Patients in the control group were screened daily, but did not undergo trials of spontaneous breathing. All decisions about patient care were made by the attending physician.

Results.—Patients in the intervention group had more severe disease, but received mechanical ventilation for a mean of 4.5 days, compared to 6 days for patients in the control group. The mean interval between when a patient met screening criteria for discontinuation of ventilation and actual discontinuation was 1 day for the intervention group and 3 days for the control group. Controls had significantly higher incidence of: removal of the breathing tube by the patient, reintubation, tracheostomy, and mechanical ventilation for more than 21 days, compared to the intervention group (41% vs. 20%). There were no between-group differences in the number of days in the intensive care and hospital (Table 2), but costs for these services were significantly lower: $15,740 vs. $20,890 for intensive care and $26,229 vs. $29,048 for hospitalization.

Conclusion.—Notifying physicians regarding results of spontaneous breathing in mechanically ventilated medical patients resulted in earlier removal (about 2 days) of mechanical ventilation and a 25% reduction in intensive care costs.

A Randomized, Controlled Trial of Protocol-directed Versus Physician-directed Weaning From Mechanical Ventilation

Kollef MH, Shapiro SD, Silver P, et al (Washington Univ, St Louis; Barnes-Jewish-Christian Hosp Health System, St Louis)
Crit Care Med 25:567–574, 1997   60–3

Introduction.—The gradual reduction of ventilatory support and its replacement with spontaneous ventilation is the definition of weaning from mechanical ventilation, yet there is controversy on how it should be performed. The efficacy and efficiency of a protocol to wean patients from mechanical ventilation was compared to the traditional practice of physician-directed weaning. Using the protocol guidelines, it was hypothesized that nurses and respiratory therapists could safely and effectively wean most patients from mechanical ventilation.

Methods.—There were 357 patients requiring mechanical ventilation; 179 were randomized into the protocol-directed group and 178 were randomized into the physician-directed weaning from mechanical ventilation group. The duration of mechanical ventilation from tracheal intubation until discontinuation of mechanical ventilation was measured. Need for reintubation, length of hospital stay, hospital mortality rate, and hospital costs were also analyzed.

Results.—For the protocol-directed group, the median duration of mechanical ventilation was 35 hours compared to 44 hours for the physician-directed group. Significantly shorter durations of mechanical ventilation were seen with the patient randomized to protocol-directed weaning when compared to those randomized to physician-directed weaning. The rate of successful weaning was significantly greater for patients receiving protocol-directed weaning compared with those receiving physician-directed weaning. For the 2 treatment groups, the hospital mortality rates were similar, with the protocol-directed group having a 22.3% mortality rate and the physician-directed group having a 23.6% mortality rate. Patients in the protocol-directed group saved $42,9609 on hospital costs in comparison to the patients in the physician-directed group.

Conclusion.—Extubation occurred more rapidly with protocol-guided weaning of mechanical ventilation, as performed by nurses and respiratory therapists, than with physician-directed weaning.

▶ These 2 studies demonstrate that protocol-directed assessment of eligibility for liberation from mechanical ventilation leads to earlier extubation and decreased cost of hospitalization without adverse outcome with regard to reintubation, length of stay, and mortality (see Table 2, Abstract 60–2). The study by Ely et al. (see Abstract 60–2) was conducted primarily in the medical intensive care unit (MICU) and more rigidly controlled. The study by Kollef et al. (see Abstract 60–3) involve patients in 4 intensive care units (ICUs), 2 MICUs and 2 surgical intensive care units (SICUs). In the Kollef study, one of the ICUs have a part time critical care physician and no critical care fellows. Another difference with the Kollef study was that each of the 4 ICUs had their own "unique" weaning protocol that involved either continuous positive airway pressure with pressure support (PS), intermittent mandatory ventilation with PS, or PS alone. This may have introduced an additional set of variables that affected the analysis of the data. Despite these limitations, it appears that protocol-directed weaning protocols are advantageous in both the SICU as well as the MICU.

P. Strollo, M.D.

61 Sleep

Risk of Traffic Accidents in Patients With Sleep-disordered Breathing:
Reduction With Nasal CPAP
Cassel W, Ploch T, Becker C, et al (Klinikum der Philipps-Universität, Marburg, Germany)
Eur Respir J 9:2606–2611, 1996   61–1

Introduction.—Sleep-related factors are involved in many types of accidents, and several studies report an elevated risk for traffic accidents in patients with sleep-related breathing disorders (SRBD). The most common treatment of SRBD, nasal continuous positive airway pressure (nCPAP), appears to reduce the accident rate in patients with obstructive sleep apnea. A study of patients with SRBD was conducted to determine whether their rate of traffic accidents would be reduced after 1 year of treatment with nCPAP.

Methods.—Study participants were 78 men aged 25 to 65. All had been referred to a sleep disorders clinic and reported excessive daytime sleepiness. Exclusion criteria included a diagnosis of narcolepsy, chronic medical illnesses, and alcohol and drug abuse. Patients underwent polysomnographic sleep studies to confirm the presence of SRBD and the indication for nCPAP. Before treatment, participants completed a questionnaire dealing with alertness-related problems while driving and underwent an 80-minute vigilance test and the Multiple Sleep Latency Test. These evaluations were repeated after 1 year of nCPAP treatment.

Results.—Patients initially enrolled in the study had a mean age of 48.1 and a mean body mass index of 31 $kg \cdot m^{-2}$. Fifty-nine patients completed the study. The 44 patients with timing meter data available had an objective average nightly use of nCPAP of 6.1 hours (minimum 4 hours and maximum 8.3 hours nightly use). Among patients completing the study, the traffic accident rate was significantly decreased from 0.8 per 100,000 in the 5 years before nCPAP treatment to 0.15 per 100,000 km in the treatment year (Fig 1). Treatment also improved sleeping spells, fatigue, vigilance test reaction time, and daytime sleep latency, all factors likely to increase accident risk.

Conclusion.—The treatment of SRBD with nCPAP for 12 months significantly reduced the accident rate of patients, improved their vigilance, and decreased daytime sleepiness. Identification and treatment of patients

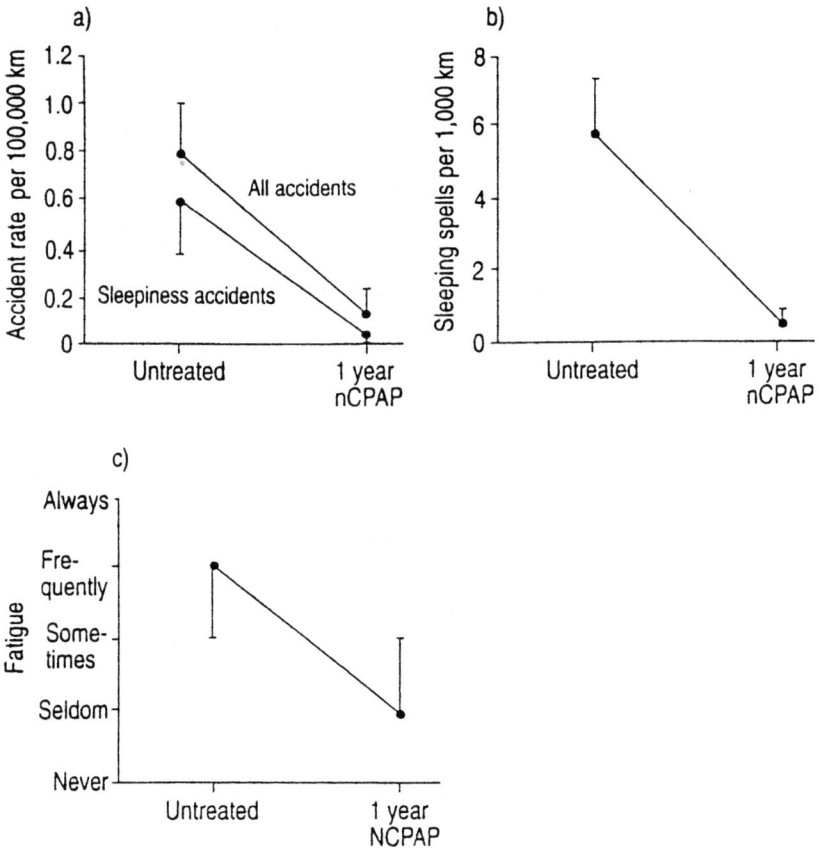

FIGURE 1.—Alertness-related problems while driving. a) Accident rate per 100,000 km (+SEM) before and after 1 year of nCPAP treatment, and sleepiness accident rate per 100,000 km (−SEM) (accidents rated by patients to be caused by falling asleep, fatigue or inability to maintain a sufficient level of concentration) before and after 1 year of nCPAP treatment. b) Mean frequency of dozing off or startling per 1,000 km (+SEM) before and after 1 year of nCPAP treatment. c) Median rating of severe fatigue/decreases in alertness whilst driving, before and after 1 year of nCPAP treatment ±1 quartile (untreated: 75% quartile =median; 1 year nCPAP: 25% quartile = median). *Abbreviation: nCPAP,* nasal continuous positive airway pressure. (Courtesy of Cassel W, Ploch T, Becker C, et al: Risk of traffic accidents in patients with sleep-disordered breathing: Reduction with nasal CPAP. *Eur Respir J* 9:2606–2611, 1996.)

with SRBD would have a positive cost-benefit effect, and would also reduce accidents in the workplace.

▶ Obstructive sleep apnea (OSA) has been linked to an increased risk of auto crashes. The risk is felt to be related to impaired vigilance. This report by Cassel et al. represents the first citation in the English literature demonstrating a favorable treatment effect with nasal continuous positive airway pressure (nCPAP). Of the patients enrolled (n = 78), 59 patients completed the study. Objective compliance with nCPAP was quite good at 6.1 + 0.16 hr/night (range, 4.0–8.3 hr/night). On the basis of a questionnaire, complaints of fatigue, sleeping spells per 1,000 km, and the accident rate per 100,000 km driven were all favorably influenced (Fig 1). This improvement was paralleled by improvement in vigilance testing. Of interest, the multiple sleep latency tests (MSLT) improved with treatment (12 + 0.67 vs. 16.8 + 0.71 min), despite the fact that the baseline tests did not reflect what would be considered significant sleepiness. This suggests that a "normal" MSLT does not guarantee adequate driving performance, possibly because of the inability to assess the presence of "micro-sleep" on this test.

P. Strollo, M.D.

PART EIGHT

THE DIGESTIVE SYSTEM
RICHARD W. MCCALLUM, M.D.

62 Diagnostic Testing

Importance of Adenomas 5 mm or Less in Diameter That Are Detected by Sigmoidoscopy
Read TE, Read JD, Butterly LF (Lahey-Hitchcock Med Ctr, Burlington, Mass)
N Engl J Med 336:8–12, 1997   62–1

Background.—Authorities disagree on the need for colonoscopy in patients with adenomas 5 mm or less in diameter that are detected by sigmoidoscopy. In the current prospective study, the prevalence of proximal colonic neoplasms was determined in a large group of asymptomatic patients at average risk for colorectal cancer and with diminutive benign adenomatous polyps on screening flexible sigmoidoscopy.

Methods.—A total of 3,496 consecutive patients underwent sigmoidoscopy, 311 of whom were found to have neoplastic rectosigmoid polyps. One hundred eight were excluded because of a history of colonic neoplasia, symptoms, previous colonic assessment, or incomplete followup data. The remaining 203 patients underwent colonoscopy. Rectosigmoid adenomas 5 mm or less in diameter were designated diminutive; 6–10 mm, small; and 11 mm or greater, large.

Findings.—Neoplasms were detected in the proximal colon of 29% of the 137 patients with diminutive index polyps, 29% of the 52 patients with small index polyps, and 57% of the 14 patients with large index polyps. Advanced neoplasms were detected in 6%, 10%, and 29%, respectively. Two patients with diminutive index polyps had proximal carcinoma in situ. Another 2 in this group had proximal stage I carcinomas. Proximal stage III carcinoma was found in a patient with a large index polyp.

Conclusions.—The prevalence of proximal colonic neoplasms, including advanced lesions, in asymptomatic average-risk patients with rectosigmoid adenomas 5 mm or less in diameter is substantial. Thus colonoscopy is warranted in these patients.

▶ This article details the importance of adenomas that are 5 mm or less in diameter and detected by flexible sigmoidoscopy. Read et al. indicate that when one finds rectosigmoid lesions of 5 mm or less in diameter, colonoscopy is warranted because there is a substantial prevalence of proximal colonic neoplasms, including advanced lesions, in asymptomatic average-risk patients. It is important to re-emphasize that these lesions are actually adenomatous and not hyperplastic. Neoplasms were found in the proximal colon in 29% of patients with the diminutive index polyps. In the patients having small polyps of 6–10 mm, 29% had a lesion and in patients having polyps greater than 10 mm, 57% had a lesion. Although other studies have looked at this, none have done compulsive biopsies. It is felt that hyperplastic polyps do not have this kind of potential, so adenomatous polyps documented by biopsy portend a different prognosis and, when combined with the genetic profile that is now being evolved in the literature, would help to identify the crucial patient subsets to focus on initially for colonoscopy and then long-term surveillance postpolypectomy as well.

R.W. McCallum, M.D.

Endoscopic Ultrasound-guided Fine-needle Aspiration Biopsy Using Linear Array and Radial Scanning Endosonography
Gress FG, Hawes RH, Savides TJ, et al (Indiana Univ, Indianapolis)
Gastrointest Endosc 45:243–250, 1997   62–2

Introduction.—The accuracy of endoscopic US (EUS) for staging esophageal, gastric, rectal, and pancreatic carcinoma has been well documented. A major disadvantage of the method is its limited ability to differentiate between inflammatory and neoplastic processes. Recent developments have made it possible to perform EUS-guided fine-needle aspiration (FNA) biopsy, and studies report a high sensitivity and specificity for the technique. Endoscopic US-guided FNA was evaluated in a study of 208 patients with suspected gastrointestinal or mediastinal masses.

Methods.—The patients, 119 men and 89 women, had a mean age of 61 years. A total of 705 FNA passes were performed for a mean of 3.39 passes per patient. Most of the lesions sampled were pancreatic masses (58%). Submucosal lesions of the gastrointestinal tract wall accounted for 13%, mediastinal lymph nodes or masses for 21%, intra-abdominal lymph nodes for 6%, and perirectal lesions for 2%. The procedure was performed using radial scanning or linear array endosonography and a 23-gauge 4-cm needle or a 22-gauge, 12-cm needle.

Results.—Adequate specimens were obtained in 90% of patients. Endoscopic US-guided FNA had an overall diagnostic accuracy of 87%, a sensitivity of 89%, and a specificity of 100%. Diagnostic accuracy was 95% for the mediastinal lymph node subgroup, 85% for the intra-abdominal lymph node subgroup, 85% for pancreatic masses, 84% for submucosal lesions, and 100% for perirectal masses. The 2 types of endosonography yielded similar results. Immediate complications were recorded in 4 (2%) patients, all with pancreatic lesions. Bleeding occurred in 2 of these cases and episodes of pancreatitis in 2.

Conclusion.—The overall diagnostic accuracy of EUS-guided FNA was 87%. This technique was safe and highly accurate for detecting mediastinal lymph node metastasis and diagnosing perirectal and pancreatic masses. A single procedure can confirm the presence of a mass, obtain a tissue diagnosis, and identify potentially resectable malignant lesions.

Staging of Ampullary and Pancreatic Carcinoma: Comparison Between Endosonography and Surgery
Tio TL, Sie LH, Kallimanis G, et al (Georgetown Univ, Washington DC; Academic Med Ctr, Amsterdam)
Gastrointest Endosc 44:706–713, 1996   62–3

Introduction.—Endoscopic US (EUS), or endosonography, can accurately stage biliary and pancreatic carcinomas because of its ability to image both the ductal and parenchymal abnormality. In an update of previously published data, the clinical TNM staging of ampullary and pancreatic carcinoma by endoscopy was compared with surgical or histologic findings or both.

Methods.—Endosonography was performed before surgery in 102 patients, 70 with pancreatic cancer and 32 with ampullary carcinoma. Diagnosis was obtained by endoscopic retrograde cholangiopancreatography and EUS, or determined before surgery with endoscopic biopsy or cytology during endoscopic retrograde cholangiopancreatography (30 patients), EUS-guided cytology (1 patient), transcutaneous US-guided cytology (3 patients), or previous laparotomy (1 patient).

Results.—Pancreatic carcinomas could be assessed histologically in 52 patients and at autopsy in 1 case; ampullary tumors were able to be assessed in all 32 patients histologically. Endosonography was accurate in staging the depth of tumor invasion and distinguished early-stage carcinomas from advanced cancers. Using real-time US, tumor nonresectability was accurately assessed on the basis of vascular involvement. Imaging with EUS was unable to diagnose tumor compression resulting from peritumoral pancreatitis and direct tumor invasion into the base of the mesocolon. Endosonography achieved an overall accuracy of 83.6% in tumor staging for pancreatic cancer and 84.4% for ampullary carcinoma. Regional lymph node metastases were accurately diagnosed with EUS, but the technique failed to define nonmetastatic lymphadenopathy and distant metastases.

Conclusion.—Pancreatic carcinoma has a highly malignant nature and a poor prognosis, whereas ampullary carcinoma is less aggressive and has a more favorable prognosis. It is important to distinguish the 2 tumors before surgery. In this series of patients, endosonography was accurate in assessing the tumor category of pancreatic and ampullary carcinoma, staging the tumors, and defining lymph node metastases.

▶ The article by Tio et al. describes the role of EUS vs. surgery in trying to stage ampullary and pancreatic cancer accurately. The EUS was accurate in staging the tumor and the lymph node metastases. The level of accuracy was 83% to 94% in pancreatic and ampullary cancer, respectively. This evolving technique of EUS is more and more becoming clearly associated with pancreatic cancer, whether it be adenocarcinoma or islet cell cancer, and also defining lymph node metastases. Its other potential use is in guiding an FNA biopsy technique as discussed by Gress et al. again in gastrointestinal endoscopy, where it can be a very important guide for FNA biopsy of suggested gastrointestinal and mediastinal lesions. The technique provided an adequate specimen in 90% of patients, and complication rates were only 2% in a series of 208 patients. This further defines an important role for EUS, a clinical tool that has perhaps been loitering in the wings waiting for a more meaningful career.

R.W. McCallum, M.D.

In Vitro and Clinical Studies of Image Acquisition in Breath-hold MR Cholangiopancreatography: Single-shot Projection Technique Versus Multislice Technique
Yamashita Y, Abe Y, Tang Y, et al (Kumamoto Univ, Japan)
AJR 168:1449–1454, 1997   62–4

Introduction.—Patients with pancreaticobiliary disease participated in a study designed to compare the in vitro and clinical value of 2-dimensional multislice breath-hold MR cholangiopancreatography with a single-shot projection technique using a half-Fourier acquisition single-shot turbo spin-echo sequence.

Methods.—Study participants were 108 consecutive patients, 76 men and 32 women, who were prospectively examined between October 1995 and March 1996. All underwent endoscopic retrograde cholangiopancreatography or percutaneous transhepatic cholangiography or both, and these images were used as the standard. In the multislice technique, 9 contiguous slices were obtained in an interleaved fashion with a thickness of 5 mm; the projection technique obtained a single slice with a thickness of 30, 50, or 70 mm. Each acquisition time was 2 seconds. Coronal and paracoronal projections were acquired for each patient. The 2 acquisition techniques were compared for detection of normal structures and diseases.

Results.—Most of the pancreatic duct and common bile duct was demonstrated on 54% and 100% of the projection images, respectively, and on 35% and 98% of the multislice images, respectively. Contrast-to-noise ratio was significantly higher with the multislice technique and decreased as slice thickness increased with the projection technique. Because of this decrease with the projection technique, large slice thickness did not markedly increase the frequency of visualization of the pancreatic duct in the tail of the pancreas. The 2 imaging techniques were equivalent in their ability to reveal dilatation and occlusion of the pancreaticobiliary tree. Projection images were superior at demonstrating abnormalities in the periampullary region and anomalies in the pancreaticobiliary tree. Source images acquired by the multislice technique were superior in showing stones in the common bile duct, gallbladder, or intrahepatic bile duct.

Conclusion.—Half-Fourier acquisition single-shot turbo spin-echo MR cholangiopancreatography, using the projection technique at 30- or 50-mm slice thickness, provides excellent visualization of the main pancreatic duct and common bile duct. This is achieved because of the absence of misregistration and fast image acquisition time of the technique. Source images acquired by the multislice technique are superior for stone evaluation.

▶ This study deals with a very important and evolving area where MR cholangiopancreatography may be replacing endoscopic retrograde cholangiopancreatography. The studies here indicated that using a projection technique, and achieving 30- or 50-mm slice thickness, there was excellent visualization of the main pancreatic duct and the common bile duct, and stones in the bile duct could actually be evaluated. This area is a rapidly growing and important development.

R.W. McCallum, M.D.

Helical CT Angiography in Gastrointestinal Bleeding of Obscure Origin
Ettore GC, Francioso G, Garribba AP, et al (Univ of Bari, Italy)
AJR 168:727–730, 1997   62–5

Introduction.—Endoscopy and barium studies are able to establish the source and nature of gastrointestinal bleeding in approximately 76% to 90% of all causes of such bleeding. In some cases, however, the origin of bleeding cannot be identified with visceral angiography. Eighteen patients with gastrointestinal bleeding of obscure origin were studied to assess the value of helical CT angiography in this setting.

Methods.—The methodology is based on a helical CT of the abdomen after catheterization of the abdominal aorta. Images are obtained before and after intra-arterial injections of a contrast medium. The site of hemorrhage is revealed as an extravasation of contrast medium, resulting in a hyperdense area in the intestinal lumen. All patients underwent conventional angiography after helical CT angiography. When helical CT angiography had indicated the bleeding source, a selective angiogram of the mesenteric superior or inferior artery involved was performed.

Results.—Helical CT angiography diagnosed gastrointestinal bleeding in 13 (72%) patients. Conventional angiography confirmed the helical CT findings in only 11 cases, but revealed an angiodysplasia of the jejunum and of the colon with active bleeding in 2 cases with negative helical CT findings. Overall, active bleeding was diagnosed in 15 (83%) patients, 11 of whom underwent surgery and had the bleeding site confirmed. No patients experienced local complications or allergic reactions as a result of the angiographic procedures.

Conclusion.—A fast and accurate diagnosis of the source of gastrointestinal bleeding allows therapy to be initiated promptly and improves prognosis. Helical CT angiography should be considered as a possible diagnostic tool for the identification of gastrointestinal bleeding of unknown origin. The technique is faster and easier than conventional angiography and may be useful as a guide for subsequent selective conventional angiography.

▶ Helical CT allows for the acquisition of volumetric data with brief scanning times, making it very important in evaluation of the chest and abdomen and for mini-evaluation of vascular dynamics. Therefore, in this study, the combination of abdominal and helical CT with catheterization of the abdominal aorta enabled a fast and more accurate diagnosis to be obtained. This report indicated that it could be a much more rapid and easier technique to identify obscure gastrointestinal bleeding sites and then be a further guide for using selective conventional angiography. This should augment a very difficult area of clinical diagnosis and can be complementary to the article by Schmit that addressed push-enteroscopy (see following abstract).

R.W. McCallum, M.D.

Diagnostic Efficacy of Push-enteroscopy and Long-term Follow-up of Patients With Small Bowel Angiodysplasias
Schmit A, Gay F, Adler M, et al (Erasme Univ, Brussels, Belgium)
Dig Dis Sci 41:2348–2352, 1996   62–6

Introduction.—Despite extensive investigations, the cause of gastrointestinal bleeding remains undiagnosed in approximately 5% of patients. The most common cause of obscure chronic digestive blood loss, gastrointestinal angiodysplasias (AD), presents a diagnostic and therapeutic problem. Eighty-three patients with anemia of obscure origin and no identified bleeding site were examined with push-enteroscopy.

Methods.—The patients were 38 women and 45 men, all with hemoglobin levels less than 10 g/100 mL and positive hemoccult tests; 28 required blood transfusions. At least 1 esophagogastroduodenoscopy and 1 colposcopy was performed in each patient; 50% had small bowel barium studies. A 240-cm Olympus push-enteroscope was used to detect bleeding sites.

Results.—The examination required a mean of 35 minutes. Six patients had to be sedated with propofol. Progression of the scope was considered successful in 86 of 90 examinations. Forty-nine patients (59%) had a potential bleeding site identified. The most common lesions, found in 33 patients, were AD. The 3 small bowel tumors that were detected had been missed on barium studies. No lesions were found in 30 (36%) patients. Biopsies, obtained in 16 patients, yielded diagnoses of Crohn's disease and ulcerative jejunitis. Patients with or without melena had a similar percentage of potential hemorrhagic lesions (37.8% and 34.8%, respectively). Patients with AD were significantly older than those without AD (71.4 years vs. 57.2 years). Fourteen patients underwent endoscopic treatment of AD by electrocoagulation, and hormonal treatment was proposed for patients with at least 5 AD; in some cases, both therapies were used. Twelve of 25 patients with small bowel AD had a good outcome, with no recurrence of anemia or need for transfusion.

Conclusion.—Push-enteroscopy proved to be a safe and useful diagnostic modality for patients with obscure digestive bleeding. Most of the 90 examinations were well tolerated and none led to complications. Almost 60% of patients had a potential source of bleeding identified. Treatment, however, was successful in only 50% of patients.

▶ A major challenge is investigation of patients with mysterious sites of gastrointestinal bleeding. This is a very important article because push-enteroscopy is now being done in clinical centers in gastroenterology. It indicates that up to 240 cm of endoscope can be inserted over a period of 20–45 minutes and that a diagnostic yield can be obtained. However, it did indicate that endoscopic cautery or hormonal therapy did not always seem to make a difference as far as final clinical outcome is concerned when compared to no treatment, nevertheless, this is an ongoing important area of investigation.

R.W. McCallum, M.D.

63 Inflammatory Bowel Disease

Long-term Outcome After Ileocecal Resection for Crohn's Disease
Kim NK, Senagore AJ, Luchtefeld MA, et al (Ferguson-Blodgett Digestive
Disease Inst, Grand Rapids, Mich; Michigan State Univ, East Lansing)
Am Surg 63:627–633, 1997   63–1

Background.—Concerns about early recurrence and the potential for
multiple small bowel resections, resulting in gastroenterologic crippling,
usually affect the decision to operate on patients with ileocecal Crohn's
disease. However, delaying surgical treatment may unnecessarily prolong a
patient's disease state and increase the risk of complications from medication or unchecked disease. The long-term clinical outcomes of patients
undergoing ileocecal resection for Crohn's disease between 1970 and 1993
were reported.

Methods and Findings.—One hundred eighty-one patients undergoing
ileocecal resection for Crohn's disease were reviewed. Median follow-up
was 14.3 years. Mean age at first resection was 32.7 years. Initial resection
was indicated by intractability in 68.4% of patients, obstruction in 25.9%,
enteric fistula in 15.5%, perforation in 9.2%, intraabdominal abscess in
4%, and hemorrhage in 2.9%. Postoperative complications included prolonged ileus in 7.5% of patients, pneumonia/atelectasis in 8.6%, wound
infection in 6.3%, urinary tract infection in 5.7%, intraabdominal abscess
in 4%, and wound dehiscence in 0.6%. No operative deaths occurred.
Recurrence necessitating additional surgery occurred in 30.9% of patients,
at a mean interval of 72.3 months. A second recurrence developed in
10.5% of patients, at a mean interval of 52.3 months. The sites of first
recurrences were the preanastomotic ileum in 87.5% of patients, postanastomotic colon in 17.9%, other colonic sites in 28.6%, other small
bowel sites in 3.6%, and other sites in 7.1%. Types of resection for first
recurrences were ileal in 50% of patients, right hemicolectomy in 30.4%,
segmental colectomy in 10.7%, total proctocolectomy in 5.4%, and proximal small bowel resection in 3.6%. By the end of follow-up, 69.1% of
patients had only 1 resection, 20.4% had 2, 8.3% had 3, and 2.2% had 4.

Conclusions.—Ileocecal resection of Crohn's disease is associated with a
high rate of disease control, with low morbidity, and with a low frequency

of 3 or more bowel resections. Thus surgical resection of ileocecal Crohn's disease should not be delayed unduly because of concerns about the possibility of short bowel syndrome. Earlier resection should minimize overall disease-related patient morbidity by avoiding long periods of chronic disease.

▶ Kim et al. show that an ileocecal resection of Crohn's disease has a high rate of disease control, and that 30% of patients developed a recurrence requiring further surgery, with a mean interval of 6 years between the initial resection and the first operation. The most frequent site of recurrence is well known and was reconfirmed here in 88% of patients limited to the immediate preanastomotic ileum and the remaining recurrences were in the immediate postanastomotic colon. The authors should be congratulated for trying to reassure us that short-bowel syndrome from chronic recurrent surgery is not really a great risk and that it should not deter the first procedure, which optimally is for severe stricturing when a minimal or limited amount of bowel to be resected.

R.W. McCallum, M.D.

Neoplastic Transformation of the Pelvic Pouch Mucosa in Patients With Ulcerative Colitis

Gullberg K, Ståhlberg D, Liljeqvist L, et al (Huddinge Univ, Sweden; Karolinska Inst, Stockholm; Univ Hosp Malmö Allmänna Sjukhus, Sweden)
Gastroenterology 112:1487–1492, 1997   63–2

Background.—Persistent severe villous atrophy develops in the pouch mucosa of some patients receiving an ileal pelvic pouch with ileoanal anastomosis (IPAA) for ulcerative colitis (UC). Whether mucosal atrophy is a risk factor for subsequent neoplastic transformation of the ileal pouch mucosa was studied.

Methods.—Seven patients with UC, an IPAA, and persistent severe atrophy (type C) and 14 control patients with no or only slight atrophy (type A) were studied prospectively. Flexible videoendoscopy was performed with multiple biopsies to assess possible neoplastic changes.

Findings.—In both groups, the median time of the pouch in function was 9 years. Dysplasia occurred in 5 of 7 patients (71%) in the type C group and in none of the type A group. Four patients had low-grade dysplasia. One patient had sequential multifocal development into high-grade dysplasia. Two patients had multifocal DNA aneuploidy—low-grade in 1 and high-grade in 1.

Conclusions.—The development of persistent severe mucosal atrophy in patients with UC and a long-standing IPAA indicates a risk of neoplastic transformation of the pouch mucosa. Thorough follow-up with long-term endoscopic surveillance, including multiple biopsy samples for the assessment of possible dysplastic development, would be prudent. Flow-cytometric analysis may also be useful for detecting DNA aneuploidy.

▶ Gullberg et al. show that there can be neoplastic transformation of the pelvic pouch mucosa in patients with ulcerative colitis. There has been a great deal of interest in the role of the ileal pelvic pouch following an ileoanal anastomosis because there is restoration of the integrity of the gut without the patient's having to retain an ostomy bag. These patients who are at risk tend to have frequent attacks of severe "pouchitis" and that leads to atrophy and perhaps neoplastic change. Therefore, some endoscopic follow-up in these pouches is indicated, and the average time involved in this study was around 9 years.

R.W. McCallum, M.D.

Transdermal Nicotine for Mildly to Moderately Active Ulcerative Colitis: A Randomized, Double-blind, Placebo-controlled Trial
Sandborn WJ, Tremaine WJ, Offord KP, et al (Mayo Clinic and Found, Rochester, Minn)
Ann Intern Med 126:364–371, 1997   63–3

Introduction.—The knowledge that ulcerative colitis is infrequently seen in current smokers prompted trials on the effect of transdermal nicotine. To confirm the findings of uncontrolled trials, a randomized trial was conducted to determine the efficacy of transdermal nicotine for controlling clinical disease activity in patients with active ulcerative colitis.

Methods.—The 64 nonsmoking patients who entered the double-blind trial had mildly to moderately active ulcerative colitis. After stratification on the basis of smoking history, extent of disease, and concomitant medical therapy, 31 patients were randomly assigned to daily treatment with

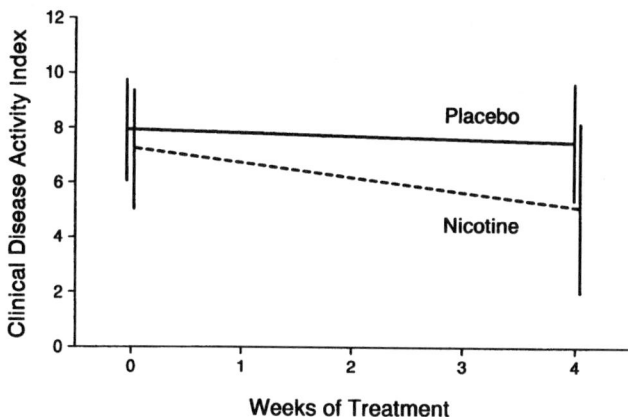

Weeks of Treatment

FIGURE 2.—Mean scores on the ulcerative colitis clinical disease activity index for each treatment group at each study visit. *Vertical bars* at 0 and 4 weeks represent SDs. $P = 0.009$ (2-sample rank-sum test) for scores in the nicotine group at week 4 compared with scores in the placebo group at week 4 (2-sample rank-sum test). $P = 0.001$ (1-sample signed-rank test) for scores in the nicotine group at baseline compared with those at week 4. (Courtesy of Sandborn WJ, Tremaine WJ, Offord KP, et al: Transdermal nicotine for mildly to moderately active ulcerative colitis: A randomized, double-blind, placebo-controlled trial. *Ann Intern Med* 126:364–371, 1997.)

transdermal nicotine at the highest tolerated dose (11 mg for 1 week, then 22 mg or less for 3 weeks) and 33 were randomly assigned to placebo. Patients were evaluated at study entry and after 4 weeks for disease activity, adverse reactions, extent of remission, and concentrations of serum nicotine and plasma cotinine.

Results.—The active treatment and placebo groups were similar in demographic characteristics, concomitant drug therapy, and disease severity. At 4 weeks, clinical improvement was present in 39% of patients who received nicotine vs. 9% who were given placebo. Clinical disease activity scores improved significantly in the nicotine group and showed no significant change in the placebo group (Fig 2). Side effects, including contact dermatitis, nausea, and acute pancreatitis, led 4 patients to discontinue nicotine treatment. At the end of the trial, the nicotine group had a mean trough serum nicotine concentration of 11.3 ng/mL and a mean trough plasma cotinine concentration of 192 ng/mL. Plasma concentrations of cotinine showed no significant correlation with change in disease activity.

Conclusion.—As suggested by results of previous studies, transdermal nicotine administered at the highest tolerated dosage (22 mg or less/day) for 4 weeks controlled the clinical manifestations of mildly to moderately active ulcerative colitis. Patients had all continued with their previous therapy (5-aminosalicylate compounds or oral corticosteroids or both).

▶ This article showed that transdermal nicotine patches administering the highest tolerated dose, approximately 22 mg/day for 4 weeks, was efficacious for controlling the clinical manifestations of mildly to moderately active ulcerative colitis. This comes out of the background of our knowledge that nonsmokers who have ulcerative colitis and begin smoking can actually go into remission, and although obviously not offering encouragement as far as beginning to smoke is concerned, this research using transdermal nicotine is exciting because of its mechanistic implications. It is interesting that in Crohn's disease, nicotine actually worsens the disease. The patients studied here were nonsmokers. An important aspect to remember in reading this article is that in actual fact these patients were receiving 5-aminosalicylate compounds or oral steroids or both and that transdermal nicotine patches did not induce remission in these nonsmokers.

R.W. McCallum, M.D.

A Trial of Zileuton Versus Mesalazine or Placebo in the Maintenance of Remission of Ulcerative Colitis
Hawkey CJ, Dube LM, Rountree LV, et al (Univ Hosp, Nottingham, England; Abbott Labs Ltd, Chicago)
Gastroenterology 112:718–724, 1997   63–4

Introduction.—Studies in animal models and human beings suggest that leukotriene B$_4$ may be a therapeutic target for the maintenance of remission in patients with ulcerative colitis. A phase III double-blind study was designed to compare the efficacy of zileuton, an active 5-lipoxygenase inhibitor, with mesalazine and placebo.

Methods.—The 6-month, multinational study randomized 305 patients with ulcerative colitis in remission: 113 received zileuton (600 mg 4 times daily), 99 were treated with mesalazine (400 mg 4 times daily), and 111 were given placebo. All patients took 3 capsules at 7 AM, 1 PM, 6 PM, and 11 PM. Evaluations were scheduled for days 1 and 14 and at weeks 8, 16, and 26 of treatment. Patients underwent sigmoidoscopy and rectal biopsy

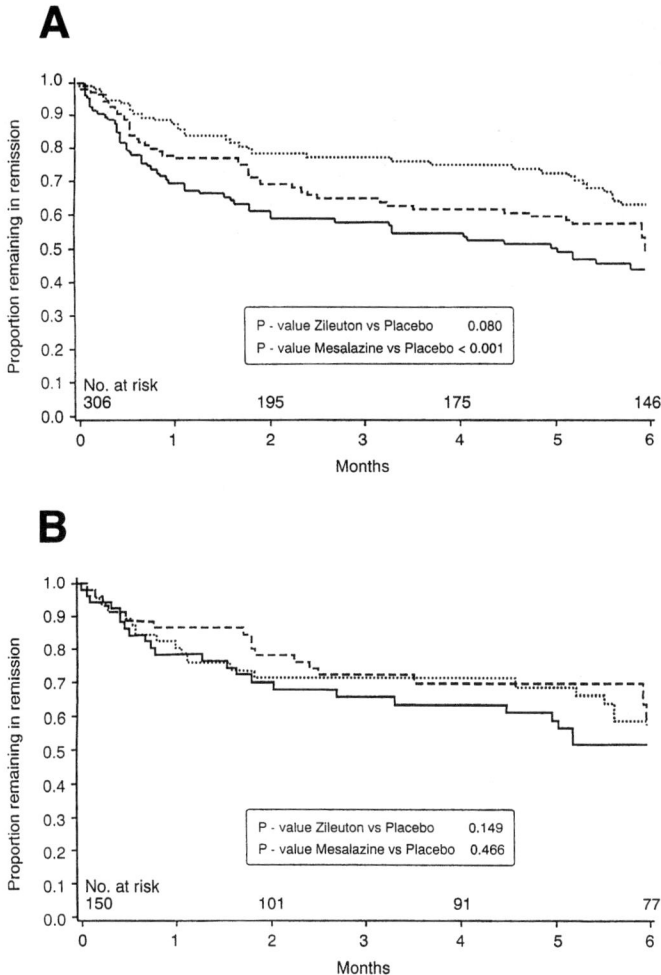

FIGURE 2.—Estimated distributions of time until relapse. Proportion of patients who had a relapse by treatment group for **(A)** all evaluable patients and **(B)** evaluable patients not taking mesalazine within 30 days before the first dose of study drug. *Solid line*, placebo; *dotted line*, mesalazine; *dashed line*, zileuton. (Courtesy of Hawkey CJ, Dube LM, Rountree LV, et al: A trial of zileuton versus mesalazine or placebo in the maintenance of remission of ulcerative colitis. *Gastroenterology* 112:718–724, 1997.)

before study entry and at weeks 8 and 26 or at relapse. Maintenance of remission was the primary efficacy end point.

Results.—At the end of 6 months, remission had been maintained in 43% of patients in the placebo group, 54% in the zileuton group, and 63% in the mesalazine group. Differences between the 2 active treatments were not significant, but relapse rates were significantly lower for mesalazine than for placebo. Life-table analysis of Kaplan-Meier estimates yielded similar results (Fig 2). Other variables significantly influencing remission were reported extent of disease, duration of current remission, multiple vs. single episodes, steroid use up to 30 days before study entry, and mesalazine vs. placebo. All treatments were well tolerated. Headache, the most commonly reported adverse event, occurred less often with zileuton than with mesalazine and placebo.

Conclusion.—Although there was a trend toward improved outcome in patients receiving zileuton, the difference between this drug and placebo was not statistically significant. Zileuton may be of limited potential in the maintenance of remission of ulcerative colitis.

▶ This is a very important negative result showing that leukotriene B_4, a major neutrophil chemoattractant, can be inhibited by zileuton, an active 5-lipoxygenase inhibitor, and yet this does not really offer any clinical improvement compared to placebo and seems to actually be less than what may be achieved with mesalazine. The relapse rates with Mesalazine were also significantly lower than with a placebo. This just continues to add to the problems with inflammatory bowel disease. Although we have exciting theories about how the cascade of inflammation is perpetuated and maintained, inhibiting or impacting on this cycle or cascade has not been that clinically productive or applicable. Clearly, the goal is discovery of the etiologic agent, stimulant, catalyst, or trigger. This remains the elusive target, which hopefully will be attained in the near future.

R.W. McCallum, M.D.

64 Hepatology— Hepatitis

Prophylaxis in Liver Transplant Recipients Using a Fixed Dosing Schedule of Hepatitis B Immunoglobulin

Terrault NA, Zhou S, Combs C, et al (Veterans Affairs Med Ctr, San Francisco; Univ of California, San Francisco)

Hepatology 24:1327–1333, 1996   64–1

Background.—In liver-transplant recipients who are positive for hepatitis B (HB) surface antigen, prophylactic hepatitis B immunoglobulin (HBIg) reduces the incidence of recurrent hepatitis B virus infection and improves survival. The long-term effects of HBIg and an optimal schedule for its administration have yet to be defined; the efficacy of one protocol is described.

Methods.—Participating in the trial were 52 patients receiving liver transplants who were positive for HB surface antigen at the time of transplant. Twenty-four patients received HBIg prophylaxis at a fixed dose of 10,000 IU monthly and 28 were given no specific therapy. Mean duration of follow-up was 28.9 months.

Results.—Two-year recurrence rate (reappearance of HB surface antigen) for treated patients was 19% and for control patients, 76%. Titer of antibody to HB surface antigen varied significantly both over time and among patients in the treated group, raising concern about the antigen's usefulness in guiding therapy. Nine patients remained negative for HB surface antigen after being treated with HBIg for at least 1 year; hepatitis B virus DNA could be detected by polymerase chain reaction in the sera of 67% of patients, the lymphocytes of 50%, and the liver of 57%.

Conclusions.—These data suggest that, even in patients with indications of active viral replication before transplantation, a fixed monthly dose of HBIg can reduce the recurrence of HB surface antigenemia. Long-term administration of HBIg may be necessary, as evidenced by the presence of residual virus in the majority of treated patients. Larger, even longer-term studies may be needed to show a survival benefit.

▶ This article shows that the major challenge of hepatitis B liver transplantation involves reducing the recurrence of hepatitis B antigenemia. The cost of this study was about $53,000 for the first year posttransplant and $35,000 for each subsequent year. This is a huge commitment and I ask how many centers could really be entertaining this kind of protocol.

R.W. McCallum, M.D.

Long-term Efficacy of Ribavirin Plus Interferon Alfa in the Treatment of Chronic Hepatitis C

Lai M-Y, Kao J-H, Yang P-M, et al (Natl Taiwan Univ, Taipei)
Gastroenterology 111:1307–1312, 1996   64–2

Introduction.—Although 24 weeks of treatment with interferon alfa can normalize serum alanine aminotransferase (ALT) levels in approximately 50% of patients with chronic hepatitis C, fewer than 25% will have a sustained ALT response. Whether the combination of interferon alfa and ribavirin induces a better sustained efficacy than interferon alone was investigated.

Methods.—Sixty patients with chronic hepatitis C were enrolled in the study. All had elevated serum ALT, positive antibody to hepatitis C virus (HCV), and a histologic diagnosis of chronic hepatitis without cirrhosis. None had previously received interferon therapy. Patients were randomly assigned to 3 groups: 1,200 mg of oral ribavirin daily plus 3 million units of recombinant interferon alfa 2a, 3 times a week for 24 weeks (group 1); the same dose of interferon alfa alone for 24 weeks (group 2); no treatment (group 3). Patients were then followed up for an additional 96 weeks to determine the nature and duration of response.

Results.—The 3 groups were similar in baseline characteristics. Fifty-nine (98%) patients were positive for serum HCV RNA. In no patient was hepatocellular carcinoma diagnosed during the 2-year follow-up period. The only death was the result of a traffic accident. A complete response, defined as the normalization of serum ALT levels and absence of serum HCV RNA, was achieved after 24 weeks in 76% of group 1 patients and in 32% of those in group 2; untreated patients had no complete responses. At 96 weeks, the rate of complete, sustained response was higher for the combination treatment group (43%) than for the interferon alone group (6%). Twenty-eight patients who received treatment underwent a second biopsy of the liver. Seven of these patients were among those with a sustained complete response, and their livers showed nearly normal histologic features.

Conclusion.—The combination of ribavirin and interferon was confirmed to be more effective than interferon alone for the treatment of chronic hepatitis C. With 2 years of follow-up after 24 weeks of therapy, about one half of treated patients had sustained biochemical and virologic responses.

▶ This very important article shows that combined treatment with ribavirin and interferon alfa 2a for 24 weeks using 200 mg of ribavirin daily plus 3 million units of recombinant interferon thrice weekly for 24 weeks is more effective than interferon alone for 24 weeks in the treatment of hepatitis C. The biochemical and virologic responses have been sustained in about half the patients treated for at least 2 years after the therapy was stopped. The authors admit here that the optimal dose and the duration of studies have yet to be achieved or defined. This is a very active area of research, and I predict that in next year's YEAR BOOK, this area will be very actively represented. Although we have somewhat of a limited eradication and cure rate for hepatitis C, it does seem that the combination therapy adds the best chance of some kind of sustained response and perhaps reduces the side-effect profile of interferon as well by reducing the doses that may be required.

R.W. McCallum, M.D.

Acute Non-A–E Hepatitis in the United States and the Role of Hepatitis G Virus Infection

Alter MJ, for the Sentinel Counties Viral Hepatitis Study Team (Ctrs for Disease Control and Prevention, Atlanta, Ga; Genelabs Technologies, Redwood City, Calif)
N Engl J Med 336:741–746, 1997   64–3

Introduction.—Non-A–E hepatitis is said to be present in patients who have parenterally transmitted non-A, non-B hepatitis but no evidence of hepatitis C virus. The recently discovered hepatitis G virus (HGV) is related to hepatitis C virus. Surveillance data were used to study the possible role of HGV in acute non-A–E hepatitis.

Methods.—The study included patients with acute viral hepatitis who were reported to the Sentinel Counties surveillance system during 2 periods: 1985–1986 and 1991–1995. Of more than 10,500 patients reported to this system from 1982–1995, 48% had hepatitis A, 34% had hepatitis B, 15% had hepatitis C, and 3% had non-A–E hepatitis. In the study groups, polymerase chain reaction was used to test serum samples for HGV RNA. Clinical outcome data were evaluated as well.

Findings.—The study included sera from 100 patients each with hepatitis A and B, 45 patients with non-A–E hepatitis, and 116 patients with hepatitis C. Hepatitis G virus RNA was found in 25% of patients with hepatitis A, 32% of those with hepatitis B, 23% of those with hepatitis C, and 9% of those with non-A–E hepatitis. Hepatitis G virus was significantly more prevalent among patients with hepatitis B than among those with hepatitis C or non-A–E hepatitis. There were 4 patients infected with HGV only; none had evidence of chronic hepatitis during a follow-up period of 1–9 years.

Conclusions.—Although HGV RNA can be detected in the sera of many patients with acute viral hepatitis, it does not appear to be a causative agent of non-A, non-B hepatitis. Rather than being a hepatotropic agent, HGV may lead to hepatitis only when certain other circumstances are present, as observed with other viruses such as cytomegalovirus and yellow fever virus. Although HGV is clearly a unique virus that can be transmitted by blood, its link with disease remains uncertain.

The Incidence of Transfusion-associated Hepatitis G Virus Infection and Its Relation to Liver Disease

Alter HJ, Nakatsuji Y, Melpolder J, et al (NIH, Bethesda, Md; Genelabs Technologies, Redwood City, Calif)

N Engl J Med 336:747–754, 1997   64–4

Background.—Hepatitis C virus (HCV) is not involved in perhaps 20% of cases of community-acquired hepatitis nor in 10% of cases of transfusion-acquired hepatitis. Molecular amplification and cloning studies have led to the discovery of the hepatitis G virus (HGV). The role of HGV in transfusion-related hepatitis was studied.

Methods.—Four groups of serum samples were studied: 357 from transfusion recipients, 157 from controls who had not received transfusions, 500 from randomly selected blood donors, and 230 from donors who gave blood to a patient with transfusion-associated HGV infection. Polymerase chain reaction assays were used to test these samples for HGV RNA. Also studied were pretransfusion and posttransfusion samples from 79 patients with transfusion-related non-A, non-B hepatitis.

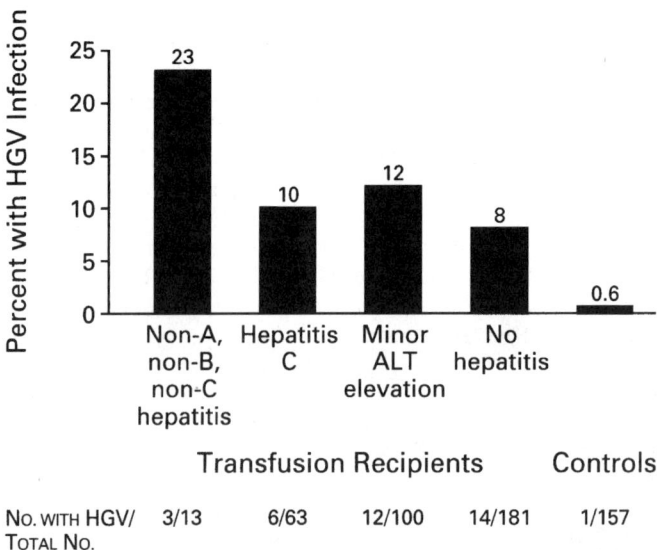

	No. WITH HGV/ TOTAL No.
Non-A, non-B, non-C hepatitis	3/13
Hepatitis C	6/63
Minor ALT elevation	12/100
No hepatitis	14/181
Controls	1/157

FIGURE 3.—Frequency of HGV infection in transfusion recipients with and without hepatitis and in controls who did not receive transfusions. (Reprinted by permission of *The New England Journal of Medicine* from Alter HJ, Nakatsuji Y, Melpolder J, et al: The incidence of transfusion-associated hepatitis G virus infection and its relation to liver disease. *N Engl J Med* 336:747–754, copyright 1997, Massachusetts Medical Society. All rights reserved.)

Results.—Eighty percent of patients with transfusion-associated hepatitis had HCV infection, and another 4% had pre-existing HCV infection and no apparent cause of the acute hepatitis episode. This left 13 patients, 3 of whom had acute HGV infection and 10 of whom had an unidentified infecting agent. Ten percent of patients infected with HCV also had HGV infection. Hepatitis was mild for the 3 patients with HGV infection only; none had jaundice, and their mean peak alanine aminotransferase level was 198 U/L. The severity of hepatitis was not strongly related to the level of HGV RNA. Patients with combined HCV–HGV infection had no more severe hepatitis than those with HCV infection only.

Of the transfusion recipients studied, 10% had HGV infection, but less than 1% had HGV as their sole viral marker. Hepatitis G virus RNA was detected in 1.4% of random blood donors (Fig 3). There were 8 testable patients with acute HGV infection after transfusion; all had received blood from at least 1 donor with HGV-positive status.

Conclusions.—Hepatitis G virus is demonstrated in 1% of a random sample of blood donors. This virus can be transmitted by transfusion, although most such infections do not lead to hepatitis. When a patient infected with HCV is infected with HGV, a worsened severity of hepatitis does not occur. This study finds no evidence that the so-called HGV actually causes hepatitis.

▶ Miriam Alter et al. look at the role of hepatitis G as an etiologic agent in patients with non-A–E hepatitis. They found that persistent infection of hepatitis G is common but it does not lead to chronic liver disease and does not affect the clinical course of patients with hepatitis A, B, or C. It's presumed that hepatitis G is transmitted by a transfusion or by blood-borne transmission from inoculation and/or birth or perhaps even dialysis. Hepatitis G is found in approximately 2% of blood donors and 14%-52% of patients with various types of viral hepatitis. However, Harvey Alter et al. indicate that hepatitis G can be transmitted by transfusion; but it was not associated with hepatitis C infections. In addition, hepatitis G did not tend to worsen the cause of concurrent hepatitis C infection.

R.W. McCallum, M.D.

Hepatitis G Virus Co-infection in Liver Transplantation Recipients With Chronic Hepatitis C and Nonviral Chronic Liver Disease
Fried MW, Khudyakov YE, Smallwood GA, et al (Emory Univ, Atlanta, Ga; Viral Hepatitis Branch, Ctrs for Disease Control, Atlanta, Ga; Roche Molecular Systems, Branchburg, NJ)
Hepatology 25:1271–1275, 1997   64–5

Introduction.—The newly described hepatitis G virus (HGV) has been found in up to 1.7% of volunteer blood donors in the United States and in approximately 10% to 20% of IV drug users at risk for parenterally transmitted viral infections. The prevalence rate of HGV co-infection and its clinical impact after liver transplantation in patients with chronic hepatitis C and patients receiving transplants for nonviral chronic liver disease was determined.

Methods.—The 53 patients included in the study group were positive for HCV RNA before and after transplantation; 22 control subjects were negative for HCV RNA and hepatitis B surface antigen. Polymerase chain reaction was used to measure HGV RNA in pre- and posttransplantation sera collected from both groups of patients. Survival curves were generated using Kaplan-Meier methods and compared for the HGV-positive and HGV-negative patients.

Results.—Paired sera from both before and after transplantation were available from 31 patients; 20 had only posttransplantation and 2 had only pretransplantation sera available. Posttransplantation sera were obtained an average of 228 days after the operation in the study group and an average of 370 days in the control group. The HCV-positive cohort had a 20.7% prevalence rate of HGV RNA. Among those with paired sera, 4 of 31 were positive for HGV RNA before transplantation and 2 became positive after transplantation. There was a positive correlation between serum levels of HGV RNA and levels of HCV RNA. The HGV-positive and HGV-negative groups were similar in mean serum alanine aminotransferase activity, hepatic histologic activity, and patient and graft survival. Transplanted controls had a 64% prevalence rate of HGV RNA, and the rate of acquisition of HGV infection after transplantation was significantly higher than that of patients with chronic hepatitis C (53% vs. 7.4%). Mean serum alanine aminotransferase activity was significantly lower in controls with HGV infection alone after transplanation than in patients co-infected with hepatitis C (37 vs. 70 U/L).

Conclusion.—Although HGV is often found in liver transplant recipients co-infected with HCV, the presence of HGV appears to have little clinical impact. And although a high rate of HGV acquisition is seen after transplantation in patients with nonviral causes of end-stage liver disease, acquisition of the virus does not appear to predispose to chronic hepatitis. Findings raise questions as to whether HGV is a true hepatotropic virus.

▶ This study shows that although hepatitis G is very common and it may often be acquired at the time of transplantation of livers, it does not appear to play a very important clinical role in predisposing to chronic hepatitis. This is very good news and the career of hepatitis G is only beginning and will be closely monitored.

R.W. McCallum, M.D.

65 Hepatology—General

Beta-adrenergic Antagonists in the Prevention of Gastrointestinal Rebleeding in Patients With Cirrhosis: A Meta-analysis
Bernard B, Lebrec D, Mathurin P, et al (Hôpital Pitié-Salpêtrière, Paris; INSERM, Clichy, France; CNRS URA, Paris)
Hepatology 25:63–70, 1997   65–1

Introduction.—All of the 7 meta-analyses conducted to assess the efficacy of beta-blockers in the prevention of gastrointestinal rebleeding confirm that these agents significantly reduce the risk of variceal rebleeding, but only 1 found propranolol to have a significant positive effect on long-term survival. The impact of beta-blocker treatment on rebleeding and long-term survival was examined in a meta-analysis of 12 selected randomized trials.

Methods.—Both MEDLINE and a manual search were used to identify randomized clinical trials (RCTs) in English, French, German, and Spanish, general reviews, and references. Events chosen as end points were rebleeding from any cause, first rebleeding from esophageal varices, death, death from bleeding, and the incidence of adverse events. Analyses were performed according to the intention-to-treat method. Sensitivity analyses, performed when a significant difference was identified, employed stratification according to treatment duration, cause of initial bleeding, placebo use, type of beta-blocker, type of publication, certainty of randomization, severity of cirrhosis, interval between index bleed and randomization, and methodologic quality.

Results.—Except in 1 RCT, all patients in the 12 trials that met selection criteria had cirrhosis. With the exception of 3 RCTs, initial bleeding before randomization was variceal in all cases. Control groups in 8 of the 12 RCTs received placebo. Treatment with beta-blockers significantly increased the mean percentage of patients free of rebleeding (21% mean improvement rate), the mean percentage of patients free of variceal rebleeding (20% mean improvement rate), mean survival rate (5.4% mean improvement rate), and mean percentage of patients free of bleeding death (7.4%). The improvement in long-term survival rate after beta-blocker treatment was most pronounced in the most severely affected patients.

Conclusion.—For the first time, this analysis showed that beta-blockers, effective in preventing rebleeding, also significantly increase long-term survival in patients with cirrhosis. The 5% increase in survival is clinically relevant because of the high prevalence of patients with cirrhosis and bleeding.

▶ Finally, I bring to the attention of the readers an article by Bernard et al., which complements the article by Teran et al. that I also reviewed (see Abstract 65–2). Here, the authors found, using a meta-analysis approach, that beta-adrenergic antagonists significantly increased the mean percentage of patients free of rebleeding, and actually the mean survival rate at 2 years in patients with cirrhosis who had bled once and were rebleeding. This study, by adding survival to the statistical significance, is very impressive.

R.W. McCallum, M.D.

Primary Prophylaxis of Variceal Bleeding in Cirrhosis: A Cost-effectiveness Analysis
Teran JC, Imperiale TF, Mullen KD, et al (MetroHealth Med Ctr, Cleveland, Ohio; Case Western Reserve Univ, Cleveland, Ohio)
Gastroenterology 112:473–482, 1997   65–2

Introduction.—Because patients with cirrhosis and esophageal varices have a higher rate of mortality than those without varices, there is considerable interest in preventing the occurrence of the first episode of variceal bleeding (VB). The cost-effectiveness of 3 prophylactic therapies was examined in a hypothetical cohort of patients stratified according to bleeding risk.

Methods.—A Markov model was used to determine which type of patients would benefit most from prophylaxis, which outcomes are affected, and whether these prophylactic therapies for VB are cost-effective. Results were analyzed in terms of VB incidence, VB mortality, total mortality, life expectancy, and quality-adjusted life expectancy. Four main therapeutic possibilities for patients with nonbleeding varices were included in the Markov decision tree: observation, propranolol, sclerotherapy, and shunt surgery. Costs for the therapies were obtained from the billing department of the study institution.

Results.—The cost-effectiveness of propranolol exceeded that of the other therapeutic possibilities because this agent prevented VB, and the costs of VB are greater than those of propranolol therapy. Sclerotherapy achieved only borderline savings in certain subgroups of patients, and shunt surgery was not effective in any subgroup because of its high costs and association with a decreased quality-adjusted life expectancy in some subgroups.

Conclusion.—Depending upon an individual patient's bleeding risk, propranolol was estimated to result in cost savings ranging between $450 and $14,600 over a 5-year period. This drug also increased the quality-adjusted life expectancy by 0.1 to 0.4 years. Whatever a patient's bleeding risk, propranolol is the most cost-effective therapy for prophylaxis against initial VB. The therapy may have to continue for life.

▶ In an important article dealing with the economics of treatment, Dr. Teran et al. showed that propranolol is the only cost-effective form of prophylactic therapy for preventing an initial variceal bleed in patients with cirrhosis who have varices and are thought to be at high risk for bleeding. It was felt that propranolol results in a cost savings ranging from $450 to $14,600 over a 5-year period when compared to sclerotherapy and shunt surgery. Based on this it would certainly favor a more aggressive use of propranolol in the average cirrhotic patient who has not yet bled. In patients who have lung disease and have a contraindication to propranolol, we would recommend isosorbide nitrate to replace propranolol in this particular setting.

R.W. McCallum, M.D.

Double-blind Randomized Controlled Trial Comparing Terlipressin and Somatostatin for Acute Variceal Hemorrhage
Feu F, del Arbol LR, Bañares R, et al (Univ of Barcelona; Univ of Alcalá de Henares, Madrid; Universidad Complutense, Madrid; et al)
Gastroenterology 111:1291–1299, 1996   65–3

Introduction.—Despite advances in treatment, the mortality rate remains high among patients with cirrhosis and variceal hemorrhage. Somatostatin and terlipressin, both of which decrease portal pressure, have been used successfully to treat this complication, but only terlipressin was shown to reduce mortality from variceal hemorrhage in placebo-controlled trials. The 2 drugs were compared for efficacy and safety in a double-blind trial with a large series of patients.

Methods.—The study, conducted at 4 teaching hospitals in Spain, randomized 80 patients to terlipressin (2 mg/4hr, IV) and 81 to somatostatin (IV injection of 250 μg, followed by a continuous infusion of 250 μg/hr). Inclusion criteria were clinical evidence of bleeding within the 24 hours before admission, endoscopically proven hemorrhage from esophageal varices, and no previous use of vasopressin or somatostatin or both to control the bleeding episode. Therapeutic success was defined as a 24-hour bleeding-free period within 48 hours from randomization.

Results.—Control of bleeding was achieved in 64 patients (80%) in the terlipressin group and in 68 patients (84%) in the somatostatin group. The 2 groups were similar in mean interval required for cessation of bleeding (5.7 and 4.7 hours, respectively). In patients with Child's class A and B disease, terlipressin and somatostatin were effective in an equal percentage of patients (87%). Success rates in class C were 60% and 77%, respectively. Rebleeding rates were similar in the 2 treatment groups, and 13 patients in each group died. The incidence of side effects, however, was significantly higher in the terlipressin group (38.8%) than in the somatostatin group (23.5%), and terlipressin was associated with significantly more cardiovascular events.

Conclusion.—Both terlipressin and somatostatin are highly effective in controlling acute variceal hemorrhage and maintaining a low mortality rate. Results of the 2 agents compare quite well with those obtained with emergency sclerotherapy. Although patients treated with terlipressin had a high incidence of side effects, there were few severe side effects in either group.

▶ This important study comparing a new vasopressin agent, terlipressin, and somatostatin for acute variceal hemorrhage shows that both agents were equally effective as first-line therapy of variceal hemorrhage in cirrhotic patients, but the lack of side effects suggests that octreotide may also be maintained for longer periods and could therefore also prevent rebleeding. I believe that, with longer treatment periods, the problem will be cost—somatostatin (octreotide) can be quite expensive—and this will need to be addressed. However, at the ICU level or in the acute setting it is pleasing to know that both agents are valuable. The long-acting vasopressin agent terlipressin did have a significantly more frequent prevalence of cardiovascular events, and I think that will still be a concern, which may favor Octreotide for use in the long-term future in this area.

R.W. McCallum, M.D.

Total Volume Paracentesis Decreases Variceal Pressure, Size, and Variceal Wall Tension in Cirrhotic Patients
Kravetz D, Romero G, Argonz J, et al (Hosp de Gastroenterologia "Dr. Bonorino Udaondo," Buenos Aires, Argentina)
Hepatology 25:59–62, 1997   65–4

Introduction.—Patients with cirrhosis and tense ascites can be effectively managed using total volume paracentesis (TVP) with volume replacement. Because ascites may be a risk factor for variceal bleeding, there is interest in the effects of TVP on hepatic hemodynamics. A group of patients with cirrhosis took part in a study of the effects of TVP on variceal pressure, size, and tension.

Methods.—Patients eligible for the study had esophageal varices size grade 2 or greater, a prothrombin time of 40% or higher, and a platelet count of 40,000/mL or more. Excluded were patients with hepatocarcinoma, portal thrombosis, heart failure, or respiratory insufficiency and current evidence of encephalopathy, active gastrointestinal bleeding, or infection. Studies were carried out before sclerotherapy. Twelve patients had measurements obtained at basal conditions and after TVP: inferior vena cava pressure, esophageal pressure, intravariceal pressure (IVP), and variceal size at endoscopy. Six patients served as controls and had the same measurements performed at basal condition and 1 hour later without TVP. The variceal pressure gradient was calculated as the difference in pressures between IVP and esophageal pressure. Variceal wall pressure was also determined. A direct puncture was used to obtain paracentesis and intraabdominal pressure.

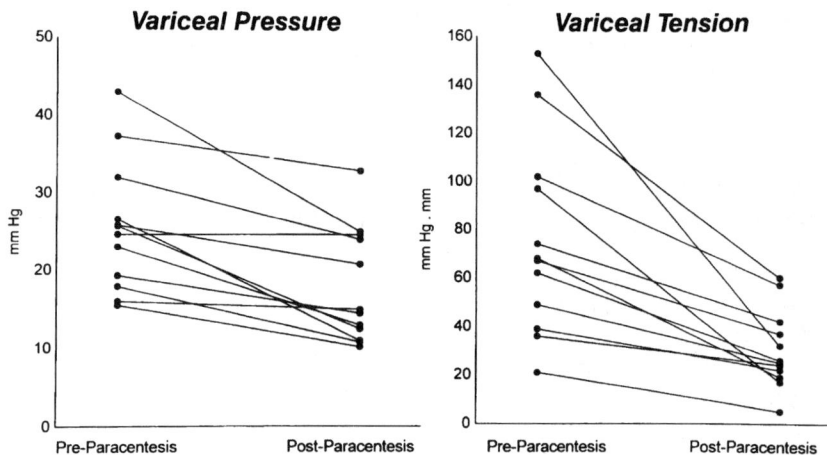

FIGURE 2.—Individual values of variceal pressure and variceal wall tension in basal condition and after total volume paracentesis in cirrhotic patients with tense ascites. (Courtesy of Kravetz D, Romero G, Argonz J, et al: Total volume paracentesis decreased variceal pressure, size, and variceal wall tension in cirrhotic patients. *Hepatology* 25:59–62, 1997.)

Results.—The 2 groups of patients were similar in age, sex, disease etiology, and laboratory data. All in the study group had tense ascites, but only 3 in the control group had mild ascites. The mean volume of ascites removed was 8 L. Paracentesis produced a significant reduction of IVP (from a mean of 25.6 to a mean of 17.9 mm Hg) and of the variceal pressure gradient (from a mean of 16.6 to a mean of 10.8 mm Hg) (Fig 2). Both variceal size and wall tension were reduced by TVP (38% and 60%, respectively). There was a decrease in mean intra-abdominal pressure (from 18 to 4 mm Hg) and in mean inferior vena cava pressure (from 15.5 to 5.7 mm Hg). Mean arterial pressure and heart rate were unaffected. Measurements in the control group did not differ significantly from those in the study group.

Conclusion.—Total volume paracentesis significantly reduces variceal pressure, variceal pressure gradient, and variceal wall tension in patients with severe ascites. This finding suggests that the procedure could be used to treat acute variceal bleeding in patients with cirrhosis and portal hypertension.

▶ The authors review a very popular technique: large volume paracentesis, which is being used in patients with severe ascites. Kravetz et al. demonstrate that large volume paracentesis significantly decreased IVP and tension and, therefore, the extrapolation is that ascites should be removed in patients where variceal bleeding is a real risk. In the past, it was thought that large volume paracentesis had a cosmetic role and an important role in improving respiration and overall patient mobility and comfort. The mean volume removed was 8 L with a range of 4.6 to 11.51 L. The effects of this paracentesis are decreased pressure in the abdomen and plasma volume re-expansion after paracentesis. This article may give further incentive for aggressive treatment of ascites in patients who have already bled or have broken through a program of prophylaxis (as already described in previous articles).

R.W. McCallum, M.D.

Endoscopic Variceal Ligation Is Superior to Combined Ligation and Sclerotherapy for Esophageal Varices: A Multicenter Prospective Randomized Trial

Saeed ZA, Stiegmann GV, Ramirez FC, et al (Baylor College of Medicine, Houston; Univ of Colorado, Denver)

Hepatology 25:71–74, 1997   65–5

Introduction.—Rebleeding is common among patients who have survived a first episode of variceal hemorrhage. Methods used to lower the rate of rebleeding include sclerotherapy and rubber band ligation. Whether the combination of ligation and sclerotherapy would eradicate varices faster than either modality alone was studied.

Methods.—The multicenter, prospective trial enrolled 47 patients with bleeding esophageal varices. Twenty-seven were randomly assigned to endoscopic variceal ligation (EVL) alone and 22 to the combination therapy. Those in the combination group underwent distal ligation of each variceal column, followed by an injection of 1 mL of ethanolamine proximal to each ligated site. Treatment sessions continued at 7- to 14-day intervals until the varices were eradicated. Each technique was studied for its efficiency in eradicating esophageal varices, the incidence of recurrence, the development of gastric varices, its ability to control active bleeding, the rate of recurrent hemorrhage, and survival. Patients were followed up for up to 30 months.

Results.—The 2 patient groups were similar in clinical and endoscopic characteristics. Seven patients in the EVL group and 4 in the combination group were actively bleeding at the time of endoscopy. During follow-up, active bleeding was controlled in 100% of patients in the EVL group and 75% of those in the combination group, not a significant difference. The mean number of sessions required to eradicate varices was similar in the EVL (3.3) and combination (4.1) groups. Rates of survival, rebleeding, and varix recurrence were also similar. Four patients in the EVL group and 8 in the combination therapy group died. Significantly more complications occurred after combination therapy.

Conclusion.—Sclerotherapy combined with ligation was not superior to ligation alone in eradicating esophageal varices, controlling active bleeding, or improving survival. Combination therapy was associated with a higher rate of complications and is likely to be more costly than ligation alone.

▶ Saeed et al. showed that ligation of the varices is better than ligation plus sclerotherapy and that there's no real need for the combination of the 2 procedures, mainly because the combination involves complications induced by sclerotherapy. Ligation tends to be gaining popularity around the country and really is best used electively in the setting of post acute bleeding. Sometimes during acute endoscopy when there is too much bleeding, appropriate visualization cannot be obtained to perform ligation and here sclerotherapy might be favored as the first approach.

R.W. McCallum, M.D.

The Natural History of Portal Hypertension After Transjugular Intrahepatic Portosystemic Shunts
Sanyal AJ, Freedman AM, Luketic VA, et al (Virginia Commonwealth Univ, Richmond)
Gastroenterology 112:889–898, 1997   65–6

Introduction.—Transjugular-intrahepatic-portosystemic shunt (TIPS) functions like side-to-side surgical portacaval shunts in patients with portal hypertension, but avoids the risks of major surgery. One hundred consecutive patients undergoing TIPS were studied prospectively to define the effects of the procedure on portal pressures and flow, variceal resolution, and hepatic function.

Methods.—The patients underwent TIPS for a variety of indications, including refractory ascites and prevention of recurrent variceal hemorrhage. Patients were studied after TIPS placement by clinical assessment, angiography, Doppler US, and endoscopy. Liver function was assessed by a battery of tests. Stent dysfunction was defined for recurrent portal hypertension, stent occlusion, stent thrombosis, and stent stenosis.

Results.—Patients were 68 men and 32 women with a mean age of 49 years. Thirty-one had Child's class B cirrhosis and 61 had Child's class C cirrhosis. The most common causes of liver disease were alcoholism (45 patients) and hepatitis C virus (40 patients). After the TIPS procedure, the mean portosystemic gradient decreased significantly from 24 to 11 mm Hg. Recurrent portal hypertension caused by stent stenosis occurred in 51 patients by 6 months; 5 additional cases were caused by stent thrombosis and 2 by stent retraction. During a median follow-up of 1,050 days, mean survival after TIPS was 72% at 1 year, 68% at 3 years, and 50% at 5 years. Risk factors for recurrent hemorrhage were systemic venous pressures of more than 15 mm Hg, stent dysfunction, and continued alcoholism. The best method for detection of recurrent portal hypertension was angiography, followed by endoscopy and Doppler sonography.

Conclusion.—Treatment with TIPS leads to complex changes in portal pressures, portal flow, varices, hepatic blood flow, and liver function. Shunt patency is an important determinant of the long-term outcome of portal pressures. Although stent stenosis is common, this problem is usually amenable to dilation. Fundic gastric varices often persist after TIPS.

▶ This article addresses the natural history of portal hypertension after TIPS. The group from Medical College of Virginia (Dr. Sanyal et al.) show that in 100 consecutive patients studied over a period of 5 years, recurrent portal hypertension caused by stent stenosis does occur commonly in the first 2 years after TIPS. In addition, fundic varices do not generally improve, and, finally, the effect of TIPS on liver function is unpredictable. An important take-home message in this article is that the economics of TIPS is very, very significant. In the first weeks and months of the follow-up of the procedure, abdominal US was done routinely and commonly, and it is generally the initial study when the patient returns for any complication of liver disease, including varices or worsening of ascites. This was not built into the study, but from my own experience, this aspect is a very significant and continuing economic factor. It may be another reason in the future why US will also be in the possession of hepatologists who can use this appropriately in patients being seen in their clinic for routine evaluation to prevent some of the higher costs engendered by radiology referrals.

R.W. McCallum, M.D.

Randomised Trial of Transjugular-Intrahepatic-Portosystemic Shunt Versus Endoscopy Plus Propranolol for Prevention of Variceal Rebleeding
Rössle M, Deibert P, Haag K, et al (Univ of Freiburg, Germany; Gen Hosp of Offenburg; Gen Hosp of Rastatt, Germany)
Lancet 349:1043–1049, 1997   65–7

Introduction.—The transjugular-intrahepatic-portosystemic shunt has become widely accepted over the past decade, despite a lack of studies comparing this treatment for portal hypertension with conventional therapies. The shunt was compared with endoscopic treatment plus propranolol in the prevention of recurrent variceal bleeding in a randomized study.

Methods.—The 126 patients, all with liver cirrhosis, were treated between March 1993 and March 1996. Sixty-one were randomly assigned to transjugular shunt and 65 to endoscopic treatment. The 2 groups were similar in baseline clinical characteristics. At the time of shunt placement, 31 patients in this group underwent simultaneous transjugular-variceal embolization. Patients assigned to endoscopic treatment had sclerotherapy or banding ligation or both combined with propranolol.

Results.—The transjugular-intrahepatic-portosystemic shunt was implanted successfully in all patients. During follow-up ranging from 8 to 25 months, the cumulative 1-year rate of variceal bleeding was 15% in patients with implanted shunt and 41% in endoscopically treated patients; 2-year rates were 21% and 52%, respectively. Overall, 15 patients who received shunts and 33 endoscopically treated patients had 19 and 100 upper gastrointestinal rebleedings, respectively. Endoscopic treatment failed in 9 (12%) patients, all of whom then received the shunt treatment. One- and 2-year survival rates were similar for the 2 groups. The shunt group, however, had twice the rate of clinically significant hepatic encephalopathy (Fig 4) after 1 year (36%) compared to the endoscopically treated group (18%). There was a trend toward a reduction in hospital stay and outpatient visits in the shunt group.

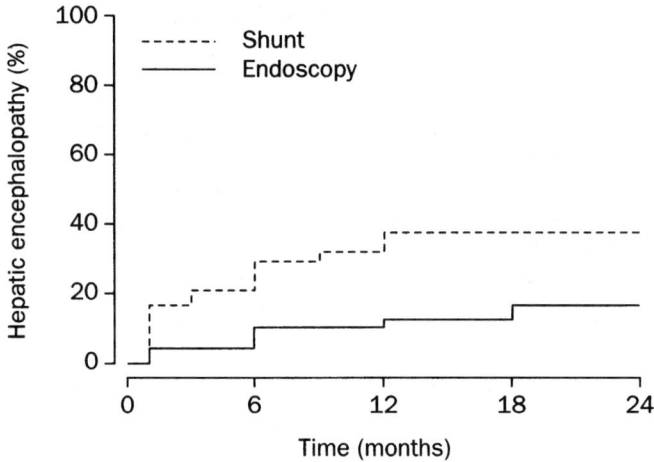

Patients at risk

Shunt	61	37	23	12	8
Endoscopy	65	51	37	23	15

FIGURE 4.—Estimated probability of the development of hepatic encephalopathy according to intention-to-treat. The difference between the groups is statistically significant ($P = 0.011$). (Courtesy of Rössle M, Deibert P, Haag K, et al: Randomised trial of transjugular-intrahepatic-portosystemic shunt versus endoscopy plus propranolol for prevention of variceal rebleeding. *Lancet* 349:1043–1049, 1997. Copyright 1997 by The Lancet Ltd.)

Conclusion.—Shunt treatment was found to be more effective than endoscopic treatment for the prevention of variceal rebleeding. Although 1- and 2-year survival rates were similar in the 2 groups, the shunt carries a considerable risk of hepatic encephalopathy.

▶ Rössle et al. showed that transjugular-intrahepatic-portosystemic shunt is more effective than endoscopy in sclerosis in the prevention of bleeding, but with some risk (20%) for hepatic encephalopathy, and with an overall survival was similar in the 2 groups.

R.W. McCallum, M.D.

Transjugular Intrahepatic Portosystemic Shunts Compared With Endoscopic Sclerotherapy for the Prevention of Recurrent Variceal Hemorrhage: A Randomized, Controlled Trial
Sanyal AJ, Freedman AM, Luketic VA, et al (Med College of Virginia, Richmond)
Ann Intern Med 126:849–857, 1997   65–8

Introduction.—For patients with recurrent variceal hemorrhage, transjugular intrahepatic portosystemic shunts (TIPS) help to avoid the risks associated with anesthesia and major surgery by functioning as side-to-side portacaval shunts. The efficacy of TIPS has not been compared with that of other treatments in controlled trials. In a prospective, randomized, controlled trial, the efficacy and safety of TIPS were compared with those of endoscopic sclerotherapy in the prevention of recurrent variceal hemorrhage.

Methods.—One hundred patients with cirrhosis were assessed at a mean of 10 days after an episode of acute variceal bleeding. Six patients had to be excluded for portal venous thrombosis, 3 for hepatoma, 6 for florid alcoholic hepatitis, and 5 for refusal to give consent. Forty-one patients underwent TIPS and 39 underwent sclerotherapy by freehand injections of 5% sodium morrhuate at 2- to 3-week intervals. Patients were followed for rebleeding and survival (primary endpoints) and complications and rates of rehospitalization (secondary endpoints). Patients receiving sclerotherapy who rebled from varices were offered TIPS.

Results.—At a mean of 1,000 days, recurrent gastrointestinal bleeding resulted from variceal hemorrhage for 9 patients in the TIPS group and 8 patients in the sclerotherapy group, portal gastropathy for 1 patient in each group, and gastric lipoma for 1 patient in the sclerotherapy group. Mortality was significantly higher in the TIPS group than in the sclerotherapy group. Causes of death were variceal bleeding for 5 patients in the TIPS group and 3 patients in the sclerotherapy group, sepsis (3 and 2 patients, respectively), liver failure (2 patients in each group), hepatoma (1 and 0 patients, respectively), and hemoperitoneum (1 and 0 patients, respectively). The most common complications in the TIPS and sclerotherapy groups were encephalopathy (12 patients) and pain (10 patients), respectively. There were no between-group differences in rates of rehospitalization.

Conclusion.—Long-term incidence of rebleeding was similar for patients in the TIPS and sclerotherapy groups. Survival was significantly better for sclerotherapy patients than for TIPS patients.

▶ Through a randomized, controlled trial, Dr. Sanyal and colleagues concluded that endoscopic sclerotherapy and TIPS are actually equivalent with respect to rebleeding developing over a follow-up period of about a year, but did find that sclerotherapy may be superior to TIPS regarding survival. However, as the authors point out, there may be a learning curve to the procedure of TIPS. Nevertheless, it seems reasonable that endoscopic sclerotherapy be the treatment of choice as first-line therapy and that TIPS be reserved for patients who have failed sclerotherapy attempts to obliterate their varices.

R.W. McCallum, M.D.

Endoscopic Sclerotherapy Compared With Percutaneous Transjugular Intrahepatic Portosystemic Shunt After Initial Sclerotherapy in Patients With Acute Variceal Hemorrhage

Cello JP, Ring EJ, Olcott EW, et al (Univ of California, San Francisco; Stanford Univ, Calif; Veterans Affairs Med Ctr, San Francisco)
Ann Intern Med 126:858–865, 1997   65–9

Background.—Endoscopic sclerotherapy became the preferred treatment for acute variceal hemorrhage during the past 15 years, but its status in the long-term management of patients with bleeding varices has been questioned. Newer techniques, such as band ligation and pharmacologic agents, are also selected over surgical shunting. In a recent study, however, surgical portacaval shunting was associated with a significantly reduced need for rehospitalization for recurrent variceal hemorrhage when compared with sclerotherapy. The efficacy of each of these 2 treatment methods was assessed in a randomized, controlled trial.

Methods.—Study participants were 49 adults hospitalized at 3 teaching hospitals from November 1991 to December 1995. All received endoscopic sclerotherapy at the time of diagnosis. Twenty-five were assigned to sclerotherapy and 24 to transjugular intrahepatic portosystemic shunt (TIPS), a nonsurgical procedure in which an expandable metal prosthesis is used to connect an intrahepatic portal vein with an adjacent hepatic vein. These therapies were compared for their success in preventing recurrent variceal hemorrhage.

Results.—The 2 groups were similar in pretreatment clinical and laboratory variables, except that the TIPS group had a worse Child-Pugh score and higher blood transfusion requirements before randomization. Mean follow-up was 567 days in the sclerotherapy group and 575 days in the TIPS group. Varices were obliterated more reliably in the TIPS group, and patients who underwent TIPS were significantly less likely to rebleed from esophageal varices than patients receiving sclerotherapy (3 of 24 vs. 12 of 25, respectively). The other follow-up measures, including index hospitalization survival, duration of hospitalization for variceal bleeding, blood transfusion needs after randomization, and total health care costs, did not differ significantly between groups. After 2 years there was a trend toward improved survival with TIPS.

Conclusion.—Although TIPS was more effective than sclerotherapy in obliterating esophageal varices and reducing rebleeding events, morbidity and health care costs did not differ significantly between the 2 therapies. There was slightly better survival in patients treated with TIPS.

▶ Cello et al. found in a randomized double-blind controlled trial that TIPS was more effective than sclerotherapy in obliterating varices and reducing rebleeding. However, TIPS did not have a decreased morbidity after randomization, nor did it improve the health-care costs. It did seem to produce better survival, but this was not quite statistically significant.

R.W. McCallum, M.D.

66 Helicobacter Pylori

► *Helicobacter* remains an extremely important and active area in gastro-enterology this year. Following are a number of the articles that are very relevant and contribute new concepts.

R.W. McCallum, M.D.

Management Strategies for *Helicobacter pylori*-seropositive Patients With Dyspepsia: Clinical and Economic Consequences
Ofman JJ, Etchason J, Fullerton S, et al (Univ of California, Los Angeles; Emory Univ, Atlanta, Ga; RAND, Santa Monica, Calif)
Ann Intern Med 126:280–291, 1997   66–1

Introduction.—Up to 40% of the adult population in the United States is affected by dyspepsia, or epigastric pain or discomfort represented by a gnawing or burning sensation. This condition results in indigestion with belching, bloating, and fullness, and is relieved by food, antacids, or antisecretory drugs. Ulcer therapy has been revolutionized with recognition of the role of *Helicobacter pylori* (*H pylori*) in the pathogenesis of peptic ulcer disease. The role of anti-*H pylori* therapy in the management of nonulcer dyspepsia is being debated, because the association between *H pylori* gastritis and nonulcer dyspepsia is equivocal and dyspeptic symptoms have not been alleviated consistently by antibiotic treatment. Initial anti-*H pylori* therapy is the alternative to initial endoscopy in *H-pylori*-seropositive patients; however, the costs and benefits of these alternative strategies are still unknown.

Methods.—In *H pylori*-seropositive patients with dyspepsia, the costs and outcomes of initial anti-*H pylori* therapy and initial endoscopy were compared with decision analysis. The initial endoscopy strategy entailed biopsy and a rapid urease test of all ulcers. Patients with nonulcer dyspepsia received a trial of ranitidine, 150 mg twice daily, for 8 weeks. Patients with esophagitis received omeprazole, 20 mg twice daily for 12 weeks. Surgery was performed on patients with gastric cancer.

Results.—Initial anti-*H pylori* therapy averages $820 per patient, compared with $1,276 per patient for initial endoscopy, an average savings of $456 per patient. The financial effect of a 252% increase in the use of antibiotics for initial *H pylori* therapy is offset by reduction of the endos-

TABLE 4.—Results of Base-Case Analysis

Variable	Initial Endoscopy	Initial Anti-Helicobacter pylori Therapy	Difference
Cost/patient, $	1276.00	820.00	456.00
Endoscopies/1000 patients, n	1050	492	Reduction of 53%
Courses of antibiotics/1000 patients, n	314	1105	Increase of 252%

(Courtesy of Offman JJ, Etchason J, Fullerton S, et al: Management strategies for *Helicobacter pylori*-seropositive patients with dyspepsia: Clinical and economic consequences. *Ann Intern Med* 126:280–291, 1997.)

copy workload by 53% (Table 4). Before the 2 strategies become equally cost-effective, endoscopy-related costs must be reduced by 96%. Varying the rates of *H pylori* eradication, the complications of antibiotics, or the response of symptoms did not substantially affect the financial benefits of initial anti-*H pylori* therapy in patients with nonulcer dyspepsia.

Conclusion.—The most cost-effective management strategy is initial anti-*H pylori* therapy in *H pylori*-seropositive patients with dyspepsia. This strategy can be used as a basis for management and policy decisions about *H pylori*-seropositive patients with dyspepsia, unless physicians are concerned about resistance to antimicrobial agents or the lack of proven benefit of anti-*H pylori* therapy in nonulcer dyspepsia. Randomized studies of the strategies that evaluate outcomes and patient preferences are needed to optimize management decisions.

▶ The consensus conference of National Institutes of Health in 1994 concluded that dyspepsia was still really not a valid indication for using *H pylori* eradication therapy and this area or indication remained on a wait-and-see status. This, nevertheless, has brought up a number of discussions and many, many debates about the role of screening for *H pylori* and/or treating for *H pylori* in patients presenting with the diffuse upper gastrointestinal symptom spectrum that is referred to as dyspepsia. In this article, the authors use a technique of decision analysis to compare the costs and outcomes that would be incurred by an initial anti-*H pylori* therapy approach and by initial endoscopy. In patients who are seropositive with dyspepsia, and initial eradication of *H pylori* was the most cost-effective management strategy. This, of course, implies that randomized trials must be done, but nevertheless the authors provide a very impressive list of costs that could be prevented or limited by empiric therapy.

If we assume that approximately 20% or more of patients with dyspepsia will have an impressive turnaround in the symptoms and/or total resolution after eradication of *H pylori*, then approximately 75% of patients will not. They may have remaining symptoms that need other therapies including prokinetics. However, we know that these patients can rest assured that they don't have a risk factor for cancer, that indeed long-term surveillance and screening won't be a problem, and that there won't be concerns about gastric cancer. I believe the strategy described here has great merit and will be of course the subject of many good long-term clinical trials in the future. Here, "long-term" is critical because we are now learning that after perhaps 6–12 months of eradication in dyspepsia patients, we are starting to see a change in quality of life and an overall improvement in symptom status. This is not appreciated in the first 3–4 months and probably indicates that gastritis and more serious histological changes take some months, perhaps even years, to be fully resolved. Stay tuned.

R.W. McCallum, M.D.

▶ Certainly on a therapeutic basis a huge amount of attention is being focused on where percutaneous transjugular intrahepatic porto systemic shunt now stands in managing complicated or end-stage liver disease. Three articles (Abstracts 66–2 to 66–4) address the role of this procedure in controlling the bleeding from esophageal varices and compare it to other modalities.

Richard W. McCallum, M.D.

Curing *Helicobacter pylori* Infection in Patients With Duodenal Ulcer May Provoke Reflux Esophagitis

Labenz J, Blum AL, Bayerdörffer E, et al (Elisabeth Hosp, Essen, Germany; Centre Hospitalier Universitaire Vaudois, Lausanne, Switzerland; Otto-von-Guericke Univ, Magdeburg, Germany; et al)
Gastroenterology 112:1442–1447, 1997   66–2

Introduction.—Although the cure for *Helicobacter pylori* reduces ulcer recurrences, there is a question as to whether successful antimicrobial treatment also cures reflux esophagitis. Reflux disease was found to develop in some patients cured of *H. pylori* infection, suggesting that the cure may actually increase the risk of reflux esophagitis. In a prospective, controlled study, the long-term outcome of patients who received antimicrobial treatment for duodenal ulcer disease was assessed.

Methods.—Patients who entered the study had a history of relapsing or complicated duodenal ulcer disease but were free of concomitant reflux esophagitis at the time of *H. pylori* treatment. They were studied prospectively after cure of the infection or after diagnosis of persisting infection. Endoscopy was performed at 1-year intervals or when upper gastrointestinal symptoms recurred. Biopsy specimens obtained at endoscopy were assessed for *H. pylori* by rapid urease test and histology.

Results.—Cure of *H. pylori* infection was achieved in 244 patients; 216 remained *H. pylori*-positive. An endoscopically proven ulcer relapse was documented in 126 (58%) of *H. pylori* positive patients. The rate of endoscopically proven reflux esophagitis during follow-up was 25.8% in patients cured of the infection and 12.9% in those with ongoing infection (Fig 1). Patients in whom reflux esophagitis developed after cure of *H.*

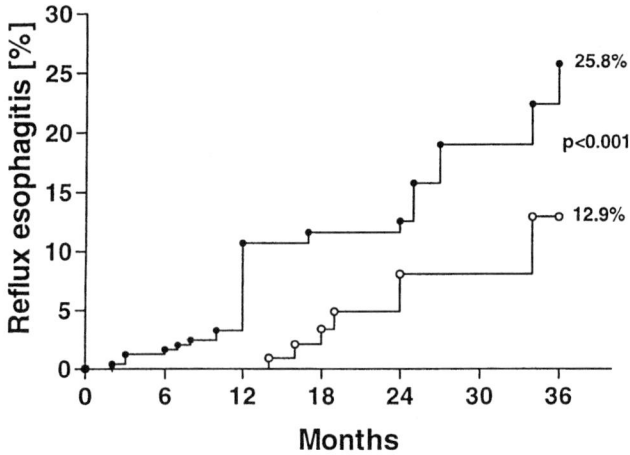

FIGURE 1.—Life-table analysis; incidence of reflux esophagitis in patients with duodenal ulcer with cured *Helicobacter pylori* infection (*filled circles*; n = 244) and in patients with duodenal ulcer with ongoing infection (*open circles*; n = 216). (Courtesy of Labenz J, Blum AL, Bayerdörffer E, et al: Curing *Helicobacter pylori* infection in patients with duodenal ulcer may provoke reflux esophagitis. *Gastroenterology* 112:1442–1447, 1997.)

pylori had a higher score of body gastritis before ulcer treatment, more frequently gained weight after the cure, and were predominantly men. And compared to patients without endoscopic evidence of reflux esophagitis during follow-up, they were more likely to be alcohol drinkers.

Conclusion.—Reflux esophagitis develops in about 25% of patients with duodenal ulcer with cured *H. pylori* infection in the 3 years after the cure. The risk factors for reflux esophagitis in this setting are male sex, weight gain, and severity of corpus gastritis. Some patients with high gastric acid secretion may be protected from reflux esophagitis when a duodenal ulcer develops after infection by *H. pylori*. Once the infection is cured, an ammonia buffer produced by *H. pylori* disappears and reflux esophagitis can occur.

▶ This provocative article by Labenz et al. has resulted in a lot of discussion throughout the world. The authors noticed gastroesophageal reflux symptoms in patients with duodenal ulcer disease or after *H. pylori* was eradicated. It was related in some cases to the severity of the gastritis in the body of the stomach as well as weight gain and being a male. The hypothesis that the authors put forward is that perhaps the ammonia buffer produced by *H. pylori* actually somehow neutralizes or protects the esophagus from the reflux material during the *H. pylori* infection. When this infection is eradicated, this buffering is lost. Personally, I don't like this explanation, but rather the explanation I would put forward is that it depends on the stage of disease progression in the patient when *H. pylori* is eradicated. If there is indeed significant gastritis in the body of the stomach to the point of severe metaplasia that no gastric acid production really remains, then at that point it probably won't matter whether you eradicate *H. pylori* or not — there is probably irreversibly severe gastric atrophy. This is typically very late in the course of the *H. pylori* infection and could represent patients who are much older. However, if *H. pylori* were to be eradicated in a middle-aged or younger patient, perhaps with only a few years of *H. pylori* gastritis, then the body of the stomach may be relatively preserved and gastric acid production would be restored after *H. pylori* is eradicated because the inflammation would not be so severe that it would be irreversible. Hence, acid production returns for the first time in some years and in turn will reflux up into the esophagus. This will begin a new set of symptoms that had previously not been appreciated by the patient.

This is a very pertinent observation, because, in Asia, with the eradication of *H. pylori*, heartburn is being appreciated as a new disease. This brings up the quotation that is often being used at meetings and conferences around the world now that perhaps not all good *H. pylori* are dead *H. pylori*, i.e., live *H. pylori* may have had some protective mechanisms in the past in protecting against gastroesophageal reflux and maybe even protecting against Barrett's esophagus, so by disturbing the environment or by eradicating *H. pylori* in certain countries or settings, perhaps we are setting the stage for a new set of symptoms or new problems that have been dormant in the past in those populations. This is a very interesting observation and certainly is going to stimulate a lot of discussion, particularly about the etiologic implications of these observations.

R.W. McCallum, M.D.

Gastric Mucosa During Treatment With Lansoprazole: *Helicobacter pylori* Is a Risk Factor for Argyrophil Cell Hyperplasia
Eissele E, Brunner G, Simon B, et al (Philipps Univ, Marburg, Germany; Med School of Hannover, Germany; Univ of Pavia, Italy)
Gastroenterology 112:707–717, 1997   66–3

Introduction.—A group of patients who had been treated daily with lansoprazole for up to 5 years was evaluated for serum gastrin levels, fundic gastritis, gastric endocrine cell proliferation, and *Helicobacter pylori* infection. The hypothesis that *H. pylori* is a risk factor for both gastritis and argyrophil cell hyperplasia in patients undergoing long-term treatment with proton pump inhibitors was examined.

Methods.—Forty-two patients, 31 men and 11 women with a mean age of 54 years, were enrolled in the study. Forty agreed to enter a 5-year maintenance therapy with lansoprazole after their acid-related disorders failed to respond to ranitidine treatment. During long-term treatment, the dose of lansoprazole was adjusted up to 90 mg/day according to endoscopic and clinical findings. Thirty-eight patients were followed up for more than 1 year, 37 for 2 years, and 28 for 5 years.

Results.—In the 38 nonantrectomized patients, serum gastrin levels increased from a median of 76 pg/mL to 163 pg/mL within 3 months. Significant increases were seen as well in antral gastrin cell density (from a mean of 175 to 267 cells/mm²) and in fundic argyrophil cell density (from a mean of 83 to 149 cells/mm²). Before lansoprazole treatment, *H. pylori* infection was identified histologically in 36 patients. In the long-term study, the infection disappeared in 22 patients and was persistent in 14. Only patients with *H. pylori* showed a worsening of chronic inflammation, activity, and atrophy of the oxyntic mucosa. Whereas only 2.6% of patients had received a diagnosis of linear or micronodular argyrophil cell hyperplasia or both before lansoprazole, 29.2% had this finding after 5 years of treatment. There was a significant relationship between these changes and serum gastrin levels, *H. pylori* infection, chronic inflammation, and atrophy of the oxyntic mucosa.

Conclusion.—Infection with *H. pylori* was confirmed to be an important factor for the progression of fundic gastritis and the development of argyrophil cell hyperplasia during long-term lansoprazole therapy. Eradication of the infection before long-term treatment with proton pump inhibitors may prevent these changes.

▶ The authors show that during long-term treatment with lansoprazole for up to 5 years in a dose of 30–90 mg/day, *Helicobacter pylori* represented an important factor for the progression of fundic gastritis into argyrophil cell hyperplasia. This is thought to definitely be related to the consequences of the induced hypergastrinemia. The implication here is to eradicate *H. pylori* before long-term treatment with a proton pump inhibitor is contemplated. At the present time, there has been no clinically assignable risk as far as cancer development is concerned, although this obviously begs the question in patients for whom 10–20 years of long-term therapy with a proton pump inhibitor could be contemplated.

R.W. McCallum, M.D.

Helicobacter pylori Infection in Spouses of Patients With Duodenal Ulcers and Comparison of Ribosomal RNA Gene Patterns

Georgopoulos SD, Mentis AF, Spiliadis CA, et al (Gen Hosp of Athens, Greece; Hellenic Pasteur Inst, Athens, Greece)
Gut 39:634–638, 1996   66–4

Introduction.—Although *Helicobacter pylori* infection is mainly acquired in childhood, some reports suggest that infection may also appear in adulthood. Sixty-four patients with duodenal ulcer and their spouses were studied to determine whether intra-familial spread of the microorganism does occur.

Methods.—Participants underwent endoscopy after an overnight fast. Eight biopsy specimens were obtained in each participant, 6 from the antrum and 2 from the corpus. Two antrum specimens and the 2 corpus specimens were used for histologic examination, 2 were used for culture, and 2 for the CLO test. Patients were considered to be *H. pylori* positive if at least 2 methods yielded positive results and *H. pylori* negative if all tests gave negative results. *Helicobacter pylori* isolates were compared on the basis of their rRNA gene patterns (ribopatterns) after digestion of chromosomal DNA by the restriction endonucleases *Hae*III or *Hind*III.

Results.—Fifty-four patients with duodenal ulcer were *H. pylori* positive, and most (78%) of the spouses in this group were also positive. Ten patients were *H. pylori* negative, and only 2 (20%) of their partners were infected. Ribopatterns of *H. pylori* strains were obtained in 18 couples; both partners in 8 couples were colonized by a single strain and each partner by a distinct strain in 10 couples.

Conclusion.—A certain percentage of *H. pylori* infection is acquired in adulthood. This study of cohabiting married couples showed a significantly higher prevalence of *H. pylori* infection in spouses of *H. pylori* positive patients with duodenal ulcer than in spouses of *H. pylori* negative patients. Person-to-person transmission within couples appears to be a common source of the infection.

Prevalence of *Helicobacter Pylori* Infection and Related Gastroduodenal Lesions in Spouses of *Helicobacter Pylori* Positive Patients With Duodenal Ulcer

Parente F, Maconi G, Sangaletti O, et al (L Sacco Univ Hosp, Milan, Italy)
Gut 39:629–633, 1996 66–5

Background.—Very few studies to date have assessed the risk of infection among spouses of patients positive for *Helicobacter pylori* (*H pylori*). Furthermore, the studies that do exist have yielded conflicting findings.

Methods.—One hundred twenty-four spouses (52% female) of patients with duodenal ulcer were seen consecutively during 10 months. The spouses were screened for serum immunoglobulin G anti-*H pylori* antibodies and completed a questionnaire eliciting information on the presence of chronic or recurrent dyspepsia. The control group consisted of 249 volunteer blood donors matched for age, sex, origin, and socio-economic status.

Findings.—The seroprevalence of *H pylori* infection was significantly higher in spouses than in control subjects, the rates being 71% and 58%, respectively. Thirty-four percent of the 88 seropositive spouses reported dyspeptic symptoms, compared with only 12% of the 34 seronegative spouses. Ninety-eight percent of the 49 seropositive spouses undergoing endoscopy had confirmation of *H pylori* infection. Among those spouses, endoscopic findings demonstrated active duodenal ulcer in 17%, duodenal scar and cap deformity in 4%, active gastric ulcer in 4%, erosive duodenitis in 6%, antral erosions in 4%, antral erosions plus duodenitis in 1 patient, and peptic esophagitis in 1 patient. Compared with spouses who had never been symptomatic, symptomatic spouses had a significantly greater prevalence of major endoscopic lesions.

Conclusions.—Spouses of *H pylori*-positive patients with duodenal ulcer may be at increased risk for *H pylori* colonization and possibly for peptic ulcer disease. Thus there may be a need for serologic screening of the cohabiting partners of such patients.

▶ These 2 articles (Abstracts 66–4 and 66–5) regarding patterns of infection and transmission of *Helicobacter pylori* are very interesting because they both deal with spouses. Parente et al. find that being the spouse of an *H. pylori* positive patient with duodenal ulcer disease does increase the risk of *H. pylori* colonization in that spouse and perhaps of later having peptic ulcer disease, and raises the question as to whether serologic screening of cohabiting partners of *H. pylori* positive patients with duodenal ulcer may be indicated. This particular study, I think, is relevant in the situation where having eradicated *H. pylori* in a patient with peptic ulcer disease or with another appropriate clinical setting, there seems to be a recurrence after a few months or a few years. Once eradication is demonstrated, it is believed that recurrence or reinfection is less than 1% per year. When reinfection does occur, it could bring up the possibility that in close household contacts, potential fecal-oral spread or even transmission through saliva or kissing can be hypothesized, e.g., a spouse situation.

This concept is further explored in the article published by the group headed by Georgopoulos in which their data showed or supported the suggestion that spouses of *H. pylori* positive patients with duodenal ulcer constitute a high-risk group for colonization of *H. pylori* and subsequent development of either duodenal or gastric ulcer disease. These data would also suggest person-to-person transmission within couples or that exposure to a common source of infection is quite possible and common.

R.W. McCallum, M.D.

MALT-Type Lymphoma of the Stomach Is Associated With *Helicobacter pylori* Strains Expressing the CagA Protein

Eck M, Schmausser B, Haas R, et al (Universität Würzburg, Germany; Max-Planck Institut für Biologie, Tübingen, Germany)
Gastroenterology 112:1482–1486, 1997   66–6

Introduction.—Infection of the stomach by *Helicobacter pylori* is thought to be involved in the pathogenesis of gastric lymphoma of mucosa-associated lymphoid tissue (MALT) type, a concept supported by 2 large studies that found the bacterium in almost all gastric MALT-type lymphomas. Strains of *H. pylori* have been subdivided into 2 major types according to the expression of cytotoxin associated antigen (CagA). Predominantly CagA+ strains appear to be responsible for the development of gastroduodenal diseases. Sera of patients with gastric MALT-type lymphoma were examined for the presence of *H. pylori* and the incidence of CagA+ strains.

Methods.—Sera from 68 patients had been collected between 1992 and 1996. Gastric MALT-type lymphoma was classified as low grade in 22 cases, high grade in 36, and secondary high grade in 10. The serologic response to CagA was studied by immunoblotting, using a purified recombinant CagA protein, a CagA+ strain, and the corresponding isogenic CagA− mutant. The specificity and sensitivity of the immunoblot were determined using sera of control patients.

Results.—Sixty-seven (98.5%) patients with MALT-type lymphoma were *H. pylori* seropositive. The bacterium was detected histologically in the only seronegative patient by Warthin-Starry staining. Overall, 95.5% of seropositive patients had serum immunoglobulin G antibodies to CagA. In a *H. pylori*-positive control group with chronic active gastritis, 33 of 49 patients (67%) had antibodies to CagA. All patients with high-grade or secondary high-grade MALT-type lymphoma had serum antibodies specific for *H. pylori* infection.

Conclusion.—Previous studies have demonstrated an association between CagA+ strains of *H. pylori* and severe active gastritis, duodenal ulceration, and gastric adenocarcinoma. The finding of CagA+ strains in almost all patients with MALT-type lymphoma supports a role for these apparently more virulent strains in the pathogenesis of the disease.

▶ This article addresses the fact that besides gastritis and adenocarcinoma, another scenario of chronic *Helicobacter pylori* infection is the development of gastric lymphoma of mucosa-associated lymphoid tissue (MALT) type. Infection with *H. pylori* triggers the acquisition of gastric MALT and may then provide the background for a development of MALT-type lymphoma, which becomes invasive. Most gastric low-grade MALT-type lymphomas have been shown to regress after eradication of the *H. pylori*. In studying patients with MALT-type lymphomas, the authors found that *H. pylori* infection with the CagA-positive *H. pylori* strains is present in almost all patients, and this indicates that perhaps the CagA protein may be a marker or may play a crucial role in the evolution of gastric MALT-type lymphoma.

R.W. McCallum, M.D.

Clinical and Pathological Importance of Heterogeneity in *vacA*, the Vacuolating Cytotoxin Gene of *Helicobacter pylori*
Atherton JC, Peek RM Jr, Tham KT, et al (Univ Hosp, Nottingham, England; Vanderbilt Univ, Nashville, Tenn; Veterans Affairs Med Ctr, Nashville, Tenn)
Gastroenterology 112:92–99, 1997   66–7

Introduction.—Infection with *Helicobacter pylori* is quite common, but most individuals with the bacterium do not experience clinical sequelae of infection. Certain strains linked to pathogenicity produce a vacuolating cytotoxin (*vacA*) and exhibit *CagA*. Both characteristics are significant risk factors for peptic ulceration, and the latter for atrophic gastritis and gastric adenocarcinoma. Biopsy specimens from 61 dyspeptic patients were examined to define whether *vacA* genotype had any independent association with inflammation and to study its association with gastric epithelial damage.

Methods.—Patients underwent endoscopy and gastric biopsy. All specimens obtained were processed for *H. pylori* culture and 52 were also processed for histology. Polymerase chain reaction and colony hybridization were used to type *H. pylori vacA*. A HeLa cell vacuolation assay assessed cytotoxin activity. Peptic ulcer disease was defined as active peptic ulceration seen during the study or a diagnosis of peptic ulceration by a previous endoscopy or upper gastrointestinal series.

Results.—Twenty-three patients (37%) had duodenal ulcer disease alone, 5 (8%) had gastric ulcer disease alone, and 2 (3%) had both. Forty-two patients tested positive for *H. pylori* and 19 tested negative. Of the patients with complete sets of biopsy specimens taken for histologic analysis, 34 were infected and 18 were not infected. Strains of *H. pylori* with *vacA* signal sequence type s1a were associated with greater antral mucosal neutrophil and lymphocyte infiltration than s1b or s2 strains. Both midregion and signal sequence were associated with cytotoxin activity in vitro. The incidence of duodenal ulcer disease was 89% in patients with s1a strains, 29% in those with s1b strains, 20% in those with s2 strains, and 16% in uninfected patients.

Conclusion.—Infection with *vacA* strains of *H. pylori* leads to more gastric inflammation than infection with s1b or s2 strains. Gastric epithelial injury was more closely associated with *vacA* midregion type m1. Infection with *vacA* s2 strains appears relatively benign.

▶ Patients with CagA positive *Helicobacter pylori* infection can also have or produce a vacuolating cytotoxin. This gene encoding the cytotoxin is called *vacA*. Gastric inflammation and epithelial damage are believed to be very important in peptic ulcer pathogenesis, but the relationship of *vacA* genotype in this setting has not been studied. The article by Atherton et al. from the laboratory of Dr. Martin Blaser at Vanderbilt University addresses this issue and finds that *H. pylori* strains of *vacA* signal sequence type s1a are associated with an enhanced gastric inflammation and duodenal ulceration as a scenario, whereas *vacA* s2 strains are associated with less inflammation and a lower prevalence of ulcer. Again, we are seeing in these ongoing studies of strains and genotype characteristics, an attempt to try to ferret out the markers that might designate why certain patients will have a complicated outcome as in peptic ulcer disease, whereas others may have more benign problems, including dyspepsia, or perhaps no symptoms at all.

R.W. McCallum, M.D.

Risk for Gastric Cancer in People With CagA Positive or CagA Negative *Helicobacter pylori* Infection

Parsonnet J, Friedman GD, Orentreich N, et al (Stanford Univ, Calif; Kaiser Permanente Care Program, Oakland, Calif; Orentreich Found, Cold-Spring-on-Hudson, NY)
Gut 40:297–301, 1997   66–8

Introduction.—Infection with *Helicobacter pylori* is a strong risk factor for gastric cancer, but it is not known why some individuals will have these cancers and others will not. A previous study suggested that antibodies to the CagA gene, a gene associated with cytotoxic expression, are more common in *H. pylori*-infected patients with gastric malignancy than in infected patients without such malignancy. Whether the CagA phenotype of *H. pylori* infection is an independent risk for cancer was investigated.

Methods.—In a group of 242 patients who participated in an earlier nested case-control study of gastric cancer, 179 (90 cases and 89 controls) were infected with *H. pylori* and 63 (13 cases and 50 controls) were uninfected. Serum samples were confirmed positive for *H. pylori* antibodies by enzyme linked immunosorbent assay (ELISA). The samples, obtained a mean of 14.2 years before diagnosis of gastric cancer in cases, were tested by ELISA for IgG antibodies against the CagA gene product of *H. pylori*. Testing for pepsinogen I, a low concentration of which was previously found to greatly increase cancer risk, had also been performed. The risk for gastric cancer was compared among infected patients with CagA antibodies, infected patients without CagA antibodies, and uninfected individuals.

Results.—Compared to uninfected individuals, those infected with *H. pylori* and exhibiting the presence of CagA antibodies had a 5.8-fold increased risk for the development of gastric cancer. This increased risk was true for both intestinal (odds ratio 5·1) and diffuse type (odds ratio 10·1) cancers. Patients with *H. pylori* but no CagA antibodies had only a slight, nonsignificant increase in risk. The presence of low concentrations (less than 50 ng/mL) of pepsinogen I significantly increased risk for both intestinal and diffuse type cancers in those with *H. pylori* infection, but lessened the degree of association between CagA and cancer.

Conclusion.—Inflammatory changes that occur with *H. pylori* infections have been linked to an increased risk for intestinal and diffuse types of gastric adenocarcinoma. The risk is greatest among patients infected with CagA-positive *H. pylori*, which leads to greater inflammation than CagA-negative *H. pylori*. The latter strain may only be associated with diffuse type disease.

▶ *Helicobacter pylori* at the phenotypic level has strains that can be characterized in 2 types: those that contain a gene associated with cytotoxin expression or the so-called CagA gene, and those that do not. Expression of the CagA protein can be sensitively and specifically diagnosed by detecting antibodies to it. Therefore, in the article by Parsonnet et al, the conclusions were that persons infected with CagA positive *H. pylori* are at considerably increased risk of gastric cancer, whereas infections with CagA-negative *H. pylori* are less strongly linked to malignancy and may only be associated with diffuse type gastritis. This is a very important concept as far as the potential for surveillance and screening in the future is concerned, and it may foster intervention strategies to prevent the slow evolution to malignancy in the subset of patients with CagA-positive *H. pylori* infection.

R.W. McCallum, M.D.

67 Gastrointestinal Motility

> ► The next series of articles was chosen to review the spectrum of gastrointestinal motility, which was a very active area of publication in the gastrointestinal literature in 1997. I'd say the single biggest development in gastric motility is the understanding now that the interstitial cells of Cajal actually control gut motility and that they are the site where the basal electrical rhythm emanates from, and that these interstitial cells are intimately connected and woven into the myenteric plexus and into the smooth muscle of the gut. This is well described and discussed in a review article by Hagger et al. (Abstract 67–1). which builds on primary work done by the groups of Kent Sanders and Jan Huizinga. It opens up a huge area for discussion. One could argue about whether abnormal function of these cells may be amenable to pharmacologic intervention. Regarding the concept of electrical dysrhythmias of the stomach and gut and how they relate to abnormalities in the interstitial cells of Cajal: Could pacing of the gut, and in particular gastric pacing, reorganize and improve the electromechanical coupling from these cells? And how does that impact on the connection to the smooth muscle and the release of neuronal transmitters such as nitric oxide and astrocholine from the neuronal network?
>
> **R.W. McCallum, M.D.**

Role of the Interstitial Cells of Cajal in the Control of Gut Motility

Hagger R, Finlayson C, Jeffrey I, et al (St George's Hosp, London)
Br J Surg 84:445–450, 1997   67–1

Background.—It has been suggested that the interstitial cells of Cajal (ICCs) may play a role in controlling gut motility. Current knowledge of these cells is reviewed, including the evidence for the role as pacemakers of gut motility and as the intermediaries of neural control of gut muscular activity.

The ICCs and Control of Gut Motility.—Light microscopic examination of the ICCs shows large oval nuclei, little perinuclear cytoplasm, and a spindle or stellate cell shape (Fig 1). Their ultrastructural findings vary

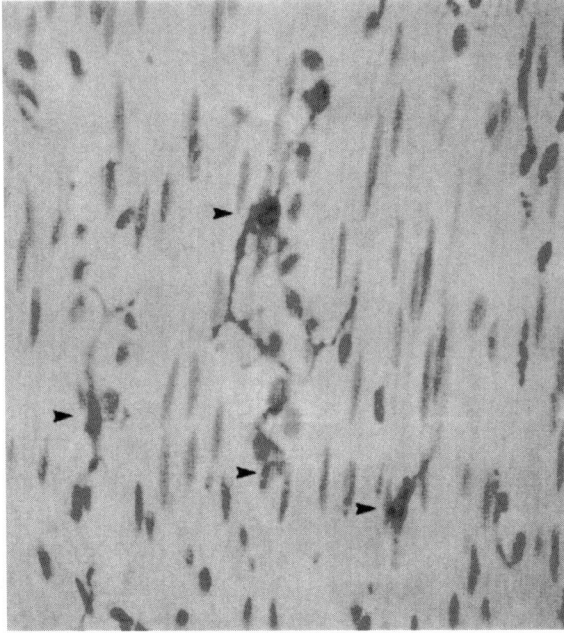

FIGURE 1.—Interstitial cells of Cajal (*arrowed*) in the circular muscle of the sigmoid colon (original magnification ×400). Immunohistochemistry using an anti-c-*kit* antibody. (Courtesy of Hagger R, Finlayson C, Jeffrey I, et al: Role of the interstitial cells of Cajal in the control of gut motility. *Br J Surg* 84:445–450, 1997, Blackwell Science Ltd.)

between species and location within the gut. These cells are sometimes difficult to identify because of their similarities to other types of cells; electron microscopy is needed for definitive identification. An anti-c-*kit* antibody is now available for selective immunocytochemical labeling of ICCs. Most areas of the human gastrointestinal (GI) tract have been found to contain ICCs. They are found only in the circular muscle layer of the gastric fundus and in the circular muscle layer and myenteric plexus of the gastric body and antrum. They are found in the deep muscular plexus, circular muscle, and myenteric plexus of the small intestine and in the submucous plexus, circular muscle, myenteric plexus, and longitudinal muscle of the colon.

It has been suggested that the ICCs act as pacemakers for the GI tract and as intermediaries in the control of muscle activity by the enteric nervous system. In their pacemaker role, it has been suggested that the ICCs are responsible for generating the rhythmic oscillations of membrane potential known as slow waves. Most of the evidence for this function comes from animal studies; blockade of ICC development leads to severe abnormalities of gut motility in mice. The ICCs are closely innervated and associated with nerve plexi. In the dog colon, ICCs are in close contact with neurones and connected to smooth muscle cells via gap junctions; however, there are no specialized contacts between neurones and smooth muscle cells. Experiments have shown that neural modulation of ICC activity affects gut motility. When the development of ICCs is impaired, the response of intestinal smooth muscle to neural stimulation is reduced but not abolished. Little is known about the development of ICCs in the GI tract, though they are thought to be of mesenchymal origin.

Discussion.—Current knowledge of the ICCs and their roles in controlling gut motility is reviewed. Diseases involving abnormal gut motility may involve abnormal ICC distribution or function. However, more complete information on the distribution of these cells in the normal human GI tract is needed before this hypothesis can be tested. Abnormal distribution of ICCs could become a useful marker for diagnosis and surgical planning.

Interstitial Cells of Cajal Mediate Inhibitory Neurotransmission in the Stomach

Burns AJ, Lomax AEJ, Torihashi S, et al (Univ of Nevada, Reno; Nagoya Univ, Japan)
Proc Natl Acad Sci U S A 93:12008–12013, 1996   67–2

Introduction.—Previous studies have demonstrated close structural relationships between the interstitial cells of Cajal (ICC), varicose nerve fibers, and the smooth muscle cells of the gastrointestinal tract. These findings suggest a possible role of ICC in governing enteric neurotransmission. Recent experiments have shown that mutations in the c-*kit* proto-oncogene can cause developmental defects in some classes of ICC. The role of these cells in neurotransmission in the stomach was studied using mice with such a mutation.

Methods and Results.—Through morphologic studies and analysis of immunoreactivity to antibodies against c-kit receptors, the investigators identified 2 classes of ICC in the mouse stomach. A network of ICC with multiple processes was found in the myenteric plexus region, extending from the corpus to the pylorus. Throughout the stomach, the circular and longitudinal muscle layers (IC-IM) were found to contain spindle-shaped ICC, with the greatest density in the circular and longitudinal muscle layers. The IC-IM, which ran along nerve fibers, were closely related to nerve terminals and smooth muscle cells.

Mice with a c-*kit* mutation that led to failure of IC-IM development were studied to evaluate the role of these cells in mediating neural inputs in the gastric fundus muscles. The stomachs of mutant mice showed normal distribution of inhibitory nerves. They also had great reductions in nitric oxide-dependent inhibitory neuroregulation. Administration of sodium nitroprusside caused relaxation of smooth muscle tissues in the mutant mice, though the membrane potential effects of sodium nitroprusside were reduced.

Conclusions.—In mice, ICC located within the circular and longitudinal muscle layers appear to play a critical serial role in nitric oxide–dependent neurotransmission. These cells may provide the cellular mechanism by which nitric oxide is transduced into electrical responses. Mutant mice without IC-IM demonstrate loss of electrical responsiveness and markedly reduced responses to nitrergic nerve stimulation.

▶ These authors show that the ICC actually play a critical role in nitric oxide–dependent neurotransmission. They go on to suggest that these cells may selectively express the iron channels or the second messenger systems necessary to transduce nitric oxide signals into electrical responses in postjunctional cells.

R.W. McCallum, M.D.

[¹³C]Octanoic Acid Breath Test for Gastric Emptying of Solids: Accuracy, Reproducibility, and Comparison With Scintigraphy
Choi M-G, Camilleri M, Burton DD, et al (Mayo Clinic and Found, Rochester, Minn)
Gastroenterology 112:1155–1162, 1997   67–3

Introduction.—Alternatives have been sought for the use of scintigraphy as a means of measuring gastric emptying. A promising alternative is the *C-substrate breath test, the advantages of which include simplicity, safety, and the potential for widespread clinical application when gamma camera facilities are not available. The accuracy of a nonradioactive breath test using the stable isotope [¹³C]octanoic acid for measuring gastric emptying of solids was evaluated.

Methods.—Fifteen healthy volunteers with a mean age of 41 years participated in the study. All underwent simultaneous scintigraphy and [¹³C]octanoic acid breath test. Scans and breath samples were obtained

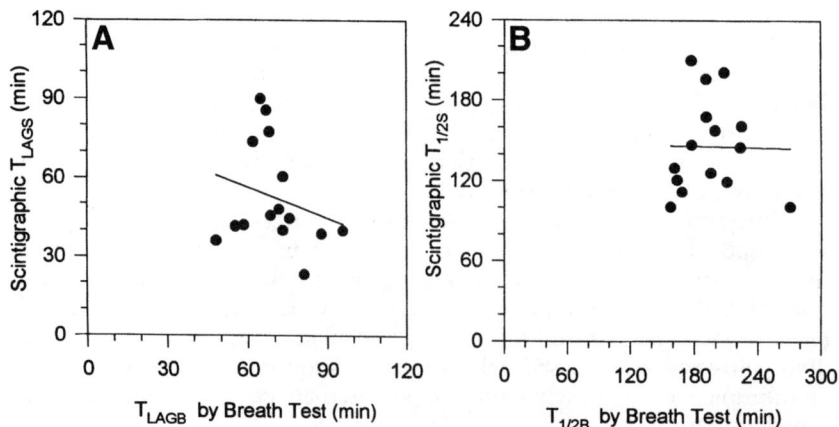

FIGURE 4.—Regression analysis of (A) lag phase and (B) half emptying time for scintigraphy on breath test values. Note the lack of any significant correlation between the 2 methods. (Courtesy of Choi M-G, Camilleri M, Burton DD, et al: [¹³C]Octanoic acid breath test for gastric emptying of solids: Accuracy, reproducibility, and comparison with scintigraphy. *Gastroenterology* 112:1155–1162, 1997.)

every 15 minutes for 4 and 6 hours, respectively. To evaluate intraindividual variability of gastric emptying parameters, the breath test was repeated on 2 other occasions within a 3-week period.

Results.—No significant correlations were observed for parameters from scintigraphy and the breath test. There was a significant difference in the lag phase and the half-gastric emptying time for solid meals as determined from the breath tests compared with those from scintigraphy, and the differences were highly variable rather than constant. At octanoic acid breath test (OCT) 6 hours, lag phase and half-gastric emptying time were not significantly correlated with those from scintigraphy in these normal individuals (Fig 4). Examination of the reproducibility of the OCT found no significant differences in the lag phase and half-gastric emptying times. Median values for delta (differences between pairs of studies) were close to zero.

Conclusion.—Scintigraphy is the gold standard test for measuring gastric emptying, but patients are exposed to gamma radiation and a well-equipped laboratory is required. Most nonscintigraphic techniques are most effective in evaluating the emptying of liquids. The [^{13}C]octanoic acid breath test for gastric emptying of solids appears to be useful for intraindividual comparisons, but further validation is required before it can substitute for scintigraphy as a diagnostic test.

▶ This article, published by a group at the Mayo Clinic, describes an innovative technique for measuring gastric emptying. This study further extends the concepts that were first published by Ghoos and colleagues at the University of Leuven who described this breath test,[1] which is a noninvasive method with no radiation using the stable isotope carbon 13. Although it has been more accepted in Europe, there are still concerns about the extrapolations and assumptions made about the absorption and timing of this process, which is crucial to the calculations that are made. The Mayo Clinic group concluded that this type of breath test for gastric emptying of solids requires further validation before it can really be a substitution for scintigraphy as a diagnostic test. I think this is a very wise, conservative, and prudent conclusion. The scintigraphic test involving the egg meal typically has been universally accepted throughout the world and standardizations have been achieved to a large extent. Visually, it is very important in many cases to understand where the isotope is moving as far as the intragastric distribution is concerned, and finally how it is moving through the small bowel and perhaps even achieving a colonic transit component by the end of the study. This is all denied in a noninvasive test. The stimulus for the carbon 13 test was that normal patients or subjects could be studied extensively with many dose responses or pharmacologic agents being investigated for gastric motility. This indeed is probably a very desirable goal of safety and repetitive testing, which is not possible with radioactive material. However, in the clinical setting where less repetitive studies may be done and where a visible reproduction or appreciation of the movement of a meal can be achieved, the impetus to move to a stable isotope that is noninvasive is really not very great. I believe that the extrapolation of noninvasive breath testing to a local community hospital will not be straightforward and that the impetus may be best used in research studies while further work and evolution takes place.

R.W. McCallum, M.D.

Reference

1. Ghoos YF, Maes BD, Geypens BJ, et al: Measurement of gastric emptying rate of solids by means of a carbon-labeled octanoic acid breath test. *Gastroenterology* 104:1640–1647, 1993.

Analysis of Fasting Antroduodenal Manometry in Children

Tomomasa T, DiLorenzo C, Morikawa A, et al (Gunma Univ, Japan; Children's Hosp of Pittsburgh, Pa; Univ of Iowa, Iowa City; et al)
Dig Dis Sci 41:2195–2203, 1996   67–4

Objective.—Intraluminal pressures in the distal stomach and duodenum can be measured by antroduodenal manometry. This technique has provided useful information on the pathophysiologic findings associated with signs and symptoms of gastrointestinal motility disorders. However, the unavailability of data on the findings of antroduodenal manometry in normal children has limited its diagnostic value. The results of antroduodenal manometry in children with and without upper GI motility disturbances are presented.

Methods.—The study included 95 patients with symptoms of GI motility disorder, as well as 20 controls without upper GI disease. Some of the patients required no nutritional support therapy, some required occasional IV and/or gastrostomy or jejunostomy feedings to relieve their GI symptoms, and others required central parenteral nutrition at least occasionally. The results of antoduodenal manometry were compared for the 2 groups in an attempt to define normal and abnormal findings.

Results.—The patients with GI motility disturbances exhibited phase III of the migrating motor complex (MMC) less frequently than controls did. This was especially true of patients who required total parenteral nutrition. The patients also more frequently had abnormal migration of phase III and short intervals between phase IIIs. During phase II, the children who were dependent on parenteral nutrition showed persistent low-amplitude contractions and sustained tonic-phasic contractions. Other manometric findings, including short or prolonged phase III, absence of phase I following phase III, tonic contractions during phase III, low amplitude of phase III contractions in a single recording, and clusters of contractions or prolonged propagating contractions during phase II, were no more commonly found in patients than in controls.

Conclusions.—This study identifies several findings of antroduodenal manometry that are associated with GI motility disorders in children. The abnormal findings are absence of phase III of the MMC, abnormal migration of phase III, short intervals between phase III episodes, persistent low-amplitude contractions, and sustained tonic-phasic contractions. The findings, though incomplete, should help to increase the clinical applicability of antroduodenal manometry in children.

▶ This article relates to how to investigate the symptoms of nausea, vomiting, and abdominal pain in children and the use of the antroduodenal motility study. Tomomasa et al. found that there are a number of specific manometric features that can be identified in pediatric GI motility disorders. These are actually very similar to adult observations and probably emphasize that there are limited ways in which the gut can react or change or respond, whether it be in children or adults.

R.W. McCallum, M.D.

Role of Plasma Vasopressin as a Mediator of Nausea and Gastric Slow Wave Dysrhythmias in Motion Sickness
Kim MS, Chey WD, Owyang C, et al (Univ of Michigan, Ann Arbor)
Am J Physiol 272:G853–G862, 1997   67–5

Objective.—Experimental studies of motion sickness have shown disturbances in the rhythm of the gastric pacemaker activity known as the slow wave. The mechanisms of these gastric dysrhythmias are unclear, but recent studies suggest that release of vasopressin into the peripheral circulation may play a role. The role of vasopressin in mediation of human motion sickness and gastric slow wave dysrhythmias was evaluated.

Methods.—The study included 14 healthy volunteers with a history of motion sickness but no gastrointestinal diseases. Circular vection studies were performed to induce motion sickness, with and without infusion of atropine (a muscarinic receptor antagonist) and pretreatment with indomethacin (a prostaglandin synthesis inhibitor). Vasopressin infusion studies were performed as well. During both circular vection and vasopressin infusion studies, cutaneous electrogastrography was performed to assess the presence of gastric dysrhythmias. The signal percentage exceeding 4.5 cycles/min was used to express the extent of tachygastria.

Results.—Ten subjects became nauseated during circular vection, with a mean nausea score of 2.6 on a scale of 0 to 3. This group showed increases in tachygastric activity, from 15% to 45%, and in plasma vasopressin, from 4.5 to 8.4 pg/mL. Atropine blocked these responses, but indomethacin did not. The other 4 subjects did not become nauseated and did not have increased tachygastria or vasopressin release. Vasopressin infusion to achieve a plasma level of 322 pg/mL caused nausea and increased tachyarrhythmic activity (Fig 9). Atropine reduced these responses, but indomethacin did not. Subjects with and without nausea in response to circular vection were no different in their responses to vasopressin infusion.

Conclusions.—In subjects prone to motion sickness, circular vection leads to nausea, dysrhythmias, and vasopressin release. These effects take

A

B

C

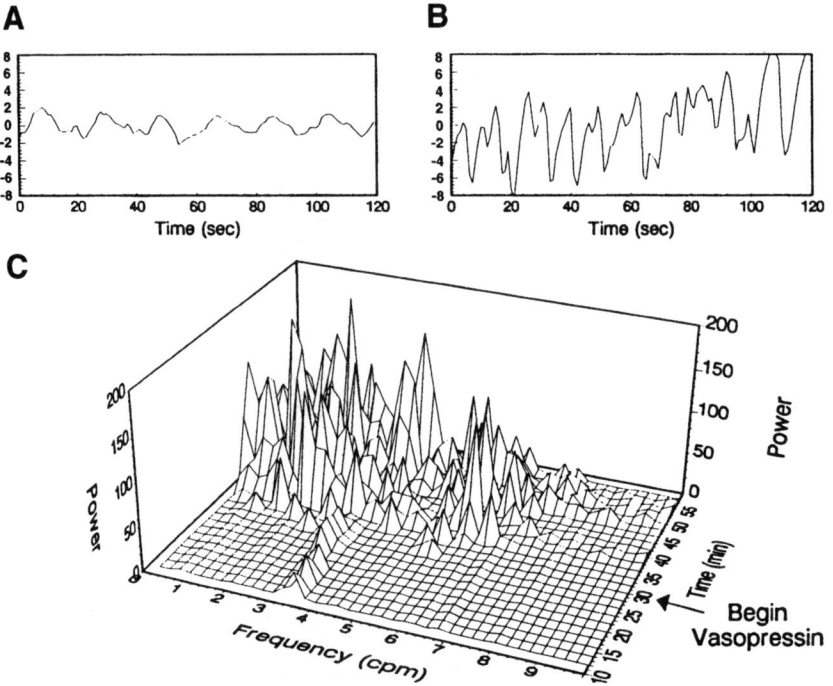

FIGURE 9.—Raw electrogastrographic signals and running spectral analysis of the waveform from a representative vasopressin infusion study are shown. Under basal conditions, the raw slow wave exhibits a regular oscillation with a period of ~20 sec (**A**). With vasopressin infusion (0.2 U/min), there is degeneration of slow wave rhythmicity with replacement by a high-amplitude waveform with a period of ~10 sec (**B**). Spectral analysis of the raw signal shows a predominance of 3 cpm activity (**C**). With vasopressin infusion, the total signal power increases markedly with a relative increase in power in the 4.5 to 9.0 cpm frequency range. Thus vasopressin produced a gastric slow wave tachyarrhythmia in this individual. (Courtesy of Kim MS, Chey WD, Owyang C, et al: Role of plasma vasopressin as a mediator of nausea and gastric slow wave dysrhythmias in motion sickness. *Am J Physiol* 272:G853–G862, 1997, copyright The American Physiological Society.)

place through cholinergic prostaglandin-independent pathways. Nausea and dysrhythmias occur through similar pathways in subjects in response to supraphysiologic vasopressin infusion, with no difference between subjects who are and are not susceptible to motion sickness. Vasopressin appears to have peripheral actions that play a role in the nausea and slow wave disruption occurring in response to circular vection. Atropine reduces the release and activity of vasopressin, which may account for its effectiveness in patients with motion sickness.

The Effect of Intravenous Vasopressin on Gastric Myoelectrical Activity in Human Subjects

Caras SD, Soykan I, Beverly V, et al (Univ of Kansas, Kansas City)
Neurogastroenterol Motil 9:151–156, 1997 67–6

Purpose.—There are unanswered questions about the physiologic events leading to nausea. There is evidence that vasopressin may play a role. This study used electrogastrography (EGG) to study the effects of IV vasopressin on gastric myoelectrical activity.

Methods.—Five healthy subjects were studied under fasting conditions. After baseline EGG recordings, the subjects received a 1-hr infusion of vasopressin, 0.15 or 0.30 U kg^{-1} hr^{-1}. Repeated measurements of serum vasopressin were made during the infusion, and symptoms of nausea, cramping, retching, vomiting, and bloating were assessed. The same assessments were made during 1-hr infusion of normal saline solution.

Results.—The percentage of normal slow waves was reduced by a mean of 29% at the lower vasopressin dose and 43% at the higher dose. Reductions in the EGG dominant frequency were 0.2 and 0.8 cpm, respectively (Fig 2). In patients receiving the higher dose of vasopressin, bradycardia < 2.4 cpm was the main abnormality noted, as opposed to tachygastria >3.7 cpm. At both vasopressin doses, the subjects reported

RUNNING POWER SPECTRA

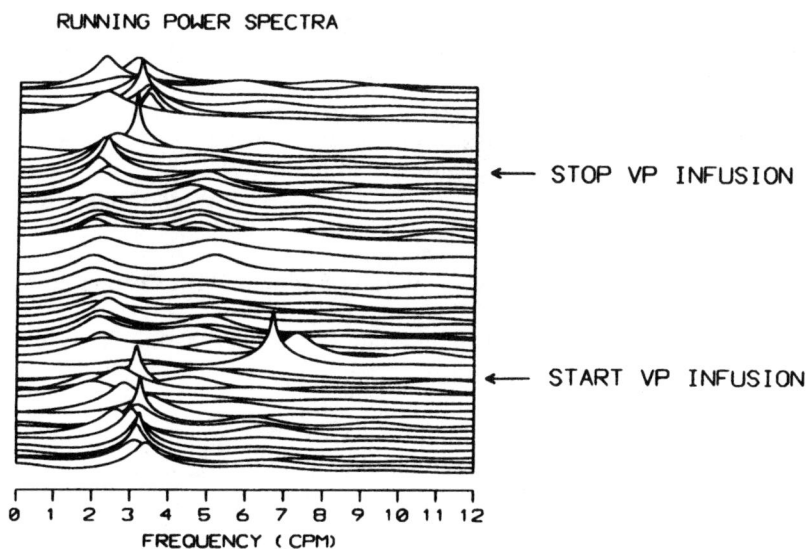

FIGURE 2.—An example of a running power spectra of an EGG signal recorded from a subject at baseline, during vasopressin infusion, and washout period. Each spectrum represents analysis of serial 2-min periods of EGG data. Regular 3-cpm waves were seen before vasopressin infusion. They changed to bradygastria during vasopressin infusion. Note the change of bradygastria again to regular 3-cpm waves immediately after stopping vasopressin infusion. (Courtesy of Caras SD, Soykan I, Beverly V, et al: The effect of intravenous vasopressin on gastric myoelectrical activity in human subjects. *Neurogastroenterol Motil* 9:151–156, 1997 by permission of Blackwell Science Ltd.)

significant nausea and abdominal cramping, though none had vomiting or retching. Nausea and cramping scores were greater with the higher dose.

Conclusions.—Supraphysiologic vasopressin infusion causes nausea, but not vomiting or retching, in most normal subjects. High-dose vasopressin infusion is associated with predominant bradygastria. Higher vasopressin levels lead to greater symptoms of nausea. Vasopressin release appears to play an important role in the development of gastric arrhythmia and nausea.

▶ Kim et al. address the evolving concept of electrogastrography as a cutaneous study reflecting the intrinsic electrical rhythm of the stomach. This is equivalent to the cardiogram of the stomach, if you like. These investigators show in a very well controlled setting and with sophisticated methodology that vasopressin, a peptide released in patients with motion sickness, in this case induced by a vector motion method, was being released by a cholinergic prostaglandin-independent pathway. They also concluded that a central but not peripheral action of vasopressin may contribute to nausea and in turn slow wave disruption during vection. They also explain why simple motion sickness medications that are often anticholinergic and/or antiemetic work, because these agents block the release of vasopressin and the dysrhythmic effects well. This article relates to the one by Caras et al. What they showed is that at supraphysiologic doses vasopressin did induce nausea but did not go on to induce retching or vomiting despite the presence of dysrhythmias. Increasing vasopressin levels did correlate with increasing nausea. These 2 articles indicate that vasopressin is a marker for nausea, perhaps of any source, particularly motion related, and/or dysrhythmia of the stomach. In the future, it's conceivable that pharmacologic agents that suppress vasopressin could actually have a therapeutic role in the treatment of some states of nausea.

R.W. McCallum, M.D.

Impaired Gastric Myoelectrical Activity in Patients With Chronic Renal Failure
Lin X, Mellow MH, Southmayd L III, et al (Integris Baptist Med Ctr, Oklahoma City, Okla)
Dig Dis Sci 42:898–906, 1997   67–7

Background.—Previous reports have described gastric dysmotility and delayed emptying in patients with chronic renal failure (CRF). These symptoms are commonly associated with abnormal gastric myoelectric activity. Electrogastrography (EGG) was performed in patients with CRF.

Methods.—The study included 24 patients with symptomatic CRF and 12 healthy controls. Fifteen of the patients with CRF had diabetes. All subjects underwent two 30-min EGG recordings, before and after a standard meal. The recordings were analyzed by spectral analysis. The study sought to identify gastric myoelectrical dysrhythmia in patients with CRF, including possible EGG differences in patients with and without diabetes.

Results.—The percentage of normal 2 to 4 cpm slow waves was significantly lower in the CRF group vs. controls: 63% vs. 89% on the fasting studies and 62% vs. 90% in the fed studies. Values for diabetic CRF patients were 67% and 65%, respectively. Abnormal EGG, defined as <70% 2 to 4 cpm slow waves, was significantly more frequent in the CRF groups than in the control group: 56% of nondiabetic CRF patients and 60% of diabetic CRF patients vs. 8% of controls in the fasting state; 56% and 53% vs. 0%, respectively, in the fed state. The 2 CRF groups were not significantly different in the regularity of gastric slow waves. In the controls, the standard meal was followed by a significant increase in the dominant EGG power and frequency. This response did not occur in the CRF groups.

Conclusions.—This study presents EGG evidence of abnormal gastric myoelectrical activity in patients with CRF. These patients show impaired regularity of the gastric slow wave with a failed increase in EGG power at 3 cpm. The findings of EGG are similar in patients with CRF with and without diabetes. Gastric motility can be noninvasively assessed in patients with CRF by means of EGG.

Regional Cerebral Activity in Normal and Pathological Perception of Visceral Pain
Silverman DHS, Munakata JA, Ennes H, et al (Univ of California, Los Angeles; West Los Angeles VA Med Ctr, Calif; Univ of California, Irvine)
Gastroenterology 112:64–72, 1997   67–8

Introduction.—Little is known about how the brain processes visceral pain. In many common gastrointestinal conditions, including irritable bowel syndrome (IBS), chronic visceral hyperalgesia may occur in the absence of detectable organic disease. This study used ^{15}O-water positron emission tomography (PET) to study the relationship between visceral pain and regional cerebral activity in subjects with and without IBS.

Methods.—The study included 6 patients with IBS and 6 healthy controls. In each subject, regional brain activity was studied using ^{15}O-water PET at baseline, during a balloon catheter rectal pressure stimulus, and during simulated delivery of the rectal pressure stimulus. Statistical parametric mapping and region of interest methods were used to analyze changes in regional cerebral blood flow.

Results.—During actual and simulated delivery of the painful stimulus, the control subjects showed significant activity of the anterior cingulate cortex (ACC). Nonpainful stimuli produced no ACC response. Patients in the IBS group had no ACC response to the same stimuli; however, they did show significant activation of the left prefrontal cortex.

Conclusions.—Acute rectal pain is associated with activation of the ACC in healthy subjects, as this PET study demonstrates. For patients with

IBS, an aberrant pattern of brain activation is noted during both rectal pressure stimulus and anticipation of rectal pain. The findings support exaggerated activation of a central vigilance network in anticipation of rectal pain, along with failure to activate brain regions associated with endogenous pain inhibition. Functional brain imaging studies can demonstrate specific CNS changes in patients with functional GI disorders.

▶ The article by Lin et al. in Oklahoma City continues the theme related to the electrogastrogram and indicates that in patients with chronic renal failure there are frequently abnormalities found in the gastric myoelectric activity, as measured by the EGG. It is also known that patients with chronic renal failure often have nausea, and we believe that centrally acting antiemetics can relieve this nausea. It would be interesting to know, in this latter paper, why gastric emptying studies were not performed. It would no doubt have shown that indeed many patients can have normal gastric emptying and still have abnormal EGG findings, indicative that dysrhythmias can be associated with a spectrum of gastric symptoms and that gastric motor failure is only a part of the spectrum and not always present when gastric symptoms begin. Another area that's very topical in the field of dyspepsia and/or nausea and indigestion symptoms is the area of visceral sensitivity or hyperalgesia of the gut. The study by Silverman et al. extends this concept to a new dimension. They found that the perception of acute rectal pain is associated with activation of the anterior singulate cortex and the prefrontal cortex, regions of the brain that are believed to play a role in the processing of affective components of the pain experience. The rectal pain was induced by balloon distention, a similar technique used throughout the gut, whether it be the esophagus, stomach, small bowel, or colon. Hence a model could be proposed that includes the fact that there could be some sort of exaggerated activation of the central vigilance network, that is, the prefrontal cortex, in anticipation of rectal pain, and an associated failure to activate brain regions associated with inhibition of endogenous pain. Hence, in patients with functional gut disease and unexplained or exaggerated pain responses to physiologic events such as eating, gastrocolic reflux, and defecation, then imbalance is indeed in place. These are fascinating studies that only further enhance the concept of the brain-gut connection so prevalent in GI neuromuscular disorders.

R.W. McCallum, M.D.

Oesophageal Motility Disorders in Patients With Psychiatric Disease
Roland J, Dhaenen H, Ham HR, et al (Free Univ of Brussels, Belgium)
Eur J Nucl Med 23:1583–1587, 1996   67–9

Background.—Even in healthy subjects, emotional stimuli can affect esophageal motility. Some clinical observations linking esophageal motility disorders to psychologic disorders have been reported as well. A previous study showed an elevated prevalence of psychiatric disorders among patients with abnormal distal esophageal contraction on manometry. This study evaluated the incidence of esophageal contractility abnormalities among patients with psychiatric disorders.

Methods.—The study included 51 consecutive patients admitted to a hospital psychiatric department. Most had affective disorders, and all had digestive symptoms consistent with possible esophageal illness. All patients underwent a krypton 81m esophageal transit study, performed during a psychotropic drug washout period. Patients with abnormal results were studied with manometry and endoscopy. The Hamilton Depression Scale and the Hamilton Anxiety Rating Scale were used to assess levels of these symptoms.

Results.—Thirteen of the 51 patients had abnormal results on esophageal transit studies. Eleven patients went on to undergo receive manometric studies, the other 2 refusing. Ten of the patients undergoing manometry were found to have functional motor abnormalities. All 10 of these patients underwent endoscopy, with normal results in every case.

Conclusions.—Many psychiatric patients with anxiety and/or depression have esophageal contractility abnormalities, this study suggests. The impairment can be demonstrated with scintigraphic as well as manometric studies. However, in the authors' series, all patients had normal endoscopic findings. Thus the esophageal contraction abnormalities demonstrated in psychiatric patients seem likely to represent a functional motor impairment.

▶ This article further extends an original observation by Clouse and Lustman[1] showing that in patients who had esophageal manometry abnormalities, a higher prevalence of psychiatric disorders were found. Roland et al. report that in patients who were seeing psychiatrists and who had no intentions of undergoing esophageal motility studies, when indeed they did submit to an esophageal motility study, a high percentage of esophageal contraction and disturbances was found in those psychiatric patients complaining of anxiety and/or depression. For those of us who are very interested in gastrointestinal motility studies and in particular have observed the evolution of esophageal motility disorders in patients with noncardiac chest pain, these observations continue to be very important. What they indicate is that, indeed, the finding of depression and anxiety is really a marker or a footprint for esophageal abnormalities, and may be found even in patients who don't have specific symptoms at the time. This very much complicates the interpretation of esophageal motility studies in patients referred to a diagnostic motility unit. It is a reminder and a reaffirmation of the fact that microscopically measuring esophageal contractions and trying to extrapolate to a disease is not profitable. Rather, it points out that such patients with anxiety and depression may be very prone to afferent visceral sensitivity, and the esophagus may be reactive to any insult, be it stress, eating or acid pepsin/bile reflux. Hence, the concept that in patients who have gastroesophageal reflux disease and degrees of chest pain not responding to standard therapy, the use of tricyclic antidepressants, pioneered by Clouse and Lustman,[2] is a very real and relevant approach.

R.W. McCallum, M.D.

Reference

1. Clouse RE, Lustman PJ: Psychiatric illness and contraction abnormalities of the esophagus. *N Engl J Med* 309:1337–1342, 1983.
2. Clouse RE, Lustman PJ, Eckert TC, et al: Low-dose trazodone for symptomatic patients with esophageal contraction abnormalities: A double blind, placebo-controlled trial. *Gastroenterology* 92:1027–1036, 1987.

Laparoscopic Surgical Treatment of Achalasia

Holzman MD, Sharp KW, Ladipo JK, et al (Vanderbilt Univ, Nashville, Tenn; Veterans Administration Med Ctr, Nashville, Tenn)

Am J Surg 173:308–311, 1997   67–10

Objective.—Though effective surgical and nonsurgical treatments for achalasia exist, there is debate as to which treatment is best. The advent of minimally invasive surgery provides the opportunity for good surgical results with minimal discomfort and quick recovery. An experience with thoracoscopic and laparoscopic esophagomyotomy for the treatment of achalasia is reported.

Methods.—Over a 3-year period, the investigators performed surgery using minimally invasive techniques in 10 patients with achalasia, mean age 50. The first 3 patients were treated with a transthoracic approach. For several reasons, including experience with laparoscopic antireflux procedures, instrumentation concerns, and ease of access to the lower esophageal sphincter, a transabdominal approach was used in the remaining 7 patients. Intraoperative endoscopy was performed to facilitate dissection, to demonstrate division of the lower esophageal sphincter, and to help determine the length of the myotomy.

Results.—Just 1 patient received IV and IM narcotics for longer than 24 hr after surgery, and 2 required no postoperative narcotics. Mucosal perforation necessitated conversion to open thoracotomy for 1 patient. For procedures completed endoscopically, the average hospital stay was 2 days. A second laparoscopic myotomy was performed in 1 patient with recurrent dysphagia at 3 months. At follow-up, all patients had relief of dysphagia. The results were considered excellent in 8 patients, good in 1, and fair in 1.

Conclusions.—The authors present their experience with minimally invasive surgery for achalasia. They prefer a laparoscopic approach over a thoracoscopic approach because it simplifies anesthetic and surgical management. Laparoscopic myotomy provides a simple and effective alternative to open myotomy or dilation for patients with achalasia.

▶ This article by Bill Richards' group at Vanderbilt is timely because of concerns about other therapies for achalasia. This shows that a so-called Heller myotomy performed by the laparoscopic technique can actually be very, very effective. The authors could avoid the need for fundoplication, in their view, by doing simultaneous endoscopy. Transillumination of the mucosa by the endoscopic light assured adequate division of the lower esophageal sphincter, thus preventing a lengthy extension of the myotomy into the stomach, which is why they thought reflux was not a problem. I personally believe that this very, very simple approach to surgery for achalasia will become extremely attractive and probably will become the treatment of choice at all levels of care. If the esophagus is developing a sigmoid deformity and has become extremely tortuous, then more than just a laparoscopic approach will be required as far as straightening and changing the angulation of the esophagus as well as doing a myotomy.

R.W. McCallum, M.D.

Anti-myenteric Neuronal Antibodies in Patients With Achalasia: A Prospective Study

Verne GN, Sallustio JE, Eaker EY (Univ of Florida, Gainesville)
Dig Dis Sci 42:307–313, 1997   67–11

Introduction.—Patients with idiopathic achalasia have functional obstruction resulting from esophageal aperistalsis with incomplete relaxation of the lower esophageal sphincter. Previous studies have demonstrated loss of inhibitory neurons in the distal esophagus in patients with this condition. Though the pathogenesis of idiopathic achalasia is unknown, there is evidence to suggest an autoimmune mechanism. The possible involvement of antimyenteric antibodies in idiopathic achalasia was analyzed.

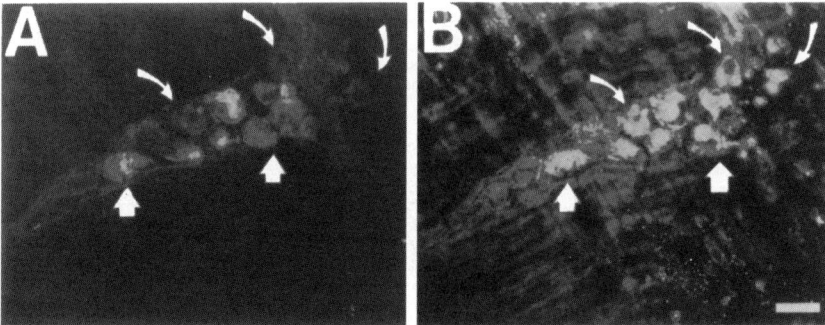

FIGURE 2.—Representative double-labeled indirect immunofluorescence microscopy of rat ileum. A and B, corresponding double-labeled views of the same longitudinal section of ileum. A, The tissue is stained with neurofilament antibody (1:200) to allow localization of the myenteric neurons. B, Sera from an achalasia patient (1:200) stains neurons that are both neurofilament positive (*curved arrows*) and neurofilament negative (*large arrows*). Bar = 20 μm. (Courtesy of Verne GN, Sallustio JE, Eaker EY: Anti-myenteric neuronal antibodies in patients with achalasia: A prospective study. *Dig Dis Sci* 42:307–313, 1997, Plenum Publishing Corporation.)

Methods.—The prospective study included 18 patients with clinically, radiologically, and manometrically established achalasia. Serum samples were collected for these patients and analyzed for the presence of antimyenteric neuronal antibodies. The specificity of these antibodies was determined by analyzing sera from patients with gastroesophageal reflux disease and from disease-free controls. Immunofluorescence studies were performed by double-labeling sections of rat esophagus and intestine with patient sera, prepared in dilutions of 1:50 to 1:400, and with neurofilament antibody to localize neurons.

Results.—Sera from 39% of the achalasia group stained the majority of neurons within plexi in the esophageal and intestinal sections. This included neurons that were both positive and negative for NADPH diaphorase (nitric oxide synthase) (Fig 2). Staining did not occur with sera from any patients in the gastroesophageal reflux or control groups.

Conclusions.—This study demonstrates the presence of antimyenteric neuronal antibodies in patients with achalasia. The results suggest a possible immune basis for this diffuse, idiopathic disease. However, there are no differences in the clinical characteristics of patients with achalasia with and without antimyenteric antibodies.

Untoward Effects of Esophageal Botulinum Toxin Injection in the Treatment of Achalasia
Eaker EY, Gordon JM, Vogel SB (Univ of Florida, Gainesville; VA Med Ctr, Gainesville, Fla)
Dig Dis Sci 42:724–727, 1997   67–12

Objective.—Some authors have suggested injection of botulinum toxin into the lower esophageal sphincter (LES) as a treatment for achalasia. This technique appears to have minimal side effects and complications, compared with surgery or dilation. Some previous unreported side effects of esophageal botulinum toxin injection are reported.

> *Case.*—Man, 63, was evaluated for symptoms of achalasia. He had a history of pulmonary valve stenosis, pulmonary hypertension, and congestive heart failure. The patient was selected for participation in a prospective study of botulinum toxin esophageal injection for high-risk patients. Pretreatment endoscopy showed mild esophageal dilatation without any stricture or mucosal abnormalities in the distal esophagus or proximal stomach. At endoscopy, the region of the LES was injected with a total of 80 units of botulinum toxin. There were no immediate complications, but 2 weeks later, hematemesis developed. Ulceration of the distal esophagus was noted at endoscopy. The patient was started on omeprazole, 20 mg twice daily; he had no further hematemesis, but achalasia symptoms were unchanged. Further studies showed persis-

tent distal esophageal ulcers, aperistalsis, and significant reflux without omeprazole. Eventually, because of severe reflux and persistent hypertensive LES, the patient underwent transabdominal surgery, including myotomy carried into the gastric cardia and a loose Nissen fundoplication. Surgery demonstrated dense adhesions around the distal esophagus, with thickening of the distal esophageal wall and loss of normal tissue planes. Results of barium swallow study were normal postoperatively, and symptoms were significantly improved at 3 weeks' follow-up.

Discussion.—This patient had gastroesophageal reflux, esophageal ulceration and hemorrhage, and extraluminal esophageal inflammation after botulinum toxin injection of the LES for achalasia. The findings suggest the need for caution with this treatment option, which is generally regarded as a safe alternative to dilation or myotomy.

▶ These 2 articles (Abstracts 67–11 and 67–12) deal with the entity of achalasia, and both involve Dr. E. Y. Eaker and his group at Florida University and also the University of Kansas Medical Center, where he currently is located. He first of all showed, in the paper entitled "Anti-myenteric Neuronal Antibodies in Patients with Achalasia," that neuronal antibodies are definitely present in achalasia and could provide a very attractive hypothesis to explain a possibly immune–mediated or immune-based disorder. He used the double-label previously. Anti-myenteric neuronal antibodies have been described in patients with small cell lung cancer,[1] and studies by Caras et al.[2] indicate that such antibodies can actually inhibit myenteric reflexes in the guinea pig myenteric plexus. This observation by Eaker et al. extends the spectrum of understanding about achalasia. As one can imagine, this is a primary failure of neuronal migration from the dorsal motor crest, beginning in childhood, where there's a deficit of neuronal function that finally fails at some point in adulthood. On the other hand, whether the concentrations of neurons is imparted by an immune mediated event, be it neural or otherwise, that could indeed stimulate these antibodies to in turn inhibit and induce degeneration and/or failure and atrophy of these neurons. This may explain why achalasia can present anywhere from childhood to the 10th decade.

The other article addresses the need for caution in the treatment of achalasia with botulinum toxin, an attractive way of treating some patients. The complication here involves gastroesophageal reflux disease with esophageal ulceration and hemorrhage and actually extraluminal inflammation suggesting a microperforation at the time of injection. This is a timely reminder that, although botulinum toxin is being used extensively in patients who usually aren't surgery candidates and/or would not tolerate pneumatic dilation, they should still be carefully monitored, and further follow-up studies are required in order to ascertain its true safety.

R.W. McCallum, M.D.

References

1. Lennon VA, Sas DF, Busk MF, et al: Enteric neuronal autoantibodies in pseudo-obstruction with small-cell carcinoma. *Gastroenterology* 100:137–142, 1991.
2. Caras SD, Brashear HR, McCallum RW, et al: Effect of human antineuronal antibodies on the ascending excitatory reflex in the isolated guinea-pig ileum: An enteric motor disorder? *Am J Gastroenterol* 90:1631, 1995.

Chronic Constipation: Is the Work-up Worth the Cost?
Rantis PC Jr, Vernava AM III, Daniel GL, et al (Saint Louis Univ)
Dis Colon Rectum 40:280–286, 1997   67–13

Introduction.—Patients with chronic constipation who fail to respond to lifestyle interventions or conservative medical treatment may be referred for extensive diagnostic studies. In some cases, however, even a thorough workup fails to identify a specific cause for the condition. A study of 51 outpatients referred for evaluation of chronic constipation sought to determine the cost of the workup and subsequent outcome.

Methods.—Patients included in the study had undergone barium enema or colonoscopy to rule out colorectal neoplasia. Chronic constipation was defined as less than 2 bowel movements per week, difficulty with evacuation, cathartic- or enema-dependence, or abdominal symptoms associated with infrequent bowel movements. Patient records were reviewed for the costs and results of tests, treatment, and eventual outcome.

Results.—The patients were 29 women and 22 men with a mean age of 54 years. All required laxative or enema assistance or both for evacuation. The average duration of symptoms was 5 years. Colonoscopy, performed in 44 patients, yielded normal findings or diverticula in 93%. Barium enema studies were performed in 37 patients, 86% of whom had normal findings or had only diverticula. Colonic transit studies and defecography showed abnormal findings in 25% and 46%, respectively, of patients who underwent these tests. Overall, 16% of patients received diagnoses of outlet obstruction, 24% of colonic inertia, and 61% of constipation of uncertain etiology. The overall mean cost of diagnosis was $2,752. Thirty-three of 51 patients were managed successfully with fiber, cathartics, or biofeedback therapy. Twelve of the remaining 18 patients underwent surgery, which was successful in 10; 8 patients have remained constipated.

Conclusion.—The total cost of diagnostic tests for this group of patients was $140,369. Only 12 (23%) patients benefited specifically by receiving surgery or biofeedback. Constipation was resolved in most cases by conservative therapies. An algorithm is proposed for the management of chronic constipation.

▶ Dr. Rantis, Jr, et al. concluded that at a cost of $1,140,369 expended on extensive diagnostic testings, only 23% of the patients actually benefited.

They go into detail about what a reasonable diagnostic algorithm would be. It is a useful, practical outline of how patients do respond to medical therapy, but, also, how some patients deservedly go on to surgery because of refractory constipation and can greatly benefit from this approach.

R.W. McCallum, M.D.

68 Gastroesophageal Reflux Disease

Prospective Long-term Endoscopic and Histological Follow-up of Short Segment Barrett's Esophagus: Comparison With Traditional Long Segment Barrett's Esophagus
Weston AP, Krmpotich PT, Cherian R, et al (Veterans Administration Med Ctr, Kansas City, Mo; Univ of Kansas, Kansas City)
Am J Gastroenterol 92:407–413, 1997   68–1

Introduction.—Adenocarcinoma of the cardia and esophagus is associated with Barrett's esophagus (BE), regardless of the extent of esophageal involvement. However, the risk of dysplasia and adenocarcinoma associated with short-segment BE (SSB), arbitrarily defined as involvement of <2 cm of the distal tubular esophagus, is unknown. This study compared the prevalence and incidence of dysplasia and adenocarcinoma in patients with SSB and traditional long-segment BE.

Methods.—The study included 74 patients with SSB and 78 with traditional BE. All patients were studied with elective upper esophagogastroduodenoscopy over a 40-month period. The 2 groups were similar in terms of age and sex, though patients with SSB were more likely to be African-American. Follow-up endoscopic examinations were performed yearly or as indicated. The risk for dysplasia and esophageal/gastroesophageal junction/cardia adenocarcinoma for each group was assessed at diagnosis and during follow-up.

Results.—At diagnosis, 8% of the SSB group and 24% of the BE group had dysplasia. None of the patients in the SSB group had adenocarcinoma at diagnosis. Prospective follow-up data lasting 12 to 40 months were analyzed for 26 patients with SSB and 29 with traditional BE. The rate of dysphagia during follow-up was 8% in the SSB group and 21% in the BE group. None of the SSB patients was found to have high-grade dysplasia or cancer during follow-up. At last follow-up, patients with traditional BE continued to have a higher frequency of dysplasia than did those with SSB. On histologic examination, biopsy specimens from the SSB group frequently showed an absence of goblet cells, compared with those from patients with traditional BE.

Conclusions.—Compared with patients with traditional, long-segment BE, those with SSB have a lower prevalence of dysplasia or adenocarcinoma and a lower incidence of dysplasia. This follow-up study shows no high-grade dysplasia or adenocarcinoma developing in patients with SSB.. Prospective follow-up studies will be needed to assess the true incidence of adenocarcinoma in patients with SSB.

► Dr. Allan P. Weston and colleagues from the University of Kansas Medical Cancer and the Kansas City VA Medical Center addressed the evolving concept of SSB esophagus (<2 cm in size) when compared with traditional long-segment BE during a follow-up period that ranged from 12 to 40 months. This paper showed that the prevalence of dysplasia or adenocarcinoma in patients with traditional BE is significantly higher than in patients with SSB. However, I think the authors will be the first to reiterate the fact that further surveillance will be required to really appreciate whether this is going to hold up in the long run. I think a fair comment at this point about the evolving concept of SSB is perhaps not focusing so much on whether it's <2 cm or <3 cm, but more importantly that endoscopists appreciate the fact that elongated tongues at the point of the Z-line (gastroesophageal histologic junction) is the area of suspicion where the early stages of so-called SSB begins. Nevertheless, this tissue has to show true specialized epithelium that involves villous architecture and goblet cells, and without that the diagnosis of any kind of BE cannot be sustained.

R.W. McCallum, M.D.

Intestinal Metaplasia of the Gastric Cardia

Morales TG, Sampliner RE, Bhattacharyya A (Arizona Health Sciences Ctr, Tucson)

Am J Gastroenterol 92:414–418, 1997   68–2

Objective.—As the U.S. incidence of adenocarcinoma of the stomach decreases, the incidence of cancers arising from the gastric cardia has increased. Most cases of esophageal carcinoma involve the intestinal metaplasia (IM) of Barrett's esophagus. It is uncertain whether there is any such premalignant lesion for adenocarcinoma of the gastric cardia. Patients undergoing upper endoscopy were studied to assess the prevalence of IM involving the cardia and the factors associated with this finding.

Methods.—The study included 104 patients undergoing elective upper endoscopy at a VA medical center over a 7-month period. The patients were 99 men and 5 women, mean age 62. Symptoms of gastroesophageal reflux disease, and smoking and alcohol history were assessed before endoscopy. The presence of esophagitis, hiatus hernia, and Barrett's mucosa was evaluated during the procedure. The investigators obtained 7 biopsy specimens from 6 specific sites in the antrum, angularis, cardia, and esophageal gastric junction (EGJ), defined as the end of the tubular esophagus meeting the proximal heads of the gastric folds. After staining with a combination of hematoxylin and eosin and Alcian blue at a pH of 2.5, the specimens were evaluated for evidence of IM, defined as columnar-type epithelium with goblet cells. The presence of *Helicobacter pylori* infection was assessed histologically and serologically.

Results.—Intestinal metaplasia of the gastric cardia was found in 23% of patients, none of whom had dysplasia. Barrett's esophagus was present in 11 patients, only 2 of whom also had IM of the cardia. However, 9 of 24 patients with IM of the cardia also had IM elsewhere in the stomach. *H. pylori* infection was identified in 47% of patients; this finding was significantly associated with IM of the gastric cardia.

Conclusions.—This study demonstrates IM of the gastric cardia in nearly one fourth of patients undergoing elective upper endoscopy. This finding is significantly associated with *H. pylori* infection. The study identifies no cases of dysplasia associated with IM of the cardia. However, the true incidence of associated dysplasia or adenocarcinoma must be evaluated in long-term follow-up studies.

▶ Dr. Sampliner and his group from the University of Arizona in Tucson conclude that IM of the gastric cardia is a common problem and was present in 23% of patients undergoing routine endoscopy. In addition, 11% of patients had Barrett's esophagus, but only 2 had the crossover of Barrett's and IM. On the other hand, the presence of *H. pylori* did significantly correlate with the finding of IM of the gastric cardia. No dysplasia was identified at any time. I believe that this study starts to address some of the concerns related to the increasing diagnosis of adenocarcinoma of the body of the esophagus and the fundus. One review would have it that IM of the cardia and fundus induced by *H. pylori* or perhaps idiopathic in turn can evolve into tongues of IM that would be called short segment Barrett's, which in turn could evolve into long segment Barrett's with a greater cancer risk. On the other hand, there would be those investigators who would say that IM of the gastric cardia and fundus is a purely *H. pylori* mediated event and there is not any relationship at all to events above the gastroesophageal junction, and that perhaps we should start to think about fundic adenocarcinoma as a different entity than the Barrett's epithelium related to years of chronic gastroesophageal reflux disease. Certainly the screening procedures being used in Barrett's esophagus still leave a lot to be desired, but one important observation by the group from Houston was that Younes et al. found that the p53 protein, which is a tumor suppressor gene located on the short arm of chromosome 17, appears to play an important role in cellular growth control. p53 accumulation is more specific and a better predictor for the development of high-grade dysplasia in carcinoma than just simply the finding of some degree of low-grade dysplasia, and special stainings with p53 would be and should be used routinely to start to identify this subgroup of patients with Barrett's esophagus who may need more intensive surveillance, while other Barrett's patients could be screened with less frequency and more economically.

R.W. McCallum, M.D.

Role of Acid and Duodenogastroesophageal Reflux in Gastroesophageal Reflux Disease

Vaezi MF, Richter JE (Univ of Alabama, Birmingham; Cleveland Clinic Found, Ohio)
Gastroenterology 111:1192–1199, 1996   68–3

Purpose.—In patients with gastroesophageal reflux disease (GERD), acid and pepsin are known to play an important role in causing esophagitis. There is debate, however, regarding the role of duodenogastroesophageal reflux (DGER) across the spectrum of GERD. The Bilitec 2000 is a

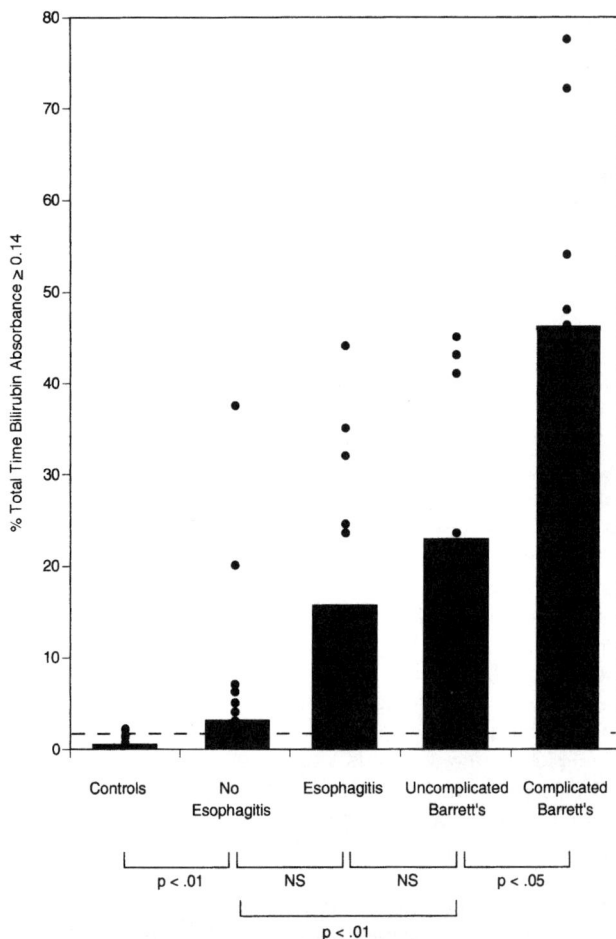

FIGURE 3.—Data for percentage total time bilirubin absorbance level was ≥0.14 for the 5 study populations. *Bold bars* represent the median data. The *horizontal dashed line* across the 5 groups represents the upper limits of normal DGER. Bile reflux showed a graded increase across the groups. Patients with Barrett's esophagus had the highest amount of DGER and the controls the least degree of DGER. (Courtesy of Vaezi MF, Richter JE: Role of acid and duodenogastroesophageal reflux in gastroesophageal reflux disease. *Gastroenterology* 111:1192–1199, 1996.)

new fiberoptic system for spectrophotometric detection of DGER, based on the optical property of bilirubin pigment in detecting bile and independent of pH. This approach was used to study the relationship between pH, DGER, and fasting bile acid concentrations in the development of esophageal damage in patients with GERD.

Methods.—The study included 30 patients with GERD, mean age 41; 20 patients with Barrett's esophagus, mean age 58; and 20 healthy controls. Some of the patients with GERD had had esophageal mucosal injury, and some did not; some of the patients with Barrett's esophagus had complications, and others did not. All subjects were studied with ambulatory esophageal pH monitoring and ambulatory DGER monitoring using the Bilitec 2000 system. Fasting gastric bile acid concentrations were measured as well.

Results.—In the patients with GERD, the percentage total time pH was <4 and the bilirubin level was ≥0.14 (Fig 3). Fasting gastric bile acid concentration in this group varied across the spectrum of GERD. In both patient groups, the most commonly observed reflux pattern was esophageal exposure to both acid and DGER. This pattern was present in all patients with complicated Barrett's esophagus, 89% of patients with uncomplicated Barrett's esophagus, 79% of patients with esophagitis, and 50% of patients without esophagitis. Seventy percent to 90% of episodes of DGER occurred at pH <4. On linear regression analysis, the percentage of time at pH <4 was significantly correlated with the percentage of time at a bilirubin absorbance level of ≥0.14.

Conclusions.—In patients representing the spectrum of GERD, exposure to acid and DGER both increase in severity, leading to increased esophageal mucosal damage. Most episodes of reflux involve simultaneous acid reflux and DGER, the results indicate. Patients with more severe GERD (those with esophagitis and Barrett's esophagus) have greater simultaneous exposure to both acid and bile than do those with less severe disease (those without esophagitis).

▶ This article relates to the observation by Joel Richter's group in Alabama and Cleveland that in severe reflux disease there is increased amount of bile accompanying acid and pepsin in the esophagus. It is believed that this combination may be quite vicious and dangerous, compared with acid and pepsin alone, and could explain the more aggressive presentation of reflux in some patients with stricture and Barrett's esophagus. Two major points in this study: (1) Even when the pH is 4, which is the indication of acid pepsin reflux, bile is refluxing at the same time based on the Bilitec measurement of bile acids, and hence pH measurements alone cannot predict when bile is refluxing. (2) The other aspect is that there is no connection that is known yet about the prevalence of bile in the esophagus and the evolution toward dysplasia, but perhaps this is an area that needs to be considered as a more virulent and aggressive form of Barrett's and/or go on to high-grade dysplasia. Therapeutics were not addressed in this study, but it does beg the question, of course, that a prokinetic agent that begins to prevent bile reflux at the level of the duodenum and the pylorus and through gastric emptying would be a very effective therapy. At the same time, a proton pump inhibitor, by blocking acid secretion, would make the bile somewhat impotent in the esophagus and would also have a role.

R.W. McCallum, M.D.

Comparison of Total Versus Partial Laparoscopic Fundoplication in the Management of Gastroesophageal Reflux Disease

Karim SS, Panton ON, Finley RJ, et al (Vancouver and Delta Hosp, Delta, BC, Canada)

Am J Surg 172:375–378, 1997   68–4

Introduction.—For patients with gastroesophageal reflux disease (GERD), laparoscopic fundoplication has been proven a safe and effective procedure. Before the laparoscopic era, the most effective technique for controlling GERD symptoms was total (360-degree) fundoplication. However, this procedure caused considerable dysphagia and gas bloating. Partial fundoplication was developed in an attempt to avoid these symptoms and has been modified for laparoscopic use. The results of laparoscopic total (LTF) and partial fundoplication (LPF) were compared.

Methods.—The study included 89 patients undergoing attempted laparoscopic fundoplication over a 4-year period. Six patients required conversion to open surgery; thus, the analysis included 48 LTFs and 35 LPFs, including 25 anterior and 10 Toupet procedures. The LTF and LPF groups were compared in terms of operating room times, conversion rates, and incidence of perioperative complications. At mean follow-up intervals of 6 and 15 months, the results were compared in terms of patient satisfaction, symptom control, and late complication rate.

Results.—The preoperative Demeester score was 44 in the LTF group and 39 in the LPF group. Operative times were 2.9 and 2.5 hours, respectively. The LTF group was hospitalized for 3.6 days, compared with 4.1 days for the LPF group. The rate of in-hospital complications was 25% with LTF vs. 1% with LPF. None of the patients died.

At 6 months' follow-up, 17% of the LTF group and 8% of the LPF group had new-onset dysphagia; the difference was nonsignificant. Almost all patients in both groups had complete relief of symptoms. At 15 months' follow-up, heartburn was eliminated or improved in 76% of the LTF group and 87% of the LPF group; regurgitation was eliminated or improved in 93% of both groups. The patient satisfaction rate was 93% with LTF and 97% with LPF. There was no difference in the rate of persistent dysphagia (7.3% and 10.3%, respectively). However, 56% of patients in the LTF group reported early satiety, compared with 83% of the LPF group.

Conclusion.—In patients with GERD, LTF and LPF appear to be equally effective in terms of symptom control and patient satisfaction, at least through 15 months' follow-up. Patients undergoing LTF may have a higher incidence of new-onset dysphagia at 6 months' follow-up, but this difference resolves by 15 months. For patients with GERD plus abnormal esophageal motility, LPF appears to control GERD with no higher incidence of dysphagia and other symptoms than in patients with normal motility undergoing a total wrap.

Outcome of Laparoscopic Nissen Fundoplication in Patients With Disordered Preoperative Peristalsis
Baigrie RJ, Watson DI, Myers JC, et al (Royal Adelaide Hosp, South Australia)
Gut 40:381–385, 1997   68–5

Objective.—Laparoscopic antireflux surgery is an established treatment for reflux disease. Debate continues over the use of a 360-degree wrap, or Nissen fundoplication, in patients with disordered peristalsis. To prevent the complication of dysphagia, some surgeons recommend the use of a partial or modified wrap. The results of Nissen fundoplication in patients with disordered peristalsis were investigated, including the symptomatic and manometric outcomes.

Methods.—Thirty-one patients with disordered peristalsis were identified from a prospectively studied series of 345 patients. According to the results of preoperative manometry, 8 patients had equivocal primary peristalsis, 4 had abnormal primary peristalsis, 13 had abnormal maximal contraction pressure, and 6 had abnormal primary peristalsis and maximal contraction pressure. The postoperative results were analyzed in blinded fashion, including the findings after a barium meal, esophageal manometric examination, and standardized clinical review.

Results.—All patients said they would undergo the procedure again, and 80% reported a satisfaction score of ≥8 on a 10–point scale. Dysphagia scores of >4 were recorded for 48% of patients preoperatively, compared with 6% at 1 year postoperatively. The postoperative manometric studies showed improvements in peristalsis for 78% of patients. Mean lower esophageal sphincter pressure improved from 6.6 mm Hg before surgery to 19.0 mm Hg postoperatively. The results were comparable to those achieved in the overall group of 345 patients.

Conclusions.—Laparoscopic Nissen fundoplication gives good results in patients with reflux who have disordered preoperative peristalsis. This procedure is not contraindicated in patients with disordered peristalsis, or even those with absent peristalsis. The authors' technique included 360-degree fundoplication performed over a large bougie, with or without division of the short gastric vessels.

Laparoscopic Treatment of Gastroesophageal Reflux Disease
Alexander HC, Hendler RS, Seymour NE, et al (Univ of Texas, Dallas)
Am Surg 63:434–440, 1997   68–6

Background.—The laparoscopic approach to surgery has made surgical treatment for gastroesophageal reflux disease (GERD) more acceptable to patients and health care providers alike. Multicenter trials have shown excellent results with open Nissen fundoplication, as long as certain operative principles are adhered to. The results in 59 patients with GERD managed by a standardized technique of laparoscopic Nissen fundoplication are presented.

Methods.—The patients were 35 men and 23 women, mean age 54, treated at 3 Dallas institutions. All patients had clinical evidence of GERD and continued to have mild to severe symptoms despite treatment with omeprazole. Eighty-four percent had heartburn, and 2% had laryngitis; 15% of patients could not tolerate or would not take omeprazole. The standardized technique emphasized a loose wrap to reduce the risk of postfundoplication dysphagia and gas bloating. Esophageal manometric studies were performed in all patients, and 24–hr pH studies in two thirds. Lower esophageal sphincter pressure was <15 mm Hg in 76% of patients. Five patients with esophageal body peristaltic pressures <35 mm Hg were managed by Toupét partial fundoplication; the rest underwent Nissen fundoplication. One-year follow-up data were available for 45 patients.

Results.—The operations lasted a mean of 158 min. Conversion to an open procedure was necessary in 5% of patients. The operative complication rate was 13%, but all complications were minor. In the follow-up group, 98% of patients had resolution of heartburn. Mild dysphagia was noted at 1 month in 70% of patients, and severe dysphagia in 19%. Most severe cases responded to nonoperative dilation, though 2 of 9 patients had continued symptoms of mild dysphagia. In 2 patients with severe dysphagia, the laparoscopic procedure was converted from Nissen to Toupét fundoplication, improving the symptoms considerably. Though 45% of patients had early symptoms of gas bloating, this rate decreased to 5% by 1 year.

Conclusions.—For patients with GERD, laparoscopic surgery is a safe and effective treatment for reflux symptoms. This study demonstrates very good results with a standardized technique of laparoscopic Nissen fundoplication. Mild dysphagia may occur postoperatively, but is usually transient. If dysphagia becomes severe, nonoperative dilation or laparoscopic partial fundoplication can be performed without interfering with the antireflux characteristics of the wrap.

▶ Interesting articles (Abstracts 68–4, 68–5, and 68–6) by Karim et al., Baigrie et al., and Alexander et al. all focus on the very important issue of, Can a total wrap, or 360-degree fundoplication, be safely performed in the setting of GERD and concomitant impairment of contraction amplitudes in the distal body of the esophagus and/or accompanying dysphagia, and can this partial wrap or very loose wrap, as the case may be, sustain an effective and competent antireflux barrier? The paper from Australia by Baigrie's group dealing with the outcome of laparoscopic Nissen fundoplication in patients with impaired preoperative peristalsis is indeed a surprising one, in that using a 52F bougie (171/3 mm in diameter), the authors reported that in an overall group of 345 patients studied prospectively, 31 patients actually underwent surgery where there was some impairment of peristalsis. While patients with impaired contraction amplitudes (in their hands, <25 mm Hg) may be candidates for surgery, it had been thought that when there is <50% of swallows being propagated, then outcome is not predictable and generally would militate against surgery. This group has a long history of expertise in this type of surgery, and this has to be considered when extrapolating these data to general practice and the average community hospital settings. The other 2 papers, i.e., those of Karim et. al. and Alexander et. al., may be a little more practical for the average laparoscopic surgeon addressing GERD. Here the concept of a Toupét fundoplication is addressed by Alexander, and the concept of a partial wrap (some patients had the 200-degree wrap or the Dor and the other patients had the Toupét or posterior 240-degree wrap). All the techniques gave a similar efficacy regarding improvement in heartburn and regurgitation. The total wraps gave a higher incidence of early dysphagia, but after 15 months there were no significant differences. The other paper by Alexander et al. showed that when contraction amplitudes are decreased to <35 mm Hg but are still peristaltic, then a partial fundoplication using the Toupét procedure seems to be better than the total wrap, and this could be particularly relevant to the average surgeon again who is not in a major academic center.

R.W. McCallum, M.D.

Choice of Long-term Strategy for the Management of Patients With Severe Esophagitis: A Cost-Utility Analysis

Heudebert GR, Marks R, Wilcox CM, et al (Univ of Alabama, Birmingham)
Gastroenterology 112:1078–1086, 1997   68–7

Objective.—Gastroesophageal reflux disease, which affects 10% of the population, progresses to erosive esophagitis in 40% of these patients. Proton pump inhibitors (PPIs), such as omeprazole, and fundoplication procedures have lowered morbidity, but have never been compared in a clinical trial. Using a decision analytic modeling technique, a cost-utility analysis was performed to determine which therapeutic approach is more efficacious, cost-effective, and safe, and what factors influence the choice of therapy.

Methods.—A Markov-cycle tree simulation model followed 10,000 patients for 5 years to compare laparoscopic Nissen fundoplication (LNF) vs. omeprazole for the management of patients with erosive esophagitis. The health state of patients was determined every 3 months for a total of 20 cycles. Transitional probabilities from 1 state to another were calculated from literature values or expert opinion. For each cycle, quality of life and cost for each patient were determined, accumulated, and discounted at 3% per year. Adjusted population-based mortality rates were obtained from published U.S. Vital Statistics. A 1-way sensitivity analysis was performed on appropriate variables.

Results.—The cost per patient was $6,043 for PPI and $9,426 for surgery. The number of quality-adjusted life years was 4.334 for LNF and 4.332 for PPI. The cost-effectiveness was $1,398 for PPI and $2,186 for LNF. When the time horizon was extended to 10 years, the cost per patient for the strategies was approximately equal, although the marginal cost-effectiveness of LNF was more than $300,000. Sensitivity analyses of efficacy for PPI did not significantly change the results. Effectiveness estimates were very sensitive to changes in quality of life.

Conclusion.—Surgical and PPI strategies for treatment of erosive esophagitis in gastroesophageal reflux disease are equally effective for most patients. Long-term effects on quality of life are an important consideration in making the initial decision, and cost is the most significant parameter in the model. Both aspects should be major factors in the design of any randomized clinical trial.

Long-term Comparison of Antireflux Surgery Versus Conservative Therapy for Reflux Esophagitis
Isolauri J, Luostarinen M, Viljakka M, et al (Univ of Tampere, Finland)
Ann Surg 225:295–299, 1997   68–8

Objective.—Endoscopic examination revealed that approximately 50% of patients with gastroesophageal reflux disease have erosive esophagitis. The course of endoscopically proven esophagitis treated surgically or conservatively and the possible predictive factors of long-term outcome were examined.

Methods.—Between 1982 and 1983, 120 patients (39 women), aged 36.1 to 82.5, with severe reflux symptoms and endoscopically proven erosive esophagitis, were treated with conservative management ($n = 81$) or antireflux surgery ($n = 37$) (Nissen fundoplication). Standardized interviews, conducted with 105 patients who were followed for 9.1–13.4 years, assessed symptoms, time of referral, and endoscopic observations.

Results.—Most of the 37 patients who had undergone the Nissen procedure without mortality or morbidity had failed conservative treatment within 6–14 months ($n = 31$). Six patients had failed conservative treatment within 19–78 months. At follow-up, 84% of surgically treated patients had mild or no heartburn, and 89% had no erosive esophagitis, whereas with conservatively treated patients, 53% were heartburn free and only 45% no longer had erosive esophagitis. Five percent of surgically treated patients were using deuterium antagonists or omeprazole, whereas 21% of conservatively treated patients used such drugs. The surgically treated group had a significantly greater change in symptom score than the conservatively treated group (5.7 vs. 1.7). At baseline, Barrett's metaplasia was diagnosed in 5 patients who later had surgery and in no patients treated conservatively. At follow-up, Barrett's metaplasia was diagnosed in 12 surgery patients and in 8 conservatively managed patients. Severity of esophagitis or presence of hiatal hernia at baseline was not a predictor of esophagitis or symptoms at follow-up.

Conclusion.—Surgery rather than conservative management yielded improved results for patients with gastroesophageal reflux disease. There were no significant predictors of outcome.

▶ Articles by Heudebert et al. (Abstract 68–7) and Isolauri et al. (Abstract 68–8) deal with the long-term comparison of antireflux surgery vs. conservative medical therapy in reflux esophagitis. Heudebert et al. from Birmingham show that certainly for the first 10 years a PPI therapy for gastroesophageal reflux disease was less expensive than a laparoscopic Nissen fundoplication. However, after 10 years the results were similar, indicating that in young patients and patients with a long life expectancy quality of life issues are important. In patients who cannot be tapered from a PPI after 10 years, surgery would be appropriate. In the other article from Finland by Isolauri et al., a standard Nissen fundoplication without a laparoscopic approach was used for 37 patients and the remaining 68 had medical therapy consisting of deuterium antagonists or omeprazole. Follow-up was for a median of 10.9 years and showed that the change in symptoms in the surgery group was significantly greater than in the medical therapy group. These articles should be compared to a recent study done by Dr. Stewart Spechler in the United States and published as an abstract in *Gastroenterology* in 1993, Volume 1 of 4, abstract A5, showing that a lifetime course of surgical treatment was more effective than medical management in men younger than 49 and women younger than 56. Both these articles are very important because the concerns of long-term PPI therapy relate not only to expense but also to the unknown, namely the effects of chronic atrophic gastritis, enterochromaffin-like (ECL) cell hyperplasia, and the concern about carcinoid and/or other cancers when lifetime therapy is being entertained. I personally believe that the laparoscopic role for surgery in patients, who cannot taper PPIs and more specifically require them every day, is going to become a major alternative. However, in many cases the PPI and/or prokinetic therapy that is being used on a long-term basis can be tapered or used intermittently when and if needed, for larger meals and other provocative events, and at that time an operation would not be appropriate. One must also remember that the informed consent for surgery does mention an 0.1% or even an .05% chance of death, and as far as we know at the present time, death is not likely to occur during chronic prokinetic and/or omeprazole therapy, at least as the current follow-up data stands.

R.W. McCallum, M.D.

Subject Index

A

Abciximab
before and during coronary intervention in refractory unstable angina, 201
Abdominal
abscess after ileocecal resection for Crohn's disease, 605
pain after cabergoline in prolactinoma, 271
Abscess
intraabdominal, after ileocecal resection for Crohn's disease, 605
Abuse
diuretic, longtime, causing premenopausal tophaceous gout, 487
Acarbose
in diabetes, type I, 342
Accidents
traffic, risk in patients with sleep-disordered breathing, 591
Achalasia
antibodies in, anti-myenteric neuronal, 655
botulinum toxin injection for, untoward effects of, 656
laparoscopic surgical treatment of, 654
Acid
-base, 439
status improvement and nutrition in patients on continuous ambulatory peritoneal dialysis, 435
reflux, role in gastroesophageal reflux, 664
Acquired immunodeficiency syndrome (see AIDS)
Acromegaly
lanreotide in, 3-year follow-up, 265
ACTH
low plasma, in adrenal incidentalomas, 275
Acyclovir
in herpes zoster, 34
in lymphoproliferative disorders, posttransplant T cell, 117
Addison's disease
new immunoprecipitation test for 21-hydroxylase autoantibodies in, 277
ADE
vs. DAT induction chemotherapy in acute myeloid leukemia, 97
Adenocarcinoma
antigen, potential anticancer vaccine KH-1, total synthesis of, 153

prevalence and incidence in patients with short segment Barrett's esophagus, 661
Adenoma
rectosigmoid, 5 mm or less in diameter, detected by sigmoidoscopy, importance of, 597
Adiposity
leptin and gender, 351
Adolescent
female, diabetes mellitus in, insulin-dependent, and eating disorders and microvascular complications, 335
hypereosinophilic syndrome and myocardial infarction in, 91
Adrenal(s), 275
hypothalamo-pituitary-adrenal axis, inhaled beclomethasone suppresses in dose dependent manner, 287
insufficiency
hydrocortisone replacement therapy in, optimal, 280
during megestrol therapy, 279
secondary, perioperative steroid requirements in, 283
mass, incidentally discovered, investigation and management of, 275
Adriamycin (see Doxorubicin)
Advance directives
attitudes of pulmonary rehabilitation patients toward, 534
African Americans (see Blacks)
Age
aortic valve disease and, calcific, 223
influence on outcome of autologous bone marrow transplant procedures for hematologic malignancies, 126
AIDS
(See also HIV)
candidiasis in, fluconazole-resistant, 22
cryptococcal infection in, low-dose fluconazole as primary prophylaxis for, 19
opportunistic infections, 19
retinitis in, cytomegalovirus, cidofovir for, 23, 24
Airway
pressure, continuous positive, nasal, in sleep-disordered breathing, effect on risk of traffic accidents, 591
Alcohol
consumption, moderate, and risk for angina pectoris or myocardial infarction, 163

Alendronate
in prevention of nonvertebral fractures, 319
Allergic
children, immunotherapy for asthma in, 544
Allopurinol
for intradermal urate tophi, 489
Amino acid
profile in patients on continuous ambulatory peritoneal dialysis, 434
Aminooxypentane
-RANTES, potent inhibition of HIV-1 infectivity in macrophages and lymphocytes by, 13
Amiodarone
effect on mortality in patients with left ventricular dysfunction after recent myocardial infarction, 241
Amoxicillin
in sinusitis, acute maxillary, 43
Ampullary
carcinoma, staging of, endosonography vs. surgery in, 599
Amyloidosis
primary, trial of three regimens for, 119
Androgen
excess, prostate-specific antigen in female serum as potential new marker of, 327
Anemia
aplastic, acquired, primary treatment of, 81
Fanconi's, and myelodysplasia, donor leukocyte infusions for relapse after allogeneic bone marrow transplantation in, 128
hemolytic, in Canale-Smith syndrome, 120
Angina
with aortic stenosis and normal coronary arteries, mechanisms and pathophysiological concepts of, 221
heparin in, low-molecular-weight vs. unfractionated, 173
postprandial, and exercise tolerance, 187
prognosis in, long-term, and serum cholesterol, in middle-aged men, 166
risk, and moderate alcohol consumption, 163
unstable, refractory, abciximab before and during coronary intervention in, 201
Angiodysplasias
small bowel, diagnostic efficacy of push-enteroscopy in, 602

Angiography
coronary, immediate, in survivors of out-of-hospital cardiac arrest, 200
CT
helical, in gastrointestinal bleeding of obscure origin, 601
spiral, validation in pulmonary embolism, 565
Angioplasty
coronary
in angina, refractory unstable, abciximab before and during, 201
volume-outcome relationships for hospitals and cardiologists, 199
vs. stenting for isolated stenosis of proximal left anterior descending coronary artery, 203
Angiotensin
-converting enzyme inhibitors, effect on progression of nondiabetic renal disease, 408
receptor, subtype 2, mediates renal production of nitric oxide (in rat), 421
Anion
production, glomerular superoxide, induced by lipoprotein(a) (in rat), 406
Annexin
V and pregnancy loss in antiphospholipid antibody syndrome, 468
Anorexia
nervosa and premenopausal tophaceous gout due to longtime diuretic abuse, 487
Anthrax
as biological warfare agent, clinical recognition and management of patients exposed to, 71
Antibiotics
combination, after exposure to brucellosis as biological warfare agent, 72
after infected pacemaker lead removal, 249
macrolide, after exposure to Q fever as biological warfare agent, 72
in sinusitis, acute maxillary, 43
Antibody(ies)
anti-DNA, peptide inhibition of glomerular deposition of, 365
anti-glutamic acid decarboxylase, in insulin-dependent diabetes with onset before and after age 40 years, 337
anti-myenteric neuronal, in achalasia, 655

antineutrophil cytoplasmic, in
  connective tissue disease, 472
antinuclear, in healthy individuals, range
  of, 474
antiphospholipid
  clinical associations of, 465
  syndrome, pregnancy loss in, 468
anti-tyrosine phosphatase, in
  insulin-dependent diabetes with
  onset before and after age 40 years,
  337
Chlamydia pneumoniae, and serum
  lipids, 68
islet cell, measurement in
  insulin-dependent diabetes with
  onset before and after age 40 years,
  337
therapy after exposure to viral
  hemorrhagic fevers as biological
  warfare agents, 76
Anticancer
  vaccine KH-1 adenocarcinoma antigen,
    potential, total synthesis of, 153
Anticoagulation
  low-dose, effect on saphenous vein
    coronary artery bypass graft
    obstructive changes, 192
  therapy
    oral, duration after second episode of
      venous thromboembolism, 563
    in prevention of thromboembolism in
      chronic atrial flutter, 233
Antidiuretic
  hormone, syndrome of inappropriate
    secretion of, OPC-31260 in, 272
Anti-DNA
  antibody, peptide inhibition of
    glomerular deposition of, 365
Antigen
  adenocarcinoma, potential anticancer
    vaccine KH-1, total synthesis of,
    153
  cytotoxin associated
    positive or negative *Helicobacter
      pylori* infection, risk of gastric
      cancer in people with, 639
    protein, expression by *Helicobacter
      pylori* strains in MALT-type gastric
      lymphoma, 636
  prostate-specific, in female serum, as
    potential new marker of androgen
    excess, 327
Anti-glutamic acid
  decarboxylase antibodies in
    insulin-dependent diabetes with
    onset before and after age 40 years,
    337

Antihypertensive
  drugs in elderly with isolated systolic
    hypertension, prevention of heart
    failure by, 208
  treatment-induced fall in glomerular
    filtration rate, short-term, predicts
    long-term stability of renal
    function, 417
Anti-inflammatory
  drugs, nonsteroidal, risk of acute renal
    failure with, 399
Antimicrobial
  prophylaxis prior to shock wave
    lithotripsy in patients with sterile
    urine before treatment, 396
Antineutrophil
  cytoplasmic antibodies in connective
    tissue disease, 472
Antinuclear
  antibodies in healthy individuals, range
    of, 474
Antiphospholipid
  antibody(ies)
    clinical associations of, 465
    syndrome, pregnancy loss in, 468
Antireflux
  surgery *vs.* conservative therapy for
    reflux esophagitis, long-term
    comparison of, 670
Antiretroviral
  therapy for HIV infection in 1997,
    updated recommendations of
    International AIDS Society–USA
    panel, 17
Antithrombotic
  therapy in congestive heart failure,
    effect on risk of sudden coronary
    death, 216
Anti-tyrosine phosphatase
  antibodies in insulin-dependent diabetes
    mellitus with onset before and after
    age 40 years, 337
Antroduodenal
  manometry, fasting, in children, 646
AOP-RANTES
  potent inhibition of HIV-1 infectivity in
    macrophages and lymphocytes by,
    13
Aortic
  arch atherosclerosis, vascular events
    during follow-up of, 247
  stenosis, normal coronary arteries, and
    angina, mechanisms and
    pathophysiological concepts of, 221
  valve disease, calcific, clinical factors
    associated with, 223

Apheresis
  of low-density lipoprotein, effect on
    peripheral vascular disease in
    hypercholesterolemic patients with
    coronary artery disease, 190
Aphthous
  ulcers, oral, in HIV patients,
    thalidomide for, 26
Aplastic
  anemia, acquired, primary treatment of,
    81
Apnea
  sleep, obstructive, and risk of traffic
    accidents, 591
Apoptosis
  in failing heart, 207
  resistance caused by *PIG-A* gene
    mutations in paroxysmal nocturnal
    hemoglobinuria, 82
Aquaporin-2
  water channel expression, upregulation
    in chronic heart failure (in rat), 440
Aquaresis
  acute, by OPC-31260 in syndrome of
    inappropriate secretion of
    antidiuretic hormone, 272
Arbutamine
  vs. exercise echocardiography in
    diagnosing myocardial ischemia,
    229
L-Arginine
  depletion in acute peritonitis in patients
    on continuous ambulatory
    peritoneal dialysis, 434
  vascular effects of, 419
Argyrophil
  cell hyperplasia, *Helicobacter pylori* as
    risk factor for, during lansoprazole
    treatment, 633
Arrhythmia, 233
  ventricular, implanted defibrillator in
    patients with coronary disease at
    high risk for, 243
Arteriolar
  sclerosis and myofibroblasts in diabetic
    nephropathy, 372
Arteritis
  temporal, color duplex ultrasound in
    diagnosis, 491
Artery
  coronary (*see* Coronary, artery)
  renal, stenosis, in patients with
    myocardial infarction, prevalence
    and predictors of, 390
Arthritis
  crystal-associated, 487
  infectious, 499

osteoarthritis of knee, and quadriceps
    weakness, 509
  reactive, 477
  rheumatoid, 451
    antineutrophil cytoplasmic antibodies
      in, 472
    corticosteroids in, low-dose, spinal
      bone loss secondary to, calcium
      and vitamin D₃ supplementation
      prevents, 452
    cyclosporine combined with
      methotrexate in, 451
    early, minocycline in, 460
    gamma-linolenic acid treatment of,
      458
    interferon-gamma in, 451
    irradiation in, total lymphoid, 456
    methotrexate in, lung injury due to,
      predictors of, 451
    tumor necrosis factor receptor
      (p75)-Fc fusion protein in,
      recombinant human, 462
Arthropathy
  chronic, persistence of parvovirus B19
    DNA in synovial membranes in,
    501
Aspiration
  biopsy, endoscopic ultrasound-guided
    fine-needle, using linear array and
    radial scanning endosonography,
    598
Aspirin
  inflammation and risk of cardiovascular
    disease, 169
  vs. clopidogrel in patients at risk of
    ischemic events, 196
Asthma, 543
  beclomethasone in, inhaled,
    hypothalamo-pituitary-adrenal axis
    suppressed in dose dependent
    manner by, 287
  in elderly, incidence and outcomes, 546
  exacerbation
    acute, changes in peak flow, symptom
      score, and use of medications
      during, 543
    during reduction of high-dose inhaled
      corticosteroid prevented by
      leukotriene antagonist, 549
  immunotherapy for, in allergic children,
    544
  mortality, stabilization of, 552
  salmeterol in, long-term, 547
Atelectasis
  after ileocecal resection for Crohn's
    disease, 605

Atenolol
-induced fall in glomerular filtration
rate, short-term, predicts long-term
stability of renal function, 417
in noncardiac surgery, effect on
mortality and cardiovascular
morbidity, 252
Atheroma
cardiovascular, specificity of detection of
Chlamydia pneumoniae in, 67
Atherosclerosis
aortic arch, vascular events during
follow-up of, 247
Atrial
fibrillation (*see* Fibrillation, atrial)
flutter, chronic, thromboembolism in,
233
natriuretic peptide levels after
radiocontrast exposure, 401
Atrioventricular
node, radiofrequency modification in
atrial fibrillation, long-term
follow-up, 238
Attitudes
regarding advance directives among
pulmonary rehabilitation patients,
534
Autoantibodies
21-hydroxylase, measurements with
new immunoprecipitation assay,
277
ribosomal P, in systemic lupus
erythematosus, 470
Autoimmune
manifestations of Canale-Smith
syndrome, 120
polyglandular syndrome type I and II,
new immunoprecipitation test for
21-hydroxylase autoantibodies in,
277
Azathioprine
in Behçet's syndrome, effect on
long-term prognosis, 493

B

B cell
abnormalities after total lymphoid
irradiation in rheumatoid arthritis,
457
lymphoma, polymorphic, in bone
marrow transplant recipients, 135
Babesia microti
infection simultaneous with *Borrelia
burgdorferi* infection, 507
Back
injuries, low, educational program to
prevent, 509

Bacteremia
microbiology, epidemiology, and
outcome of, 47
Bacterial
infections, 47, 581
pneumonia in HIV infection, 577
Balloon
mitral commissurotomy, percutaneous,
4-year follow-up, 224
Barbiturates
myocardial infarction risk with, 168
Barrett's esophagus
short segment, long-term endoscopic
and histological follow-up, 661
Bartter's syndrome
Gitelman's syndrome as variant of,
maps to thiazide-sensitive
cotransporter gene locus on
chromosome 16q13, 381
Beclomethasone
inhaled
high-dose, leukotriene antagonist
prevents exacerbation of asthma
during reduction of, 549
suppresses
hypothalamo-pituitary-adrenal axis
in dose dependent manner, 287
Behçet's syndrome
azathioprine in, effect on long-term
prognosis, 493
Benazepril
effect on progression of nondiabetic
renal disease, 410
Beta-adrenergic
antagonists in prevention of
gastrointestinal rebleeding in
cirrhotics, 617
Bilitec 2000
in gastroesophageal reflux disease, 665
Biologic
terrorism and warfare, 71
warfare agents, clinical recognition and
management of patients exposed
to, 71
Biopsy
aspiration, endoscopic
ultrasound-guided fine-needle, using
linear array and radial scanning
endosonography, 598
Blacks
asthma death rates in, 552
glomerulonephritis in, immune complex,
and coinfection with HIV and
hepatitis C virus, 369
nephrosclerosis in, hypertensive,
accuracy of diagnosis, 415

Bleeding (*see* Hemorrhage)
Bleomycin
in MACOP-B regimen in diffuse
large-cell lymphoma, late relapse
with, 113
in MOPP-ABVD regimen, primary, in
Hodgkin's disease, outcome of
patients after failing, 118
in ProMACE-CytaBOM regimen in
aggressive non-Hodgkin's
lymphoma, 110
Blood
cell
progenitor, peripheral, transplantation
with, with high-dose chemotherapy,
and treatment-related mortality,
123
red, 81
white (*see* White cell)
cord
stem cells from, extensive
amplification and self-renewal of,
132
transplantation from related and
unrelated donors, outcome of, 130
cultures, positive, clinical significance in
1990s, 47
peripheral, micrometastases in,
detection in breast cancer patients
with immunohistochemistry and
reverse transcriptase polymerase
chain reaction for keratin 19, 141
pressure, increased, and thrombolytic
therapy in myocardial infarction,
176
Bone, 305, 443
density
in elderly, effect of calcium and
vitamin D supplementation on, 317
in postmenopausal women, effect of
hormone replacement therapy on,
312
loss
in older women not associated with
low thyrotropin levels, 300
spinal, corticosteroid-induced, in
rheumatoid arthritis, calcium and
vitamin D_3 supplementation
prevents, 452
marrow
micrometastases in, detection in
breast cancer patients with
immunohistochemistry and reverse
transcriptase polymerase chain
reaction for keratin 19, 141
transplantation (*see* Transplantation,
bone marrow)

mass after 8 years of hormonal
replacement therapy, 315
Borrelia burgdorferi
infection and reinfection,
culture-confirmed, 499
Borreliosis
Lyme (*see* Lyme disease)
Botulinum
toxin(s)
as biological warfare agents, clinical
recognition and management of
patients exposed to, 76
injection for achalasia, untoward
effects of, 656
Bovine
spongiform encephalopathy causing new
variant Creutzfeldt-Jakob disease,
39
Bowel
disease, inflammatory, 605
small, angiodysplasias, diagnostic
efficacy of push-enteroscopy in,
602
Brain
serotonin neurotoxicity from
fenfluramine and dexfenfluramine,
568
Brca2
mice lacking, embryonic lethality and
radiation hypersensitivity mediated
by Rad51 in, 152
Breast
cancer (*see* Cancer, breast)
carcinoma (*see* Cancer, breast)
-preserving surgery
for ductal carcinoma in situ, national
trends for, 142
for early-stage cancer, routine
radiotherapy after, patient
preferences concerning trade-off
between risks and benefits of, 153
Breath
-hold MR cholangiopancreatography, in
vitro and clinical studies of image
acquisition in, 600
test, [^{13}C]octanoic acid, for gastric
emptying of solids, 644
Breathing
sleep-disordered, and risk of traffic
accidents, 591
spontaneous, effect on duration of
mechanical ventilation in
identifying patients capable of, 587
Bromocriptine
in acromegaly, 266
in hyperprolactinemia in
postmenopausal women, 268

vs. cabergoline in women with microprolactinomas or idiopathic hyperprolactinemia, 271

Bronchitis
acute, in HIV infection, 577

Bronchogenic
carcinoma, changing radiographic presentation with reference to cell types, 523

Brucellosis
as biological warfare agent, clinical recognition and management of patients exposed to, 71

Brush
method, endoluminal, for diagnosis of catheter-related sepsis, 56

Bupropion
sustained-release, for smoking cessation, 518

Bursitis
proximal, in active polymyalgia rheumatica, 454

Bypass
coronary artery
prediction of ventricular function improvement after, FDG SPECT *vs.* dobutamine echocardiography in, 227
saphenous vein, obstructive changes in grafts, effect of low-density lipoprotein cholesterol lowering and low-dose anticoagulation on, 192
survival after, effect of estrogen replacement therapy on, 204

C

Cabergoline
in prolactinoma, 269
vs. bromocriptine in women with microprolactinomas or idiopathic hyperprolactinemia, 271

CagA
positive or negative people with *Helicobacter pylori* infection, risk for gastric cancer in, 639
protein, *Helicobacter pylori* strains expressing, in MALT-type gastric lymphoma, 636

Cajal
interstitial cells of
mediation of inhibitory neurotransmission of stomach by (in mice), 643
role in control of gut motility, 641

Calcaneus
ultrasound of bone predicts fractures in older women, 311

Calcific
aortic valve disease, clinical factors associated with, 223

Calcitonin
serum, interest in routine measurement of, 302

Calcium, 443
antagonist felodipine added to enalapril therapy in chronic heart failure, 214
commissural, echocardiographic assessment of, 230
intake, dietary
kidney stones and, in women, 444
optimal, in primary hyperparathyroidism, 307
-receptor agonist in primary hyperparathyroidism, short-term inhibition of parathyroid hormone secretion by, 309
supplementation
effect on bone density in elderly, 317
kidney stones and, in women, 444
in prevention of bone loss in spine secondary to low-dose corticosteroids in rheumatoid arthritis, 452

Canale-Smith syndrome
Fas gene mutations in, 120

Cancer, 141
breast
ductal in situ, national treatment trends for, 142
early-stage, patient preferences concerning trade-off between risks and benefits of routine radiation therapy after conservative surgery for, 153
megestrol in, and adrenal insufficiency, 279
metastatic, double dose-intensive chemotherapy with autologous stem cell support for, 145
micrometastases in peripheral blood and bone marrow in, detection with immunohistochemistry and reverse transcriptase polymerase chain reaction for keratin 19, 141
patients with negative nodes and estrogen receptor-positive tumors, tamoxifen in, 5 *vs.* more than 5 years of, 143

centers, community, treatment-related mortality in patients receiving high-dose chemotherapy and peripheral blood progenitor cell transplantation in, 123
colorectal, prognosis, and DCC protein, 149
gastric, risk in people with CagA positive or negative *Helicobacter pylori* infection, 639
hematologic
  advanced, allogeneic peripheral blood stem cell *vs.* marrow transplantation in, 129
  bone marrow transplantation in, autologous, influence of age on outcome, 126
hereditary, risk notification and testing, 151
lung, 523
  peripheral, screening and detection with low-dose spiral CT *vs.* radiography, 524
  small cell, dose-intense therapy with etoposide, ifosfamide, cisplatin, and epirubicin in, 148
ovarian, high-dose chemotherapy with hematopoietic rescue in, long-term results, 146
patients, thrombopoietin in, single-dose recombinant human, effect on megakaryocyte and platelet production, 87
relapsed, after allogeneic bone marrow transplantation, donor leukocyte infusions in, 127
solid, after bone marrow transplantation, 134
susceptibility testing, informed consent for, 151
Candida
  albicans, fluconazole-resistant, in HIV patients, 20
  infection, fluconazole-resistant, in AIDS, 22
Candidiasis
  mucosal, in HIV-infected women, weekly fluconazole for prevention of, 21
  oropharyngeal, in HIV patients, detection and significance of fluconazole resistance in, 20
Captopril
  effect on progression of nondiabetic renal disease, 410
  vs. losartan in heart failure, in elderly, 212

Carbohydrate
  high-carbohydrate meal and angina, 187
  metabolism, 335
Carbon-13
  octanoic acid breath test for gastric emptying of solids, 644
Carboplatin
  in dose-intense therapy for small cell lung cancer, 148
  melphalan after
    with autologous stem cell support for metastatic breast cancer, 145
    high-dose, with hematopoietic rescue in ovarian cancer, 146
Carcinoma
  ampullary, staging of, endosonography *vs.* surgery in, 599
  breast (*see* Cancer, breast)
  bronchogenic, changing radiographic presentation with reference to cell types, 523
  pancreatic, staging of, endosonography *vs.* surgery in, 599
  thyroid, medullary, serum calcitonin measurement in detection of, 302
Cardia
  gastric, intestinal metaplasia of, 662
Cardiologists
  coronary angioplasty volume-outcome relationships for, 199
Cardiomyopathy, 207
  hypertrophic, dual-chamber pacing for, 255
Cardiovascular
  atheroma, specificity of detection of *Chlamydia pneumoniae* in, 67
  disease
    Chlamydia pneumoniae and, 67
    risk, and inflammation and aspirin, 169
  morbidity after noncardiac surgery, effect of atenolol on, 252
  testing, noninvasive, 227
Cardioversion
  in atrial fibrillation lasting less than 48 hours, and risk for clinical thromboembolism, 234
  guided by transesophageal echocardiography, 236
Carditis
  in rheumatic fever, acute, in adults, 511
Care
  intensive care medicine, 585
  patient, in community teaching hospital, effects of medical intensivist on, 585

β-Carotene
supplements, effect on incidence of major coronary events in men with previous myocardial infarction, 194
Carvedilol
in heart failure due to ischemic heart disease, 209
in myocardial infarction, 177
Catheter
infection, triple-lumen, diagnosis of, 50
-related sepsis, diagnosis with endoluminal brush method, 56
CCR5
antagonist, novel, potent inhibition of HIV-1 infectivity in macrophages and lymphocytes by, 13
CD4
counts, low, as predictor for *Pneumocystis carinii* pneumonia in HIV infection, 579
CD4+
T cells, CD28 costimulation of, differential regulation of HIV-1 fusion cofactor expression by, 12
CD28
costimulation of CD4+ T cells, differential regulation of HIV-1 fusion cofactor expression by, 12
Cefaclor
in sinusitis, acute paranasal, in children, 42
Cefepime
for *Enterobacter* infections, multiply resistant, 55
Ceftriaxone
vs. doxycycline for acute disseminated Lyme disease, 505
Cell(s)
argyrophil, hyperplasia, *Helicobacter pylori* as risk factor for, during lansoprazole treatment, 633
B
abnormalities after total lymphoid irradiation in rheumatoid arthritis, 457
lymphoma, polymorphic, in bone marrow transplant recipients, 135
blood (*see* Blood, cell)
interstitial cells of Cajal
mediation of inhibitory neurotransmission of stomach by (in mice), 643
role in control of gut motility, 641
islet cell antibody measurement in insulin-dependent diabetes with onset before and after age 40 years, 337

mesangial, exposed to high glucose concentrations, effect of enalaprilat on hydrogen peroxide production by (in mice), 388
polarity, intercalated, in vitro plasticity of, role of hensin in, 439
red, 81
stem
from cord blood, extensive amplification and self-renewal of, 132
transplantation (*see* Transplantation, stem cell)
T
CD28 costimulation of, differential regulation of HIV-1 fusion cofactor expression by, 12
lymphoproliferative disorders, posttransplant, 116
Cellular
telephones, interference with pacemakers by, 254
Central nervous system
viral infections of, diagnosis, 36
Cerebral
activity, regional, and visceral pain, 651
Chemotherapy
of breast cancer, metastatic, double dose-intensive chemo with autologous stem cell support, 145
high-dose, with peripheral blood progenitor cell transplantation, and treatment-related mortality, 123
in Hodgkin's disease, primary MOPP-ABVD regimen, outcome of patients after failing, 118
induction with DAT *vs.* ADE in acute myeloid leukemia, 97
of lung cancer, small cell, with dose-intense therapy with etoposide, ifosfamide, cisplatin, and epirubicin, 148
of lymphoma
diffuse large-cell, MACOP-B regimen, late relapse in, 113
non-Hodgkin's, aggressive, CHOP *vs.* ProMACE-CytaBOM regimen, 110
non-Hodgkin's, aggressive, in elderly, CVP *vs.* CTVP regimen, 114
non-Hodgkin's, aggressive, poor-risk, sequential chemo *vs.* autologous marrow transplantation, 111
of lymphoproliferative disorders, posttransplant T cell, 117
of ovarian cancer, high-dose chemo with hematopoietic rescue, 146

Chemstrips
  combined with sulfosalicylic acid testing
    for microalbuminuria, 412
Chest
  radiography in coccidioidomycosis in
    HIV infection, 26
Children
  adolescent
    female, diabetes mellitus in,
      insulin-dependent, and eating
      disorders and microvascular
      complications, 335
    hypereosinophilic syndrome and
      myocardial infarction in, 91
  allergic, immunotherapy for asthma in,
    544
  antroduodenal manometry in, fasting,
    646
  interferon-gamma receptor gene
    mutation and susceptibility to
    mycobacterial infection in, 6
  leukemia in, acute myeloid, DAT vs.
    ADE as induction chemotherapy in,
    97
  parvovirus B19 DNA persistence in
    synovial membranes of, in patients
    with and without chronic
    arthropathy, 501
  Salmonella Marina infection in, and
    iguanas, 62
  sinusitis in, acute paranasal, ten-day
    mark as practical diagnostic
    approach for, in children, 42
  Streptococcus pneumoniae in,
    drug-resistant, 581
Chills
  in coccidioidomycosis in HIV infection,
    26
Chlamydia pneumoniae
  antibodies and serum lipids, 68
  in cardiovascular atheroma, specificity
    of detection of, 67
  cardiovascular disease and, 67
  as new source of infectious outbreaks in
    nursing homes, 45
Chloramphenicol
  after exposure to plague as biological
    warfare agent, 72
2-Chlorodeoxyadenosine
  in lymphoma, follicular, previously
    untreated, 108
Chlorthalidone
  in prevention of heart failure in elderly
    with isolated systolic hypertension,
    208
Cholangiopancreatography
  breath-hold MR, in vitro and clinical
    studies of image acquisition in, 600

Cholesterol
  low-density lipoprotein (see
    Lipoprotein, low-density)
  -lowering therapy as primary prevention
    against first myocardial infarction,
    167
  reduction, effect on myocardial ischemia
    in coronary disease, 188
  serum, long-term prognosis in
    middle-aged men with myocardial
    infarction and angina and, 166
CHOP regimen
  vs. ProMACE-CytaBOM regimen in
    aggressive non-Hodgkin's
    lymphoma, 110
Chromosome
  5q35, NPT2 gene localized to, 446
  9q34, identification of tuberous sclerosis
    gene TSC1 on, 395
  16q13, Gitelman's syndrome maps to
    thiazide-sensitive cotransporter
    gene locus on, 381
Cidofovir
  for cytomegalovirus retinitis in AIDS,
    23, 24
Cigarette
  smoking (see Smoking)
Cilazapril
  effect on progression of nondiabetic
    renal disease, 410
Ciprofloxacin
  IV, after exposure to anthrax as
    biological warfare agent, 71
Cirrhosis
  gastrointestinal rebleeding in,
    beta-adrenergic antagonists in
    prevention of, 617
  variceal bleeding in, primary
    prophylaxis of, 618
  variceal pressure, size, and wall tension
    in, total volume paracentesis
    decreases, 620
Cisplatin
  in dose-intense therapy for small cell
    lung cancer, 148
Clopidogrel
  vs. aspirin in patients at risk of ischemic
    events, 196
Clothing
  insulin injection through, safety of, 341
Coagulase
  -negative staphylococci causing
    bacteremia, 49
Coccidioidomycosis
  in HIV infection, 25
Colchicine
  in amyloidosis, primary, 119

Colitis
  ulcerative
    active, mildly to moderately,
      transdermal nicotine for, 607
    neoplastic transformation of pelvic
      pouch mucosa in, 606
    remission maintenance in, zileuton *vs.*
      mesalazine in, 608
Collagen
  type I, N-telopeptide of, urinary
    excretion, therapeutic response of
    hormone replacement therapy in
    postmenopausal women monitored
    by, 312
  type III, urinary and serum, as markers
    of renal fibrosis, 410
Colony stimulating factor
  granulocyte-, in diabetic foot infections,
    349
Colorectal
  cancer prognosis and DCC protein, 149
Commissural
  calcium, echocardiographic assessment,
    as predictor of outcome after
    percutaneous mitral balloon
    valvotomy, 230
Commissurotomy
  mitral, percutaneous balloon, 4-year
    follow-up, 224
Computed tomography
  angiography
    helical, in gastrointestinal bleeding of
      obscure origin, 601
    spiral, validation in pulmonary
      embolism, 565
  in lung disease, diffuse, diagnostic
    accuracy of, 557
  lung nodule enhancement at, 525
  single-photon emission, FDG, *vs.*
    dobutamine echocardiography in
    prediction of ventricular function
    improvement after
    revascularization, 227
  spinal, low-dose, *vs.* radiography in
    screening and detection of
    peripheral lung cancer, 524
Connective tissue
  disease, antineutrophil cytoplasmic
    antibodies in, 472
Consent
  informed, for cancer susceptibility
    testing, 151
Constipation
  chronic, is work-up worth the cost? 658
COPD (*see* Lung, disease, chronic
    obstructive)
Cord
  blood

    stem cells from, extensive
      amplification and self-renewal of,
      132
    transplantation from related and
      unrelated donors, outcome of, 130
Coronary
  angiography, immediate, in survivors of
    out-of-hospital cardiac arrest, 200
  angioplasty (*see* Angioplasty, coronary)
  artery
    bypass (*see* Bypass, coronary artery)
    descending, proximal left anterior,
      isolated stenosis of, coronary artery
      stenting *vs.* angioplasty for, 203
    disease (*see below*)
    normal, with angina and aortic
      stenosis, mechanisms and
      pathophysiological concepts of, 221
    stenting *vs.* angioplasty for isolated
      stenosis of proximal left anterior
      descending coronary artery, 203
  artery disease
    (*See also* Heart, disease, coronary)
    chronic, 185
    in hypercholesterolemia patients,
      effect of apheresis of low-density
      lipoprotein on peripheral vascular
      disease in, 190
    myocardial ischemia in, effect of
      cholesterol reduction on, 188
    risk factors for, 163
    stable, myocardial ischemia in, silent
      vs. symptomatic exercise-induced,
      clinical implications of, 185
    unstable, heparin in,
      low-molecular-weight *vs.*
      unfractionated heparin, 173
  death, sudden, risk in congestive heart
    failure, effect of antithrombotic
    therapy on, 216
  events, major, incidence in men with
    previous myocardial infarction,
    effect of α-tocopherol and
    β-carotene supplements on, 194
  heart disease (*see* Heart, disease,
    coronary)
  intervention
    in angina, refractory unstable,
      abciximab before and during, 201
    procedures, 199
  revascularization, prediction of
    ventricular function improvement
    after, FDG SPECT *vs.* dobutamine
    echocardiography in, 227
  syndromes, acute, 173

Corticosteroid(s)
-induced bone loss in spine in
rheumatoid arthritis, calcium and
vitamin D_3 supplementation
prevents, 452
-induced osteoporosis, prevention with
intermittent etidronate, 320
inhaled high-dose, leukotriene
antagonist prevents exacerbation of
asthma during reduction of, 549
in nephropathy, adult-onset
minimal-change, 367
in severe illness, 509
therapy
in COPD, adverse effects of, 535
in sarcoidosis, and relapse, 559
Corticotropin
low plasma, in adrenal incidentalomas,
275
-releasing hormone, lack of ACTH
response to, in adrenal
incidentalomas, 275
Cortisol
hypersecretion in adrenal
incidentalomas, 275
Cost
-effective analysis of antimicrobial
prophylaxis prior to shock wave
lithotripsy in patients with sterile
urine before treatment, 396
-effectiveness
of antibiotic therapy, oral *vs.* IV, for
acute disseminated Lyme disease,
506
of prophylaxis of variceal bleeding in
cirrhosis, primary, 618
of treating nicotine dependence, 517
of streptokinase *vs.* urokinase in
complicated parapneumonic
effusions, 584
-utility analysis of long-term
management strategy in severe
esophagitis, 669
of work-up for chronic constipation,
658
Cough
in *Chlamydia pneumoniae* infection in
nursing homes, 46
in coccidioidomycosis in HIV infection,
26
CPAP
nasal, in sleep-disordered breathing,
effect on risk of traffic accidents,
591
Crackles
inspiratory, in idiopathic pulmonary
fibrosis, 555

C-reactive protein
aspirin and risk of cardiovascular
disease and, 169
Creutzfeldt-Jakob disease
new variant, due to bovine spongiform
encephalopathy, 39
Crohn's disease
ileocecal resection for, long-term
outcome, 605
Cryptococcal
infection in AIDS, low-dose fluconazole
as primary prophylaxis for, 19
Crystal
-associated arthritis, 487
Crystalluria
indinavir-associated, 392
CT (*see* Computed tomography)
CTVP regimen
in lymphoma, aggressive
non-Hodgkin's, in elderly, 114
Culture
blood, positive, clinical significance in
1990s, 47
-confirmed infection and reinfection
with *Borrelia burgdorferi*, 499
Cushing's disease
irradiation in, pituitary, after
unsuccessful transsphenoidal
surgery, long-term outcome, 285
Cutaneous
carriage of *Staphylococcus aureus* in
hemodialysis patients, 52
CVP regimen
in lymphoma, aggressive
non-Hodgkin's, in elderly, 114
Cyclophosphamide
in CHOP *vs.* ProMACE-CytaBOM
regimen in aggressive
non-Hodgkin's lymphoma, 110
in CVP *vs.* CTVP regimen in aggressive
non-Hodgkin's lymphoma, in
elderly, 114
in MACOP-B regimen in diffuse
large-cell lymphoma, late relapse
with, 113
melphalan after
high-dose, with hematopoietic rescue
in ovarian cancer, 146
with stem cell support for metastatic
breast cancer, autologous, 145
in nephropathy, adult-onset
minimal-change, 367
Cyclosporiasis
outbreak associated with imported
raspberries in 1996, 59
Cyclosporine
in lupus erythematosus, systemic,
long-term treatment, 465

/methotrexate in rheumatoid arthritis,
451
Cyst
renal, and endothelin-1 (in mice), 387
Cystic
fibrosis, prognostic model for prediction
of survival in, 536
Cytarabine
in ADE *vs.* DAT induction
chemotherapy in acute myeloid
leukemia, 97
/interferon alfa-2b in chronic
myelogenous leukemia, 101
in ProMACE-CytaBOM regimen in
aggressive non-Hodgkin's
lymphoma, 110
Cytomegalovirus
infection, severe, in immunocompetent
patients, 38
retinitis in AIDS, cidofovir for, 23, 24
Cytoplasmic
antibodies, antineutrophil, in connective
tissue disease, 472
Cytotoxin
-associated antigen
positive or negative *Helicobacter
pylori* infection, risk of gastric
cancer in people with, 639
protein expressed by *Helicobacter
pylori* strains in MALT-type gastric
lymphoma, 636
gene, vacuolating, of *Helicobacter
pylori,* heterogeneity in, clinical and
pathological importance of, 637

D

Dacarbazine
in MOPP-ABVD regimen, primary, in
Hodgkin's disease, outcome of
patients after failing, 118
Dactylitis
toe, in spondyloarthropathy, 479
Dalteparin
vs. unfractionated heparin in unstable
coronary artery disease, 173
DAT
vs. ADE induction chemotherapy in
acute myeloid leukemia, 97
Daunorubicin
in ADE *vs.* DAT induction
chemotherapy in acute myeloid
leukemia, 97
DCC protein
prognosis in colorectal cancer and, 149
Death
(*See also* Mortality)

causes of, in families with factor V
mutation, 90
coronary, sudden, risk in congestive
heart failure, effect of
antithrombotic therapy on, 216
sudden, in severe heart failure, and
nonsustained ventricular
tachycardia, 239
Debridement
for *Staphylococcus aureus* prosthetic
joint infection, 54
Defibrillator
implanted, in patients with coronary
disease at high risk for ventricular
arrhythmia, 243
Dengue
fever in U.S. military personnel in Haiti,
31
Depression
psychotropic medication in, and risk of
myocardial infarction, 167
Development
megakaryocyte growth and development
factor, pegylated recombinant
human, effect on functional platelet
production, 85
Dexamethasone
suppressibility in adrenal
incidentalomas, 275
Dexfenfluramine
brain serotonin neurotoxicity and
primary pulmonary hypertension
from, 568
Diabetes mellitus, 335
corticosteroid therapy in COPD and,
535
foot infections in, granulocyte-colony
stimulating factor for, 349
insulin-dependent
acarbose in, 342
eating disorders and microvascular
complications in, in young women,
335
insulin-analog treatment of, effect on
postprandial hyperglycemia and
frequency of hypoglycemia, 339
islet transplantation in, 343
in normotensives with
microalbuminuria, lisinopril in, 344
onset before and after age 40, genetic
and immunological features of, 337
nephropathy in
myofibroblasts and arteriolar sclerosis
in, 372
progression of renal disease in, effect
of angiotensin-converting enzyme
inhibitors on, 410
non–insulin-dependent

estrogen replacement therapy and, postmenopausal, 347
leptin concentration in, plasma, and gender, 353
renal production of transforming growth factor-β1 increased in, 373
ovarian hyperthecosis and hirsutism in postmenopausal women, 329
type I (*see* insulin-dependent *above*)
type II (*see* non–insulin-dependent *above*)
Diagnostic
testing in digestive disorders, 597
Dialysis, 429
peritoneal, continuous ambulatory amino acid profile and nitric oxide pathway in patients on, 434
role of improvement in acid-base status and nutrition in patients on, 435
Diarrhea
after ceftriaxone in acute disseminated Lyme disease, 506
after clopidogrel in prevention of ischemic events, 197
Escherichia coli O157:H7, clinical and epidemiologic features, in U.S., 60
Dicumarol
therapy, duration after second episode of venous thromboembolism, 563
Diet
cholesterol-lowering, effect on myocardial ischemia in coronary disease, 188
Digestive
disorders, diagnostic testing in, 597
Digoxin
withdrawal, worsening of mild heart failure during, 213
Directives
advance, attitudes of pulmonary rehabilitation patients toward, 534
Disease
mechanisms of, 5
Diuretic
abuse, longtime, causing premenopausal tophaceous gout, 487
use, chronic, and internal urate tophi, 489
Dizziness
after cabergoline in prolactinoma, 271
DNA
anti-DNA antibody, peptide inhibition of glomerular deposition of, 365
parvovirus B19, persistence in synovial membranes of young patients with and without chronic arthropathy, 501

Dobutamine
echocardiography *vs.* FDG SPECT in prediction of ventricular function improvement after revascularization, 227
Doxorubicin
in CHOP *vs.* ProMACE-CytaBOM regimen in aggressive non-Hodgkin's lymphoma, 110
in MACOP-B regimen in diffuse large-cell lymphoma, late relapse with, 113
in MOPP-ABVD regimen, primary, in Hodgkin's disease, outcome of patients after failing, 118
Doxycycline
in Lyme borreliosis simultaneous with granulocytic ehrlichiosis, 507
vs. ceftriaxone for acute disseminated Lyme disease, 505
Drug(s)
antihypertensive, in elderly with isolated systolic hypertension, prevention of heart failure by, 208
anti-inflammatory, nonsteroidal, risk of acute renal failure with, 399
psychotropic, for depression, and risk of myocardial infarction, 167
-resistant *Streptococcus pneumoniae*, continued emergence in U.S., 581
use during acute exacerbations of asthma, changes in, 543
users, IV, and immune complex glomerulonephritis and coinfection with HIV and hepatitis C virus, in blacks, 369
Duodenal
gastroduodenal lesions related to *Helicobacter pylori* infection in spouses of patients with duodenal ulcer, prevalence of, 635
ulcer (*see* Ulcer, duodenal)
Duodenogastroesophageal
reflux, role in gastroesophageal reflux, 664
Dyspepsia
patients, *Helicobacter pylori*-seropositive, management of, 629
Dysphagia
after fundoplication, laparoscopic Nissen, 668
Dysplasia
prevalence and incidence in patients with short segment Barrett's esophagus, 661

Dysrhythmias
gastric slow wave, in motion sickness, role of plasma vasopressin as mediator of, 647

E

Eating
disorders and microvascular complications in young women with insulin-dependent diabetes, 335
Echocardiography
arbutamine *vs.* exercise, in diagnosing myocardial ischemia, 229
in assessment of commissural calcium, 230
dobutamine, *vs.* FDG SPECT in prediction of ventricular function improvement after revascularization, 227
transesophageal, cardioversion guided by, 236
Economic
consequences of management strategies for *Helicobacter pylori*-seropositive patients with dyspepsia, 629
Educational
program to prevent low back injuries, 509
Effusions
pleural
malignant, thoracoscopic talc poudrage pleurodesis for, 529
parapneumonic, complicated, streptokinase *vs.* urokinase in, 583
Ehrlichiosis
granulocytic, simultaneous with Lyme borreliosis, 507
Elastase
neutrophil, in crescentic glomerulonephritis, 377
Elderly
aortic valve disease in, calcific, clinical factors associated with, 223
asthma in, incidence and outcomes, 546
bone density in, effect of calcium and vitamin D supplementation on, 317
bone loss in, no association with low thyrotropin levels, in women, 300
COPD in, outcomes after acute exacerbation, 531
fracture occurrence in, broadband ultrasound attenuation predicts, in women, 311
heart disease in, coronary, and serum lipids, 164

heart failure in, losartan *vs.* captopril in, 212
hypertension in, isolated systolic, prevention of heart failure by antihypertensive drug treatment in, 208
hypothyroidism in, subclinical, effect of L-thyroxine on health status in, 297
lymphoma in, aggressive non-Hodgkin's, 114
myocardial infarction outcome in, and specialty of admitting physician, 183
pseudogout in, intramuscular triamcinolone acetonide in, 489
Electrocoagulation
in bowel angiodysplasias, small, long-term follow-up, 602
Electrogastrography
for effects of IV vasopressin on gastric myoelectrical activity, 649
for gastric myoelectrical impairment in chronic renal failure, 650
Electrolytes, 439
Emboli
pleural, 563
Embolism
pulmonary
thrombolytic therapy and prognosis in hemodynamically stable patients with, 566
validation of spiral CT angiography in, 565
thromboembolism (*see* Thromboembolism)
Embryonic
lethality and radiation hypersensitivity mediated by Rad51 in mice lacking *Brca2,* 152
Emphysema
lung volume reduction surgery in (*see* Lung, volume reduction surgery in emphysema)
Empyema
pleural, streptokinase *vs.* urokinase in, 583
after thoracoscopic talc poudrage pleurodesis for malignant effusions, 529
Enalapril
effect on progression of nondiabetic renal disease, 410
with felodipine in chronic heart failure, 214
-induced fall in glomerular filtration rate, short-term, predicts long-term stability of renal function, 417

Enalaprilat
  inhibits hydrogen peroxide production
    by mesangial cells exposed to high
    glucose concentrations (in mice),
    388
Encephalitides
  viral, as biological warfare agents,
    clinical recognition and
    management of patients exposed
    to, 76
Encephalopathy
  bovine spongiform, causing new variant
    Creutzfeldt-Jakob disease, 39
  liver, risk with transjugular intrahepatic
    portosystemic shunts, 625
Endocarditis
  on pacemaker leads, systemic infection
    related to, 248
Endoluminal
  brush method for diagnosis of
    catheter-related sepsis, 56
Endoscopic
  follow-up of short segment Barrett's
    esophagus, long-term, 661
  sclerotherapy vs. transjugular
    intrahepatic portosystemic shunt
    after initial sclerotherapy in acute
    variceal hemorrhage, 627
  for prevention of variceal rebleeding,
    625
  treatment plus propranolol vs.
    transjugular intrahepatic
    portosystemic shunt for prevention
    of variceal rebleeding, 624
  ultrasound (see Ultrasound, endoscopic)
  variceal ligation for esophageal varices,
    622
Endosonography
  linear array and radial scanning,
    endoscopic ultrasound-guided
    fine-needle aspiration biopsy using,
    598
  vs. surgery in staging of ampullary and
    pancreatic carcinoma, 599
Endothelin
  levels after radiocontrast exposure, 401
  production, renal, in type II diabetes,
    373
Endothelin-1
  glomerulosclerosis, interstitial fibrosis,
    and renal cysts and (in mice), 387
Energy
  expenditure, leptin, and gender, 351
Enterobacter
  infections, multiply resistant, cefepime
    for, 55
Enterococcus
  bacteremia due to, 49

Enteroscopy
  push-, diagnostic efficacy in small bowel
    angiodysplasias, 602
Enterotoxin
  B, staphylococcal, as biological warfare
    agent, clinical recognition and
    management of patients exposed
    to, 76
Enterovirus
  infection of central nervous system,
    diagnosis of, 36
Enzyme
  inhibitors, angiotensin-converting, effect
    on progression of nondiabetic renal
    disease, 408
Epidermal
  growth factor-like growth factor,
    heparin-binding, production in
    early phase of regeneration after
    acute renal injury (in rat), 400
Epirubicin
  in dose-intense therapy for small cell
    lung cancer, 148
Epstein-Barr virus
  infection of central nervous system,
    diagnosis of, 36
Erythromycin
  -resistant *Streptococcus pneumoniae*,
    continued emergence in U.S., 581
Escherichia coli
  bacteremia due to, 49
  O157:H7 diarrhea, clinical and
    epidemiologic features, in U.S., 60
Esophagitis
  reflux
    curing *Helicobacter pylori* infection in
      duodenal ulcer may provoke, 631
    therapy for, conservative, long-term
      comparison with antireflux surgery,
      670
    severe, choice of long-term management
      strategy, 669
Esophagomyotomy
  laparoscopic, for achalasia, 654
Esophagus
  Barrett's, short segment, long-term
    endoscopic and histological
    follow-up, 661
  botulinum toxin injection for achalasia,
    untoward effects of, 656
  gastroesophageal reflux (see Reflux,
    gastroesophageal)
  motility disorders and psychiatric
    disease, 652
  ulcer after botulinum toxin injection in
    achalasia, 656
  varices (see Varices)

Estrogen
-progestin *vs.* simvastatin for
hypercholesterolemia in
postmenopausal women, 355
receptor-positive breast cancer, 5 *vs.*
more than 5 years of tamoxifen
therapy for, 143
replacement therapy
effect on survival after coronary
artery bypass, 204
postmenopausal (*see* Hormone,
replacement therapy,
postmenopausal)
Ethambutol
in tuberculosis with and without HIV
infection, in 6-month supervised
intermittent therapy, in Haitians,
575
Ethnicity
ribosomal P autoantibodies in systemic
lupus erythematosus and, 470
Etidronate
intermittent, in prevention of
corticosteroid-induced osteoporosis,
320
Etoposide
in dose-intense therapy for small cell
lung cancer, 148
in induction chemotherapy regimen in
acute myeloid leukemia, 97
in ProMACE-CytaBOM regimen *vs.*
CHOP regimen in aggressive
non-Hodgkin's lymphoma, 110
Euthanasia
physician desire for, 155
Exercise
capacity, effect of long-term
levothyroxine on, 299
-induced myocardial ischemia,
symptomatic *vs.* silent, clinical
implications in stable coronary
disease, 185
responses, effect of rhinovirus-caused
upper respiratory illness on, 41
tolerance and postprandial angina, 187
vs. arbutamine echocardiography in
diagnosing myocardial ischemia,
229
Expiratory
flow, peak, changes during acute
exacerbations of asthma, 543

F

Factor
V

gene mutation causing activated
protein C resistance in chronic
venous leg ulcers, 88
Leiden mutation, mortality and
causes of death in families with, 90
Fanconi's anemia
myelodysplasia and, donor leukocyte
infusions for relapse after
allogeneic bone marrow
transplantation in, 128
Fas
gene mutations in Canale-Smith
syndrome, 120
Fat
high-fat meal and angina, 187
FDG
SPECT *vs.* dobutamine
echocardiography in prediction of
ventricular function improvement
after revascularization, 227
Felodipine
with enalapril in chronic heart failure,
214
Fenfluramine
brain serotonin neurotoxicity and
primary pulmonary hypertension
from, 568
-phentermine associated with valvular
heart disease, 569
Fever
in *Chlamydia pneumoniae* infection in
nursing homes, 46
in coccidioidomycosis in HIV infection,
26
dengue, in U.S. military personnel in
Haiti, 31
/gastroenteritis outbreak due to *Listeria
monocytogenes* in milk, 64
inhibition by virus, mechanism for, 8
Q, as biological warfare agent, clinical
recognition and management of
patients exposed to, 72
rheumatic, acute, in adults, 511
after thoracoscopic talc poudrage
pleurodesis for malignant effusions,
529
viral hemorrhagic, as biological warfare
agent, clinical recognition and
management of patients exposed
to, 76
Fibrillation
atrial
cardioversion in, transesophageal
echocardiography-guided, 236
lasting less than 48 hours, conversion
to sinus rhythm in, and risk of
clinical thromboembolism, 234

radiofrequency modification of
atrioventricular node in, long-term
follow-up, 238
ventricular, in-hospital, effect on
prognosis after myocardial
infarction, 178
Fibromyalgia
syndrome, overdiagnosis of, 477
Fibrosis
cystic, prognostic model for prediction
of survival in, 536
interstitial, and endothelin-1 (in mice),
387
portal, non-cirrhotic, increased
incidence of glomerulonephritis
after spleno-renal shunt surgery in,
375
pulmonary, idiopathic
pulmonary function tests in, 556
smoking as risk factor for, 555
renal, urinary and serum type III
collagen as markers of, 410
Filgrastim
in diabetic foot infection, 349
FK-506
rescue therapy for renal allograft
rejection, 425
Fluconazole
low-dose, as primary prophylaxis for
cryptococcal infection in AIDS, 19
resistance in oropharyngeal candidiasis
in HIV patients, detection and
significance of, 20
-resistant *Candida* infection in AIDS, 22
weekly, for prevention of mucosal
candidiasis in HIV-infected women,
21
Fludarabine
in leukemia, refractory chronic
lymphocytic, 98
in lymphoma, low-grade follicular, 99
Fluorine-18
FDG SPECT *vs.* dobutamine
echocardiography in prediction of
ventricular function improvement
after revascularization, 227
Fluorodeoxyglucose
SPECT *vs.* dobutamine
echocardiography in prediction of
ventricular function improvement
after revascularization, 227
Flushing
method of diagnosis of triple-lumen
catheter infection, 50
Flutter
atrial, chronic, thromboembolism in,
233

Follicular
lymphoma (*see* Lymphoma, follicular)
Foot
infections, diabetic, granulocyte-colony
stimulating factor in, 349
Foscarnet
in cytomegalovirus infection in
immunocompetent patients, 38
Fracture
nonvertebral, prevention by
alendronate, 319
occurrence in older women, broadband
ultrasound attenuation predicts,
311
Friction
rub, palpable tendon, in systemic
sclerosis, 483
Fundoplication
laparoscopic
Nissen, in esophagitis, severe,
cost-utility analysis of, 669
Nissen, in gastroesophageal reflux
disease, 668
Nissen, outcome in patients with
disordered preoperative peristalsis,
667
total *vs.* partial, 666
Nissen, in reflux esophagitis, long-term
comparison with conservative
therapy, 670
Fungal
infections, 47
Fungemia
microbiology, epidemiology, and
outcome of, 47
Fusion protein
tumor necrosis factor receptor (p75)-Fc,
recombinant human, in rheumatoid
arthritis, 462

G

Gamma-linolenic acid
treatment of rheumatoid arthritis, 458
Ganciclovir
in cytomegalovirus infection in
immunocompetent patients, 38
Gastric
(*See also* Gastrointestinal; Stomach)
cardia, intestinal metaplasia of, 662
emptying of solids, [^{13}C]octanoic acid
breath test for, 644
lymphoma, MALT-type, *Helicobacter
pylori* strains expressing CagA
protein in, 636
mucosa during treatment with
lansoprazole, 633
myoelectrical activity

effect of IV vasopressin on, 649
impairment in chronic renal failure, 650
slow wave dysrhythmias in motion sickness, role of plasma vasopressin as mediator of, 647
Gastroduodenal
lesions related to *Helicobacter pylori* infection in spouses of patients with duodenal ulcer, prevalence of, 635
Gastroenteritis
/fever outbreak due to *Listeria monocytogenes* in milk, 64
Gastroesophageal
reflux (*see* Reflux, gastroesophageal)
Gastrointestinal
(*See also* Gastric; Stomach)
bleeding of obscure origin, helical CT angiography in, 601
discomfort, upper, after clopidogrel in prevention of ischemic events, 197
hemorrhage after clopidogrel in prevention of ischemic events, 197
infections, 59
masses, biopsy of, endoscopic ultrasound-guided fine-needle aspiration, 598
motility, 641
rebleeding in cirrhotics, beta-adrenergic antagonists in prevention of, 617
symptoms after long-term cyclosporin A in systemic lupus erythematosus, 467
Gender
cystic fibrosis survival and, 537
differences in relation of leptin to adiposity, insulin sensitivity, and energy expenditure, 351
male, and calcific aortic valve disease, 223
Gene(s)
Brca2, mice lacking, embryonic lethality and radiation hypersensitivity mediated by Rad51 in, 152
cytotoxin, vacuolating, of *Helicobacter pylori,* heterogeneity in, clinical and pathological importance of, 637
factor V
Leiden, mutation, mortality and causes of death in families with, 90
mutation, causing activated protein C resistance in chronic venous leg ulcers, 88
Fas, mutations in Canale-Smith syndrome, 120

HSV-TK, transfer into donor lymphocytes for control of allogeneic graft-*vs.*-leukemia, 137
interferon-gamma receptor, mutation, and susceptibility to mycobacterial infection, 6
locus, thiazide-sensitive, on chromosome 16q13, Gitelman's syndrome maps to, 381
NPT2, localization to chromosome 5q35, 446
patterns, rRNA, and *Helicobacter pylori* infection in spouses of patients with duodenal ulcers, 634
PIG-A, mutations in paroxysmal nocturnal hemoglobinuria causing resistance to apoptosis, 82
products of PKD1 and PKD2, homo- and heterodimeric interactions between, 394
therapy, 123
in vivo, complete short-term correction of hemophilia A by, 138
TSC1, identification on chromosome 9q34, 395
Genetic
features in patients with onset of insulin-dependent diabetes before and after age 40 years, 337
Genital
herpes simplex virus 2 shedding, frequent, in immunocompetent women, 32
Gentamicin
after exposure to plague as biological warfare agent, 72
after exposure to tularemia as biological warfare agent, 72
Gingival
hyperplasia after long-term cyclosporin A in systemic lupus erythematosus, 467
Gitelman's syndrome
maps to thiazide-sensitive cotransporter gene locus on chromosome 16q13, 381
Globulin
immune (*see* Immunoglobulin)
Glomerular
basement membrane nephropathy, thin, and hypertension and late onset renal failure, 370
deposition of anti-DNA antibody, peptide inhibition of, 365
disease, 363

filtration rate, short-term
    antihypertensive treatment-induced
    fall in, predicts long-term stability
    of renal function, 417
    superoxide anion production induced by
    lipoprotein(a) (in rat), 406
Glomerulonephritis
    crescentic, neutrophil elastase in, 377
    immune complex, in patients coinfected
    with HIV and hepatitis C virus,
    368
    increased incidence after spleno-renal
    shunt surgery in non-cirrhotic
    portal fibrosis, 375
Glomerulosclerosis
    endothelin-1 and (in mice), 387
Glucose
    concentrations, high, mesangial cells
    exposed to, enalaprilat inhibits
    hydrogen peroxide production by
    (in mice), 388
    homeostasis in postmenopausal women
    with non–insulin-dependent
    diabetes, effect of estrogen
    replacement therapy on, 347
    tolerance, impaired, plasma leptin
    concentration in, and gender, 353
Glutamic acid
    decarboxylase antibodies in
    insulin-dependent diabetes mellitus
    with onset before and after age 40
    years, 337
Glycoprotein
    Tamm-Horsfall, localization of single
    binding site for immunoglobulin
    light chains on, 382
Gold
    miners, silica-exposed, end-stage renal
    disease among, 384
Gout
    tophaceous, premenopausal, due to
    longtime diuretic abuse, 487
Graft
    -vs.-leukemia, HSV-TK gene transfer
    into donor lymphocytes for control
    of, 137
Gram's stain
    sputum, in community-acquired
    pneumococcal pneumonia, 44
Granulocyte
    -colony stimulating factor in diabetic
    foot infection, 349
Granulocytic
    ehrlichiosis simultaneous with Lyme
    borreliosis, 507
Growth
    factor

epidermal growth factor-like growth
    factor, heparin-binding, production
    in early phase of regeneration after
    acute renal injury (in rat), 400
    megakaryocyte growth and
    development factor, pegylated
    recombinant human, effect on
    production of functional platelets,
    85
    transforming growth factor-β1
    production, renal, increase in type
    II diabetes, 373
    hormone, recombinant human, effects
    on muscle protein turnover in
    malnourished hemodialysis
    patients, 431
Guatemalan raspberries
    1996 cyclosporiasis outbreak associated
    with, 59
Guideline
    practice, reducing length of stay for
    patients hospitalized with
    exacerbation of COPD, 533

H

Haiti
    dengue fever in U.S. military personnel
    in, 31
Health
    effects of HTLV-I, 37
    status in middle-aged and older adults
    with subclinical hypothyroidism,
    effect of L-thyroxine on, 297
Heart
    arrest, out-of-hospital, immediate
    coronary angiography in survivors
    of, 200
    disease
    coronary (See also Coronary, artery
    disease)
    coronary, implanted defibrillator in
    patients at high risk for ventricular
    arrhythmia with, 243
    coronary, incidence, and serum lipids,
    in elderly, 164
    ischemic, causing heart failure,
    carvedilol in, 209
    valvular, 221
    valvular, associated with
    fenfluramine-phentermine, 569
    failing, apoptosis in, 207
    failure, 207
    chronic, enalapril with felodipine in,
    214
    chronic, upregulation of aquaporin-2
    water channel expression in (in
    rat), 440

congestive, antithrombotic therapy in, effect on risk of sudden coronary death, 216
ischemic heart disease causing, carvedilol in, 209
losartan *vs.* captopril in, in elderly, 212
mild, worsening during digoxin withdrawal, 213
prevention by antihypertensive drugs in elderly with isolated systolic hypertension, 208
severe, nonsustained ventricular tachycardia in, 239
reserve, effect of long-term levothyroxine on, 299
transplantation in patients over 54 years of age, 217
Helicobacter pylori, 629
gene, vacuolating cytotoxin, heterogeneity in, clinical and pathological importance of, 637
infection
in duodenal ulcer, curing may provoke reflux esophagitis, 631
intestinal metaplasia of gastric cardia and, 663
in spouses of patients with duodenal ulcer, and ribosomal RNA gene patterns, 634
in spouses of patients with duodenal ulcer, prevalence of, 635
as risk factor for argyrophil cell hyperplasia during lansoprazole treatment, 633
-seropositive patients with dyspepsia, management of, 629
strains expressing CagA protein in MALT-type gastric lymphoma, 636
Hematemesis
after botulinum toxin injection in achalasia, 656
Hematologic
malignancies
advanced, allogeneic peripheral blood stem cell *vs.* marrow transplantation in, 129
bone marrow transplantation in, autologous, influence of age on outcome, 126
Hematopoietic
rescue after high-dose chemotherapy in ovarian cancer, long-term results, 146
Hemodialysis
dose and patient mortality, 429
patients
leptin in, elevated plasma, 432

malnourished, effects of recombinant human growth hormone on muscle protein turnover in, 431
nasal and cutaneous carriage of *Staphylococcus aureus* in, 52
Hemoglobinuria
paroxysmal nocturnal, resistance to apoptosis caused by *PIG-A* mutations in, 82
Hemolytic
anemia in Canale-Smith syndrome, 120
Hemophilia
A, complete short-term correction by in vivo gene therapy (in dog), 138
Hemorrhage
gastrointestinal
after clopidogrel in prevention of ischemic events, 197
of obscure origin, helical CT angiography in, 601
intracranial, after clopidogrel in prevention of ischemic events, 197
repeat (*see* Rebleeding)
after thrombolytic therapy in pulmonary embolism, 567
variceal (*see under* Variceal)
Hemorrhagic
fevers, viral, as biological warfare agents, clinical recognition and management of patients exposed to, 76
Hemostasis, 81
Hensin
role in in vitro plasticity of intercalated cell polarity, 439
Heparin
-binding epidermal growth factor-like growth factor production in early phase of regeneration after acute renal injury (in rat), 400
low-molecular-weight
in stroke, ischemic, 175
in venoembolic disease, 175
vs. unfractionated, in unstable coronary artery disease, 173
Hepatic (*see* Liver)
Hepatitis, 611
B
immunoglobulin, fixed dosing schedule, as prophylaxis in liver transplant recipients, 611
transmission to patients from four infected surgeons without hepatitis B e antigen, 30
C

chronic, effect of hepatitis G virus
infection on severity of liver disease
and response to interferon-α in
patients with, 29
chronic, ribavirin plus interferon alfa
in, long-term efficacy of, 612
virus co-infection with hepatitis G
virus in liver transplant recipients,
615
virus co-infection with HIV, and
immune complex
glomerulonephritis, 368
G virus
in bone marrow transplant recipients
and patients treated for acute
leukemia, 139
co-infection in liver transplant
recipients with chronic hepatitis C
and nonviral chronic liver disease,
615
infection, effect on severity of liver
disease and response to
interferon-α in chronic hepatitis C
patients, 29
infection, role in acute non-A–E
hepatitis, 613
infection, transfusion-associated,
incidence and relation to liver
disease, 614
non-A–E, acute, role of hepatitis G
virus infection in, 613
Hepatology, 611
Hepatomegaly
poor survival in cystic fibrosis and, 537
Hepatosplenomegaly
in Canale-Smith syndrome, 120
Hereditary
cancer risk notification and testing, 151
Herpes
simplex virus
infection of central nervous system,
diagnosis of, 36
thymidine kinase gene transfer into
donor lymphocytes for control of
graft-vs.-leukemia, 138
type 2 shedding, frequent genital, in
immunocompetent women, 32
zoster, acyclovir in, 34
Heterodimeric
interactions between gene products of
PKD1 and PKD2, 394
Hirsutism
ovarian hyperthecosis and diabetes in
postmenopausal women, 329
Histologic
features of lymphoproliferative
disorders in bone marrow
transplant recipients, 135

follow-up of short segment Barrett's
esophagus, long-term, 661
HIV, 9, 577
(See also AIDS)
infection
antiretroviral therapy for, in 1977,
updated recommendations of
International AIDS Society–USA
panel, 17
aphthous ulcers in, oral, thalidomide
for, 26
candidiasis in, mucosal, weekly
fluconazole for prevention of, in
women, 21
candidiasis in, oropharyngeal,
fluconazole resistance in, detection
and significance of, 20
coccidioidomycosis in, 25
hepatitis C virus coinfection and, and
immune complex
glomerulonephritis, 368
indinavir in, crystalluria and urinary
tract abnormalities associated with,
392
interleukin-2 therapy in, controlled
trial of, 14
interleukin-2 therapy in, daily low
dose, 14
pneumonia in, *Pneumocystis carinii*,
predictors of, 578
respiratory disease trends in
pulmonary complications of, 577
tuberculosis and, 6-month supervised
intermittent therapy in, in Haitians,
575
tuberculosis and, 575
type 1
concentration reduction in semen
after urethritis treatment, 11
disease, acute, as mononucleosis-like
illness, 9
fusion cofactor expression by CD28
costimulation of CD4+ T cells,
differential regulation of, 12
infected compartments, decay
characteristics during combination
therapy, 16
infectivity in macrophages and
lymphocytes, potent inhibition by
novel CCR5 antagonist, 13
Hoarseness
in *Chlamydia pneumoniae* infection in
nursing homes, 46
Hodgkin's disease
bone marrow transplantation in
allogeneic, donor leukocyte infusions
for relapse after, 128

autologous, influence of age on
outcome of, 126
chemotherapy failure in, primary
MOPP-ABVD, outcome after, 118
Home
nursing, *Chlamydia pneumoniae* as new
source of infectious outbreaks in,
45
Homeless
rifampin preventive therapy for
tuberculosis in, 572
Homocysteinemia
vascular disease in end-stage renal
disease and, 405
Homodimeric
interactions between gene products of
PKD1 and PKD2, 394
Hormone
antidiuretic, syndrome of inappropriate
secretion of, OPC-31260 in, 272
corticotropin-releasing, lack of ACTH
response to, in adrenal
incidentalomas, 275
growth, recombinant human, effects on
muscle protein turnover in
malnourished hemodialysis
patients, 431
parathyroid, short-term secretion
inhibition by calcium-receptor
agonist in primary
hyperparathyroidism, 309
replacement therapy, postmenopausal
in diabetics, non–insulin-dependent,
347
effects on bone mass after 8 years of,
315
therapeutic response monitored by
urinary excretion of N-telopeptide,
312
women's beliefs and decisions about,
328
therapy of small bowel angiodysplasias,
long-term follow-up, 602
Hospital(s)
coronary angioplasty volume-outcome
relationships for, 199
length of stay for exacerbation of
COPD, reduction using practice
guideline, 533
teaching, community, effects of medical
intensivist on patient care in, 585
HSV-TK
gene transfer into donor lymphocytes
for control of allogeneic
graft-*vs.*-leukemia, 137
HTLV-I
health effects of, 37

Human immunodeficiency virus (*see* HIV)
Hydration
IV, with cidofovir for cytomegalovirus
retinitis in AIDS, 23, 24
Hydrocortisone
replacement therapy, optimal,
assessment of, 280
Hydrogen
peroxide production by mesangial cells
exposed to high glucose
concentrations, effect of enalaprilat
on (in mice), 388
Hydroxychloroquine
retinopathy, rarity of, 451
21-Hydroxylase
autoantibodies, measurements with new
immunoprecipitation assay, 277
Hyperandrogenicity
effect of estrogen replacement therapy
on, in postmenopausal women with
non–insulin-dependent diabetes,
347
Hypercholesterolemia
patients with coronary artery disease,
effect of apheresis of low-density
lipoprotein on peripheral vascular
disease in, 190
in postmenopausal women,
estrogen-progestin *vs.* simvastatin
for, 355
Hypereosinophilic
syndrome and myocardial infarction in
15-year-old, 91
Hyperglycemia
postprandial, in insulin-dependent
diabetics, effect of insulin-analog
treatment on, 339
Hyperostosis
skeletal, diffuse idiopathic, clinical
features of, 481
Hyperparathyroidism
primary
calcium intake in, optimal dietary,
307
calcium-receptor agonist in,
short-term inhibition of
parathyroid hormone secretion by,
309
rise and fall of, 305
Hyperplasia
argyrophil cell, *Helicobacter pylori* as
risk factor for, during lansoprazole
treatment, 633
gingival, after long-term cyclosporin A
in systemic lupus erythematosus,
467

Hyperprolactinemia
  idiopathic, cabergoline *vs.*
    bromocriptine in, in women, 271
  in postmenopausal women, 267
Hypertension, 415
  aortic valve disease and, calcific, 223
  after cyclosporin A in systemic lupus
    erythematosus, long-term, 467
  lead-induced, effect of lazaroid therapy
    on altered nitric oxide metabolism
    and increased oxygen free radical
    activity in (in rat), 423
  nephropathy and, thin glomerular
    basement membrane, 370
  nephrosclerosis due to, accuracy of
    diagnosis in African Americans,
    415
  portal, after transjugular intrahepatic
    portosystemic shunts, natural
    history of, 623
  pulmonary, primary, from fenfluramine
    and dexfenfluramine, 568
  -related symptoms in incidentally
    discovered pheochromocytoma,
    290
  systolic, isolated, prevention of heart
    failure by antihypertensive drugs in,
    in elderly, 208
  tophi and, intradermal urate, 489
Hyperthecosis
  ovarian, and diabetes and hirsutism in
    postmenopausal women, 329
Hypertrichosis
  after cyclosporin A in systemic lupus
    erythematosus, long-term, 467
Hypertrophic
  cardiomyopathy, dual-chamber pacing
    for, 255
Hypoglycemia
  in insulin-dependent diabetics, effect of
    insulin-analog treatment on
    frequency of, 339
Hypogonadism
  hypogonadotropic, adult-onset, 331
Hypogonadotropic
  hypogonadism, adult-onset, 331
Hyponatremia
  in SIADH improved with OPC-31260,
    272
Hypotension
  postural, after cabergoline in
    prolactinoma, 271
Hypothalamo
  -pituitary-adrenal axis, inhaled
    beclomethasone suppresses in dose
    dependent manner, 287

Hypothyroid
  tissue, estimation by new clinical score,
    293
Hypothyroidism
  levothyroxine products in,
    bioequivalence of generic and
    brand-name, 295
  subclinical, effect of L-thyroxine on
    health status in middle-aged and
    older adults with, 297

I

Ibuprofen
  in sepsis, effects on physiology and
    patient survival, 5
Idarubicin
  with all-*trans* retinoic acid in
    PML/RARα-positive acute
    promyelocytic leukemia, 95
Ifosfamide
  in dose-intense therapy for small cell
    lung cancer, 148
Iguanas
  Salmonella Marina infection in children
    and, 62
Ileocecal
  resection for Crohn's disease, long-term
    outcome, 605
Ileus
  prolonged, after ileocecal resection for
    Crohn's disease, 605
Illness
  severe, corticosteroids in, 509
Image
  acquisition in breath-hold MR
    cholangiopancreatography, in vitro
    and clinical studies of, 600
Imaging
  magnetic resonance
    of bursitis, proximal, in active
      polymyalgia rheumatica, 454
    of toe dactylitis in
      spondyloarthropathy, 479
Immune
  complex glomerulonephritis in patients
    coinfected with HIV and hepatitis
    C virus, 368
  globulin (*see* Immunoglobulin)
Immunobiologic
  features of lymphoproliferative
    disorders in bone marrow
    transplant recipients, 135
Immunoblastic
  lymphoma, malignant, in bone marrow
    transplant recipients, 135

Immunocompetent
  patients, severe cytomegalovirus
    infection in, 38
  women, frequent genital herpes simplex
    virus 2 shedding in, 32
Immunodeficiency
  syndrome, acquired (*see* AIDS)
  virus, human (*see* HIV)
Immunogenetic
  analysis of relapsing polychondritis, 496
  associations of ribosomal P
    autoantibodies in systemic lupus
    erythematosus, 470
Immunoglobulin
  A nephropathy, predicting renal
    outcome in, 363
  hepatitis B, fixed dosing schedule, as
    prophylaxis in liver transplant
    recipients, 611
  IV, high-dose, and response to
    splenectomy in idiopathic
    thrombocytopenic purpura, 84
  light chains, localization of single
    binding site on Tamm-Horsfall
    glycoprotein, 382
Immunohistochemistry
  detection of micrometastases in
    peripheral blood and bone marrow
    of breast cancer patients with, 141
Immunologic
  features in patients with onset of
    insulin-dependent diabetes before
    and after age 40 years, 337
Immunoprecipitation
  assay, new, for 21-hydroxylase
    autoantibodies, 277
Immunosuppressive therapy
  in anemia, acquired aplastic, outcomes
    of, 81
Immunotherapy
  for asthma in allergic children, 544
Incidentaloma
  adrenal, investigation and management
    of, 275
  thyroid, 260
Indinavir
  crystalluria and urinary tract
    abnormalities associated with, 392
Infarction
  myocardial (*see* Myocardial, infarction)
Infection
  foot, diabetic, granulocyte-colony
    stimulating factor in, 349
  systemic, related to endocarditis on
    pacemaker leads, 248
Infectious
  arthritis, 499

outbreaks in nursing homes, *Chlamydia
    pneumoniae* as new source of, 45
Inflammation
  aspirin and risk of cardiovascular
    disease, 169
Inflammatory
  bowel disease, 605
  myositis, antineutrophil cytoplasmic
    antibodies in, 472
Informed consent
  for cancer susceptibility testing, 151
Injection
  insulin, through-clothing, safety of, 341
Injuries
  back, low, educational program to
    prevent, 509
Inspiratory
  crackles in idiopathic pulmonary
    fibrosis, 555
Insulin
  -analog treatment, effect on
    postprandial hyperglycemia and
    frequency of hypoglycemia in
    insulin-dependent diabetics, 339
  -dependent diabetes mellitus (*see*
    Diabetes mellitus,
    insulin-dependent)
  endogenous, and vascular effects of
    L-arginine, 419
  injection through clothing, safety of,
    341
  insensitivity, leptin, and gender, 351
Intensive care
  medicine, 585
Intensivist
  medical, effects on patient care in
    community teaching hospital, 585
Intercalated
  cell polarity, in vitro plasticity of, role
    of hensin in, 439
Interferon
  alfa
    in hepatitis C, chronic, effect of
      hepatitis G virus infection on, 29
    in lymphoma, low-tumor-burden
      follicular, 107
    ribavirin with, in chronic hepatitis C,
      long-term efficacy of, 612
  alfa-2b with cytarabine *vs.* interferon
    alone in chronic myelogenous
    leukemia, 101
  gamma
    receptor gene mutation and
      susceptibility to mycobacterial
      infection, 6
    in rheumatoid arthritis, 451
Interleukin
  -2 therapy in HIV infection

controlled trial of, 14
daily low dose, 14
International AIDS Society–USA panel
updated recommendations for
antiretroviral therapy for HIV
infection in 1997, 17
Interstitial cells of Cajal
mediation of inhibitory
neurotransmission of stomach by
(in mice), 643
role in control of gut motility, 641
Intestinal
(*See also* Gastrointestinal)
metaplasia of gastric cardia, 662
Intraabdominal
abscess after ileocecal resection for
Crohn's disease, 605
Intracranial
hemorrhage after clopidogrel in
prevention of ischemic events, 197
Intradermal
urate tophi, 487
Intrahepatic
portosystemic shunt, transjugular (*see*
Shunt, portosystemic, transjugular
intrahepatic)
Irradiation (*see* Radiation)
Ischemia
myocardial (*see* Myocardial, ischemia)
Ischemic
events, clopidogrel *vs.* aspirin in
patients at risk of, 196
heart disease causing heart failure,
carvedilol in, 209
stroke, low-molecular weight heparin
in, 175
Islet
cell antibody measurement in
insulin-dependent diabetes with
onset before and after age 40 years,
337
transplantation in insulin-dependent
diabetics, 343
Isoniazid
in tuberculosis with and without HIV
infection, in 6-month supervised
intermittent therapy, in Haitians,
575

J

Joint
prosthetic, *Staphylococcus aureus*
infection, treatment with
debridement and prosthesis
retention, 54
Juvenile
(*See also* Children)

leukemia, myelogenous, donor
leukocyte infusions for relapse after
allogeneic bone marrow
transplantation in, 128

K

Keratin 19
polymerase chain reaction for, reverse
transcriptase, detection of
micrometastases in peripheral
blood and bone marrow of breast
cancer patients with, 141
Ketoconazole
after pituitary irradiation in Cushing's
disease, 286
Ketorolac
parenteral, risk for acute renal failure
with, 399
KH-1
adenocarcinoma antigen, potential
anticancer vaccine, total synthesis
of, 153
Kidney
(*See also* Renal)
collecting duct protein hensin, role in in
vitro plasticity of intercalated cell
polarity, 439
cysts and endothelin-1 (in mice), 387
disease, 381
end-stage, among silica-exposed gold
miners, 384
end-stage, due to renal artery
stenosis, 392
end-stage, homocysteinemia and
vascular disease in, 405
nondiabetic, progression of, effect of
angiotensin-converting enzyme
inhibitors on, 408
polycystic, gene products of PKD1
and PKD2, homo- and
heterodimeric interactions between,
394
failure
acute, 399
acute, risk with parenteral ketorolac,
399
chronic, 405
chronic, gastric myoelectrical activity
impairment in, 650
late onset, and thin glomerular
basement membrane nephropathy,
370
function, long-term stability of,
short-term antihypertensive
treatment-induced fall in
glomerular filtration rate predicts,
417

insufficiency and intradermal urate
tophi, 489
role in clearing leptin from circulation,
432
stones in women, and calcium intake,
444
transplantation (*see* Transplantation,
kidney)
Klebsiella pneumoniae
bacteremia due to, 49
Knee
osteoarthritis, and quadriceps weakness,
509

L

Laboratory
evaluation in Lyme disease diagnosis,
499
Lamivudine
with nelfinavir and zidovudine, decay
characteristics of HIV-1–infected
compartments during, 16
Lanreotide
in acromegaly, 3-year follow-up, 265
Lansoprazole
treatment, gastric mucosa during, 633
Laparoscopic
fundoplication (*see* Fundoplication,
laparoscopic)
surgical treatment of achalasia, 654
Lead
-induced hypertension, effect of lazaroid
therapy on altered nitric oxide
metabolism and increased oxygen
free radical activity in (in rat), 423
Leads
pacemaker, systemic infection related to
endocarditis on, 248
Leg
ulcers, chronic venous, activated protein
C resistance due to factor V gene
mutation in, 88
Length of stay
for exacerbation of COPD, reduction
using practice guideline, 533
Leptin
concentration, plasma, sexual
dimorphism in, 353
metabolic significance of, 351
plasma, partly cleared by kidney and
elevated in hemodialysis patients,
432
Leukemia, 95
acute, treatment, hepatitis G virus after,
139

bone marrow transplantation in,
allogeneic, with donors other than
HLA-identical siblings, results of,
124
graft-*vs.*-leukemia, HSV-TK gene
transfer into donor lymphocytes for
control of, 137
lymphoblastic, acute, allogeneic bone
marrow transplantation in, donor
leukocyte infusions for relapse
after, 128
lymphocytic, chronic
bone marrow transplantation in,
allogeneic, donor leukocyte
infusions for relapse after, 128
refractory, fludarabine in, 98
splenectomy in, 100
myelogenous
acute, bone marrow transplantation
in, allogeneic, donor leukocyte
infusions for relapse after, 128
acute, bone marrow transplantation
in, autologous, influence of age on
outcome of, 126
chronic, bone marrow transplantation
in, allogeneic, donor leukocyte
infusions for relapse after, 128
chronic, interferon alfa-2b combined
with cytarabine *vs.* interferon alone
in, 101
juvenile, bone marrow
transplantation in, allogeneic,
donor leukocyte infusions for
relapse after, 128
myeloid, acute, induction chemotherapy
in, DAT *vs.* ADE as, 97
promyelocytic, PML/RARα-positive
acute, all-*trans* retinoic acid and
idarubicin in, 95
Leukocyte (*see* White cell)
Leukotriene
antagonist prevents exacerbation of
asthma during reduction of
high-dose inhaled corticosteroid,
549
Levothyroxine
effect on health status in middle-aged
and older adults with subclinical
hypothyroidism, 297
long-term, effect on cardiac reserve and
exercise capacity, 299
products in hypothyroidism treatment,
bioequivalence of generic and
brand-name, 295
Levoxine
bioequivalence with generic
levothyroxine products, 296

Levoxyl
  bioequivalence with generic
    levothyroxine products, 296
Lipid(s)
  metabolism, 351
  plasma, in postmenopausal women with
    non–insulin-dependent diabetes,
    effect of estrogen replacement
    therapy on, 347
  serum
    Chlamydia pneumoniae antibodies
      and, 68
    incidence of coronary heart disease
      and, in elderly, 164
Lipoprotein
  (a)
    glomerular superoxide anion
      production induced by (in rat), 406
    levels and calcific aortic valve disease,
      223
  low-density
    aortic valve disease and, calcific, 223
    apheresis of, effect on peripheral
      vascular disease in
      hypercholesterolemic patients with
      coronary artery disease, 190
    lowering, effect on saphenous vein
      coronary artery bypass graft
      obstructive changes, 192
Lisinopril
  in diabetics, insulin-dependent
    normotensive, with
    microalbuminuria, 344
Listeria monocytogenes
  in milk causing outbreak of
    gastroenteritis and fever, 64
Lithium
  myocardial infarction risk with, 168
Lithotripsy
  shock wave, antimicrobial prophylaxis
    prior to, in patients with sterile
    urine before treatment, 396
Liver
  disease
    chronic, nonviral, and hepatitis G
      virus infection in liver transplant
      recipients, 615
    hepatitis G virus infection related to,
      transfusion-associated, 614
    severity in chronic hepatitis C virus
      infection, effect of hepatitis G virus
      infection on, 29
  encephalopathy risk with transjugular
    intrahepatic portosystemic shunts,
    625
  transplantation recipients

hepatitis G virus co-infection in
    recipients with chronic hepatitis C
    and nonviral chronic liver disease,
    615
  prophylaxis with fixed dosing
    schedule of hepatitis B
    immunoglobulin, 611
Losartan
  vs. captopril in heart failure, in elderly,
    212
Lovastatin
  effect on myocardial ischemia in
    coronary disease, 188
  effect on obstructive changes in
    saphenous vein coronary bypass
    grafts, 193
Lung
  (See also Pulmonary)
  cancer (see Cancer, lung)
  disease
    chronic obstructive, 531
    chronic obstructive, corticosteroid
      therapy in, adverse effects of, 535
    chronic obstructive, exacerbation of,
      practice guideline reducing length
      of stay for patients hospitalized
      with, 533
    chronic obstructive, severe, outcomes
      after acute exacerbation, 531
    diffuse, diagnostic accuracy of CT in,
      557
    interstitial, 555
  injury, methotrexate-induced, in
    rheumatoid arthritis, predictors of,
    451
  nodule enhancement at CT, 525
  volume reduction surgery in
    emphysema, 539
    bilateral, median sternotomy vs.
      thoracoscopic approach, 540
    bilateral, results of, 539
Lupus
  erythematosus, systemic, 465
    antineutrophil cytoplasmic antibodies
      in, 472
    cyclosporin A in, long-term, 465
    ribosomal P autoantibodies in, 470
Lyme disease
  acute disseminated, ceftriaxone vs.
    doxycycline for, 505
  diagnosis, laboratory evaluation in, 499
  risk in endemic areas, duration of tick
    attachment as predictor of, 503
  simultaneous granulocytic ehrlichiosis
    and, 507
Lymph node(s)
  enlargement in coccidioidomycosis in
    HIV infection, 26

negative, in breast cancer patients, and
5 *vs.* more than 5 years of
tamoxifen therapy, 143
Lymphadenopathy
in Canale-Smith syndrome, 120
Lymphoblastic
leukemia, acute, allogeneic bone
marrow transplantation in, donor
leukocyte infusions for relapse
after, 128
Lymphocyte(s)
CD4, low counts, as predictor of
Pneumocystis carinii pneumonia in
HIV infection, 579
-depleted marrow grafts in
myelodysplastic syndromes,
outcome of, 103
donor, HSV-TK gene transfer into, for
control of graft-*vs.*-leukemia, 137
HIV-1 infectivity in, potent inhibition
by novel CCR5 antagonist, 13
Lymphocytic
leukemia (*see* Leukemia, lymphocytic)
Lymphoid
irradiation, total, in rheumatoid
arthritis, 456
Lymphoma
B cell, polymorphic, in bone marrow
transplant recipients, 135
follicular
low-grade, fludarabine in, 99
low-tumor-burden, no treatment *vs.*
prednimustine or interferon alfa in,
107
previously untreated,
2-chlorodeoxyadenosine in, 108
gastric MALT-type, *Helicobacter pylori*
strains expressing CagA protein in,
636
immunoblastic, malignant, in bone
marrow transplant recipients, 135
large-cell, diffuse, late-relapse after
MACOP-B treatment, 113
non-Hodgkin's
aggressive, CHOP *vs.*
ProMACE-CytaBOM in, 110
aggressive, in elderly, 114
aggressive, poor-risk, autologous
marrow transplantation *vs.*
sequential chemotherapy in, 111
bone marrow transplantation in,
allogeneic, donor leukocyte
infusions for relapse after, 128
bone marrow transplantation in,
autologous, durability of remission
after, 115

bone marrow transplantation in,
autologous, influence of age on
outcome of, 126
Lymphoproliferative
disorders, 107
posttransplant, in bone marrow
recipients, adverse histologic and
immunobiologic features of, 135
T cell, posttransplant, 116
Lymphotropic
T-lymphotropic virus type I, human,
health effects of, 37

M

MACOP-B
regimen in lymphoma, diffuse large-cell,
late relapse with, 113
Macroadenoma
hyperprolactinemia due to, in
postmenopausal women, 268
Macrolide
antibiotics after exposure to Q fever as
biological warfare agent, 72
Macrophage
HIV-1 infectivity in, potent inhibition
by novel CCR5 antagonist, 13
Magnetic resonance
cholangiopancreatography, breath-hold,
in vitro and clinical studies of
image acquisition in, 600
imaging
of bursitis, proximal, in active
polymyalgia rheumatica, 454
of toe dactylitis in
spondyloarthropathy, 479
Malignancy (*see* Cancer)
Malnourished
hemodialysis patients, effects of
recombinant human growth
hormone on muscle protein
turnover in, 431
MALT-type lymphoma
gastric, *Helicobacter pylori* strains
expressing CagA protein in, 636
Mannitol
during kidney transplantation in
reduction of delayed graft function,
427
Manometry
antroduodenal, fasting, in children, 646
Marrow
micrometastases in, detection in breast
cancer patients with
immunohistochemistry and reverse
transcriptase polymerase chain
reaction for keratin 19, 141

transplantation (*see* Transplantation, bone marrow)

Maxillary
sinusitis, acute, antibiotics in, 43

Meal
composition, postprandial angina, and exercise tolerance, 187

Mechlorethamine
in MOPP-ABVD regimen, primary, in Hodgkin's disease, outcome of patients after failing, 118

Mediastinal
masses, biopsy of, endoscopic ultrasound-guided fine-needle aspiration, 598

Medical
intensivist, effects on patient care in community teaching hospital, 585

Medicare
patients, myocardial infarction outcome in, and specialty of admitting physician, 183

Medications (*see* Drugs)

Medicine
intensive care, 585

Megakaryocyte
growth and development factor, pegylated recombinant human, effect on functional platelet production, 85
stimulation by single dose of recombinant human thrombopoietin in cancer patients, 87

Megestrol
adrenal insufficiency in patients on, 279

Melphalan
high-dose
after carboplatin plus cyclophosphamide with hematopoietic rescue in ovarian cancer, 146
after cyclophosphamide, thiotepa, and carboplatin with autologous stem cell support for metastatic breast cancer, 145
/prednisone *vs.* melphalan/prednisone/colchicine in primary amyloidosis, 119

Menses
secondary sexual characteristics and, in young girls, 325

Meprobamates
myocardial infarction risk with, 168

Mesalazine
vs. zileuton in maintenance of remission of ulcerative colitis, 608

Mesangial
cells exposed to high glucose concentrations, effect of enalaprilat on hydrogen peroxide production by (in mice), 388

Metabolic
significance of leptin, 351

Metabolism
carbohydrate, 335
lipid, 351
nitric oxide, altered, in lead-induced hypertension, effect of lazaroid therapy on (in rat), 423

Metaplasia
intestinal, of gastric cardia, 662

Metastases
breast cancer, double dose-intensive chemotherapy with autologous stem cell support for, 145
micrometastases in peripheral blood and bone marrow of breast cancer patients, detection with immunohistochemistry and reverse transcriptase polymerase chain reaction for keratin 19, 141

Methicillin
-resistant *Staphylococcus aureus,* emergence of high-level mupirocin resistance in, 53

Methotrexate
/cyclosporine in rheumatoid arthritis, 451
-induced lung injury in rheumatoid arthritis, predictors of, 451
in MACOP-B regimen in diffuse large-cell lymphoma, late relapse with, 113
in ProMACE-CytaBOM regimen in aggressive non-Hodgkin's lymphoma, 110

Micral-Test
in microalbuminuria screening, 412

Microalbuminuria
in normotensives with insulin-dependent diabetes, lisinopril in, 344
simplified screening for, 412

Microbiology
of bacteremia and fungemia, 47
of *Candida,* fluconazole-resistant, in AIDS, 22

Micrometastases
detection in peripheral blood and bone marrow of breast cancer patients with immunohistochemistry and reverse transcriptase polymerase chain reaction for keratin 19, 141

Microprolactinoma
  cabergoline *vs.* bromocriptine in, in
    women, 271
Microvascular
  complications and eating disorders in
    young women with
    insulin-dependent diabetes, 335
Military
  personnel, U.S., in Haiti, dengue fever
    in, 31
Milk
  Listeria monocytogenes in, causing
    outbreak of gastroenteritis and
    fever, 64
Miners
  gold, silica-exposed, end-stage renal
    disease among, 384
Minocycline
  in rheumatoid arthritis, early, 460
Mitral
  commissurotomy, percutaneous balloon,
    4-year follow-up, 224
  valvotomy, percutaneous balloon,
    echocardiographic assessment of
    commissural calcium as predictor
    of outcome, 230
Model
  prognostic, for prediction of survival in
    cystic fibrosis, 536
Molecular
  remission in PML/RARα-positive
    promyelocytic leukemia by
    combined all-*trans* retinoic acid
    and idarubicin therapy, 95
Monitoring
  of Whipple's disease by polymerase
    chain reaction, 499
Mononucleosis
  -like illness, acute HIV type 1 disease
    as, 9
MOPP-ABVD regimen
  primary, in Hodgkin's disease, outcome
    of patients after failing, 118
Morbidity
  cardiovascular, after noncardiac surgery,
    effect of atenolol on, 252
  of heart transplantation in patients over
    54 years of age, 217
Mortality
  (*See also* Death)
  asthma, stabilization of, 552
  of coccidioidomycosis in HIV infection,
    26
  in families with factor V mutation, 90
  of heart transplantation in patients over
    54 years of age, 217
  hemodialysis dose and, 429

increased, in severe heart failure, and
    nonsustained ventricular
    tachycardia, 239
  after lung volume reduction surgery for
    emphysema, 539, 540
  after lymphoid irradiation, total, in
    rheumatoid arthritis, 457
  of myocardial infarction
    recent, in patients with left
      ventricular dysfunction, effect of
      amiodarone on, 241
    after thrombolytic therapy, and
      increased arterial blood pressure
      and stroke, 176
    after noncardiac surgery, effect of
      atenolol on, 252
  treatment-related, in patients receiving
    high-dose chemotherapy and
    peripheral blood progenitor cell
    transplantation, 123
Motion sickness
  role of plasma vasopressin as mediator
    of nausea and gastric slow wave
    dysrhythmias in, 647
MR (*see* Magnetic resonance)
MRI
  of bursitis, proximal, in active
    polymyalgia rheumatica, 454
  of toe dactylitis in spondyloarthropathy,
    479
Mucosa
  candidiasis in HIV-infected women,
    weekly fluconazole for prevention
    of, 21
  gastric, during treatment with
    lansoprazole, 633
  pelvic pouch, neoplastic transformation
    in ulcerative colitis, 606
Multiple sclerosis
  management of, 509
Mupirocin
  nasal, effect on nasal and cutaneous
    carriage of *Staphylococcus aureus*
    in hemodialysis patients, 52
  resistance, high-level, in
    methicillin-resistant *Staphylococcus
    aureus*, 53
Muscle
  protein turnover in malnourished
    hemodialysis patients, effects of
    recombinant human growth
    hormone on, 431
  quadriceps, weakness of, and
    osteoarthritis of knee, 509
Mycobacterial
  infection, susceptibility to, and mutation
    in interferon-gamma receptor gene,
    6

Myelodysplasia
Fanconi's anemia and, donor leukocyte infusions for relapse after allogeneic bone marrow transplantation in, 128
Myelodysplastic
syndromes, allogeneic bone marrow transplantation in
with lymphocyte-depleted marrow grafts, outcome, 103
relapse after, donor leukocyte infusions for, 128
Myelogenous
leukemia (see Leukemia, myelogenous)
Myeloid
leukemia, acute, induction chemotherapy in, DAT vs. ADE as, 97
Myeloma
bone marrow transplantation in, allogeneic, donor leukocyte infusions for relapse after, 128
multiple, 107
bone marrow transplant procedures in, autologous, influence of age on outcome of, 126
Myeloproliferative
disorders, 95
Myocardial
infarction
carvedilol in, 177
delayed hospital presentation with, 181
first, cholesterol-lowering therapy as primary prevention against, 167
heparin in, low-molecular-weight vs. unfractionated, 173
hypereosinophilic syndrome and, in 15-year-old, 91
outcome, and specialty of admitting physician, 183
previous, incidence of major coronary events in men with, effect of α-tocopherol and β-carotene supplements on, 194
prognosis after, effect of in-hospital ventricular fibrillation on, 178
prognosis in, long-term, and serum cholesterol, in middle-aged men, 166
recent, left ventricular dysfunction after, and effect of amiodarone on mortality, 241
renal artery stenosis in patients with, prevalence and predictors of, 390
risk, and alcohol consumption, moderate, 163
risk, and depression and psychotropic medication, 167
risk, clopidogrel vs. aspirin in prevention of, 196
thrombolytic therapy in, and increased arterial blood pressure, mortality and stroke, 176
ischemia
in coronary artery disease, effect of cholesterol reduction on, 188
diagnosis, arbutamine vs. exercise echocardiography in, 229
exercise-induced, silent vs. symptomatic, clinical implications in stable coronary disease, 185
Myoelectrical
activity, gastric
effect of IV vasopressin on, 649
impairment in chronic renal failure, 650
Myofibroblasts
arteriolar sclerosis in diabetic nephropathy and, 372
Myositis
inflammatory, antineutrophil cytoplasmic antibodies in, 472
Myotomy
laparoscopic, for achalasia, 654

N

Nasal
carriage of Staphylococcus aureus in hemodialysis patients, 52
CPAP in sleep-disordered breathing, effect on risk of traffic accidents, 591
Natriuretic
peptide, atrial, levels after radiocontrast exposure, 401
Nausea
after cabergoline in prolactinoma, 271
in motion sickness, role of plasma vasopressin as mediator of, 647
Nelfinavir
with zidovudine and lamivudine, decay characteristics of HIV-1–infected compartments during, 16
Neoplastic
transformation of pelvic pouch mucosa in ulcerative colitis, 606
Nephropathy
diabetic
myofibroblasts and arteriolar sclerosis in, 372
progression of renal disease in, effect of angiotensin-converting enzyme inhibitors on, 410

IgA, predicting renal outcome in, 363
minimal-change, adult-onset, long-term
outcome of, 366
thin glomerular basement membrane,
and hypertension and late onset
renal failure, 370
Nephrosclerosis
hypertensive, accuracy of diagnosis in
African Americans, 415
Nephrotoxicity
of cyclosporin A in systemic lupus
erythematosus, long-term, 467
Nervous
system, central, viral infections of,
diagnosis, 36
Neuronal
antibodies, anti-myenteric, in achalasia,
655
Neurotoxicity
brain serotonin, from fenfluramine and
dexfenfluramine, 568
Neurotransmission
in stomach, inhibitory, mediation by
interstitial cells of Cajal (in mice),
643
Neutropenia
after 2-chlorodeoxyadenosine in
previously untreated follicular
lymphoma, 109
Neutrophil
elastase in crescentic glomerulonephritis,
377
Nicotine, 517
dependence
cost-effectiveness of treating, 517
severe, 1-week inpatient treatment
for, 521
transdermal, for mildly to moderately
active ulcerative colitis, 607
Night
sweats in coccidioidomycosis in HIV
infection, 26
Nissen fundoplication (*see under*
Fundoplication)
Nitric oxide
metabolism, altered, in lead-induced
hypertension, effect of lazaroid
therapy on (in rat), 423
pathway in patients on continuous
ambulatory peritoneal dialysis, 434
production, renal, mediated by subtype
2 angiotensin receptor (in rat), 421
Nocturnal
hemoglobinuria, paroxysmal, resistance
to apoptosis caused by *PIG-A*
mutations in, 82
Nodule
lung, enhancement at CT, 525

Norepinephrine
excretion, increased urinary, in
incidentally discovered
pheochromocytoma, 290
NPT2
gene localization to chromosome 5q35,
446
Nursing
homes, *Chlamydia pneumoniae* as new
source of infectious outbreaks in,
45
Nutrients
kidney stones and, in women, 444
Nutrition
improvement in patients on continuous
ambulatory peritoneal dialysis, 435

O

Obesity, 351
Octanoic acid
breath test, [^{13}C], for gastric emptying
of solids, 644
Octreotide
in acromegaly, 267
Omeprazole
in dyspepsia in *Helicobacter
pylori*-seropositive patients, 629
in esophagitis, severe, cost-utility
analysis of, 669
Oncology
measuring accuracy of prognostic
judgments in, 154
ONO-1078
prevents exacerbation of asthma during
reduction of high-dose inhaled
corticosteroid, 549
OPC-31260
effect on aquaporin-2 water channel
expression in chronic heart failure
(in rat), 440
in syndrome of inappropriate secretion
of antidiuretic hormone, 272
Opportunistic
infections, AIDS, 19
Oral
aphthous ulcers in HIV patients,
thalidomide for, 26
Organ
solid organ transplantation,
posttransplant T cell
lymphoproliferative disorders after,
116
Oropharyngeal
candidiasis in HIV patients
detection and significance of
fluconazole resistance in, 20

women, weekly fluconazole for
prevention of, 21
Osteoarthritis
knee, and quadriceps weakness, 509
Osteoporosis
corticosteroid-induced
in COPD, 535
etidronate in prevention of,
intermittent, 320
postmenopausal, alendronate in
prevention of nonvertebral
fractures in, 319
Ovarian
cancer, high-dose chemotherapy with
hematopoietic rescue in, 146
hyperthecosis, and diabetes and
hirsutism in postmenopausal
women, 329
Oxygen
-15 PET for relation of regional cerebral
activity and visceral pain, 651
free radical activity increase in
lead-induced hypertension, effect of
lazaroid therapy on (in rat), 423

P

P autoantibodies
ribosomal, in systemic lupus
erythematosus, 470
Pacemaker
interference by cellular telephones, 254
leads, systemic infection related to
endocarditis on, 248
Pacing
dual-chamber, for hypertrophic
cardiomyopathy, 255
Pain
abdominal, after cabergoline in
prolactinoma, 271
visceral, and regional cerebral activity,
651
Pancreas
carcinoma, staging of, endosonography
vs. surgery in, 599
Paracentesis
total volume, decreases variceal
pressure, size and wall tension in
cirrhosis, 620
Paranasal
sinusitis, acute, ten-day mark as
practical diagnostic approach for,
in children, 42
Parapneumonic
effusions, complicated, streptokinase vs.
urokinase in, 583
Parathyroid
glands, 305

hormone secretion inhibition,
short-term, by calcium-receptor
agonist in primary
hyperparathyroidism, 309
Paresthesias
after cyclosporin A in systemic lupus
erythematosus, long-term, 467
Parvovirus
B19 DNA persistence in synovial
membranes of young patients with
and without chronic arthropathy,
501
Pathological
importance of heterogeneity in vacA,
637
Pathophysiological
concepts of angina in patients with
aortic stenosis and normal
coronary arteries, 221
Patient
care in community teaching hospital,
effects of medical intensivist on,
585
preferences concerning trade-off
between risks and benefits of
routine radiation therapy after
conservative surgery for early-stage
breast cancer, 153
self-interpretation of tuberculin skin
tests, 571
Peak expiratory flow
changes during acute exacerbations of
asthma, 543
Pegylated
recombinant human megakaryocyte
growth and development factor,
effect on production of functional
platelets, 85
Pelvic
pouch mucosa, neoplastic
transformation in ulcerative colitis,
606
Penicillin
-resistant Streptococcus pneumoniae,
continued emergence in U.S., 581
Peptide
atrial natriuretic, levels after
radiocontrast exposure, 401
inhibition of glomerular deposition of
anti-DNA antibody, 365
Percutaneous
balloon mitral commissurotomy, 4-year
follow-up, 224
removal of infected pacemaker leads,
249

Peristalsis
disordered preoperative, and outcome
of laparoscopic Nissen
fundoplication, 667
Peritoneal
dialysis patients, continuous ambulatory
amino acid profile and nitric oxide
pathway in, 434
role of improvement in acid-base
status and nutrition in, 435
Peritonitis
acute, L-arginine depletion in, in
patients on continuous ambulatory
peritoneal dialysis, 434
Personnel
military, U.S., in Haiti, dengue fever in,
31
PET
^{15}O, for relation of regional cerebral
activity and visceral pain, 651
Phenothiazines
myocardial infarction risk with, 168
Phentermine
-fenfluramine associated with valvular
heart disease, 569
Pheochromocytoma
incidentally discovered, 290
Phosphorus, 443
Physician
admitting, specialty of, and outcome of
myocardial infarction, 183
desire for euthanasia and assisted
suicide, 155
-directed *vs.* protocol-directed weaning
from mechanical ventilation, 588
Physiology
effects of ibuprofen in sepsis on, 5
PIG-A
gene mutations in paroxysmal nocturnal
hemoglobinuria causing resistance
to apoptosis, 82
Pirarubicin
plus CVP in aggressive non-Hodgkin's
lymphoma, in elderly, 114
Pituitary, 265
hypothalamo-pituitary-adrenal axis,
inhaled beclomethasone suppresses
in dose dependent manner, 287
radiotherapy after unsuccessful
transsphenoidal surgery in
Cushing's disease, long-term
outcome of, 285
PKD1 and PKD2
gene products of, homo- and
heterodimeric interactions between,
394

Plague
as biological warfare agent, clinical
recognition and management of
patients exposed to, 72
Plasticity
in vitro, of intercalated cell polarity,
role of hensin in, 439
Platelet(s)
functional, production of, effect of
pegylated recombinant human
megakaryocyte growth and
development factor on, 85
production stimulated by single dose of
recombinant human
thrombopoietin in cancer patients,
87
Pleural
effusions
malignant, thoracoscopic talc
poudrage pleurodesis for, 529
parapneumonic, complicated,
streptokinase *vs.* urokinase in, 583
emboli, 563
Pleurodesis
thoracoscopic talc poudrage, for
malignant effusions, 529
Pneumococcal
pneumonia, community-acquired,
sputum Gram's stain in, 44
Pneumocystis carinii
pneumonia in HIV infection, 577
predictors of, 578
Pneumonia
/atelectasis after ileocecal resection for
Crohn's disease, 605
bacterial, in HIV infection, 577
community-acquired, prediction rule to
identify low-risk patients with, 582
pneumococcal, community-acquired,
sputum Gram's stain in, 44
Pneumocystis carinii, in HIV infection,
577
predictors of, 578
Polychondritis
relapsing, clinical and immunogenetic
analysis of, 496
Polycystic
kidney disease, gene products of PKD1
and PKD2, homo- and
heterodimeric interactions between,
394
Polycystin
vascular expression of, 385
Polyglandular
syndrome, autoimmune, type I and II,
new immunoprecipitation test for
21-hydroxylase autoantibodies in,
277

Polymerase chain reaction
  diagnosis and monitoring of Whipple's
    disease by, 499
  for herpes simplex virus 2 shedding,
    frequent genital, in
    immunocompetent women, 32
  for parvovirus B19 DNA in synovial
    membranes of young patients with
    and without chronic arthropathy,
    501
  reverse transcriptase, for keratin 19,
    detection of micrometastases in
    peripheral blood and bone marrow
    of breast cancer patients with, 141
  for viral infections of central nervous
    system, 36
Polymyalgia
  rheumatica, proximal bursitis in, 454
Portal
  fibrosis, non-cirrhotic, increased
    incidence of glomerulonephritis
    after spleno-renal shunt surgery in,
    375
  hypertension after transjugular
    intrahepatic portosystemic shunts,
    natural history of, 623
Portosystemic
  shunt (*see* Shunt, portosystemic)
Positron emission
  tomography, ^{15}O, for relation of
    regional cerebral activity and
    visceral pain, 651
Postmenopausal women
  diabetes in, non–insulin-dependent, and
    estrogen replacement therapy, 347
  estrogen replacement therapy in, effect
    on survival after coronary artery
    bypass, 204
  fractures in, nonverteberal, alendronate
    in prevention of, 319
  hirsutism, ovarian hyperthecosis and
    diabetes in, 329
  hormone replacement therapy in (*see*
    Hormone, replacement therapy,
    postmenopausal)
  hypercholesterolemia in,
    estrogen-progestin *vs.* simvastatin
    for, 355
  hyperparathyroidism in, primary, effect
    of R-568 on parathyroid hormone
    secretion in, 309
  hyperprolactinemia in, 267
Postprandial
  angina and exercise tolerance, 187
  hyperglycemia in insulin-dependent
    diabetics, effect of insulin-analog
    treatment on, 339

Postural
  hypotension after cabergoline in
    prolactinoma, 271
Poudrage
  pleurodesis, thoracoscopic talc, for
    malignant effusions, 529
Practice guideline
  reducing length of stay for patients
    hospitalized with exacerbation of
    COPD, 533
Prednimustine
  in lymphoma, low-tumor-burden
    follicular, 107
Prednisone
  /acyclovir in herpes zoster, 34
  for adrenal insufficiency during
    megestrol therapy, 279
  in CHOP *vs.* ProMACE-CytaBOM
    regimen in aggressive
    non-Hodgkin's lymphoma, 110
  in CVP *vs.* CTVP regimen in aggressive
    non-Hodgkin's lymphoma, in
    elderly, 114
  -induced osteoporosis, prevention with
    intermittent etidronate, 320
  in MACOP-B regimen in diffuse
    large-cell lymphoma, late relapse
    with, 113
  /melphalan *vs.*
    prednisone/melphalan/colchicine in
    primary amyloidosis, 119
  in MOPP-ABVD regimen, primary, in
    Hodgkin's disease, outcome of
    patients after failing, 118
  requirements, perioperative, in
    secondary adrenal insufficiency, 283
  in rheumatoid arthritis, spinal bone loss
    secondary to, calcium and vitamin
    D_3 supplementation prevents, 452
  in sarcoidosis, and relapse, 559
Pregnancy
  loss in antiphospholipid antibody
    syndrome, 468
Premenopausal
  tophaceous gout due to longtime
    diuretic abuse, 487
Probenecid
  with cidofovir for cytomegalovirus
    retinitis in AIDS, 23, 24
Procarbazine
  in MOPP-ABVD regimen, primary, in
    Hodgkin's disease, outcome of
    patients after failing, 118
Progenitor
  cell transplantation, peripheral blood,
    with high-dose chemotherapy, and
    treatment-related mortality, 123

Progestin
-estrogen *vs.* simvastatin for
hypercholesterolemia in
postmenopausal women, 355
Prognostic judgments
in oncology, measuring accuracy of, 154
Prolactinoma
cabergoline in, 269
ProMACE-CytaBOM regimen
vs. CHOP regimen in aggressive
non-Hodgkin's lymphoma, 110
Promyelocytic
leukemia, PML/RARα-positive acute,
all-*trans* retinoic acid and
idarubicin in, 95
Propranolol
plus endoscopy *vs.* transjugular
intrahepatic portosystemic shunt
for prevention of variceal
rebleeding, 624
as primary prophylaxis of variceal
bleeding in cirrhosis,
cost-effectiveness of, 618
Prostate
-specific antigen in female serum as
potential new marker of androgen
excess, 327
Prosthetic
joint infection, *Staphylococcus aureus*,
treated with debridement and
prosthesis retention, 54
Protein
C, activated, resistance to
factor V gene mutation causing, in
chronic venous leg ulcers, 88
mortality and causes of death in
families with, 90
CagA, *Helicobacter pylori* strains
expressing, in MALT-type gastric
lymphoma, 636
C-reactive, and aspirin and risk of
cardiovascular disease, 169
DCC, and prognosis in colorectal
cancer, 149
fusion, tumor necrosis factor receptor
(p75)-Fc, recombinant human, in
rheumatoid arthritis, 462
muscle, turnover in malnourished
hemodialysis patients, effects of
recombinant human growth
hormone on, 431
Protocol
-directed *vs.* physician-directed weaning
from mechanical ventilation, 588
Pseudogout
triamcinolone acetonide in,
intramuscular, 489

Psychiatric
disease and esophageal motility
disorders, 652
disorders in young people with
insulin-dependent diabetes mellitus,
336
reactions, acute, to corticosteroids in
COPD, 535
Psychosis
lupus, and ribosomal P autoantibodies,
470
Psychotropic
medication for depression and risk of
myocardial infarction, 167
Puberty
onset in young girls, 325
Pulmonary
(*See also* Lung)
complications of HIV infection,
respiratory disease trends in, 577
embolism
thrombolytic therapy and prognosis
in hemodynamically stable patients
with, 566
validation of spiral CT angiography
in, 565
fibrosis, idiopathic
pulmonary function tests in, 556
smoking as risk factor for, 555
function test
effect of rhinovirus-caused upper
respiratory illness on, 41
in pulmonary fibrosis, idiopathic, 556
hypertension, primary, from
fenfluramine and dexfenfluramine,
568
infection after thoracoscopic talc
poudrage pleurodesis for malignant
effusions, 529
rehabilitation patients, attitudes
regarding advance directives
among, 534
Purpura
thrombocytopenic, idiopathic, high-dose
IV immune globulin and response
to splenectomy in, 84
Push-enteroscopy
diagnostic efficacy in small bowel
angiodysplasias, 602
Pyrazinamide
in tuberculosis with and without HIV
infection, in 6-month supervised
intermittent therapy, in Haitians,
575

Q

Q fever
  as biological warfare agent, clinical
    recognition and management of
    patients exposed to, 72
Quadriceps
  weakness and osteoarthritis of knee,
    509
Quality of life
  after heart transplantation in patients
    over 54 years of age, 217

R

R-568
  effect on parathyroid hormone secretion
    in primary hyperparathyroidism,
    309
Rad51
  embryonic lethality and radiation
    hypersensitivity in mice lacking
    Brca2 mediated by, 152
Radiation
  diagnostic (*see* Radiography)
  hypersensitivity mediated by Rad51 in
    mice lacking *Brca2*, 152
  therapeutic (*see* Radiotherapy)
Radiocontrast
  exposure, endothelin and atrial
    natriuretic peptide levels after, 401
Radiofrequency
  modification of atrioventricular node in
    atrial fibrillation, long-term
    follow-up, 238
Radiography
  chest, in coccidioidomycosis in HIV
    infection, 26
  presentation of bronchogenic
    carcinoma, changing, with
    reference to cell types, 523
  vs. low-dose spiral CT in screening and
    detection of peripheral lung cancer,
    524
Radiotherapy
  in acromegaly, 266
  lymphoid, total, in rheumatoid arthritis,
    456
  pituitary, after unsuccessful
    transsphenoidal surgery in
    Cushing's disease, long-term
    outcome of, 285
  routine, after conservative surgery for
    early-stage breast cancer, patient
    preferences concerning trade-off
    between risks and benefits of, 153

Ranitidine
  in dyspepsia in *Helicobacter
    pylori*-seropositive patients, 629
Rash
  after clopidogrel in prevention of
    ischemic events, 197
  after thalidomide for oral aphthous
    ulcers in HIV patients, 27
Raspberries
  imported, 1996 cyclosporiasis outbreak
    associated with, 59
Rebleeding
  in cirrhotics, beta-adrenergic antagonists
    in prevention of, 617
  gastrointestinal, in cirrhotics,
    beta-adrenergic antagonists in
    prevention of, 617
  variceal
    prevention with transjugular
      intrahepatic portosystemic shunts
      vs. endoscopic sclerotherapy, 625
    shunt for, transjugular intrahepatic
      portosystemic, *vs.* endoscopy plus
      propranolol, 624
Rectosigmoid
  adenomas 5 mm or less in diameter
    detected by sigmoidoscopy,
    importance of, 597
Red cells, 81
Reflux
  acid, role in gastroesophageal reflux,
    664
  duodenogastroesophageal, role in
    gastroesophageal reflux, 664
  esophagitis
    curing *Helicobacter pylori* infection in
      duodenal ulcer may provoke, 631
    therapy for, conservative, long-term
      comparison with antireflux surgery,
      670
  gastroesophageal, 661
    after botulinum toxin injection in
      achalasia, 657
    fundoplication in (*see* Fundoplication)
    role of acid and
      duodenogastroesophageal reflux in,
      664
Rehabilitation
  pulmonary, attitudes regarding advance
    directives among patients in, 534
Renal
  (*See also* Kidney)
  artery stenosis in patients with
    myocardial infarction, prevalence
    and predictors of, 390
  fibrosis, urinary and serum type III
    collagen as markers of, 410

injury, acute, production of
heparin-binding epidermal growth
factor-like growth factor in early
phase of regeneration after (in rat),
400
outcome in IgA nephropathy, predicting,
363
production
of nitric oxide mediated by subtype 2
angiotensin receptor (in rat), 421
of transforming growth factor-β1
increased in type II diabetes, 373
sodium-phosphate cotransporter gene
NPT2 localization to chromosome
5q35, 446
spleno-renal shunt surgery in
non-cirrhotic portal fibrosis,
increased incidence of
glomerulonephritis after, 375
Reproductive
system, 325
Reptile
-associated salmonellosis, increasing
incidence in U.S., 62
Respiratory
disease trends in pulmonary
complications of HIV infection,
577
illness, rhinovirus-caused upper, effect
on pulmonary function test and
exercise responses, 41
infections, 41
Reticulonodular
infiltrates on chest radiographs in
coccidioidomycosis in HIV
infection, 26
Retinitis
cytomegalovirus, in AIDS
cidofovir for, 23, 24
Retinoic acid
all-*trans,* with idarubicin in
PML/RARα-positive acute
promyelocytic leukemia, 95
Retinopathy
hydroxychloroquine, rarity of, 451
Revascularization
coronary, prediction of ventricular
function improvement after, FDG
SPECT *vs.* dobutamine
echocardiography in, 227
Rheumatic
fever, acute, in adults, 511
Rheumatoid
arthritis (*see* Arthritis, rheumatoid)
Rhinovirus
-caused upper respiratory illness, effect
on pulmonary function test and
exercise responses, 41

Ribavirin
after exposure to viral hemorrhagic
fevers as biological warfare agents,
76
plus interferon alfa in chronic hepatitis
C, long-term efficacy of, 612
Ribosomal
P autoantibodies in systemic lupus
erythematosus, 470
Rifampin
preventive therapy for tuberculosis, 572
in tuberculosis with and without HIV
infection, in 6-month supervised
intermittent therapy, in Haitians,
575
RNA
ribosomal, gene patterns, and
Helicobacter pylori infection in
spouses of patients with duodenal
ulcers, 634
Roll plate
method of diagnosis of triple-lumen
catheter infection, 50

S

Salmeterol
long-term, in asthma, 547
Salmonella
Marina infection in children, and
iguanas, 62
Saphenous
vein coronary artery bypass grafts,
obstructive changes in, effect of
low-density lipoprotein cholesterol
lowering and low-dose
anticoagulation on, 192
Sarcoidosis
outcome in, 559
review of, 509
Scintigraphy
vs. [^{13}C]octanoic acid breath test for
gastric emptying of solids, 644
Scleroderma
antineutrophil cytoplasmic antibodies
in, 472
Sclerosing
syndromes, 483
Sclerosis
arteriolar, and myofibroblasts in
diabetic nephropathy, 372
multiple, management of, 509
systemic, palpable tendon friction rub
in, 483
tuberous sclerosis gene *TSC1* on
chromosome 9q34, identification
of, 395

Sclerotherapy
combined with ligation *vs.* endoscopic
variceal ligation for esophageal
varices, 622
endoscopic, *vs.* transjugular intrahepatic
portosystemic shunt
after initial sclerotherapy in acute
variceal hemorrhage, 627
endoscopic, *vs.* transjugular intrahepatic
shunt for prevention of variceal
rebleeding, 625
surgery as primary prophylaxis of
variceal bleeding in cirrhosis,
cost-effectiveness of, 618
Semen
HIV-1 concentration in, reduction after
treatment of urethritis, 11
Sepsis
catheter-related, diagnosis with
endoluminal brush method, 56
ibuprofen in, effects on physiology and
patient survival, 5
Serotonin
neurotoxicity, brain, from fenfluramine
and dexfenfluramine, 568
Sex (*see* Gender)
Sexual
characteristics, secondary, and menses in
young girls, 325
dimorphism in plasma leptin
concentration, 353
transmission of HIV-1, prevention of,
11
Shock
wave lithotripsy in patients with sterile
urine before treatment,
antimicrobial prophylaxis prior to,
396
Shunt
portosystemic, transjugular intrahepatic
portal hypertension after, natural
history of, 623
vs. endoscopic sclerotherapy after
initial sclerotherapy in acute
variceal hemorrhage, 627
vs. endoscopic sclerotherapy for
prevention of variceal rebleeding,
625
vs. endoscopy plus propranolol for
prevention of variceal rebleeding,
624
surgery
as primary prophylaxis of variceal
bleeding in cirrhosis,
cost-effectiveness of, 618
spleno-renal, in non-cirrhotic portal
fibrosis, increased incidence of
glomerulonephritis after, 375

SIADH
OPC-31260 in, 272
Sigmoidoscopy
adenomas 5 mm or less in diameter
detected on, importance of, 597
Silica
-exposed gold miners, end-stage renal
disease among, 384
Silicosis
in the 1990s, 560
Simvastatin
apheresis of low-density lipoprotein
and, effect on peripheral vascular
disease in hypercholesterolemic
patients with coronary artery
disease, 190
vs. estrogen-progestin for
hypercholesterolemia in
postmenopausal women, 355
Single-photon emission computed
tomography
FDG, *vs.* dobutamine echocardiography
in prediction of ventricular function
improvement after
revascularization, 227
Sinus
rhythm, conversion to, in atrial
fibrillation lasting less than 48
hours, and risk for clinical
thromboembolism, 234
Sinusitis
maxillary, acute, antibiotics in, 43
paranasal, acute, ten-day mark as
practical diagnostic approach for,
in children, 42
Sjögren's syndrome
antineutrophil cytoplasmic antibodies
in, 472
Skeletal
hyperostosis, diffuse idiopathic, clinical
features of, 481
Skin
tests, tuberculin, patient's
self-interpretation of, 571
Sleep, 591
-disordered breathing and risk of traffic
accidents, 591
Sleepiness
after cabergoline in prolactinoma, 271
Smallpox
as biological warfare agent, clinical
recognition and management of
patients exposed to, 72
Smoking
aortic valve disease and, calcific, 223
cessation, sustained-release bupropion
for, 518

myocardial infarction and, previous, effect of α-tocopherol and β-carotene supplements on incidence of major coronary events in male smokers, 195
as risk factor for idiopathic pulmonary fibrosis, 555

Sodium
-phosphate cotransporter gene NPT2, renal, localization to chromosome 5q35, 446

Solids
gastric emptying of, [¹³C]octanoic acid breath test for, 644

Somatostatin
vs. terlipressin for acute variceal bleeding, 619

Somnolence
after thalidomide for oral aphthous ulcers in HIV patients, 27

Sonication
method of diagnosis of triple-lumen catheter infection, 50

Sore throat
in *Chlamydia pneumoniae* infection in nursing homes, 46

Specialty
of admitting physician and outcome of myocardial infarction, 183

SPECT
FDG, *vs.* dobutamine echocardiography in prediction of ventricular function improvement after revascularization, 227

Spine
bone loss, corticosteroid-induced, in rheumatoid arthritis, calcium and vitamin D₃ supplementation prevents, 452

Splenectomy
in leukemia, chronic lymphocytic, 100
in thrombocytopenic purpura, idiopathic, response to, and high-dose IV immune globulin, 84

Spleno-renal
shunt surgery in non-cirrhotic portal fibrosis, increased incidence of glomerulonephritis after, 375

Spondyloarthropathy, 477
toe dactylitis in, 479
vs. fibromyalgia, in women, 477

Spouses
of duodenal ulcer patients
Helicobacter pylori infection and related gastroduodenal lesions in, prevalence of, 636
Helicobacter pylori infection in, and ribosomal RNA gene patterns, 634

Sputum
Gram's stain in community-acquired pneumococcal pneumonia, 44

Stain
Gram's, sputum, in community-acquired pneumococcal pneumonia, 44

Staphylococcal
enterotoxin B as biological warfare agent, clinical recognition and management of patients exposed to, 76

Staphylococci
coagulase-negative, causing bacteremia, 49

Staphylococcus
aureus
bacteremia due to, 49
methicillin-resistant, emergence of high-level mupirocin resistance in, 53
nasal and cutaneous carriage, in hemodialysis patients, 52
prosthetic joint infection treated with debridement and prosthesis retention, 54
infection, pacemaker lead, 249

Stem cell(s)
from cord blood, extensive amplification and self-renewal of, 132
transplantation (*see* Transplantation, stem cell)

Stenosis
aortic, with normal coronary arteries and angina, mechanisms and pathophysiological concepts of, 221
coronary artery, proximal left anterior descending, isolated stenosis of, coronary artery stenting *vs.* angioplasty for, 203
renal artery, in patients with myocardial infarction, prevalence and predictors of, 390

Stenting
coronary artery, *vs.* angioplasty, for isolated stenosis of proximal left anterior descending coronary artery, 203

Sternotomy
median, as approach to bilateral lung volume reduction surgery for emphysema, 540

Steroid
corticosteroid (*see* Corticosteroid)
21-hydroxylase autoantibodies, measurements with new immunoprecipitation assay, 277

requirements, perioperative, in
secondary adrenal insufficiency, 283
Stomach
(*See also* Gastric; Gastrointestinal)
cancer risk in people with CagA
positive or negative *Helicobacter
pylori* infection, 639
inhibitory neurotransmission in,
mediation by interstitial cells of
Cajal (in mice), 643
Stones
kidney, and calcium intake, in women,
444
Streptococcus pneumoniae
drug-resistant, continued emergence in
U.S., 581
Streptokinase
vs. urokinase in complicated
parapneumonic effusions, 583
Streptomycin
after exposure to plague as biological
warfare agent, 72
after exposure to tularemia as biological
warfare agent, 72
Stroke
ischemic
clopidogrel *vs.* aspirin in patients at
risk of, 196
heparin in, low-molecular-weight, 175
after thrombolytic therapy for
myocardial infarction, and
increased arterial blood pressure,
176
Subacromial
bursitis in active polymyalgia
rheumatica, 454
Subdeltoid
bursitis in active polymyalgia
rheumatica, 454
Sudden death
coronary, risk in congestive heart
failure, effect of antithrombotic
therapy on, 216
in heart failure, severe, and
nonsustained ventricular
tachycardia, 239
Suicide
assisted, physician desire for, 155
Sulfamethoxazole
-trimethoprim–resistant *Streptococcus
pneumoniae,* continued emergence
in U.S., 581
Sulfosalicylic
acid test combined with Chemstrips in
microalbuminuria screening, 412
Superoxide
anion production, glomerular, induced
by lipoprotein(a) (in rat), 406

Surgeons
hepatitis B-infected, without hepatitis B
e antigen, transmission of hepatitis
B to patients from, 30
Surgery
noncardiac, effect of atenolol on
mortality and cardiovascular
morbidity after, 252
vs. endosonography in staging of
ampullary and pancreatic
carcinoma, 599
Sweats
night, in coccidioidomycosis in HIV
infection, 26
Syndrome of inappropriate secretion of
antidiuretic hormone
OPC-31260 in, 272
Synovial
membranes, persistence of parvovirus
B19 DNA in, in young patients
with and without chronic
arthropathy, 501
Synthroid
bioequivalence with generic
levothyroxine products, 296

T

T cell(s)
CD28 costimulation of, differential
regulation of HIV-1 fusion cofactor
expression by, 12
lymphoproliferative disorders,
posttransplant, 116
Tachycardia
ventricular, nonsustained, in severe
heart failure, 239
Tacrolimus
rescue therapy for renal allograft
rejection, 425
Talc
poudrage pleurodesis, thoracoscopic, for
malignant effusions, 529
Tamm-Horsfall glycoprotein
localization of single binding site for
immunoglobulin light chains on,
382
Tamoxifen
five *vs.* more than five years of, for
breast cancer patients with negative
nodes and estrogen
receptor-positive tumors, 143
Teaching
hospital, community, effects of medical
intensivist on patient care in, 585
Telephones
cellular, interference with pacemakers
by, 254

N-Telopeptide
urinary excretion, therapeutic response
of hormone replacement therapy in
postmenopausal women monitored
by, 312
Temporal
arteritis, color duplex ultrasound in
diagnosis, 491
Tendon
friction rub, palpable, in systemic
sclerosis, 483
Teniposide
in CVP *vs.* CTVP regimen in aggressive
non-Hodgkin's lymphoma, in
elderly, 114
Terlipressin
vs. somatostatin for acute variceal
bleeding, 619
Terrorism
biologic, 71
Tetracycline
after exposure to plague as biological
warfare agent, 72
after exposure to Q fever as biological
warfare agent, 72
Thalidomide
for oral aphthous ulcers in HIV
patients, 26
Thallium-201
/FDG SPECT *vs.* dobutamine
echocardiography in prediction of
ventricular function improvement
after revascularization, 227
Thiazide
-sensitive cotransporter gene locus on
chromosome 16q13, Gitelman's
syndrome maps to, 381
Thigh
injection of insulin, through-clothing,
safety of, 341
Thioguanine
in induction chemotherapy regimen in
acute myeloid leukemia, 97
Thiotepa
melphalan after, with autologous stem
cell support for metastatic breast
cancer, 145
Thoracoscopic
approach to bilateral lung volume
reduction surgery for emphysema,
540
talc poudrage pleurodesis for malignant
effusions, 529
Throat
sore, in *Chlamydia pneumoniae*
infection in nursing homes, 46
Thrombocytopenia
in Canale-Smith syndrome, 120

after 2-chlorodeoxyadenosine in
previously untreated follicular
lymphoma, 109
Thrombocytopenic
purpura, idiopathic, high-dose IV
immune globulin and response to
splenectomy in, 84
Thromboembolism
in atrial flutter, chronic, 233
clinical, risk with conversion to sinus
rhythm in atrial fibrillation lasting
less than 48 hours, 234
venous, duration of oral anticoagulation
after second episode of, 563
Thrombogenic
mechanism for pregnancy loss in
antiphospholipid antibody
syndrome, 468
Thrombolytic therapy
in myocardial infarction, and increased
arterial blood pressure, mortality
and stroke, 176
in pulmonary embolism, and prognosis
in hemodynamically stable patients,
566
Thrombopoietin
recombinant human, single dose, effect
on megakaryocyte and platelet
production in cancer patients, 87
Thyroid, 293
carcinoma, medullary, serum calcitonin
measurement in detection of, 302
incidentalomas, 260
Thyrotropin
levels, low, no association with bone
loss in older women, 300
Thyroxine
L- (*see* Levothyroxine)
Tick
attachment duration as predictor of risk
of Lyme disease in endemic areas,
503
Tissue
connective tissue disease, antineutrophil
cytoplasmic antibodies in, 472
hypothyroidism estimation by new
clinical score, 293
T-lymphotropic
virus type I, human, health effects of,
37
α-Tocopherol
supplements, effect on incidence of
major coronary events in men with
previous myocardial infarction, 194
Toe
dactylitis in spondyloarthropathy, 479
Tomography
computed (*see* Computed tomography)

positron emission, ^{15}O, for relation of regional cerebral activity and visceral pain, 651
Tophaceous
gout, premenopausal, due to longtime diuretic abuse, 487
Tophi
intradermal urate, 487
Toxin
botulinum
as biological warfare agent, clinical recognition and management of patients exposed to, 76
injection for achalasia, untoward effects of, 656
Traffic
accidents, risk in patients with sleep-disordered breathing, 591
Transdermal
nicotine for mildly to moderately active ulcerative colitis, 607
Transforming
growth factor-β1, increased renal production in type II diabetes, 373
Transfusion
-associated hepatitis G virus infection, incidence and relation to liver disease, 614
Transjugular
intrahepatic portosystemic shunt (*see* Shunt, portosystemic, transjugular intrahepatic)
Transplantation
blood progenitor cell, peripheral, with high-dose chemotherapy, and treatment-related mortality, 123
bone marrow, 123
allogeneic, in hematologic malignancies, advanced, comparison with peripheral blood stem cell transplantation, 129
allogeneic, in leukemia, with donors other than HLA-identical siblings, results of, 124
allogeneic, lymphoproliferative disorders after, adverse histologic and immunobiologic features of, 135
allogeneic, relapsed malignancy after, donor leukocyte infusions in, 127
allogeneic, with lymphocyte-depleted marrow grafts, outcome in myelodysplastic syndromes, 103
in anemia, acquired aplastic, outcomes of, 81
autologous, for hematologic malignancies, influence of age on outcome of, 126

autologous, in lymphoma, non-Hodgkin's, durability of remission after, 115
autologous, in lymphoma, non-Hodgkin's, poor-risk aggressive, *vs.* sequential chemotherapy, 111
autologous, in ovarian cancer, after high-dose chemotherapy, long-term results, 146
cancers after, solid, 134
hepatitis G virus after, 139
heart, in patients over 54 years of age, 217
islet, in insulin-dependent diabetics, 343
kidney, 425
cadaveric, risk factors for delayed graft function in, 427
rejection, tacrolimus rescue therapy for, 425
liver, recipients
hepatitis G virus co-infection with chronic hepatitis C and nonviral chronic liver disease in, 615
prophylaxis with fixed dosing schedule of hepatitis B immunoglobulin, 611
solid organ, posttransplant T cell lymphoproliferative disorders after, 116
stem cell
autologous, in metastatic breast cancer, with double dose-intensive chemotherapy, 145
cord blood, from related and unrelated donors, outcome of, 130
peripheral blood, allogeneic, in advanced hematologic malignancies, comparison with marrow transplantation, 129
peripheral blood, autologous, after high-dose chemotherapy for ovarian cancer, long-term results, 146
Transsphenoidal
surgery in Cushing's disease, unsuccessful, pituitary irradiation after, long-term outcome, 285
Tremors
after cyclosporin A in systemic lupus erythematosus, long-term, 467
Triamcinolone
acetonide intramuscular, in pseudogout, 489
Trimethoprim
-sulfamethoxazole–resistant *Streptococcus pneumoniae*, continued emergence in U.S., 581

Tropheryma whippelii
polymerase chain reaction for, 500
TSC1
identification on chromosome 9q34, 395
Tuberculin
skin tests, patient's self-interpretation of, 571
Tuberculosis, 571
HIV and, 575
rifampin preventive therapy for, 572
therapy, 6-month supervised intermittent, in Haitians with and without HIV infection, 575
Tuberous
sclerosis gene *TSC1* on chromosome 9q34, identification of, 395
Tularemia
as biological warfare agent, clinical recognition and management of patients exposed to, 72
Tumor
necrosis factor
-α increase after thalidomide for oral aphthous ulcers in HIV patients, 27
receptor (p75)-Fc fusion protein, recombinant human, in rheumatoid arthritis, 462
Tyrosine
phosphatase antibodies in insulin-dependent diabetes mellitus with onset before and after age 40 years, 337

U

Ulcer
aphthous, oral, in HIV patients, thalidomide for, 26
duodenal
Helicobacter pylori infection and related gastroduodenal lesions in spouses of patients with, prevalence of, 636
Helicobacter pylori infection in, curing may provoke reflux esophagitis, 631
Helicobacter pylori infection in spouses of patients with, and ribosomal RNA gene patterns, 634
esophageal, after botulinum toxin injection in achalasia, 656
leg, chronic venous, activated protein C resistance due to factor V gene mutation in, 88
Ulcerative
colitis (*see* Colitis, ulcerative)

Ultrasound
attenuation, broadband, predicts fracture occurrence in older women, 311
color duplex, in diagnosis of temporal arteritis, 491
endoscopic
biopsy guided by, fine-needle aspiration, using linear array and radial scanning endosonography, 598
linear array and radial scanning, endoscopic ultrasound-guided fine-needle aspiration biopsy using, 598
vs. surgery in staging of ampullary and pancreatic carcinoma, 599
Urate
tophi, intradermal, 487
Urethritis
treatment, reduction of HIV-1 concentration in semen after, 11
Urinary
N-telopeptide monitors therapeutic response of hormone replacement therapy in postmenopausal women, 312
tract
abnormalities, indinavir-associated, 392
infection after ileocecal resection for Crohn's disease, 605
Urine
collagen III measurement in, as marker of renal fibrosis, 410
sterile, before shock wave lithotripsy, and antimicrobial prophylaxis, 396
Urokinase
vs. streptokinase in complicated parapneumonic effusions, 583
Urolithiasis
vasectomy and, 443

V

vacA
heterogeneity in, clinical and pathological importance of, 637
Vaccine
anticancer vaccine KH-1 adenocarcinoma antigen, potential, total synthesis of, 153
Vaginal
candidiasis in HIV-infected women, weekly fluconazole for prevention of, 21

Valve
aortic, calcific disease of, clinical factors associated with, 223
mitral, percutaneous balloon commissurotomy of, 4-year follow-up, 224
Valvotomy
mitral, percutaneous balloon, echocardiographic assessment of commissural calcium as predictor of outcome, 230
Valvular
heart disease, 221
association with fenfluramine-phentermine, 569
Vanillylmandelic acid
excretion, urinary, in incidentally discovered pheochromocytoma, 290
Variceal
bleeding
acute, endoscopic therapy vs. transjugular intrahepatic portosystemic shunt after initial sclerotherapy in, 627
acute, terlipressin vs. somatostatin for, 619
in cirrhosis, primary prophylaxis of, 618
ligation, endoscopic, for esophageal varices, 622
pressure, size, and wall tension in cirrhosis, total volume paracentesis decreases, 620
rebleeding
prevention with transjugular intrahepatic portosystemic shunts vs. endoscopic sclerotherapy, 625
shunt for, transjugular intrahepatic portosystemic, vs. endoscopy plus propranolol, 624
Varicella
zoster virus infection of central nervous system, diagnosis of, 36
Vascular
cardiovascular (see Cardiovascular)
death, clopidogrel vs. aspirin in prevention of, 196
disease
peripheral, in hypercholesterolemic patients with coronary artery disease, effect of apheresis of low-density lipoprotein on, 190
in renal disease, end-stage, and homocysteinemia, 405
effects of L-arginine, 419
events during follow-up of aortic arch atherosclerosis, 247
expression of polycystin, 385
microvascular complications and eating disorders in young women with insulin-dependent diabetes, 335
Vasculitis, 491
small-vessel, review of, 491
Vasectomy
urolithiasis and, 443
Vasopressin
IV, effect on gastric myoelectrical activity, 649
plasma, role as mediator of nausea and gastric slow wave dysrhythmias in motion sickness, 647
Vein
saphenous, coronary artery bypass grafts, obstructive changes in, effect of low-density lipoprotein cholesterol lowering and low-dose anticoagulation on, 192
thromboembolism, duration of oral anticoagulation after second episode of, 563
ulcers, chronic leg, activated protein C resistance due to factor V gene mutation in, 88
Venoembolic
disease, low-molecular-weight heparin in, 175
Ventilation
mechanical
duration of, effect on identifying patients capable of breathing spontaneously, 587
weaning from, protocol-directed vs. physician-directed, 588
Ventricle
arrhythmia, implanted defibrillator in patients with coronary disease at high risk for, 243
fibrillation, in-hospital, effect on prognosis after myocardial infarction, 178
function improvement after revascularization, prediction of, FDG SPECT vs. dobutamine echocardiography in, 227
left, dysfunction after recent myocardial infarction, and effect of amiodarone on mortality, 241
tachycardia, nonsustained, in severe heart failure, 239
Video
-assisted thoracoscopic approach to bilateral lung volume reduction surgery for emphysema, 540

Vinblastine
  in MOPP-ABVD regimen, primary, in
    Hodgkin's disease, outcome of
    patients after failing, 118
Vincristine
  in CHOP *vs.* ProMACE-CytaBOM
    regimen in aggressive
    non-Hodgkin's lymphoma, 110
  in MACOP-B regimen in diffuse
    large-cell lymphoma, late relapse
    with, 113
  in MOPP-ABVD regimen, primary, in
    Hodgkin's disease, outcome of
    patients after failing, 118
Virus
  cytomegalovirus
    infection, severe, in
      immunocompetent patients, 38
    retinitis in AIDS, cidofovir for, 23, 24
  encephalitides as biological warfare
    agents, clinical recognition and
    management of patients exposed
    to, 72
  hemorrhagic fevers as biological warfare
    agents, clinical recognition and
    management of patients exposed
    to, 76
  hepatitis (*see* Hepatitis)
  herpes (*see* Herpes)
  immunodeficiency, human (*see* HIV)
  infections, 29
    of central nervous system, diagnosis
      of, 36
  mechanism for inhibition of fever by, 8
  parvovirus B19 DNA persistence in
    synovial membranes of young
    patients with and without chronic
    arthropathy, 501
  rhinovirus-caused upper respiratory
    illness, effect on pulmonary
    function test and exercise
    responses, 41
  T-lymphotropic, human, type I, health
    effects of, 37
Visceral
  pain and regional cerebral activity, 651
Vitamin
  D supplementation, effect on bone
    density in elderly, 317
  D$_3$ supplementation in prevention of
    bone loss in spine secondary to
    low-dose corticosteroids in
    rheumatoid arthritis, 452
VM-26
  in CVP *vs.* CTVP regimen in aggressive
    non-Hodgkin's lymphoma, in
    elderly, 114

W

Warfare
  biologic, 71
    agents, clinical recognition and
      management of patients exposed
      to, 71
Warfarin
  low-dose, effect on obstructive changes
    in saphenous vein coronary bypass
    grafts, 193
  therapy
    duration after second episode of
      venous thromboembolism, 563
    initiation of, comparison of 5-mg and
      10-mg loading doses in, 250
Water, 439
  channel expression, aquaporin-2,
    upregulation in chronic heart
    failure (in rat), 440
Weaning
  from mechanical ventilation,
    protocol-directed *vs.*
    physician-directed, 588
Weight
  loss in coccidioidomycosis in HIV
    infection, 26
Whipple's disease
  diagnosis and monitoring by polymerase
    chain reaction, 499
White cell(s), 81
  count, high, and poor survival in cystic
    fibrosis, 537
  infusions, donor, for relapsed
    malignancy after allogeneic bone
    marrow transplantation, 127
Women
  asthma deaths in, 552
  beliefs and decisions about hormone
    replacement therapy, 328
  elderly
    bone density in, effect of calcium and
      vitamin D supplementation on, 317
    fracture occurrence in, broadband
      ultrasound attenuation predicts,
      311
    no association of low thyrotropin
      levels with bone loss in, 300
  fibromyalgia syndrome in, overdiagnosis
    of, 477
  HIV-infected, weekly fluconazole for
    prevention of mucosal candidiasis
    in, 21
  immunocompetent, frequent genital
    herpes simplex virus 2 shedding in,
    32
  kidney stones in, and calcium intake,
    444

lung cancer in, 523
postmenopausal (*see* Postmenopausal women)
prostate-specific antigen in serum in, as potential new marker of androgen excess, 327
young, with insulin-dependent diabetes, eating disorders and microvascular complications in, 335
Wound
dehiscence after ileocecal resection for Crohn's disease, 605
infection after ileocecal resection for Crohn's disease, 605

Z

Zidovudine
with nelfinavir and lamivudine, decay characteristics of HIV-1–infected compartments during, 16
Zileuton
vs. mesalazine in maintenance of remission of ulcerative colitis, 608
Zoster
herpes, acyclovir in, 34
varicella zoster virus infection of central nervous system, diagnosis of, 36

Author Index

A

Abbi R, 207
Abe K, 272
Abe Y, 600
Adachi JD, 320
Adams KF Jr, 213
Adkinson NF Jr, 544
Adler M, 602
Al-Awqati Q, 439
Albert JM, 14
Albrecht U, 152
Alcamí A, 8
Alexander HC, 668
Al-Kharrat T, 585
Allard R, 9
Alter HJ, 614
Alter MJ, 613
Alzahabi B, 373
Amoateng-Adjepong Y, 585
Amyot KM, 91
Anderson BN, 41
Anderson JH Jr, 339
Andersson B, 347
Andree HAM, 468
Andresen S, 115
Andrews TC, 188
Andrykowski MA, 151
Angulo FJ, 62
Apperloo AJ, 417
Argonz J, 620
Arnett FC, 470
Arnould T, 394
Ashok M, 327
Assaad D, 487
Astoul P, 529
Atherton JC, 637
Atkinson EJ, 305
Auble TE, 582
Aughenbaugh GL, 557
Austin CC, 64
Ayash LJ, 145

B

Baba S, 290
Baigrie RJ, 667
Baker AM, 587
Bakir AA, 412
Bañares R, 619
Barber JP, 82
Barnish MJ, 19
Barozzi L, 479
Barreca A, 431

Barry J, 188
Barth JH, 329
Basser RL, 85
Bastion Y, 114
Basu S, 177
Bauer BA, 546
Bauer DC, 300, 311
Baumgartner KB, 555
Baumgartner SW, 462
Bavaria JE, 24, 540
Bax JJ, 227
Bayerdörffer E, 631
Becker C, 591
Belchetz PE, 329
Bell NH, 312
Belman MJ, 533
Bensen WG, 320
Bensinger WI, 129
Berezin M, 267
Bergstralh EJ, 363
Berlin JA, 399
Berman S, 19
Bernard B, 617
Bernard GR, 5
Betticher DC, 108
Beverly V, 649
Bhattacharyya A, 662
Bhuyan UN, 375
Bilezikian JP, 307
Biondi B, 299
Blay J-Y, 114
Bloigu A, 68
Blum AL, 631
Boelaert JR, 52
Boepple PA, 331
Bolwell B, 115
Bonan R, 224
Bone HG III, 309
Bonfante V, 118
Bonini C, 137
Boronat M, 285
Bouros D, 583
Boyer N, 29
Brandt CM, 54
Brandt KD, 509
Brice P, 107
Brodsky RA, 82
Brody RI, 368
Broste S, 523
Brown J, 320
Brown LR, 525
Bruce ME, 39
Brugger W, 148
Brunelle RL, 339
Brunner G, 633
Bryant J, 143
Buckley LM, 452

Bueso-Ramos C, 87
Burgart LJ, 499
Burns AJ, 643
Burton DD, 644
Butler JC, 581
Butterly LF, 597
Byrd GS, 44

C

Caccavo D, 465
Califf RM, 176
Calvert GM, 384
Camargo CA Jr, 163
Camilleri M, 644
Campbell LA, 67
Cannan CR, 230
Cantini F, 454
Cao Y, 16
Caras SD, 649
Carey RM, 421
Caron P, 265, 302
Carpenter CCJ, 17
Carpenter MT, 489
Carroll RG, 12
Cartularo KS, 452
Cassel W, 591
Caulfield TA, 234
Cello JP, 627
Cetron MS, 581
Chaisson RE, 575
Chang JH, 543
Chang YC, 472
Chan-Yeung M, 543
Charlesworth A, 187
Chaturvedi N, 344
Chauvel C, 229
Chawla H, 368
Cherian R, 661
Chesnut CH III, 312
Chey WD, 647
Choi M-G, 644
Clapham PR, 13
Clapperton M, 349
Clark BA, 401
Clark GS, 312
Clark M, 547
Clermont HC, 575
Clift R, 129
Cogne M, 265
Cohen A, 229
Cohen MS, 11
Cohn JN, 214
Colao A, 269
Colby TV, 525
Collingham KE, 139

Collins RH Jr, 127
Colp C, 571
Combs C, 611
Cone R, 32
Coniff RF, 342
Connelly S, 138
Connolly HM, 569
Connors AF Jr, 531
Connors JM, 113
Considine RV, 432
Cooper DA, 9
Cooper JD, 539
Corey L, 32
Cornel JH, 227
Cowley AJ, 187
Coxon V, 443
Crary JL, 569
Croghan IT, 517
Crum RM, 167
Cuocolo A, 299
Curhan GC, 444
Curtis RE, 134
Cusack JD, 100
Cushman M, 169

D

Dalley AJ, 410
Dalton CB, 64
Damani S, 353
Danias PG, 234
Daniel GL, 658
Daniels ER, 155
Danishefsky SJ, 153
Darling GM, 355
Dash SC, 375
Dattwyler RJ, 505
Dauplat J, 146
Dawson NV, 531
Dawson-Hughes B, 317
Dean LS, 224
Deeg HJ, 134
DeFraites RF, 31
De Heer F, 370
de Hoogt R, 395
Deibert P, 624
de Jong PE, 417
Delaney VB, 381
del Arbol LR, 619
De Leeuw P, 370
DeLong ER, 183
Dennis VW, 405
Dequeker J, 456
Deshpande PP, 153
de Souza Fonseca L, 53
de Zeeuw D, 417
Dhaenen H, 652
Di Sarno A, 269

Dignam J, 143
DiLorenzo C, 646
Dinda AK, 375
Ding Y, 423
Divine M, 114
Dobbins BM, 56
Doherty C, 247
Domanski MJ, 216
Donadio JV Jr, 363
Doney K, 81
Dong BJ, 295
dos Santos KRN, 53
Doval HC, 239
Drappa J, 120
Dries DL, 216
Drobyski WR, 127
Dube LM, 608
Duffy MC, 54
Dunagan DP, 587
Dunn HG, 91
Durham JA, 287

E

Eaker EY, 655, 656
Eck M, 636
Eddleston M, 38
Eggleston PA, 544
Eguchi K, 524
Eiken P, 315
Eisenberg SJ, 233
Eissele E, 633
Elias A, 145
Ellis AG, 45
Ely EW, 587
El-Zeky F, 204
Eney D, 544
Engelhardt R, 148
Ennes H, 651
Epstein FH, 401
Erbes R, 556
Esdaile JM, 477
Essunger P, 16
Estrada J, 285
Etchason J, 629
Ettinger B, 300
Ettore GC, 601
Evans RW, 517
Exer P, 293

F

Fahy B, 39, 534
Fairclough DL, 153, 155
Fallavollita A, 98
Fam AG, 487
Farber HW, 572

Fazio S, 299
Feek CM, 287
Feldman HI, 399
Feltkamp TEW, 474
Ferrari G, 137
Fetscher S, 148
Feu F, 619
Feuer J, 511
Filho PPG, 53
Fine MJ, 582
Finlayson C, 641
Finley RJ, 666
Fioretti PM, 227
Fischel RJ, 22
Fischi MA, 17
Fisher B, 143
Fitzcharles M-A, 477, 481
Fitzgerald JT, 341
Fleming DR, 341
Fleury J, 146
Fogo A, 415
Ford DE, 167
Fortin PR, 481
Francioso G, 601
Franz DR, 71
Fraser I, 372
Freedman AM, 623, 625
Fried MW, 615
Friedlander AM, 71
Friedman GD, 639
Frost PH, 164
Fujii T, 390
Fullerton S, 629

G

Gambertoglio JG, 295
García-Conde J, 110
Garetto L, 132
Garibotto G, 431
Garribba AP, 601
Gaspardone A, 203
Gates RH Jr, 44
Gay F, 602
Gaynor B, 365
Geibel A, 566
Gent M, 196
Georgopoulos SD, 634
Gerstein H, 297
Gertz MA, 119
Gettys TW, 351
Gheorghiade M, 213
Gianlupi A, 523
Giatras I, 408
Gingerich RL, 353
Giugliano D, 419
Glover ED, 518
Glowniak JV, 283

Gluckman E, 130
Glynn RJ, 163
Goker H, 279
Goldfarb A, 571
Goldman JM, 124
Goldstone AH, 97
Gomm J, 141
Goormastic M, 115
Gordon JM, 656
Gordts BZ, 52
Gottlieb DJ, 572
Gottlieb JE, 559
Gough A, 349
Graham RM, 381
Grande JP, 385
Grebe SKG, 287
Greenspan JS, 26
Greiber S, 406
Greipp PR, 119
Gress FG, 598
Griffin MD, 385
Guilhot F, 101
Gullberg K, 606
Gurwitz JH, 181
Guyatt G, 297

H

Haag K, 624
Haapasaari J, 501
Haas R, 636
Hagger R, 641
Hagman M, 166
Hahn L, 347
Hainsworth J, 123
Haioun C, 111
Haire CE, 460
Ham HR, 652
Hammer SM, 17
Hamuryudan V, 493
Hann IM, 97
Hannan EL, 199
Hanson MN, 116
Harris JR, 153
Harris MD, 489
Harris SS, 317
Harrison L, 250
Harrison P, 139
Hasse C, 238
Hauck WW, 295
Hawes RH, 598
Hawkey CJ, 608
Hayes DL, 254, 255
Hayllar KM, 536
Hayman JA, 153
Hazelrigg SR, 28
Heard SO, 50
Heffner JE, 39, 534
Heilman DK, 509

Heit JA, 88
Held PJ, 429
Hendler RS, 668
Heptonstall J, 30
Herman-Giddens ME, 325
Hermans C, 395
Herwaldt BL, 59
Heudebert GR, 669
Hewitson T, 372
Hikita C, 439
Hildebrandt P, 178
Hille ETM, 90
Hilling L, 534
Hizli N, 493
Hoar B, 62
Hocher B, 387
Hofmann J, 581
Hollander P, 342
Holt EA, 575
Holzman MD, 654
Homma T, 400
Hoppin FG Jr, 26
Horowitz HW, 507
Hotta O, 377
Howard OM, 155
Howlett TA, 280
Hromas RA, 135
Hsieh T-C, 507
Huang Z-Q, 382
Hurt RD, 518
Huston S, 6
Huxley CM, 6

I

Iles-Smith H, 435
Imperiale TF, 618
Inoue T, 390
Ironside JW, 39
Ishikawa S-E, 272
Isolauri J, 670
Israel HL, 559

J

Jackson LA, 67
Jacober SJ, 341
Jacobson EL, 14
Jacobson EW, 458
Jacobson JM, 26
Jaeschke R, 297
Jahrling PE, 71
Jeffery KJM, 36
Jeffrey I, 641
Jenkins M, 329
Jensen GVH, 178
Johns JA, 355

Johnson BJB, 503
Johnston M, 250
Jollis JG, 183
Joly L-M, 200
Jordan ML, 425
Julian DG, 241
Julius BK, 221
Juniper M, 38

K

Kalinowski DJ, 560
Kallimanis G, 599
Kalman JM, 233
Kaminsky LA, 41
Kaneko M, 524
Kanji A, 279
Kao J-H, 612
Karim SS, 666
Karpf DB, 319
Kasperlik-Zaluska AA, 275
Kearney MT, 187
Kennedy A, 351
Kessler RE, 55
Khosla S, 305
Khudyakov YE, 615
Kim D, 401
Kim E, 394
Kim MS, 647
Kim NK, 605
Kinman JL, 399
Kirkpatrick WR, 20
Kite P, 56
Klein AL, 236
Klein JP, 124
Klein W, 173
Klimo P, 113
Klug D, 248
Knottnerus JA, 43
Koivisto VA, 339
Kollef MH, 588
Kolthoff N, 315
Kong GK, 533
Koning OHJ, 427
Konstantinides S, 566
Kopp JB, 392
Kostis JB, 208
Kotloff RM, 540
Kovacs JA, 14
Kraft HE, 491
Krall EA, 317
Krane MC, 446
Kravetz D, 620
Kreusel M, 406
Krieger JN, 443
Krmpotich PT, 661
Kronmal RA, 443
Kroon AA, 190

Kruger KH, 141
Krum H, 209
Kunkel MJ, 505
Kuppermann BD, 23
Kusnierz-Glaz CR, 126
Kyle RA, 119

L

Labenz J, 631
LaCroix AZ, 328
Lacroix D, 248
Ladipo JK, 654
Laganà B, 465
Lai M-Y, 612
Lalezari JP, 23
Lampreabe I, 388
Laurila A, 68
Lavin P, 149
Law C, 84
Lawerence J, 25
Lebrec D, 617
Lee AYY, 113
Legros M, 146
Leib ES, 452
Leisenring W, 81
Lerner SA, 100
Leveille SG, 328
Levine BL, 12
Lewis NP, 217
Lewis RA, 24
Lightner R, 151
Liljeqvist L, 606
Lin X, 650
Lind BK, 223
Locker FG, 307
Loddenkemper R, 556
Loftus E Jr, 499
Lohmann T, 337
Lomax AEJ, 643
Loriaux DL, 283
Luchtefeld MA, 605
Luft BJ, 505
Luketic VA, 623, 625
Luostarinen M, 670

M

Mackillop WJ, 154
Maconi G, 635
Maenza JR, 22
Maffi P, 343
Mak SK, 366
Mallick NP, 366
Mandelli F, 95
Manfreda J, 543
Mangano DT, 252

Manthous CA, 585
Maor Y, 267
Marcaccio M, 84
Marcellin P, 29
Marfella R, 419
Marks R, 669
Marriott TB, 309
Martin P, 129
Martin P-Y, 440
Martinot M, 29
Massicotte MP, 250
Mata S, 481
Mathurin P, 617
Mattijssen V, 103
Mattsson L-Å, 347
Mauser A, 138
McAtee RK, 20
McCann UD, 568
McCloud PI, 355
McEvoy CE, 535
McGoon MD, 569
McLaughlin TJ, 181
McPherson JD, 446
Medsger TA Jr, 483
Melegos DN, 327
Mellow MH, 650
Melpolder J, 614
Menck HR, 142
Mentis AF, 634
Merkel PA, 472
Mermin J, 62
Merz WG, 22
Mican JM, 392
Michael B, 432
Mickel M, 224
Mielgo M, 285
Miller KD, 392
Mitterhofer AP, 465
Mitusch R, 247
Miyajima A, 290
Montserrat E, 110
Moorhouse J, 435
Morady F, 238
Morales TG, 662
Morange-Ramos I, 265
Moreland LW, 462
Morgan OSC, 37
Morikawa A, 646
Morimatsu M, 152
Morrison VA, 116
Moss AJ, 185, 243
Mount J, 138
Moutsopoulos HM, 470
Mullen KD, 618
Müller B, 293
Munakata JA, 651
Murphy EL, 37
Murray LJ, 87
Myers JC, 667

Myers JL, 557

N

Nachtigall LB, 331
Nadelman RB, 507
Nakashima J, 290
Nakatsuji Y, 614
Naraghi R, 425
'Narians CR, 185
Näyhä S, 68
Neiman RS, 135
Nevitt MC, 300
Newport MJ, 6
Newton KM, 328
Ni Z, 423
Niccoli P, 302
Nielsen SP, 315
Nieuwhof CMG, 370
Niewoehner DE, 535
Nishimura K, 37
Nishimura RA, 230, 255

O

Oda T, 377
O'Dell JR, 460
O'Donnell D, 16
O'Donnell R, 552
Offord KP, 517, 607
Ofman JJ, 629
Ohar JA, 19
Ohara M, 440
Ohmatsu H, 524
Olcott EW, 627
Olivetti G, 207
Olivieri I, 454, 479
Olmsted MP, 335
Olschewski M, 566
O'Malley CJ, 85
Orazi A, 135
Orentreich N, 639
Owyang C, 647
Özyazgan Y, 493

P

Palmer W, 460
Palu S, 384
Panton ON, 666
Parente F, 635
Parsonnet J, 639
Patsourakis G, 583
Patterson GA, 24, 539
Pattynama PMT, 565
Pavenstädt H, 406
Peacock S, 38

Pearle MS, 396
Pedagogos E, 372
Peek RM Jr, 637
Peeling RW, 45
Pegoraro A, 412
Perelson AS, 16
Peresleni T, 434
Perez MS, 277
Peterson BA, 116
Peterson ED, 183
Peto TEA, 36
Peus D, 88
Piacibello W, 132
Picard L, 13
Pierro A, 479
Pilaro F, 14
Pi-Sunyer X, 342
Pitt B, 212
Pittelkow MR, 88
Ploch T, 591
Ploeg RJ, 427
Polesky A, 572
Polisson RP, 472
Pollak MR, 381
Port FK, 429
Powell M, 277
Pralong FP, 331
Pratt LA, 167
Putterman C, 365

Q

Quaini F, 207
Quartey SM, 47
Quinn D, 523
Quirt CF, 154

R

Raad II, 50
Raby K, 188
Racz M, 199
Radford MG Jr, 363
Ramirez FC, 622
Ramzan NN, 499
Rand JH, 468
Rantis PC Jr, 658
Rapola JM, 194
Rasko JEJ, 85
Rauch AE, 91
Rauh G, 496
Raval U, 177
Read JD, 597
Read SJ, 36
Read TE, 597
Reale MA, 149
Reed CE, 546
Reed WW, 44

Reeder GS, 230
Reilly MJ, 560
Revankar SG, 20
Reveille JD, 470
Rey F, 529
Reynolds DW, 254
Richter JE, 664
Rickenbacher PR, 217
Ridker PM, 169
Riley JL, 12
Ring EJ, 627
Ripatti S, 194
Roane DW, 489
Robinson K, 405
Rodin GM, 335
Roehrborn CG, 396
Rohmeiss P, 387
Roland J, 652
Rolando N, 349
Romagnoli MJ, 22
Romero G, 620
Rosenberg A, 200
Rosengren A, 166
Rosenman KD, 560
Roslonowska E, 275
Rossetti RG, 458
Rössle M, 624
Rotger J, 337
Rountree LV, 608
Rowlings PA, 134
Rubin LJ, 568
Ruiz-Muñoz LM, 388
Russo R, 431
Ryan TJ, 199
Rydall AC, 335

S

Saad MF, 353
Sachs DPL, 518
Saeed ZA, 622
Saito T, 272
Sakai M, 400
Sallustio JE, 655
Salvarani C, 454
Salzman MB, 503
Samet JM, 555
Sampliner RE, 662
Sanavio F, 132
Sandborn WJ, 607
Sanders PW, 382
Sanders WE Jr, 55
Sangaletti O, 635
Santoro A, 118
Sanyal AJ, 623, 625
Sarnacchiaro F, 269
Savides TJ, 598
Savoye C, 248

Schaap N, 103
Schaberg T, 556
Schattenberg A, 103
Schiff MH, 462
Schiza S, 583
Schlegel PG, 126
Schmausser B, 636
Schmidt RA, 67
Schmidt WA, 491
Schmit A, 602
Schoenfeld A, 141
Schrijnemaekers VJJ, 43
Schulman S, 563
Schuman P, 21
Schwartz G, 145
Schwartzberg LS, 123
Secchi A, 343
Seiden LS, 568
Seissler J, 337
Senagore AJ, 605
Senior R, 177
Seymour JF, 100
Seymour NE, 668
Shapiro R, 425
Shapiro SD, 588
Sharan AK, 152
Sharma K, 373, 432
Sharp KW, 654
Sherertz RJ, 50
Shibata D, 50
Short CD, 366
Shpilberg O, 127
Sie LH, 599
Silver P, 588
Silverberg SJ, 307, 309
Silverman DHS, 651
Simmons G, 13
Simon B, 633
Simoons ML, 201
Singh A, 412
Singh N, 19
Singh VR, 25
Siragy HM, 421
Siscovick D, 223
Sistrunk WW, 54
Skidmore SJ, 139
Slemenda C, 509
Slora EJ, 325
Slowinska-Srzednicka J, 275
Slutsker L, 60
Sly RM, 552
Smallwood GA, 615
Smith DK, 25
Smith GL, 8
Smith KA, 14
Smoak BL, 31
Smolen JS, 474
Sobel J, 64

Socci C, 343
Söderlund M, 501
Sood SK, 503
Sorensen JM, 98
Southmayd L III, 650
Soykan I, 649
Soylemezoglu O, 410
Spaulding CM, 200
Speizer FE, 444
Spiera H, 511
Spiliadis CA, 634
Spillmann M, 221
Spritzler J, 26
Stagg RJ, 23
Ståhlberg D, 606
Stalenhoef AFH, 190
Stampfer MJ, 163, 169
Stansell JD, 578
Steen VD, 483
Steenland K, 384
Stein A, 435
Steiner RM, 559
Stevens RF, 97
Stewart BF, 223
Stidley CA, 555
Stiegmann GV, 622
Stokes MB, 368
Storb R, 81
Straub RH, 496
Strickberger SA, 238
Studts JL, 151
Subramanian S, 279
Suh H, 434
Sullivan JM, 204
Sullivan KE, 120
Sundaresan RS, 539
Swensen SJ, 557
Swenson SJ, 525
Szydlo R, 124

T

Taguma Y, 377
Takito J, 439
Tam P, 84
Tamaoki J, 549
Tan EM, 474
Tanaka H, 277
Tang Y, 600
Tenney JH, 55
Teran JC, 618
Terrault NA, 611
Tham KT, 637

Thöne-Reineke C, 387
Thomas C, 531
Thompson Coon J, 547
Tino G, 540
Tio TL, 599
Tomai F, 203
Tomomasa T, 646
Ton ERTA, 565
Torihashi S, 643
Torp-Pedersen C, 178
Torres VE, 385
Towns ML, 47
Tremaine WJ, 607
Trofa AF, 31
Troy CJ, 45
Trusty JM, 255
Tsiokas L, 394

U

Ueda D, 42
Uretsky BF, 213
Uzu T, 390

V

Vadhan-Raj S, 87
Vaezi MF, 664
Vaishnaw AK, 120
Vala MS, 82
Valadon P, 365
Valantine HA, 217
van Asten WNJC, 190
Van Bockel JH, 427
van Buchem FL, 43
Vandenbroucke JP, 90
Vander Zwaag R, 204
Vanhems P, 9
Van Landuyt HW, 52
van Rossum AB, 565
van Slegtenhorst M, 395
Vassalli G, 221
Vaziri ND, 423
Vena DA, 98
Vernava AM III, 658
Verne GN, 655
Verrazzo G, 419
Versaci F, 203
Verwilghen J, 456
Verzeletti S, 137
Viallat J-R, 529
Vidal-Vanaclocha F, 388

Viljakka M, 670
Vinõlas N, 110
Virtamo J, 194
Viviani S, 118
Vogel S, 14
Vogel SB, 656
von Essen R, 501
von Rohr A, 108
Vorpahl K, 491

W

Waclawiw MA, 216
Wadhwa N, 434
Wagner-McPherson CB, 446
Wald A, 32
Wallace JM, 577
Wang PJ, 254
Wasserman RC, 325
Watson DI, 667
Watson P, 351
Weaver CH, 123
Weber H, 229
Wedel H, 166
Wei I, 571
Weidner TG, 41
Weigner MJ, 234
Weingarten S, 533
Weinstein MP, 47
Wermers RA, 305
Westendorp RGJ, 90
Westhovens R, 456
Weston AP, 661
Whitley RJ, 34
Wilcox CM, 669
Wilcox MH, 56
Wild G, 410
Wilding P, 547
Wilks R, 37
Will RG, 39
Willett WC, 444
Williams SGJ, 536
Willison DJ, 181
Winchester DJ, 142
Winchester DP, 142
Wion-Barbot N, 302
Wise AE, 536
Wolfe RA, 429
Wong RM, 126
Wood KA, 233
Wu X-X, 468
Wucherpfennig H, 247

X

Xu D-L, 440

Y

Yamashita Y, 600
Yang P-M, 612

Yealy DM, 582
Yoto Y, 42
Yu H, 327
Yunginger JW, 546

Z

Zareba W, 185
Zeuner M, 496

Zhang M-Z, 400
Zhou S, 611
Ziyadeh FN, 373
Zucca E, 108
Zulewski H, 293
Zurier RB, 458